CLINICAL NEUROSURGERY

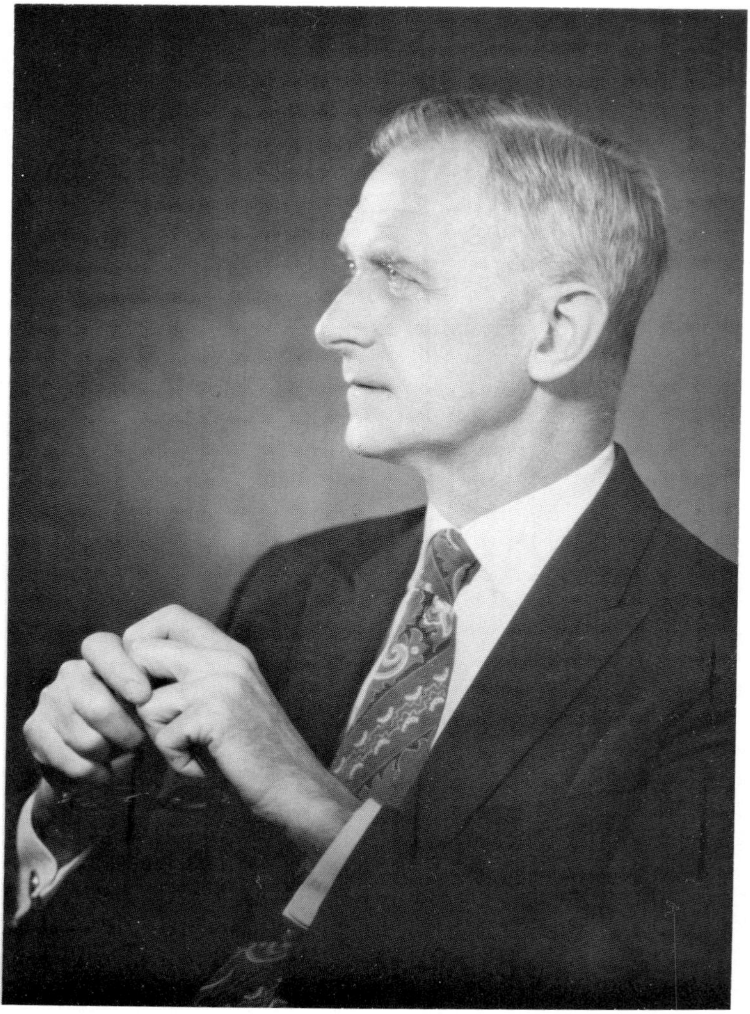

William H. Sweet, M.D., D.Sc.

CLINICAL NEUROSURGERY

Proceedings

OF THE

CONGRESS OF NEUROLOGICAL SURGEONS

Atlanta, Georgia

1975

BALTIMORE
THE WILLIAMS & WILKINS COMPANY
1976

Made in the United States of America

Library of Congress

Catalog Card Number
S4-12666
SBN 683-02010-2

COMPOSED AND PRINTED AT
WAVERLY PRESS, INC.
Mt. Royal and Guilford Aves.
BALTIMORE, MD. 21202, U.S.A.

Preface

The Congress of Neurological Surgeons respectfully dedicates this twenty-third volume of *Clinical Neurosurgery* to DR. WILLIAM H. SWEET, Honored Guest and principal speaker at the 25th Annual Meeting and Silver Anniversary of the Congress of Neurological Surgeons held in Atlanta, Georgia, October 20 through October 24, 1975.

Dr. Sweet's outstanding career is outlined in a biographical review by Dr. Robert Ojemann. Dr. Sweet's chapter, "The Difference Between Zero and One", brilliantly illustrates the value to medical progress of what can be learned from the careful study of a single case. His wide areas of interest are demonstrated by his presentations on the treatment of pain, on the surgical therapy of craniopharyngiomas, and in his timely comments on the professional malpractice problem.

Dr. James T. Robertson, President of the Congress of Neurological Surgeons, set the major theme of the meeting with his presidential address on the surgical treatment of extra-cranial occlusive disease. Other presentations published in this volume were presented by experts from various disciplines in the field of the stroke syndrome. A second major theme of the meeting and the chapters in this book is the ever important field of neurosurgical complications. A third theme on professional liability is presented by experts from disciplines of law, medicine, and insurance.

This exceptional scientific program was arranged under the direction of Dr. Robert H. Wilkins. The annual meeting was under the direction of General Chairman, Dr. William A. Buchheit.

The editor-in-chief would like to thank Dr. Wilkins, Dr. Buchheit, and the program committees for their endeavors in planning the program. He would like to thank the individual authors for preparing their manuscripts and his associate editors for collecting the manuscripts and editing the references. He would also like to acknowledge the invaluable assistance of his secretary, Miss Dorris Biggers, in the preparation of this volume. A special note of appreciation is made to the publisher and particularly to Mrs. Ruby Richardson, Mr. Stephen J. Birckhead, and Miss Jessie H. Meyer of The Williams & Wilkins Company. Finally, the editor would like to make a note of appreciation to his colleagues, Dr. Roy W. Vandiver, Dr. Ernest C. Fokes, and Dr. W. Knox Kinlaw, Jr., for allowing him time from their busy practice to carry out these editorial duties, and last but not least he would like to express appreciation to Mrs. Ann Keener who has exhibited much patience and devotion during the time spent in preparation of this volume.

ELLIS B. KEENER, M.D.
Editor-in-Chief
Associate Editors:
PETER W. CARMEL, M.D.
HARRY FRIEDMAN, M.D.
LESLIE E. GEIGER, M.D.
GAIL MAGID, M.D.
JOSEPH C. MAROON, M.D.
CLARK C. WATTS, M.D.

Honored Guests

1952—Professor Herbert Olivecrona, Stockholm, Sweden
1953—Sir Geoffrey Jefferson, Manchester, England
1954—Dr. Kenneth G. McKenzie, Toronto, Canada
1955—Dr. Carl W. Rand, Los Angeles, California
1956—Dr. Wilder G. Penfield, Montreal, Canada
1957—Dr. Francis C. Grant, Philadelphia, Pennsylvania
1958—Dr. A. Earl Walker, Baltimore, Maryland
1959—Dr. William J. German, New Haven, Connecticut
1960—Dr. Paul C. Bucy, Chicago, Illinois
1961—Professor Eduard A. V. Busch, Copenhagen, Denmark
1962—Dr. Bronson S. Ray, New York, New York
1963—Dr. James L. Poppen, Boston, Massachusetts
1964—Dr. Edgar A. Kahn, Ann Arbor, Michigan
1965—Dr. James C. White, Boston, Massachusetts
1966—Dr. Hugo A. Krayenbuhl, Zurich, Switzerland
1967—Dr. W. James Gardner, Cleveland, Ohio
1968—Professor Norman M. Dott, Edinburgh, Scotland
1969—Dr. Wallace B. Hamby, Cleveland, Ohio
1970—Dr. Barnes Woodhall, Durham, North Carolina
1971—Dr. Elisha S. Gurdjian, Detroit, Michigan
1972—Dr. Francis Murphey, Memphis, Tennessee
1973—Dr. Henry G. Schwartz, St. Louis, Missouri
1974—Dr. Guy L. Odom, Durham, North Carolina
1975—Dr. William H. Sweet, Boston, Massachusetts

Officers of the Congress of Neurological Surgeons 1975

James T. Robertson
President

Robert G. Ojemann
President-Elect

Kenneth R. Smith, Jr.
Vice-President

David L. Kelly, Jr.
Secretary

Bruce F. Sorensen
Treasurer

Executive Committee
George T. Tindall

Perry Black
William H. Buchheit
J. Fletcher Lee
Jim L. Story

John M. Tew
Robert H. Wilkins
Donald F. Dohn
Bernard S. Patrick
Albert L. Rhoton

William A. Buchheit, *Chairman, Annual Meeting Committee*
Robert H. Wilkins, *Chairman, Scientific Program Committee*

Contributors

H. J. M. BARNETT, M.D., F.R.C.P.(C), Professor and Chairman, Department of Clinical Neurological Sciences, University of Western Ontario, London, Ontario, Canada (*Chapter 41*).

DONALD P. BECKER, M.D., Professor and Chairman of Neurosurgery, Division of Neurological Surgery, Medical College of Virginia, Virginia Commonwealth University, Richmond, Virginia (*Chapter 37*).

WALTER H. BECKHAM, JR., A.B., J.D., Professor of Law, University of Miami, Of Counsel, Podhurst, Orseck & Parks, P.A., Miami, Florida (*Chapter 38*).

STEVEN BREM, M.D., Resident in Neurosurgery, Massachusetts General Hospital, Boston, Massachusetts; Instructor in Ophthalmology, Johns Hopkins University Hospital and School of Medicine, Baltimore, Maryland; Clinical Associate, National Cancer Institute, Neurosurgical Unit, Baltimore Cancer Research Center, Baltimore, Maryland (*Chapter 23*).

JEFFERSON BROWDER, M.D., Staff Physician, Veterans Administration Hospital, East Orange, New Jersey; Professor of Surgery (Neurosurgery), New Jersey Medical School, Newark, New Jersey (*Chapter 13*).

NORMAN CHATER, M.D., Associate Clinical Professor of Neurosurgery, University of California, San Francisco; Director, Microsurgical Unit, Ralph K. Davies Medical Center, San Francisco, California; Attending Neurosurgeon, San Francisco Veterans Administration Hospital (*Chapter 21*).

SHELLEY N. CHOU, M.D., Ph.D., Professor and Head, Department of Neurosurgery, University of Minnesota Medical School, Minneapolis, Minnesota (*Chapter 26*).

KEMP CLARK. M.D., Professor and Chairman, Division of Neurosurgery, Southwestern Medical School, Dallas, Texas (*Chapter 25*).

WILLIAM F. COLLINS, JR., M.D., Cushing Professor of Surgery; Chairman, Section of Neurosurgery, Yale University School of Medicine, New Haven, Connecticut (*Chapter 30*).

PAUL DIDISHEIM, M.D., Professor of Laboratory Medicine (Hematology); Director, Thrombosis Research Laboratory, Mayo Clinic, Mayo Medical School and Mayo Foundation, Rochester, Minnesota (*Chapter 10*).

THOMAS B. DUCKER, M.D., F.A.C.S., Division of Neurosurgery, University of Maryland School of Medicine, Baltimore, Maryland (*Chapter 36*).

STEWART B. DUNSKER, M.D., Mayfield Neurologic Institute; Department of Neurosurgery, Christ Hospital and Good Samaritan Hospital, Cincinnati, Ohio (*Chapter 24*).

DONALD L. ERICKSON, M.D., Assistant Professor, Department of Neurosurgery, University of Minnesota Medical School, Minneapolis, Minnesota (*Chapter 26*).

WILLIAM S. FIELDS, M.D., Professor and Chairman, Department of Neurology, University of Texas Health Science Center at Houston-Medical School, Houston, Texas (*Chapter 15*).

VALENTIN FUSTER, M.D., Assistant Professor of Medicine, Consultant, Division of Cardiovascular Diseases and Medicine, Mayo Clinic, Mayo Medical School and Mayo Foundation, Rochester, Minnesota (*Chapter 10*).

OTMAR GRATZL, M.D., Department of Neurosurgery, University of Munich, Munich, West Germany (*Chapter 20*).

JAMES LEWIS GRIFFITH, Esq., 14th Floor Packard Building, Philadelphia, Pennsylvania (*Chapter 39*).

HARRY KAPLAN, M.D., Professor of Surgery (Neurosurgery), New Jersey Medical School, Newark, New Jersey (*Chapter 13*).

EUGENE B. KERN, M.D., Consultant, Department of Otorhinolaryngology, Mayo Clinic and Mayo Foundation; Instructor in Otorhinolaryngology, Mayo Medical School, Rochester, Minnesota (*Chapter 29*).

EDWARD R. LAWS, JR., M.D., Consultant, Department of Neurologic Surgery, Mayo Clinic and Mayo Foundation; Assistant Professor of Neurologic Surgery, Mayo Medical School, Rochester, Minnesota (*Chapter 29*).

FRANK MARGUTH, M.D., Department of Neurosurgery, University of Munich, Munich, West Germany (*Chapter 20*).

WILLIAM L. MARTIN, Vice President and General Counsel, American Insurance Association, 85 John Street, New York, New York (*Chapter 40*).

FRANK H. MAYFIELD, M.D., F.A.C.S., Director, Neurosurgical Training Program, Good Samaritan Hospital-Christ Hospital; Mayfield Neurological Institute of Cincinnati, Inc., Cincinnati, Ohio (*Chapters 31 and 32*).

J. P. MOHR, M.D., Assistant Neurologist and Coordinator, Stroke Service, Massachusetts General Hospital; Assistant Professor of Neurology, Harvard Medical School, Boston, Massachusetts, (*Chapter 17*).

MARK S. O'BRIEN, M.D., Associate Professor of Surgery (Neurosurgery), Emory University School of Medicine, Atlanta, Georgia (*Chapter 35*).

ROBERT G. OJEMANN, M.D., Visiting Neurosurgeon, Massachusetts General Hospital; Associate Clinical Professor of Surgery, Harvard Medical School, Boston, Massachusetts (*Chapters 2 and 17*).

VLADIMIR OLTEANU-NERBE, M.D., Department of Neurosurgery, University of Munich, Munich, West Germany (*Chapter 20*).

AYUN KHAN OMMAYA, M.D., Surgical Neurology Branch, National Institute of Neurological and Communicative Disorders and Stroke, Bethesda, Maryland (*Chapter 27*).

NETTLETON S. PAYNE II, M.D., Assistant Professor of Surgery (Neurosurgery) Emory University School of Medicine; Chief of Neurosurgery, Veterans Administration Hospital, Atlanta, Georgia (*Chapter 35*).

S. J. PEERLESS, M.D., F.R.C.S. (C), Professor and Chairman, Division of Neurosurgery, Department of Clinical Neurological Sciences, University of Western Ontario, London, Ontario, Canada (*Chapter 19*).

DAVID G. PIEPGRAS, M.D., Consultant, Department of Neurologic Surgery, Mayo Clinic and Mayo Foundation; Instructor in Neurosurgery, Mayo Medical School; Rochester, Minnesota (*Chapter 22*).

CHARLES E. RACKLEY, M.D., Professor of Medicine, University of Alabama Medical Center, Birmingham, Alabama (*Chapter 14*).

JOSEPH S. REDDING, M.D., F.A.C.P., Division of Respiratory Therapy, Medical University of South Carolina, Charleston, South Carolina (*Chapter 36*).

O. HOWARD REICHMAN, M.D., Associate Professor, Division of Neurological Surgery, Loyola University Medical Center, Maywood, Illinois (*Chapter 23*).

JAMES C. ROBERTS, JR., M.D., Associate Clinical Professor of Pathology, University of California at Los Angeles, Rolling Hills, California; Pathologist, The Little Company of Mary Hospital, Torrance, California (*Chapter 11*).

JAMES T. ROBERTSON, M.D., Professor and Chairman, Department of Neurological Surgery, University of Tennessee College of Medicine, Memphis, Tennessee (*Chapter 1*).

JOHN F. ROCKETT, M.D., Department of Nuclear Medicine, Radiology, Baptist Memorial Hospital, Memphis, Tennessee (*Chapter 18*).

MICHAEL J. ROSNER, M.D., Neurosurgical Resident and Fellow, Division of Neurological Surgery, Medical College of Virginia, Virginia Commonwealth University, Richmond, Virginia (*Chapter 37*).

MARTIN P. SAYERS, M.D., Clinical Professor of Surgery (Neurosurgery) Ohio State University and Chief, Division of Neurosurgery, Children's Hospital, Columbus, Ohio (*Chapter 28*).

PETER SCHMIEDEK, M.D., Department of Neurosurgery, University of Munich, Munich, West Germany (*Chapter 20*).

JOHN SHILLITO, JR., M.D., Associate Professor of Surgery, Harvard Medical School; Senior Associate in Neurosurgery, Children's Hospital Medical Center; Surgeon (Neurosurgery), Peter Bent Brigham Hospital, Boston, Massachusetts (*Chapter 16*).

HARALD STEINHOFF, M.D., Department of Neurosurgery, University of Munich, Munich, West Germany (*Chapter 20*).

WILLIAM H. SWEET, M.D., D.Sc., Chief, Neurosurgical Service, Massachusetts General Hospital, and Professor of Surgery, Harvard Medical School, Boston, Massachusetts (*Chapters 3, 4, 5, 6, 7, 8, and 9*).

JOHN MCLELLAN TEW, JR., M.D., F.A.C.S., Associate Director, Neurosurgical Training Program, Good Samaritan Hospital—Christ Hospital, Cincinnati, Ohio (*Chapter 31*).

GEORGE T. TINDALL, M.D., F.A.C.S., Professor of Surgery, Chief, Division of Neurosurgery, Emory University School of Medicine, Atlanta, Georgia (*Chapter 35*).

ARTHUR G. WALTZ, M.D., Chairman, Department of Neurology, Pacific Medical Center, San Francisco, California (*Chapter 12*).

JAMES G. WEPSIC, M.D., Neurosurgical Service, Massachusetts General Hospital, Boston, Massachusetts (*Chapter 34*).

Contents

CHAPTER

1

Presidential Address: A Neurosurgical Approach to the Therapy of Extracranial Occlusive Disease

JAMES T. ROBERTSON, M.D.

Mr. Chairman, founders, members, guests, Dr. William Sweet, our Honored Guest, welcome to the Silver Anniversary Meeting of the Congress of Neurological Surgeons. It is my sincere wish this meeting will be scientifically stimulating and socially satisfying. During the last 25 years, this Society has become the largest of all neurosurgical organizations but continues to be dedicated to the education of the young neurosurgeon. It is my particular honor, an occurrence largely of chance, to serve as President for this anniversary gathering and to have as our special honored guests many founders of this Society and many former presidents. Since the founders formed the Society in St. Louis and the first meeting was held in Memphis, our meeting site is most appropriate. With pleasure, I welcome you to this gracious and exploding queen of southern cities, Atlanta. Sherman's ashes have literally turned to gold, and southern hospitality and leadership are graced by your presence.

These are trying times for the medical profession, and particuarly for neurosurgeons. The interference of government, the problems of recertification and licensure, the restrictions imposed on clinical research, and the aspects of extortion implied in current liability insurance practice concern, confuse, and frustrate everyone. Your Society, by the dedicated, unselfish hard work of the Socio-economic Committee under Dr. Ed Amyes' leadership, is educating and representing neurosurgery regarding these matters in a superb professional manner. We have combined our efforts with a similar committee of the American Association of Neurological Surgeons under Dr. Russel Patterson's chairmanship. United we stand. These positive steps should lead to honorable problem solving, but the work is expensive and demands increasing time. A central office has been established, under the direction of Dr. George Tindall, to represent neurosurgery in continuing education and to coordinate all educational seminars. In our direct negotiations with government, this office could have increasing influence of an unknown magnitude and require financing that may not be entirely tax exempt. Whatever the cost to survive, I am confident that our profession must and will stand the heat, stay in the kitchen, and preserve the free practice of medicine.

The President of this Society is allowed two special privileges. The first privilege is the selection of the Honored Guest for the Annual Meeting. Dr. William Sweet, our guest this year, is a neuroscientist of outstanding stature, a man of integrity and courage, an outstanding neurosurgeon, an excellent teacher, and a friend. The second privilege is the selection of the theme for the Annual Meeting. This year's program is dedicated to the neurosurgeon's interest in the prevention, research, and medical and surgical therapy of stroke.

If the comments I make have a bias or reflect any point of view that is worthwhile, I wish to give credit to my chief, Dr. Francis Murphy, a truly great clinical neurosurgeon, and to my colleagues in Memphis, particularly the members of the Semmes-Murphey Clinic.

Stroke due to occlusive disease is epidemic in this long living society. According to Dr. Cone Pevehouse, an excellent neurosurgical economist, stroke diagnosis and treatment constitutes a significant segment of the patient load in neurosurgical practice (21). It is a clinical challenge and the third leading cause of death in the United States (11.3%), killing at least 200,000 people per year. It is one of the leading causes of personal and family tragedy (12, 26). Stroke victims overflow our nursing homes. Stroke extracts an untold socio-economic drain on this nation. In minutes an occlusive stroke can change an active and intelligent executive into a dependent, demented, locked-in individual. Dr. Miller Fisher has appropriately defined the victim of a massive stroke as an individual in the state of "super death" (8).

Stroke demands the attention of all neurosurgeons, not only in diagnosis but in active medical and surgical therapy. It is not only a great challenge, but the results of preventive surgery are better than they are in surgical therapy of aneurysms or brain tumors. Recently, our specialty has become very aggressive in establishing neurosurgeons as stroke physicians. Due to the leadership of Dr. John Tew of Cincinnati and Dr. Thor Sundt of Rochester, a Cerebrovascular Section of the American Association of Neurological Surgeons has been formed and they will have their first meeting with the American Heart Association in Dallas in eary 1976. Dr. Steve Gurdjian, a member of the Congress and a former honored guest, has just directed an outstanding postgraduate course on the intra- and extracranial procedures for cerebral ischemia at the American College of Surgeons Meeting in San Francisco. If a few of you are less than qualified in the treatment of this very common disease entity, you are urged to attend clinics or continuing education programs or work with vascular surgeons to become expert in stroke care. Our speciality can hardly be concerned about the brain without being concerned about its blood supply. Indeed, what other speciality has the potential to deal with this problem as we do?

In the time allowed for this presentation, it is impossible to discuss all aspects of stroke therapy, but the following comments are submitted for your review and consideration:

1. More than half of all deaths are due to the combination of cerebrovascular disease, coronary artery disease, and hypertensive cardiovascular disease (12).

2. Cerebral infarction accounts for nearly two-thirds of the fatal vascular brain disorders.

3. A completed stroke is frequently (40 to 80%) preceded by warning attacks. These transient ischemic attacks are defined as the sudden onset of a focal, usually painless, neurological deficit that clears completely, often in minutes, but certainly within 24 hours (1, 3, 13, 18, 20, 24). Although an individual literally may have had a hundred attacks, there is no correlation as to the number of attacks or when the stroke will occur (8). Vertebrobasilar ischemic attacks have a better prognosis than carotid ischemic attacks. These attacks demonstrate the difference between physiological paralysis and anatomic infarction. The medical profession and the public must be educated repeatedly to recognize these warning bells and take preventive action.

4. Once transient ischemic attacks have occurred, a stroke occurs in an instance of 4 to 10% per annum (20 to 50% within 5 years) (1, 3, 9, 13, 14, 17). The prognosis is still guarded when the arteriograms are normal (16).

5. There are syndromes suggesting cerebrovascular insufficiency; for example, acceleration giddiness, difficulty in rapid thought, slowing of mental function, stepwise dementia that may be related to occlusive vascular disease both intra-and extracranially. These hypoperfusion syndromes require more study and documentation (9, 24).

6. Except in special early circumstances there is virtually no therapy for a completed cerebral infarction (9, 18, 24). Depending upon one's philosophy and the understanding that physiological paralysis may not mean anatomic infarction, there probably is a place for early surgery in symptomatic acute carotid occlusion (4 to 6 hours). Surgery in completed strokes carries a significant increased risk. All surgical and medical therapy is best administered prior to the infarction event. Essentially, therefore, stroke therapy is prophylactic.

7. Although hemodynamic factors are a cause of ischemic cerebral symptoms, emboli (usually platelet aggregates or, on occasion, choles-

terol fragments) are probably the most important cause of transient ischemic attacks (3). According to Fisher, distal emboli have not been proven to occur from the stenotic areas in intracranial vessels.

8. In the arterial system, it is generally agreed that long term anticoagulation is probably ineffective in the prevention of stroke and may carry a greater risk than no therapy at all (2, 15).

9. The dynamic role of platelets in the arterial system has provoked an intense interest in platelet-inhibiting drugs (10, 19). Platelet-inhibiting drugs are now available and fall into three categories:

A. The nonsteroidal anti-inflammatory drugs; for example, aspirin, sulfinpyrazone.
B. The pyrimido-pyrimidine compounds.
C. The tricyclic antidepressants drugs.

Preliminary studies indicate that drugs which inhibit platelet function will be effective in preventing thromboembolic states due to platelet emboli (6). Several studies are underway to test the efficacy of platelet inhibition as a therapeutic answer in the prevention of occlusive cerebral and cardiac syndromes. Should the hypothesis be proven, the benefit to the health of our senior citizens will be inestimable.

10. The present therapy of stroke, providing the patient is in a reasonably good neurological state, requires adequate cerebral arteriography (9, 24).

11. Of all the medical therapies available in the medical treatment of a transient ischemic attack, intravenous heparin is the sole dependable agent. It is best given by constant infusion (18).

12. Carotid endarterectomy has a major role in the preventive treatment of stroke. It can be done with a mortality rate of less than 2% (5, 9, 18, 20, 23, 24).

13. Vertebral endarterectomy, although occasionally indicated, has not statistically been proven to have a high patency rate and to prevent stroke (9).

14. A subclavian steal syndrome, although capable of producing symptoms, is often asymptomatic (4, 7). It is not often followed by cerebral infarction. It can be treated by simple carotid-subclavian bypass surgery (4).

15. The exact indication for surgical therapy with vertebral compression by osteophytes or in the cases of carotid kinks has not been established (9). The exact incidence and documentation of significant thromboembolism distal to small carotid ulceration without major stenosis is unknown.

16. Intracranial bypass surgery; for example, superficial temporal artery or occipital artery middle cerebral or posterior circulation anastomosis, using microsurgical techniques, is now possible with a high

patency rate. Although it is generally accepted that high grade middle cerebral or intracranial carotid stenosis that is symptomatic may be indications for the bypass procedures, they have not been proven to be of lasting benefit in a sufficient number of cases with adequate follow-up (8). However, data are accumulating that are most favorable. Chater has estimated that up to 12,000 cases per year may be available and benefited by these bypass procedures. Presently, cervical carotid-intracranial carotid bypass vein or arterial grafts, although technically possible, are not practical therapeutic measures. Endarterectomy in the intracranial carotid artery has not been of proven value.

17. Since the role of physical and rehabilitative therapy in a significant and completed stroke has not been impressive and because cerebral infarction edema has no proven therapy and may be fatal, neurosurgeons are urged to educate the public about the warning attacks of stroke.

Many of the above statements and assumptions will be discussed and challenged during the scientific sessions of this Congress. However, as a clinical neurosurgeon engaged in stroke therapy, I would like to present a few practical guidelines to the medical and surgical management of extracranial occlusive disease. In the evaluation of a patient with a stroke syndrome, the clinician should establish the temporal profile of the history. The physical examination should include careful auscultation of the cervical and upper thoracic areas but avoid palpation of the cervical carotid arteries (3, 11). The ulcerative plaques that may be contained within these arteries, covered by platelet emboli and/or clot, are extremely susceptible to trauma. Not only have emboli been dislodged, producing an immediate stroke, but, on more than one occasion, both platelet and cholesterol emboli have been seen in the retina after palpation of cervical vessels. A careful cardiac exam is mandatory. The blood pressure in both arms and with position change, if feasible, should be monitored. Additional studies should include a fasting blood sugar and 2-hour postprandial blood sugar level, thyroid studies-usually a T-3 and T-4 determination, an electrocardiogram and, if there is any question about the heart being beset by significant arrhythmias, at least a 12-hour dynamic cardiac monitor determination is indicated. In certain instances, *e.g.*, emboli that are proven or suspected and angiography proves negative, echo cardiography may be very helpful in localizing significant mural thrombi or, on occasion, an atrial myxoma. A chest and skull x-ray and spinal puncture should be routine. When possible, a technetium flow study and brain scan would be extremely helpful in indicating the presence of cerebral infarction or, more importantly as Dr. John Rockett discussed (see Chapter 18), asymmetry of cervical or middle cerebral flow or actual occlusion of a carotid artery in the neck. At least three-vessel cerebral arteriography to include arch aortography when necessary, providing the patient's condition permits, is considered mandatory. When these factors are determined, a rational medical and/or surgical therapy can proceed.

Auscultation of the cervical vessels has become routine as a result of increasing experience in stroke management. This may present the significant problem of the asymptomatic carotid bruit. Studies are available demonstrating a carotid bruit may be followed in a significant percentage of cases by transient ischemic attacks or strokes (5, 23, 24). Of real concern is the increasing pitch or high pitched bruit which usually indicates a tight stenosis. Providing the patient is otherwise in satisfactory health, it is suggested that ophthalmodynamometry or a technetium flow study should be performed. If the flow study or the retinal artery pressure is decreased on the side of the bruit, cerebral arteriography should be considered (8). If a significant stenotic lesion of 90% or more is visualized, carotid endarterectomy should be considered. The risk of carotid endarterectomy in this individual should not be more than 1% (23, 24). This is less than the risk of further difficulty from that artery.

As Dr. Miller Fisher has said, the patient with the transient cerebral ischemic attack is telling you "Doctor, I am trying to have a stroke." Since there is no way of knowing how many transient ischemic attacks a patient will have before he has a completed cerebral infarction, a patient with an attack deserves immediate attention. Providing the syndrome is clear and particularly if there is an associated appropriate carotid bruit, this patient should probably be managed by obtaining skull and chest x-rays and a spinal puncture and be placed on intravenous heparin. Continuous infusion of heparin is the best way to insure accurate heparinization. It is rare for adequate heparinization to fail to stop transient ischemic attacks (18). This therapy allows a subsequent relative elective evaluation of the stroke syndrome.

A stroke in evolution or early stroke or reversible ischemic neurological deficit is best treated with expediency. Again, angiography is the key to the understanding of the problem. Although it is realized that many vascular surgeons are less than aggressive about this high risk patient, a more appropriate approach would be to immediately render the necessary medical or surgical therapy (5, 24). This aggressive approach can be justified only by obtaining the patient within the first 4 to 6 hours of the event and rapidly determining which therapy is indicated (9). In the case of carotid occlusion with significant neurological deficit, thrombectomy and endarterectomy is recommended. If one operates on this type of patient, the high risk can be justified if the operation is done very early. If thrombectomy produces a good back flow from the internal carotid artery, operative angiography should be done to be certain that all possible clot has been removed before reconstituting flow. Hemorrhagic cerebral infarction is a definite possibility, although the exact incidence has never been proven (25). Many surgeons have had more than one case who have made dramatic improvements from a near hemiplegic state. On the other hand, in the case of the carotid thrombosis with only transient difficulty, surgery may not be indicated. Since the distal end of the clot may still be active in carotid thrombosis, heparinization for 7 to 10 days to allow the clot to organize and not propagate distally above the carotid bifurcation is recommended. Heparinization for similar time is probably indicated in vertebral thrombosis. This nonsurgical approach is based on the principle that once a vessel that is causing symptoms has become occluded, the clot has become well organized and the patient remains asymptomatic, there is little chance the patient will have difficulty from that vessel again (18). This is not to say that ischemic attacks due to further occlusive disease affecting the collateral blood supply to that hemisphere will fail to occur. Chater estimates with the passage of time, 16% of these patient with carotid thrombosis will develop ipsilateral ischemic symptoms (see Chapter 21).

There are certain circumstances in which surgery should be considered in a patient with a completed infarction. These must be individualized, but one circumstance might be illustrated as follows. A right-handed patient presents with a significant right hemiparesis but with total preservation of speech. Arteriograms reveal a high grade carotid stenosis and a partial embolic occlusion of the middle cerebral artery. The patient might be placed on heparin to prevent further emboli even though there is a risk of a hemorrhagic infarction for approximately a week or 10 days. At this point, he has a hemiparesis but essentially normal speech. He still has the capacity to worsen because another embolus may destroy speech. Additional heparin for another week is followed by arteriography and shows either a persistence or disappearance of the embolus. An acceptable approach to this case would be a left carotid endarterectomy approximately 14 to 21 days after the original completed stroke. This therapy offers preservation of speech and prevents further embolic episodes.

A special problem in surgical vs. medical therapy is often presented by the individual who has bilateral significant carotid stenosis. It is generally agreed if the carotid stenosis is 70% or more, that ultimately bilateral endarterectomy should be performed even on the asymptomatic side (9, 18). This is justified by the low mortality rate of the procedure and the preventive nature of the surgery. The procedures should be done at least 1 week apart. There is some argument in the literature about which side should be done first. Some individuals recommend the most stenotic side should be done first or the side in which cross collateral flow occurs on angiography (9). The patient's symptoms indicate the active lesion and the symptomatic side should be operated first regardless of the stenosis on the other side. Internal shunts are suggested in bilateral lesions. Prior to operating on the second side, one should document the patency of the operated side either by angiography or by the use of the technetium flow scan. The patency of the vessel can be determined by the dynamic technetium flow scan, but often it will appear to be decreased following surgery. This apparent decrease in flow will not be corroborated by angiography and returns to normal at some time greater than 1 month after surgery. The technique of carotid endarterectomy deserves comment. One must understand and be familiar with vascular surgery principles to perform this operation. This is another subject for subspecialization within neurosurgical groups. Sundt's experience, the best mortality and morbidity available for carotid endarterectomy, illustrates the value of subspecialization (22). To do an operation well, one must perform it frequently. The major problems encountered in carotid endarterectomy are failure to obtain a generous proximal and distal exposure of the affected vessel site and dislodging an embolus from the plaque. Adequate exposure is achieved by making an incision from the region at or just below the ear lobe down along the antero medial border of the sterno cleidomastoid muscle and, when necessary, dissecting up the superficial lobe of the parotid gland and retracting it superiorly. Some surgeons recommend a transversal skin incision. In addition, the patient should be positioned with a sandbag under the operative shoulder with the head turned slightly to the opposite side and the neck somewhat hyperextended. Sharp dissection is mandatory. Gentleness helps prevent dislodging an embolus. Sectioning the ansacervicalis and meticulous dissection of the XIIth nerve allows it to be moved cephalad for a significant distance. The branch of the external carotid artery that usually comes across the top of the hypoglossal nerve can be ligated and divided to allow the nerve to be moved up and insure good distal exposure of the internal carotid artery. The carotid body should be blocked with xylocaine but not disturbed any more than necessary. This is particularly important in the patient with chronic obstructive pulmonary disease (24). Ideally, EEG monitoring should be carried out during this surgery, but it is not essential. General anesthesia is preferred and halothane is the anesthetic of choice (9). Hyperventilation should be avoided. Blood pressure should be elevated slightly. Vascular clamps or ramal tourniquets are used on the distal common carotid and the proximal external carotid. It is worthwhile to use a double loop of No. 0 silk around the distal internal carotid. This allows approximately 0.5 cm. of additional operative space. After blocking the carotid body, the patient is heparinized and, although 50 mg. of heparin are used commonly, in view of Sundt's experience of finding particulate matter on internal shunts with this dose of heparin, 75 mg are recommended. Additionally, the shunt tubing can be heparinized. The internal carotid artery should be occluded first with subsequent occlusion of the external carotid and common carotid arteries. I prefer the routine use of an internal silastic shunt or Sundt's internal shunt (23). The vessel is opened usually in the common carotid artery with a No. 11 blade knife; Pott's scissors are used to section vertically through the plaque to normal distal intima. A shunt is placed in the internal carotid artery first. It should fit snugly requiring very little compression from the external tourniquet device for security. The shunt is then placed in the common carotid artery being certain to avoid air emboli. Once the shunt is in place, the operation can be done at a comfortable pace. The plaque should be sectioned sharply in the common carotid and peeled out of the external carotid and the internal carotid. At times, a tongue of atheromatous material will extend a significant distance up the posterior medial wall of the internal carotid artery. Almost invariably, the distal end of the plaque will peel out leaving a smooth intimal surface and tacking down of the intima is not carried out routinely. All debris should be removed from the endarterectomized site leaving the vessel wall as smooth as possible. If the internal artery is quite large, simple closure with 5-0 prolene running suture is adequate. However, vein or dacron patches can be used to insure a wide open lumen through the endarterectomized site. The shunt is pulled out prior to final closure of the patch, the internal carotid artery is allowed to back bleed, the external carotid artery allowed to back bleed, and finally the common carotid artery allowed to bleed. The wound is thoroughly irrigated, and final closure is effected by making certain that all of the air is out of the vessel. Then, flow is restored by opening the external, the common, and the internal carotid arteries. Without reversing the heparin, the vessel is carefully palpated and if a thrill is felt, an arteriogram is mandatory. If the arteriogram reveals an intimal flap or any debris, the vessel should be reopened and cleaned. When closure is satisfactory, there should be an excellent pulse without a thrill. Postoperative heparinization is not necessary when these principles are followed. The heparin can be completely or partially reversed at the conclusion of the procedure depending upon the operator's choice.

In summary, there are many unanswered problems in stroke therapy. These comments are presented to stimulate interest and provoke an aggressive approach to stroke therapy by neurosurgeons. There is no doubt that the quality of life can be improved by extracranial and possibly extracranial-intracranial bypass vascular surgery. Prevention of stroke and extended longevity may be forthcoming by the use of platelet-inhibiting drugs. The main issue, the central plea, is that neurosurgeons lead the way.

REFERENCES

1. Acheson, J., and Hutchinson, E. D. The natural history of focal cerebral vascular disease, Q. J. Med., *40:* 15–23, 1971.
2. Baker, R. N., Broward, J. A., Fang, H. C., Fisher, C. M., Groch, S. N., Heyman, A., Karp, H. R., McDevitt, E., Scheinberg, P., Schwartz, W., and Toole, J. F. Anticoagulant therapy in cerebral infarction. Report on cooperative study. Neurology, *12:* 823–835, 1962.
3. Barnett, H. J. M. Platelets, drugs and cerebral ischemia. *In* Platelets, Drugs and Thrombosis, Proc. of a Symp. held at McMaster University, Hamilton, Ont., Oct. 1972, edited by Hirsch, J., Cade J. F., Gallus, A. S., Schönbaum E., pp. 233–252, S. Karger, Basel, 1975.
4. Cohn, L. H., Fogarty, T. J., Daily, P. O., Silverman, J. F., and Shumway, N. E. Surgical treatment of atherosclerotic lesions of the subclavian artery. Calif. Med. *116:* 8–12, 1972.
5. Edwards, W. S., Blakeley, W. R., and Lewis, C. E., Jr. Present status of carotid surgery in stroke prevention. Am. Surg., *40:* 164–167, 1974.
6. Evans, G., and Gent, M. Effect of platelet suppressive drugs on arterial and venous thromboembolism. *In* Platelets, Drugs and Thrombosis, Proc. of a Symp. held at McMaster University, Hamilton, Ontario, Oct. 1972, edited by Hirsch, J., Cade, J. F., Gallus A. S., Schönbaum E., pp. 258–262, S. Karger, Basel, 1975.
7. Fisher, C. M. Editorial. A new vascular syndrome-the subclavian steal. N. Engl. J. Med. *265:* 912–913, 1961.
8. Fisher, C. M. Personal communication, 1974.
9. Galbraith, J. G., Extracranial arterial occlusive disease. *In* Neurological Surgery, edited by J. R. Youmans, Chapter 29. W. B. Saunders, Philadelphia, 1973.
10. Haust, M. Platelets, thrombosis and atherosclerosis *In* Platelets, Drugs and Thrombosis, Proc. of a Symp. held at McMaster University, Hamilton, Ont., Oct. 1972, edited by J. Hirsch, J. F. Cade, A. S. Gallus, E. Schönbaum, pp. 94–110, S. Karger, Basel, 1975.
11. Hollenhorst, R. W. Significance of bright plaques in the retinal arterioles. J.A.M.A. *178:* 23–29, 1961.
12. Kurtzke, J. F., and Kurland, L. T. Epidemiology of cerebrovascular disease. *In* Cerebrovascular Survey Report. Subcommittee on Cerebrovascular Disease. NINDS p. 163, 1970.
13. Marshall, J. The natural history of transient ischaemic cerebrovascular attacks. Q. J. Med., *33:* 309–324, 1964.
14. Marshall, J. and Meadows, S. The natural history of amaurosis fugax. Brain, *91:* 419–434, 1968.
15. Marshall, J., and Shaw, D. A. Anticoagulant therapy in cerebrovascular disease. Proc. R. Soc. Med., *52:* 547–549, 1959.
16. Marshall, J. and Wilkinson, I.M.S. The prognosis of carotid transient ischaemic attacks in patients with normal angiograms. Brain, *94:* 395–402, 1971.
17. Millikan, C. H. Anticoagulant therapy in cerebrovascular disease. *In* Cerebrovascular Survey Report. Subcommittee on Cerebrovascular Disease. NINDS, p. 218, 1970.
18. Murphey, F., and Maccubbin, D. A. Carotid endarterectomy. A long-term follow-up study. J. Neurosurg. *23:* 156–168, 1965; Clin. Neurosurg. *13:* 291–312, 1965.

19. Mustard, J. F. Platelets, drugs and thrombosis: the problem. *In* Platelets, Drugs, and Thrombosis, Proc. of a Symp. held at McMaster University, Hamilton, Ont., Oct. 1972, edited by J. Hirsch, J. F. Cade, A. S. Gallus, E. Schönbaum, pp. 1–14, S. Karger, Basel, 1975.
20. Ojemann, R. G. The surgical treatment of cerebrovascular disease. N. Engl. J. Med. *274:* 440–448, 1966.
21. Pevehouse, B. C.: Personal communication, 1975.
22. Sundt, T. M. Jr., Sandok, B. A. and Whisnant, J. P. Carotid endarterectomy: complications and preoperative assessment and risk, Mayo Clin. Proc., *50:* 301–306, 1975.
23. Thompson, J. E., Austin, D. J., and Patman, R. D. Carotid endarterectomy for cerebrovascular insufficiency: long-term results in 592 patients followed up to thirteen years. Ann. Surg., *172:* 663–679.
24. Wylie, E. J., and Ehrenfeld, W. K. Extracranial occlusive cerebrovascular disease. *In* Diagnosis and Management, Chapter 7. W. B. Saunders, Philadelphia 1970.
25. Wylie, E. J., Hein, M. F., and Adams, J. E. Intracranial hemorrhage following surgical revascularization for treatment of acute strokes. J. Neurosurg. *21:* 212–215, 1964.
26. Vital statistics of the United States: mortality. U. S. Dept. of Health Education and Welfare, Public Health Service, National Vital Statistics Division, Washington, D.C., 1964.

CHAPTER

2

William H. Sweet, M.D., D.Sc.: A Biographical Sketch

ROBERT G. OJEMANN, M.D.

William Herbert Sweet was born on February 13, 1910 in Kerriston, Washington, the center of the timber industry in the foothills of Mount Ranier. It was soon apparent to his father, a surgeon, and his mother, a university graduate, that their first child possessed an exceptional mind. He did the first four grades in 2 years and graduated from high school at the age of 14. During this time it was also evident that he was a gifted musician and after graduation from high school he spent a year studying piano. Realizing that he did not wish to devote his life to becoming a concert artist, and undecided about his future, he worked for a year in a sawmill in Centralia, Washington.

At this point he entered the University of Washington and in 1930 graduated summa cum laude, first in a class of 1,000 graduates. With this brilliant academic record, he was accepted into Harvard Medical School in 1930. During his second year, he received a Rhodes Scholarship and the years of 1932 to 1934 were spent at Oxford University (Magdalen College) where he did research work in neurophysiology in the department of Sir Charles Sherrington. He received his B.Sc. degree from Oxford in 1934. On the basis of subsequent research work and publications, he was awarded a D.Sc. degree from Oxford University in 1957.

Not one to waste time or remain idle for even a short period, he utilized the Oxford vacation periods to study at the University of Würzburg (Germany) Medical School. In 1934 he took (in German) and passed the German Government Written and Oral Examinations in internal medicine. He then returned to Harvard Medical School and graduated cum laude with the class of 1936.

Training in neurosurgery began at the Massachusetts General Hospital in 1936 and then was continued for the next 3 years at the University of Chicago Clinic and Billings Hospital under Dr. Percival Bailey. Upon completion of his resident training in 1940, he returned to Harvard Medical School and the Massachusetts General Hospital as a Commonwealth Fund Fellow in research and for further special training in neurosurgery, especially of the autonomic nervous system.

In the early years of World War II and long prior to the United States' entry into that war, he actively sought a means to make explicit both his appreciation of his Rhodes Scholarship and his concern over the threat to the world implicit in Hitler's Germany. This opportunity came in mid 1941 when he was asked to return to England to be the Acting Chief of the Queen Elizabeth Hospital, Birmingham, and Regional Consultant in Neurosurgery to the British Emergency Medical Service in the Midlands. He served in these capacities until June, 1945, and in recognition of his efforts, he later received His Majesty's Medal for Service in the Cause of Freedom. Returning to the Massachusetts General Hospital in 1945, he resumed his career in academic neurosurgery.

Early in the 1950's, Dr. Sweet, with the support of Dr. J. C. White, head of the neurosurgical service at that time and a former honored guest of the Congress, determined that advancement in knowledge in clinical neurosurgery would be accelerated if the neurosurgical service included a group of basic science investigators. To this end, Dr. Sweet established laboratories in the department of neurosurgery to include biophysics, neurophysiology, electromicroscopy, neurochemistry, and immunology with full-time members devoting their efforts to basic problems in the neurosurgical field. He was one of the first individuals to emphasize the importance of research training as part of the residency program.

In 1961 Dr. Sweet became chief of the neurosurgical service of the Massachusetts General Hospital and at the present time also holds the appointment of professor of surgery at Harvard Medical School.

His contributions to basic and clinical neurosurgery are numerous and wide ranging. His major areas of interest have included basic studies of the flow and formation of cerebrospinal fluid in man, application of radioactive isotopes to the investigation and treatment of central nervous system disorders, improvements in the techniques of clinical neurosurgery, treatment of extracranial and intracranial vascular disorders, treatment of pain, experimental investigations with primary malignant brain tumors, treatment of aggressive behavior disorders associated with organic brain disease, and medicolegal problems of neurosurgery.

In 1951 he established, with the help of his biophysical colleagues, one of the first brain scan research laboratories and the first such laboratory to be utilized routinely for clinical diagnosis. The use of coincidence counting of the annihilation radiation from positron-emitting isotopes for clinical localization of focal brain lesions was first brought to fruition there. With Dr. James C. White, he has published two classic texts on the neurosurgical treatment of pain.

He has been active in many other scientific endeavors which includes service on councils and committee study sections for the National Institute of Health, membership on the Science and Technology Advisory Committee in the office of Manned Space Flight, scientific trustee from Harvard of Associated Universities, Inc., and an editor of *Neurochirgia* and the series of volumes entitled *Progress in Neurological Surgery*. He was founding member of the Neurosciences Research Program and has been an active associate of the program since its inception. He is an honorary member of the leading neurosurgical societies of Great Britian, Spain and Portugal, Egypt, France, and a corresponding foreign member of Swiss, Italian, and Scandinavian neurosurgical societies, and a Fellow of the Royal Society of Medicine of England. He is a diplomate of both the American Board of Neurological Surgery and the American Board of Psychiatry and Neurology. Membership is also held in the American Academy of Neurology, American College of Surgeons, American Academy of Arts and Sciences, Biological Sciences (Vice President 1964–1967), American Academy of Neurological Surgery, American Association of Neurological Surgeons, American Neurological Association (Vice President 1971–1972), American Society of Stereotactic Surgery, American Physiologic Society, American Surgical Association, American Medical Association, Association for Research in Nervous and Mental Diseases, Research Society of Neurological Surgeons, Society for Neuroscience, Society of Neurological Surgeons (President 1969–1970), Electroencephalographic Society, Boylston Medical Society, Alsted Society, New England Neurosurgical Society (President 1957–1958), Massachusetts Medical Society, and Boston Society of Psychiatry and Neurology (President 1957–1958).

Possessing a brilliant mind, superb technical skill, and a meticulous approach to problems in the operating room, he has supplied seemingly boundless energy to a vast number of important endeavors. Neurosurgery has been fortunate in having such an individual in its ranks for 4 decades.

CHAPTER

3

Bibliography of Dr. William H. Sweet, D.SC.

1. White, J. C., Whitelaw, G. P., Sweet, W. H., and Hurwitt, E. S. Blood loss in neurosurgical operations. Ann. Surg., *107:* 287–297, 1938.
2. White, J. C., Sweet, W. H., and Hurwitt, E. S. Water balance in neurosurgical patients. Ann. Surg., *107:* 438–457, 1938.
3. Sweet, W. H. Neurosurgery: The Surgeon. (A resume of operative procedures in osteoplastic craniotomy and suboccipital craniectomy.) Am. J. Nurs., *39:* 743–747, 1939.
4. Light, G., Sweet, W. H., Livingstone, H., and Engel, R. Neurological changes following spinal anesthesia. (Review of the literature and case report.) Surgery, *7:* 138–156, 1940.
5. Bailey, P., and Sweet, W. H. Effects on respiration, blood pressure and gastric motility of stimulation of orbital surface of frontal lobe. J. Neurophysiol., *3:* 276–281, 1940.
6. Sweet, W. H. A review of dermoid, teratoid and teratomatous intracranial tumors. Dis. Nerv. Syst., *1:* 228–238, 1940.
7. Sweet, W. H. Spontaneous cerebral ventriculostium. A.M.A. Arch. Neurol. Psychiatry *44:* 532–540, 1940.
8. Sweet, W. H. Seeping intracranial aneurysm simulating neoplasm (Syndrome of the corpus callosum.) A.M.A. Arch. Neurol. Psychiatry, *45:* 86–104, 1941.
9. Sweet, W. H., and Bailey, P. Experimental production of intracranial tumors in the white rat. A.M.A. Arch. Neurol. Psychiatry, *45:* 1047–1049, 1941.
10. Sweet, W. H., Gray, S. J., and Allen, J. G. Clinical detection of hepatic disease in hepatolenticular degeneration. (Report of nine cases.) J.A.M.A. *117:* 1613–1619, 1941.
11. Bennett, H. S., and Sweet, W. H. A heated thermocouple flow-meter for recording flow in blood vessels of experimental animals. Fed. Proc., *1:* 144, 1942. (Abstract)
12. Bennett, H. S., Sweet, W. H., and Bassett, D. L. A heated thermocouple flow-meter. J. Clin. Invest., *23:* 200–208, 1944. (Appendix to Bennett, H. S., Bassett, D. L., and Beecher, H. K. Influence of anesthesia (ether, cyclopropane, sodium evipal) on the circulation under normal and shock conditions, J. Clin. Invest., *23:* 181–200, 1944.)
13. Williams, D., and Sweet, W. H. The constitutional factor in anesthetic convulsions. Lancet, *2:* 430–433, 1944.
14. Sweet, W. H. The handling of the intracranial tumor suspect. Bull. New Engl. Med. Cent., *8:* 107–112, 1946.
15. Sweet, W. H., McCulloch, W. S., and Snider, R. S. Repetitive movements on basal ganglia stimulation after transection of cerebral peduncles. Fed. Proc., *6:* 213, 1947. (Abstract)
16. Sweet, W. H. Stimulation of the sino-atrial node for cardiac arrest during operation. Bull. Am. Coll. Surg., *32:* 234, 1947. (Abstract)
17. Sweet, W. H. Relief of pain by operations on the central nervous system. Surg. Clin. North Am., *27:* 1254–1262, 1947.

18. Sweet, W. H., and Bennett, H. S. Changes in internal carotid pressure during carotid and jugular occlusion and their clinical significance. J. Neurosurg., *5:* 178–195, 1948.
19. Sweet, W. H., Cotzias, G. C., Seed, J., and Yakovlev, P. I. Gastrointestinal hemorrhages, hyperglycemia, azotemia, hyperchloremia and hypernatremia following lesions of the frontal lobe in man. *In* The Frontal Lobes, A. Research Nerv. Ment. Dis., Proc., *27:* 795–822, 1948.
20. Sweet, W. H., Soloman, A., and Selverstone, B. Studies of formation diffusion and absorption of cerebrospinal fluid. 1. Preliminary studies on Na^{24}. Trans. Am. Neurol. Assoc., *73:* 228–230, 1948.
21. Solomon, A., Selverstone, B., and Sweet, W. H. Use of isotopes in study of the nervous system. Trans. Am. Neurol. Assoc., *73:* 179, 1948.
22. Sweet, W. H. Recent impressions of medical practice in Great Britain. N. Engl. J. Med., *240:* 168–173, 1949.
23. Sweet, W. H. Cerebral lobectomy. (Functional localization in the brain with special reference to areas that may be removed with or without totally disabling sequelae). Proceedings of the First National Cancer Conference of the American Cancer Society; and the National Cancer Institute of the U.S. Public Health Service, pp. 237–239, 1949.
24. Selverstone, B., Soloman, A. K., and Sweet, W. H. Location of brain tumors by means of radioactive phosphorus. J.A.M.A., *140:* 277–278, 1949.
25. Sweet, W. H., Selverstone, B., Soloman, A. K., and Bakay, L. Studies of formation, diffusion and absorption of constituents of cerebrospinal fluid in man. 1. Studies with Na^{24}. J. Clin. Invest., *28:* 814, 1949. (Abstract)
26. Selverstone, B., Sweet, W. H., and Robinson, C. V. The clinical use of radioactive phosphorus in the surgery of brain tumors. Ann. Surg., *130:* 643–650, 1949.
27. Sweet, W. H. Medical care in England. V. Med. Mon., *76:* 491–501, 1949. (Guest Editorial)
28. Selverstone, B., Solomon, A. K., and Sweet, W. H. Localization of cerebral tumors by means of radioactive phosphorus. EEG Clin. Neurophysiol., *1:* 235, 1949.
29. Sweet, W. H., Solomon, A. K., and Selverstone, B. Studies of formation, circulation and absorption of cerebrospinal fluid employing radioactive sodium. EEG Clin. Neurophysiol., *1:* 253, 1949.
30. Sweet, W. H. Report on the British National Health Service. N. Engl. J. Med., *243:* 1060–1063, 1950.
31. Sweet, W. H. Trigeminal injection with radiographic control. Technic and results, J.A.M.A., *142:* 392–396, 1950.
32. Sweet, W. H., Sarnoff, S. J., and Bakay, L. A clinical method for recording internal carotid pressure. Significance of changes during carotid occlusion. Surg. Gynecol. Obstet., *90:* 327–334, 1950.
33. Drew, J. H., and Sweet, W. H. Complications of ligation of carotid artery in young people for treatment of intracranial aneurysm. J. Nerv. Ment. Dis., *112:* 79–82, 1950. (Abstract)
34. Yakovlev, P. I., Hamlin, H., and Sweet, W. H. Frontal lobotomy. Neuroanatomical observation. J. Neuropathol. Exp. Neurol., *9:* 250–285, 1950.
35. Sweet, W. H. Failure to demonstrate gliomas with Evans blue. Precautions in use of intravital dyes in man. J. Neurosurg., *7:* 412–413, 1950.
36. White, J. C., Sweet, W. H., Hawkins, R., and Nilges, R. G. Anterolateral cordotomy results, complications, and causes of failure. Brain, *73:* 346–367, 1950.
37. Yakovlev, P. I., Hamlin, H., and Sweet, W. H. Anatomical study of lobotomy. Survey of six specimens from 11–235 days post-operative survival. *In* Studies in Lobotomy,

edited by M. Greenblatt, R. Arnot, and H. C. Solomon, pp. 309–329, Grune & Stratton, Inc., New York, 1950.

38. Sweet, W. H., White, J. C., Selverstone, B., and Nilges, R. G. Sensory responses from anterior roots and from surface and interior of spinal cord in man. Trans. Am. Neurol. Assoc., *75:* 165–169, 1950.

39. Chapman, W. P., Livingston, R. B., Livingston, K. E., and Sweet, W. H. Possible cortical areas involved in arterial hypertension. *In* Life Stress & Bodily Disease. A. Res. Nerv. & Ment. Dis. Proc., *29:* 775–798, 1950.

40. Sweet, W. H. The uses of nuclear disintegration in the diagnosis and treatment of brain tumor. N. Engl. J. Med., *245:* 875–878, 1951.

41. Bakay, L., Selverstone, B., and Sweet, W. H. Intravascular distribution of Na^{24} injected intravenously in man. J. Lab. Clin. Med., *38:* 893–903, 1951.

42. Sweet, W. H. Large left temporal chordoma with surgical removal. J. Nerv. Ment. Dis., *114:* 544–545, 1951. (Abstract)

43. Chapman, W. P., Hamlin, H., Freshwater, D. B., Livingston, R. B., Sweet, W. H., Poppen, J. L., and Emery, F. J. Démonstration physiologique de l'éxistence des zones cérébrales du cortex cérébral prenant part a la régulation de la pression sanguine et du rythme cardiaque chez l'homme. "Present evidence concerning the relationship of the cerebral cortex and/or sub-cortical areas to the regulation of blood pressure and heart rate in man." Premier Congrés Mondial de Cardiologie. *1:* 77–78, 1951.

44. Sweet, W. H., Selverstone, B., Soloway, S., and Stetten, DeW., Jr. Studies of formation, flow and absorption of cerebrospinal fluid. 2. Studies with heavy water in the normal man. Surgical Forum. Clinical Congress of the American College of Surgeons, pp. 376–381, 1950. W. B. Saunders, Philadelphia, 1951.

45. Selverstone, B., Sweet, W. H., and Ireton, R. J. Radioactive potassium, a new isotope for brain tumor localization. Surgical Forum. Clinical Congress of the American College of Surgeons, pp. 371–375, 1950. W. B. Saunders, Philadelphia 1951.

46. Sweet, W. H., and Javid, M. The possible use of slow neutrons plus $boron^{10}$ in therapy of intracranial tumors. Trans. Am. Neurol. Assoc., *76:* 60–63, 1951.

47. White, J. C., and Sweet, W. H. Effectiveness of cordotomy in phantom pain after amputation. Trans. Am. Neurol. Assoc., *76:* 108–114, 1951.

48. Sweet, W. H., and Javid, M. The possible use of neutron-capturing isotopes such as $boron^{10}$ in the treatment of neoplasms. 1. Intracranial tumors. J. Neurosurg., *9:* 200–209, 1952.

49. Mark, V. H., and Sweet, W. H. An unusual case of unilateral eighth-nerve tumor. J. Neurosurg., *9:* 395–397, 1952.

50. Holmes, E. M., Sweet, W. H., and Kelemen, G. Hemangiomas of the frontal bone. Report of three cases. Ann. Otol. Rhinol. Laryngol., *61:* 45–61, 1952.

51. White, J. C., and Sweet, W. H. Effectiveness of chordotomy in phantom pain after amputation. A.M.A. Arch. Neurol. Psychiatry., *67:* 315–322, 1952.

52. Javid, M., Brownell, G. L., and Sweet, W. H. The possible use of neutron-capturing isotopes such as $boron^{10}$ in the treatment of neoplasms. 2. Computation of the radiation energies and estimates of effects in normal and neoplastic brain. J. Clin. Invest., *31:* 604–610, 1952.

53. Bakay, L., and Sweet, W. H. Cervical and intracranial intra-arterial pressures with and without vascular occlusion. Their significance in the treatment of aneurysms and neoplasms. Surg. Gynecol. Obstet., *95:* 67–75, 1952.

54. Bonner, F., Cobb, S., Sweet, W. H., and White, J. C. Frontal lobe surgery in the treatment of pain. Psychosom. Med., *14:* 383–405, 1952. *In* Psychiatric Treatment. A. Res. Nerv. Ment. Dis., Proc., *31:* 392–421, 1953.

55. Locksley, H. B., Powsner, H., and Sweet, W. H. A tissue-to-metal adhesive useful in Geiger counting. Science, *116:* 572–573, 1952.
56. Sweet, W. H., and White, J. C. Pain fibers in the petrosal nerves. Trans. Am. Neurol. Assoc., *77:* 87–92, 1952.
57. Bakay, L., and Sweet, W. H. Intra-arterial pressures in the neck and brain. Late changes after carotid closure, acute measurements after vertebral closure. J. Neurosurg., *10:* 353–359, 1953.
58. Sweet, W. H., and Mark, V. H. Unipolar anodal electrolytic lesions in the brain of man and cat. Report of five human cases with electrically produced bulbar or mesencephalic tractotomies. A.M.A. Arch. Neurol. Psychiatry, *70:* 224–234, 1953.
59. Brownell, G. L., and Sweet, W. H. Localization of brain tumors with positron-emitters. Nucleonics, *11:* 40–45, 1953.
60. Sweet, W. H., and Locksley, H. B. The formation, flow and reabsorption of cerebrospinal fluid in man. Proc. Soc. Exp. Biol. Med., *84:* 397–402, 1953.
61. Sweet, W. H., and White, J. C. Disposition of pain fibers in some of the sympathetic nerves of man. Trans. Am. Neurol. Assoc., *78:* 131–136, 1953.
62. Dunphy, E. B., Dreisler, K. K., Cadigan, J. B., and Sweet, W. H. The uptake of radioactive phosphorus by intraocular neoplasms. Am. J. Opthalmol. *37:* 45–54, 1954.
63. Farr, L. E., Sweet, W. H., Robertson, J. S., Foster, C. G., Locksley, H. B., Sutherland, D. L., Mendelsohn, M. L., and Stickley, E. E. Neutron-capture therapy with boron in the treatment of glioblastoma multiforme. Am. J. Roentgenol., *71:* 279–293, 1954.
64. Mark, V. H., McPherson, P. M., and Sweet, W. H. A new method for correcting distortion in cranial roentgenograms. With special reference to a new human stereotactic instrument. Am. J. Roentgenol., *71:* 435–444, 1954.
65. Sweet, W. H., and Locksley, H. Formation, flow and reabsorption of cerebrospinal fluid in man. J. Nerv. Ment. Dis., *119:* 457–461, 1954.
66. Locksley, H. B., and Sweet, W. H. Tissue distribution of boron compounds in relation to neutron-capture therapy of cancer. Proc. Soc. Exp. Biol. Med., *86:* 56–63, 1954.
67. Locksley, H. B., Sweet, W. H., Powsner, H. J., and Dow, E. Suitability of tumor-bearing mice for predicting relative usefulness of isotopes in brain tumors. Comparative clinical and laboratory study in localization and treatment of brain tumors with p^{32}, Na^{24}, K^{42}, and sodium borate, A.M.A. Arch. Neurol. Psychiatry, *71:* 684–698, 1954.
68. Farr, L. E., Sweet, W. H., Locksley, H. B., and Robertson, J. S. Neutron-capture therapy of gliomas $boron^{10}$. Trans. Am. Neurol. Assoc., *79:* 110–113, 1954.
69. Sweet, W. H., and Brownell, G. L. Localization of intracranial lesions by scanning with positron-emitting arsenic. J.A.M.A., *157:* 1183–1188, 1955.
70. White, J. C., and Sweet, W. H. *In* Pain: Its Mechanisms and Neurosurgical Control, p.736, Charles C Thomas, Springfield, 1955.
71. Lougheed, W. M., Sweet, W. H., White, J. C., and Brewster, W. R. The use of hypothermia in surgical treatment of cerebral vascular lesions. A preliminary report. J. Neurosurg., *12:* 240–255, 1955.
72. Godwin, J. T., Farr, L. E., Sweet, W. H., and Robertson, J. S. Pathological study of 8 patients with glioblastoma multiforme treated by neutron-capture therapy using $boron^{10}$. Cancer, *8:* 601–615, 1955.
73. Sweet, W. H., and Brownell, G. L. The barrier between blood and cerebrospinal fluid. Excerpta Med., *8:* Sect. VIII, 837–839, 1955. (Abstract)
74. Brownell, G. L., and Sweet, W. H. Scanning of positron-emitting isotopes in diagnosis of intracranial and other lesions. Acta Radiol. *46:* 425–434, 1956. Also printed in Radioactive Isotopes & Nuclear Radiations in Medicine, United Nations Publica-

tions, *10:* 249–254, New York, 1956. Proceedings of the International Conference on the Peaceful Uses of Atomic Energy, Geneva, Aug. 1955.

75. Sweet, W. H. Positron-emitting isotopes in diagnosis of intracranial lesions. *In* Radioactive Isotopes & Nuclear Radiations in Medicine, United Nations Publications. *10:* 399–404, New York, 1956. Proceedings of the International Conference on the Peaceful Uses of Atomic Energy, Geneva, Aug. 1955.
76. Sweet, W. H., Brownell, G. L., Scholl, J. A., Bowsher, D. R., Benda, P., and Stickley, E. E. The formation, flow and absorption of cerebrospinal fluid; newer concepts based on studies with isotopes. *In* Neurology & Psychiatry in Childhood A. Res. Nerv. Ment. Dis., Proc., *34:* 101–159, 1956.
77. Sweet, W. H., and Brownell, G. L. The use of radioactive isotopes in the detection and localization of brain tumors. *In* Radioisotopes in Medicine, pp. 211–223, edited by G. A. Andrews, M. Brucer, and E. B. Anderson. Washington, U.S. Atomic Energy Commission, 1956.
78. Sweet, W. H. Diseases of the nervous system: A. Diagnosis and localization of intracranial lesions: B. The cerebrospinal fluid. Ann. Rev. Med., *7:* 441–460, 1956.
79. Luessenhop, A. J., Sweet, W. H., and Robinson, J. Possible use of the neutron-capturing isotope Lithium[6] in the radiation therapy of brain tumors. Am. J. Roentgenol., *76:* 375–392, 1956.
80. Sweet, W. H. Progress report on research in medicine, biology, agriculture and food preservation. Statement of William H. Sweet, M. D., *In* Progress Report on Atomic Energy Research. Hearing before the Subcommittee on Research and Development of the Joint Committee on Atomic Energy, Congress of the United States, pp. 127–152, June 4–8, 1956.
81. White, J. C., Richardson, E. P., Jr., and Sweet, W. H. Upper thoracic cordotomy for relief of pain. Postmortem correlation of spinal incision with analgesic levels in 18 cases. Ann. Surg., *144:* 407–420, 1956.
82. Sweet, W. H. General surgical training for the surgical specialties. Address before the Allen O. Whipple Surgical Society, Boston, Massachusetts, January, 1957. Proceedings of a Conference on post-doctoral education and training of the surgeon, Panel III, (privately printed) pp. 40–43, 1957.
83. Sweet, W. H., Koons, R. A., and McQueen, J. D. Hypothermia and hibernation in neurosurgery. *In* Clinical Neurosurgery, Proc. of the Congress of Neurological Surgeons, Miami Beach, Florida, 1955, edited by R. K. Thompson and I. J. Jackson, Williams and Wilkins Co., Baltimore, *3:* 224–248, 1957.
84. Sweet, W. H. Cerebral studies during local and general hypothermia. *In* Cold Injury, Transactions of the Fourth Conference, Nov. 1955, Princeton, New Jersey, edited by M. I. Ferrer, pp. 329–333, Josiah Macy Jr. Foundation, New York, 1957.
85. White, J. C., Sweet, W. H., and Richardson, E. P., Jr. Cysticercosis cerebri. A diagnostic and therapeutic problem of increasing importance. N. Engl. J. Med., *256:* 479–486, 1957.
86. Sweet, W. H. Surgery of the nervous system. *In* Surgery: Principles and Practice, edited by J. G. Allen, H. N. Harkins, C. A. Moyer, and J. E. Rhoads, pp. 1396–1445, J. B. Lippincott Company, Philadelphia, 1957.
87. Sweet, W. H. Formation, absorption and flow of cerebrospinal fluid. *In* Modern Trends in Neurology, Second Series, edited by D. Williams, pp. 29–43, Butterworth and Co. Ltd., London, 1957.
88. Sweet, W. H., Brewster, W. R., Osgood, P., and White, J. C. The therapeutic use of hypothermia: Physiology of the hypothermic state. Abstracts of Reports, 1st International Congress of Neurological Surgery, Brussels, 1957, Excerpta Med., pp. 1–3, 1957.

89. Kjellberg, R. N., and Sweet, W. H. Stereotactic surgery for involuntary movements. Abstracts of Reports, 1st International Congress of Neurological Surgery, Brussels, 1957, Excerpta Med., p. 41, 1957.

90. White, J. C., Richardson, E. P., Jr., and Sweet, W. H. Upper thoracic cordotomy for relief of pain. Postmortem correlation of spinal incision and analgesia levels in 18 cases. Excerpta Med. Surg., *9.1:* 711–712, 1957.

91. Luessenhop, A. J., Gallimore, J. C., Sweet, W. H., Struxness, E. G., and Robinson, J. The toxicity in man of hexavalent uranium following intravenous administration. Am. J. Roentgenol. Radium Ther. Nucl. Med., *79:* 83–100, 1958.

92. Sweet, W. H. William Jason Mixter, 1880–1958. Harvard Medical Alumni Bulletin, pp. 36–37, Wellesley Press, Wellesley, Massachusetts, 1958.

93. Hamlin, H., Sweet, W. H., and Lougheed, W. M. Surgical reconstruction of occluded cervical carotid artery. Report of a successful case with 4-year follow up and three examples without such treatment. J. Neurosurg., *15:* 427–437, 1958.

94. Bagnall, H. J., Benda, P., Brownell, G. L., and Sweet, W. H. Positron-scanning with copper^{64} in the diagnosis of intracranial lesions. Partition of copper^{6} versenate in, and excretion from, the body. J. Neurosurg., *15:* 411–426, 1958.

95. Aronow, S., Brownell, G. L., Sweet, W. H., and Thompson, T. J. Reactor applications to brain-tumor radiation therapy. Proceedings of the 3rd International Conference on Medical Electronics, pp. 490–495, London, 1959.

96. Sweet, W. H. Discussion of Case 45031, Weekly Clinicopathological Exercises. Case Records of the Massachusetts General Hospital. N. Engl. J. Med., *260:* 132–134, 1959.

97. Brownell, G. L., and Sweet, W. H. Studies on neutron-capture therapy. Proc. of the Geneva Conference, September 1958. Progress in Nuclear Energy, Series VII, Vol. 2-Medical Sciences, pp. 114–127, 1959.

98. Sweet, W. H., Mealey, J., Jr., Brownell, G. L., and Aronow, S. Coincidence scanning with positron-emitting arsenic or copper in the diagnosis of focal intracranial disease. *In* Medical Radioisotope Scanning, pp. 163–188, A seminar jointly organized by I.A.E.A. and W.H.O., International Atomic Energy Agency, Vienna, Austria, 1959.

99. Sweet, W. H., Mealey, J., Jr., Brownell, G. L., and Aronow, S. Coincidence scanning with positron-emitting arsenic or copper in the diagnosis of focal intracranial disease. Abstracts of the Introductory Papers Presented at the International Atomic Energy Agency—World Health Organization Seminar on Medical Radioisotope Scanning Techniques and Results, Vienna, Austria, Feb. 1959. Int. J. Appl. Radiat. Isot., *5:* 152–153, 1959.

100. Mealey, J., Jr., Brownell, G. L., and Sweet, W. H. Radioarsenic in plasma, urine, normal tissues, and intracranial neoplasms. Distribution and turnover after intravenous injection in man. A.M.A. Arch. Neurol. Psychiatry, *81:* 310–320, 1959.

101. Sweet, W. H. Pain. *In* Handbook of Physiology-Neurophysiology 1, edited by H. W. Magoun, 459–506, Williams and Wilkins Co., Baltimore, 1959.

102. Sweet, W. H., Talland, G. A., and Ervin, F. R. Loss of recent memory following section of fornix. Trans. Am. Neurol. Assoc., *84:* 76–82, 1959.

103. White, J. C., Sweet, W. H., and Hackett, T. P. Electrolytic leucotomy for relief of pain. Radiofrequency coagulation of frontothalamic fibres in stages by means of in-lying electrodes. Trans. Am. Neurol. Assoc., *84:* 88–92, 1959.

104. Kjellberg, R. N. and Sweet, W. H.: Stereotactic surgery for involuntary movements. *In* Proceedings of the First International Congress of Neurological Sciences, Brussels, Belgium, 1957, (Neurological Surgery), edited by L. van Bogaert and J. Radermecker, Vol. II, pp. 56–59, Pergamon Press, New York, 1959.

105. Sweet, W. H., Brewster, W. R., Osgood, P., and White, J. C. Physiology of the hypothermic state. *In* Proceedings of the First International Congress of Neurological Sciences, Brussels, 1957, (Neurological Surgery), edited by L. van Bogaert and J. Radermecker, Vol. II, pp. 304–311, Pergamon Press, New York, 1959.

106. Brownell, G. L., Ellett, W. H., Ojemann, R. G., and Sweet, W. H. The use of short lived isotopes in the perfusion therapy of isolated organs. *In* Radioaktive Isotope in Klinik und Forschung, edited by K. Fellinger and R. Hofer, Fourth International Symposium, Bad Gastein, Austria, Urban & Schwarzenberg, Munich and Berlin, *4:* 126–141, 1960.

107. Sweet, W. H., Mark, V. H. and Hamlin, H. Radiofrequency lesions in the central nervous system of man and cat: Including case reports of eight bulbar pain-tract interruptions. J. Neurosurg., *17:* 213–225, 1960.

108. White, J. C., Sweet, W. H., and Hackett, T. P. Radiofrequency leucotomy for relief of pain. Coagulation of medial frontal white fibers in stages by means of inlying electrodes. A.M.A. Arch. Neurol., *2:* 317–330, 1960.

109. Brazier, M. A. B., Kjellberg, R. N., Sweet, W. H., and Barlow, J. S. Electrographic recording and correlation analysis from deep structures within the human brain. *In* Electrical Studies on the Unanesthetized Brain, edited by E. R. Ramey and D. S. O'Doherty, pp. 311–333, Paul C. Hoeber, New York, 1960.

110. Sweet, W. H., Soloway, A. H., and Brownell, G. L. Studies relevant to slow-neutron-capture therapy of brain tumor. Acta Union Intern. Contre le Cancer, *16:* 1216–1219, 1960.

111. Soloway, A. H., de Rougement, J. G., and Sweet, W. H. The re-establishment in dogs of the blood-brain barrier to tri-iso-propanolamine borate. Neurochirurgia, *3:* 1–5, 1960.

112. Sweet, W. H. Radioisotopes in the neurosurgical field. Address given at Sapporo Medical College, Sapporo, Japan, September 1960. Privately printed, pp. 1–17, 1960.

113. Mark, V. H. and Sweet, W. H. Ventriculo-atriostomy; a technical note: The accurate placement of the distal end of the shunt into the right atrium without X-ray control. Neurochirurgia, *3:* 115–120, 1960.

114. Field, R. A., Hall, W. A., Contreras, J. S., and Sweet, W. H. Hypophyseal-stalk section in the treatment of advancing diabetic retinopathy. Report of three cases. N. Engl. J. Med., *264:* 689–698, 1961.

115. Ojemann, R. G., Brownell, G. L., and Sweet, W. H. Possible radiation therapy of cephalic neoplasms by perfusion of short-lived isotopes. II. Dysprosium-165. Metabolism in mouse and cat. Neurochirurgia, *4:* 41–57, 1961.

116. Luessenhop, A. J., Mora, F., and Sweet, W. H. Subarachnoid hemorrhage, intracranial aneurysms and arterio-venous anomalies. Treatment by cervical carotid occlusion. *In* Pathogenesis and Treatment of Cerebrovascular Disease, Seventh Annual Scientific Meeting of the Houston Neurological Society, edited by W. S. Fields, pp. 516–556, Charles C Thomas, Springfield, Ill., 1961.

117. Sweet, W. H., Mealey, J., Jr., Aronow, S., and Brownell, G. L. Localization of focal intracranial lesions by scanning of rays from positron-emitting isotopes. *In* Clinical Neurosurgery, Proceedings of the Congress of Neurological Surgeons, Miami Beach, Florida, 1959, edited by R. G. Fisher, The Williams and Wilkins Company, Baltimore, *7:* 159–199, 1961.

118. Sweet, W. H. Surgery of the nervous system. *In* Surgery: Principles and Practice, edited by H. N. Harkins, C. A. Moyer, J. E. Rhoads, and J. G. Allen, 2nd edition (revised) pp. 1465–1515, J. B. Lippincott Company, Philadelphia, 1961.

119. Sweet, W. H., Soloway, A. H., and Brownell, G. L . Boron slow neutron-capture

therapy of operatively exposed gliomas. (Second International Congress of Neurological Surgery, Washington, D. C.) Excerpta Med., International Congress Series 36 (abstract 134), 1961.

120. Kjellberg, R. N., Mark, V. H., and Sweet, W. H. Closed chest manual systole. Two successfully treated neurosurgical patients with cardiac arrest. Neurochirurgia, *4:* 131–137, 1961.

121. Sweet, W. H. Discussion of paper by Vandewater, S. L. The use of hypotension and hypothermia in subarachnoid hemorrhage. *In* Pathogenesis and Treatment of Cerebrovascular Disease, 7th Annual Scientific Meeting of the Houston Neurological Society, 1959, edited by W. S. Fields, pp. 488–495, Charles C Thomas, Springfield, Ill., 1961.

122. Kjellberg, R. N., Todd, D. P., Schwab, R. S., England, A. C., Lance, J. W., and Sweet, W. H. Gait improvement in Parkinsonian patients by gamma motor neuron suppression. Trans. Am. Neurol. Assoc., *86:* 126–130, 1961.

123. Kjellberg, R. N., Ervin, F. R., and Sweet, W. H. Neuroelectric studies in the depths of the brain in man. Excerpta Med., International Congress Series No. 38, Abstract 85. (7th International Congress of Neurology, Rome, 1961).

124. Mark, V. H., Sweet, W. H., and McPherson, P. M. Stereotactic surgery: A note on instrumentation. J. Neurol. Neurosurg. Psychiatry., *25:* 86–89, 1962.

125. Sweet, W. H. Neurologic surgery. What's new in surgery? Surg. Gynecol. Obstet., *114:* 225–228, 1962.

126. Contreras, J. S., Field, R. A., Hall, W. A., and Sweet, W. H. Ophthalmological observations in hypophyseal stalk section. Report of eight cases of advancing diabetic retinopathy. Arch. Ophthalmol., *67:* 428–438, 1962.

127. Sweet, W. H., Soloway, A. H., and Wright, R. L. Evaluation of boron compounds for use in neutron therapy of brain tumors. II. Studies in man. J. Pharmacol., *137:* 263–266, 1962.

128. Sweet, W. H., Aronow, S. and Brownell, G. L. External localization of intracranial lesions with radioactive isotopes. Schweiz. Med. Wochenschr., *92:* 1545–1550, 1962.

129. Wright, R. L., and Sweet, W. H. Treatment of intracranial aneurysms by carotid occlusion: Correlation of late clinical follow-up with pressure recordings. Trans. Am. Neurol. Assoc., *87:* 158–162, 1962.

130. Kjellberg, R. N., Sweet, W. H., Preston, W. M., and Koehler, A. M. The Bragg peak of a proton beam in intracranial therapy of tumors. Trans. Am. Neurol. Assoc., *87:* 216–218, 1962.

131. Field, R. A., Schepens, C. L., Sweet, W. H., and Appels, A. The effect of hypophyseal stalk section on advancing diabetic retinopathy. Report of thirteen cases. Diabetes, *11:* 465–469, 1962.

132. Kjellberg, R. N., Koehler, A. M., Preston, W. M., and Sweet, W. H. Stereotaxic instrument for use with the Bragg peak of a proton beam. Confin. Neurol., *22:* 183–189, 1962. (1st International Symposium on Steteoencephalotomy, Philadelphia, 1961).

133. Sweet, W. H. The brain. *In* Surgery, edited by R. Warren, pp. 314–369. W. B. Saunders, Philadelphia, 1963.

134. Wright, R. L., and Sweet, W. H. Carotid or vertebral occlusion in the treatment of intracranial aneurysms; value of early and late readings of carotid and retinal pressures. *In* Clinical Neurosurgery, edited by W. H. Mosberg, Jr., Vol. 9, pp. 163–192, Proceedings of the Congress of Neurological Surgeons, New York, 1961, The Williams & Wilkins Co., Baltimore, 1963.

135. Sweet, W. H., Soloway, A. H., and Brownell, G. L. Boron-slow neutron capture

therapy of gliomas. Acta Radiol., *1:* 114–121, 1963.

136. Sweet, W. H., McMeel, J. W., and Field, R. A. Hypophyseal stalk section in the treatment of diabetic retinopathy. Highlights Ophthalmol., *6:* 259–283, 1963. (Symposium on Diabetic Retinopathy, Chicago Ophthalmological Society, May, 1963).

137. Field, R. A., Sweet, W. H., McMeel, J. W., Germanos, R. P., and Schepens, C. L. Influence de la section de la tige pituitaire sur la retinite diabetique hemorragique progressive. Union Med. Can., *92:* 1297–1300, 1963.

138. Ojemann, R. G., Aronow, S., and Sweet, W. H. Scanning with positron-emitting radioisotopes. Occlusive cerebral vascular disease. Arch. Neurol., *10:* 218–228, 1964.

139. Lippincott, S. W., Corcoran, C., Jansen, C. R., Jesseph, J. E., Rai, K., Aronow, S., Greene, M. W., and Sweet, W H. Labeling of globulin with I^{124} for positron scanning of neoplasms. J. Nucl. Med., *5:* 193–199, 1964.

140. Entzian, W., Aronow, S., Soloway, A. H., and Sweet, W. H. A preliminary evaluation of F^{18}-labeled tetrafluoborate as a scanning agent for intracranial tumors. J. Nucl. Med., *5:* 542–550, 1964.

141. Kjellberg, R. N., Koehler, A. M., Preston, W. M., and Sweet, W. H. Intracranial lesions made by a proton beam. *In* Response of the Nervous System in Ionizing Radiation, edited by T. J. Haley, and R. S. Snider, pp. 36–53. Little, Brown and Co., Boston, 1964, (2nd International Symposium, Los Angeles, 1963).

142. Entzian, W., Aronow, S., Soloway, A. H., and Sweet, W. H. Evaluation of fluorine-18 as a scanning agent for intracranial tumours. Med. Radioisotope Scanning, *2:* 109–120, 1964. (International Atomic Energy Agency Medical Radioisotope Scanning Symposium, April, 1964).

143. Soloway, A. H., Brownell, G. L., Ojemann, R. G., and Sweet, W. H. Boron-slow neutron capture therapy: Present status. *In* Preparation and Biomedical Application of Labeled Molecules, edited by J. Sirchis, pp. 383–403, Euratom, Brussels, 1964. (Proceedings of the International Symposium, Venice 1964).

144. Wright, R. L., and Sweet, W. H. Intraarterial pressure determinations at the time of carotid occlusion. Correlation with clinical tolerance of occlusion and subsequent subarachnoid hemorrhage. *In* Intracranial Aneurysms and Subarachnoid Hemorrhage, edited by W. S. Fields and A. L. Sahs, pp. 1–24. Charles C Thomas Co., Springfield, Ill., 1965.

145. Wilkinson, H. A., Wright, R. L., and Sweet, W. H. Correlation of reduction in pressure and angiographic cross-filling with tolerance of carotid occlusion. J. Neurosurg., *22:* 241–245, 1965.

146. Adams, R. D., Fisher, C. M., Hakim, S., Ojemann, R. G., and Sweet, W. H. Symptomatic occult hydrocephalus with "normal" cerebrospinal fluid pressure. A treatable syndrome. N. Engl. J. Med., *273:* 117–126, 1965.

147. Sweet, W. H. Some structures in man related to memory. Clin. Neurophysiol., *18:* 310, 1965. (Conference on the Neurological Basis of Behavior, Honolulu, May, 1964).

148. Ojemann, R. G., Aronow, S., and Sweet, W. H. Scanning with positron-emitting radioisotopes: Aneurysm, arteriovenous malformation, and intracerebral hemorrhage. J. Neurosurg., *22:* 489–498, 1965.

149. Sweet, W. H. Surgery of the nervous system. *In* Surgery: Principles and Practice, edited by C. A. Moyer, *et al.*, 3rd ed., pp. 1661–1715. J. P. Lippincott Co., Philadelphia, 1965.

150. Schwab, R. S., Sweet, W. H., Mark, V. H., Kjellberg, R. N., and Ervin, F. R. Treatment of intractable temporal lobe epilepsy by stereotactic amygdala lesions. Trans. Am. Neurol. Assoc., *90:* 12–19, 1965.

151. Kjellberg, R. N., Field, R. A., McMeel, J. W., and Sweet, W. H. Bragg peak pituitary

destruction for diabetic retinopathy. Excerpta Med. International Congress Series No. 93, Abstract 102. (3rd International Congress of Neurosurgery, Copenhagen, 1965).

152. Kjellberg, R. N., Koehler, A. M., Preston, W. M., and Sweet, W. H. Hemorrhagic diabetic retinopathy: Treatment by pituitary stalk section or by pituitary irradiation with protons at the Bragg peak. Neurol. Med.-Chir. (English edition), *7:* 1–13, 1966.

153. Aronow, S., Brownell, G. L., W. H., and Ojemann, R. G. Radioisotopic scanning methods. I. Use of positron-emitting isotopes in the diagnosis of intracranial disease. *In* Neurological Diagnostic Techniques, edited by W. S. Fields, pp. 190–214. Charles C Thomas, Springfield, Ill., 1966.

154. Sweet, W. H. Atypical facial neuralgia. *In* Pain: Henry Ford Hospital International Symposium, edited by R. S. Knighton and P. R. Dumke, pp. 415–420. Little, Brown and Co., Boston, 1966.

155. Hackett, T. P., White, J. C., and Sweet, W. H. Leukotomy for the relief of pain: The selection of cases and psychological hazards. *In* Pain: Henry Ford Hospital International Symposium, edited by R. S. Knighton and P. R. Dumke, pp. 461–467, Little, Brown and Co., Boston, 1966.

156. Sweet, W. H. Designated discussion of paper by Bertrand, C., Martinex, N., and Hardy, J. Frontothalamic section for intractable pain. *In* Pain: Henry Ford Hospital International Symposium, edited by R. S. Knighton and P. R. Dumke, pp. 536–539. Little Brown and Co., Boston, 1966.

157. Knighton, R. S., Owens, G., Nulsen, F. E., Nathan, P. W., Sweet, W. H., Mullan, S., and Noordenbos, W. Panel discussion; unsolved pain problems. *In* Pain: Henry Ford Hospital International Symposium, edited by R. S. Knighton and P. R. Dumke, pp. 550–560, Little, Brown and Co., Boston, 1966.

158. Entzian, W., Soloway, A. H., Raju, R., Sweet, W. H., and Brownell, G. L. Effect of neutron capture irradiation upon malignant brain tumors in mice. Acta Radiol., *5:* 95–100, 1966.

159. Sweet, W. H., Talland, G. A., and Ballantine, H. T. A memory and mood disorder associated with ruptured anterior communicating aneurysm. Trans. Am. Neurol. Assoc., *91:* 346–348, 1966.

160. Ojemann, R. G., Aronow, S., and Sweet, W. H. Scanning with positron-emitting isotopes in cerebrovascular disease. Acta Radiol., *5:* 894–905, 1966.

161. Krayenbühl, H., Maspes, P., and Sweet, W. *In* Progress in Neurological Surgery, Editorial Preface, edited by H. Krayenbühl, P. Maspes and W. Sweet. Vol. 1, Basel (Switzerland), S. Karger, New York, 1966.

162. Bogoch, S., Sachs, W., Sweet, W. H., Korsh, G., and Belval, P. C. Structure of and incorporation of (^{14}C) Glucose into isolated protein and carbohydrate macromolecules of brain subcellular membranous components in resting, training, and tumor brain tissue. *In* Protides of the Biological Fluids, edited by H. Peeters, Vol. 15, pp. 131–141, Elsevier Publishing Co., Amsterdam, 1967.

163. Sweet, W. H. Hemorrhagic diabetic retinopathy: Treatment by pituitary stalk section or by pituitary irradiation with protons at the Bragg peak. Brain Nerve (Japanese edition), *19:* 12–18, 1967.

164. Wall, P. D., and Sweet, W. H. Temporary abolition of pain in man. Science, *155:* 108–109, 1967.

165. Brownell, G. L., Soloway, A. H., and Sweet, W. H. Boron capture therapy. *In* Modern Trends in Radiotherapy, edited by T. H. Deeley and C. A. P. Wood, pp. 132–144, Butterworths, London, 1967.

166. Sweet, W. H. Neurosurgical management of pain. *In* New Concepts in Pain and Its Clinical Management, edited by E. L. Way, pp. 169–185. F. A. Davis Co., Philadelphia, 1967.

167. Hatanaka, H., Soloway, A. H., and Sweet, W. H. Incorporation of pyrimidines and boron analogues into brain tumour and brain tissue of mice: An approach to boron-neutron capture therapy. Neurochirurgia, *10:* 87–95, 1967.

168. Sweet, W. H., Kjellberg, R. N., Field, R. A., Koehler, A. M., and Preston, W. M. Time-intensity data in solar cosmic ray events; biological data relevant to their effects in man. Radiat. Res., (Suppl.), *7:* 369–383, 1967.

169. Mark, V. H., Sweet, W. H., and Ervin, F. R. Role of brain disease in riots and urban violence. J.A.M.A., *201:* 895, 1967.

170. Sweet, W. H. Designated discussion of paper by Zervas, N. T., Horner, F. G., and Gordy, P. D. Cerebellar dentatectomy in primates and humans. Trans. Am. Neurol. Assoc., *92:* 29–30, 1967.

171. Talland, G. A., Sweet, W. H., and Ballantine, H. T. Amnesic syndrome with anterior communicating artery aneurysm. J. Nerv. Ment. Dis., *145:* 179–192, 1967.

172. Sweet, W. H. Post-traumatic pain in head or neck: Possibility of neurosurgical relief. Abstracts of Papers of the 2nd Asian and Oceanian Congress of Neurology, Melbourne, p. 41, 1967.

173. Krayenbühl, H., Maspes, P. E., and Sweet, W. H. *In* Progress in Neurological Surgery, Editional preface, edited by H. Krayenbühl, P. Maspes, and W. Sweet, Vol. 2, p. V. Basel (Switzerland), S. Karger, New York, 1966.

174. Beecher, H. K., Adams, R. D., Barger, A. C., Curran, W. J., Denny-Brown, D., Farnsworth, D. L., Folch-Pi, J., Mendelsohn, E. I., Merrill, J. P., Murray, J., Potter, R., Schwab, R., and Sweet, W. H. A definition of irreversible coma: Report of the *Ad Hoc* Committee of the Harvard Medical School to examine the definition of brain death. J.A.M.A., *205:* 337–340, 1968.

175. Benda, P., Lightbody, J., Sato, G., Levine, L., and Sweet, W. H. Differentiated rat glial cell strain in tissue culture. Science, *161:* 370, 371, 1968.

176. Delgado, J. M. R., Mark, V. H., Sweet, W. H., Ervin, F. R., Weiss, G., Bach-y-Rita, G., and Hagiwara, R. Intracerebral radio stimulation and recording in completely free patients. J. Nerv. Ment. Dis., *147:* 329–340, 1968.

177. Mark, V. H., Ervin, F. R., Geschwind, N., Solomon, P., and Sweet, W. H. The neurology of behavior: Its application to human violence. Med. Op. Rev., *4:* 26–31, 1968.

178. Mark, V. H., Sweet, W. H., and Ervin, F. R. Does brain disease play a role in riots and urban violence? J.A.M.A., *203:* 368, 1968.

179. Mark, V. H., Sweet, W. H., Ervin, F. R., Solomon, P., and Geschwind, N. Brain disease and violent behavior. *In* Neuro-ophthalmology, edited by J. L. Smith, Vol. IV, pp. 282–287, C. V. Mosby, Co., St. Louis, 1968.

180. McLardy, T., Ervin, F. R., Mark, V. H., Scoville, W., and Sweet, W. H. Attempted inset-electrodes-arousal from traumatic coma: Neuropathological findings. Trans. Am. Neurol. Assoc., *93:* 25–30, 1968.

181. Roda, J. E., Soloway, A. H., Benda, P., and Sweet, W. H. Evaluation of permanganate and manganous ions as scanning agents. Neurochirugia, *11:* 246–252, 1968.

182. Schmidek, H. H., Ervin, F. R., and Sweet, W. H. Alterations in pain threshold produced by mesencephalic, thalamic, and limbic stimulation in the awake squirrel monkey (Saimiri sciureus). Fed. Proc., *27:* 518, 1968.

183. Sweet, W. H. Designated discussion of paper by Yahr, M. D., Duvoisin, R. C., Hoehn, M. M., Schear, M. J., and Barrett, R. E. L-Dopa (L-3, 4-Dihydroxyphenylalinine)

—Its clinical effects in Parkinsonism. Trans. Am. Neurol. Assoc., *93:* 61–63, 1968.
184. Sweet, W. H. Lessons on pain control from electrical stimulation. Trans. Coll. Physicians, Philadelphia *35:* 171–184, 1968.
185. Sweet, W. H. Proton radiation for acromegaly. N. Engl. J. Med., *278:* 732, 1968.
186. Sweet, W. H. Specific neural stimulation for inhibition of pain. Proc. Aust. Assoc. Neurol., *5:* 459–461, 1968.
187. Sweet, W. H. Trigeminal neuralgias. *In* Facial Pain, edited by C. C. Alling, pp. 89–106. Lea & Febiger, Philadelphia, 1968.
188. Sweet, W. H., and Wepsic, J. G. Treatment of chronic pain by stimulation of fibers of primary afferent neurone. Trans. Am. Neurol. Assoc., *93:* 103–107, 1968.
189. Ashare, A. B., Bub, B., Potsaid, M. S., Ojemann, R. G., Aronow, S., and Sweet, W. H. Comparison of brain scanning techniques: 99^m Tc using an Anger camera and ^{74}As using a positron scanner. J. Nucl. Med., *10:* 205–208, 1969.
190. Beecher, H. K., Adams, R. D., and Sweet, W. H. Procedures for the appropriate management of patients who may have supportive measures withdrawn. J.A.M.A., *209:* 405, 1969.
191. Delgado, J. M. R., Mark, V. H., Sweet, W. H., Ervin, F. R., Weiss, G., Bach-y-Rita, G., and Hagiwara, R. Stimoceiver facilitates brain study. Mod. Med., *37:* 108, 1969.
192. Ervin, F. R., Delgado, J., Mark, V. H., and Sweet, W. H. Rage: A paraepileptic phenomenon? Epilepsia, *10:* 417, 1969. (Amst.)
193. Ervin, F. R., Mark, V. H., and Sweet, W. H. Focal cerebral disease, temporal lobe epilepsy and violent behavior. Trans. Am. Neurol. Assoc., *94:* 253–256, 1969.
194. Field, R. A., McMeel, J. W., Sweet, W. H. and Schepens, C. L. Hypophyseal stalk section for angiopathic diabetic retinopathy. *In* Symposium on the Treatment of Diabetic Retinopathy, edited by M. F. Goldberg, and S. L. Fine, pp. 213–225. Public Health Service Publication No. 1890, Arlington, 1969.
195. Sweet, W. H., and Field, R. A. Pituitary stalk section for angiopathic diabetic retinopathy: Technique, mortality, morbidity, post-operative management. *In* Symposium on the Treatment of Diabetic Retinopathy, edited by M. F. Goldberg, and S. L. Fine, pp. 355–364, Public Health Service Publication No. 1890, Arlington, 1969.
196. Sweet, W. H. Summary of surgical aspects of papers on pituitary ablation. *In* Symposium on the Treatment of Diabetic Retinopathy, edited by M. F. Goldberg, and S. L. Fine, pp. 415–421. Public Health Service Publication No. 1890, Arlington, 1969.
197. Sweet, W. H., and Field, R. A. Production of hypopituitarism in the treatment of diabetes. *In* Symposium on the Treatment of Diabetic Retinopathy, edited by M. F. Goldberg and S. L. Fine, pp. 722–729. Public Health Publication No. 1890, Arlington, 1969.
198. Mark, V. H., Ervin, F. R., Sweet, W. H., and Delgado, J. M. R. Remote telemeter stimulation and recording from implanted temporal lobe electrodes. Confin. Neurol., *31:* 86–93, 1969.
199. Mark, V. H., Folkman, J., Ervin, F. R., and Sweet, W. H. Focal brain suppression by means of a silicon rubber chemode. J. Neurosurg., *30:* 195, 1969.
200. McLardy, T., Mark, V. H., Scoville, W. B., and Sweet, W. H. Pathology in diffuse projection system preventing brainstem-electrode arousal from traumatic coma. Confin. Neurol., *31:* 219–225, 1969.
201. Ojemann, R. G., Fisher, C. M., Adams, R. D., Sweet, W. H. and New, P. F. Further experience with the syndrome of "normal" pressure hydrocephalus. J. Neurosurg., *31:* 279–294, 1969.
202. Ojemann, R. G., and Sweet, W. H. Radioisotopic scanning with positron-emitting

isotopes. *In* Brain Tumor Scanning with Radioisotopes, edited by L. Bakay and D. Klein, pp. 121–139. Charles C Thomas, Springfield, 1969.

203. Roda, J. E., Soloway, A. H., Benda, P., and Sweet, W. H. Biological behavior of $K^{56}MnO_4$: Its accumulation in normal tissues and pathological brain. J. Nucl. Med., *10:* 205–208, 1969.
204. Sweet, W. H. Centenary of Cushing's birth. N. Engl. J. Med., *280:* 838, 1969.
205. Sweet, W. H. Designated discussion of paper by W. Stern: The assessment of circulatory adequacy attendant upon carotid artery occlusion. Trans. Am. Neurol. Assoc., *94:* 18–19, 1969.
206. Sweet, W. H. Lessons on pain control from electrical stimulation. Neurol. Neurosurg. (Excerpta Med.), *22:* 63, 1969.
207. Sweet, W. H. Surgical therapy in the treatment of cluster headache. *In* Research & Clinical Studies in Headache, edited by A. Freedman, Williams & Wilkins Co., Baltimore, 1969.
208. Sweet, W. H., Ervin, F. R., and Mark, V. H. The relationship of violent behaviour to focal cerebral disease. *In* Aggressive Behaviour, edited by S. Garattini and E. B. Sigg, pp. 336–352, Excerpta Med. Foundation, Amsterdam, 1969.
209. Sweet, W. H., and Wepsic, J. G. Control of pain by focal electrical stimulation for suppression. Ariz. Med., *26:* 1042–1045, 1969.
210. Sweet, W. H., and Wepsic, J. G. Treatment of pain by chronic electrical stimulation of large axons. Excerpta Med. International Congress Series No. 193. (4th International Congress of Neurological Surgery, New York, 1969).
211. White, J. C., and Sweet, W. H. Pain and the Neurosurgeon: A Forty Year Experience, Charles C Thomas, Springfield, Ill., 1969. (This is a separately bound book).
212. Krayenbühl, H., Maspes, P. F., and Sweet, W. H. *In* Progress in Neurological Surgery, Editorial Preface, edited by H. Krayenbühl, P. Maspes, and W. Sweet, Vol. 3, Basel (Switzerland), S. Karger, New York, 1969.
213. Ervin, F. R., Delgado, J., Mark, V. H., and Sweet, W. H. Rage: A paraepileptic phenomenon? Epilepsy Abstracts, *3:* 16, 1970.
214. Roda, J. E., Soloway, A. H., Benda, P. and Sweet, W. H. Biological behavior of $K^{56}MnO_4$: Its accumulation in normal tissues and pathological brain. Neurol. Neurosurg. (Excerpta Med.), *23:* 333, 1970. (Abstract)
215. Benda, P., Mori, T., and Sweet, W. H. Demonstration of an astrocyte-specific cerebroprotein by an immunofluorescence study of brain tumors. J. Neurosurg., *33:* 281–286, 1970.
216. Sweet, W. H. Designated discussion of paper by Fager, C.: Surgery of sellar and parasellar tumor. *In* Clinical Neurosurgery, edited by R. G. Ojemann, Vol. 17, p. 224, Williams and Wilkins Co., Baltimore, 1970.
217. Sweet, W. H. Book review of Pain, edited by A. Soulairac, J. Cahn, and J. Charpentier, Academic Press, London and New York, 1968. Science, *169:* 666–667, 1970.
218. Sweet, W. H. Surgery of the nervous system. *In* Surgery: Principles and Practice, edited by J. E. Rhoads, J. G. Allen, H. A. Harkins, and C. A. Moyer, 4th ed., pp. 1755–1809, J. B. Lippincott Co., Philadelphia, 1970.
219. Sweet, W. H. *In* Violence and the Brain by V. H. Mark, and F. R. Ervin p. vii, Harper & Row, New York, 1970.
220. Sweet, W. H., and Wepsic, J. G. Relation of fiber size in trigeminal posterior root to conduction of impulses for pain and touch: Production of analgesia without anesthesia in the effective treatment of trigeminal neuralgia. Trans. Am. Neurol. Assoc., *95:* 134–139, 1970.
221. Sweet, W. H., and Wepsic, J. G. Relation of fiber size in trigeminal posterior root to

conduction of impulses for pain and touch: Production of analgesia without anesthesia in the effective treatment of trigeminal neuralgia. Acta Neurol. Scand., *46:* 618–636, 1970.

222. Sweet, W. H. Designated discussion of paper by Denny-Brown, D., and Yanagisawa, N. The descending trigeminal tract as a mechanism for intersegmental facilitation. Trans. Am. Neurol. Assoc., *95:* 131, 1970.

223. Ervin, F. R., Sweet, W. H., and Mark, V. H. Amygdala function in man. The problem of violent behavior. Activ. Nerv. Suppl. (Praha), *12:* 185, 1970.

224. Krayenbühl, H., Maspes, P., and Sweet, W. *In* Progress in Neurological Surgery, Editorial Preface, edited by H. Krayenbühl, P. Maspes, and W. Sweet, Vol. 4, Basel (Switzerland), S. Karger, New York, 1971.

225. Sweet, W. H. Historical development of tracer uses in CSF dynamics. *In* Central Nervous System Investigation with Radionuclides, edited by A. J. Gilson and W. M. Smoak, pp. 39–57, Charles C Thomas, Springfield, Ill., 1971.

226. Sweet, W. H. *In* Central Nervous System Investigation with Radionuclides, edited by A. J. Gilson and W. M. Smoak, pp. ix–x, Charles C Thomas, Springfield, Ill., 1971.

227. Benda, P., Someda, I., Messer, J., and Sweet, W. H. Morphological and immunological studies of rat glial tumors and clonal strains propagated in culture. J. Neurosurg., *34:* 310–322, 1971.

228. Wright, R. L., and Sweet, W. H. Surgical treatment of intractable pain. *In* The Craft of Surgery, edited by I. Cooper, pp. 1694–1722, Little Brown and Co., Boston, 1971.

229. Sweet, W. H., and Rich, C. R. Development of criteria for the diagnosis of irreversible coma. Trans. Am. Neurol. Assoc., *96:* 314–317, 1971.

230. Sweet, W. H., and Schmidek, H. H. Case Records of the Massachusetts General Hospital. N. Engl. J. Med., *284:* 1431, 1971.

231. Sweet, W. H. and Wepsic, J. G. Destruction of pain-producing fibers by RF energy. Neuroelectric News, *2:* 3–4, 1971.

232. Schmidek, H. H., Fohanno, E., Ervin, F. R. and Sweet, W. H. Pain threshold alterations by brain stimulation in the monkey. J. Neurosurg., *35:* 715–722, 1971.

233. Sweet, W. H. Controlled thermocoagulation of trigeminal ganglion and rootlets for differential destruction of pain fibers. *In* Present Limits of Neurosurgery, edited by I. Fusek and Z. Kunc, p. 529, Avicenum, Czechoslovak Medical Press, Prague, 1972. (Fourth European Congress of Neurosurgery, Prague, 1971).

234. Sweet, W. H. Convenient protection for ultraviolet radiation. Editorial. Arch. Surg., *104:* 259, 1972.

235. Asbury, A. K., Ojemann, R. G., Nielsen, S. L., and Sweet, W. H. Neuropathologic study of fourteen cases of malignant brain tumor treated by Boron-10 slow neutron capture radiation. J. Neuropathol. Exp. Neurol., *31:* 278–303, 1972.

236. Mark, V. H., Sweet, W. H., and Ervin, F. R. The effect of amygdalotomy on violent behavior in patients with temporal lobe epilepsy. *In* Psychosurgery, pp. 139–155, Charles C Thomas, Springfield, Ill., 1972, (II International Congress of Psychosurgery, Copenhagen, 1970).

237. Mark, V. H., Ervin, F. R., and Sweet, W. H. Deep temporal lobe stimulation in man. *In* The Neurobiology of the Amygdala, edited by B. E. Eleftheriou, pp. 485–507, Plenum Publishing Corp., New York, 1972.

238. Sweet, W. H. Early uses of radioisotopic tracers in the study of CSF dynamics. *In* Radioisotopic Cisternography and Hydrocephalus, edited by J. Harbert, pp. 545–553, Charles C Thomas, Springfield, Ill., 1972.

239. Sweet, W. H. The difference between nothing and one. Arch. Suisses Neurol., Neurosurg. Psychiatry., *3:* 443–445, 1972. (70th anniversary volume in honor of Prof. H. Krayenbühl).

240. Poletti, C. E., Sujatanond, M., and Sweet, W. H. Hypothalamic, preoptic, and basal forebrain unit responses to hippocampal stimulation in awake sitting squirrel monkeys with fornix lesions. Fed. Proc., *31:* 404, 1972.

241. Poletti, C. E., Wepsic, J. G., and Sweet, W. H. Middle cerebral arterial-spasm from subarachnoid blood. Spasmolysis with topical use of nitroglycerin. Surg. Forum, *XXIII:* 449–450, 1972.

242. Hoop, B., Jr., Ames, A., Ojemann, R. G. and Sweet, W. H. Cerebral circulation in irreversible coma. Trans. Am. Neurol. Assoc., *97:* 70–73, 1972.

243. Cares, H., Hale, R., Montgomery, B., Richter, H., and Sweet, W. H. Laboratory experience with a magnetically guided intravascular catheter system. J. Neurosurg., *38:* 145–154, 1973.

244. Dagi, T., Poletti, C. E., and Sweet, W. H. Effect of hippocampal influence on unit responses in cingulate cortex of unsedated squirrel monkeys. Fed. Proc., *32:* 384, 1973.

245. Amano, K., and Sweet, W. H. α-autoradiography of ^{10}B compound distribution in tissue by use of superimposition technique. Nippon Acta Radiol., *33:* 267–272, 1973.

246. Sweet, W. H., and Wepsic, J. G. Electrical stimulation for suppression of pain in man. *In* Neural Organization and its Relevance to Prosthetics, edited by W. S. Fields, and L. A. Leavitt, pp. 219–240. Symposia Specialists, Miami, 1973, (Presented at the Houston Neurological Symposium, 1973).

247. Sweet, W. H. Special Article. Treatment of medically intractable mental disease by limited frontal leucotomy—Justifiable? N. Engl. J. Med., *289:* 1117–1125, 1973.

248. Brownell, G. L., Murray, B. W., Sweet, W. H., Wellum, G. R., and Soloway, A. H. A reassessment of neutron capture therapy in the treatment of cerebral gliomas. *In* Seventh National Cancer Conference Proceedings, pp. 827–837. J. B. Lippincott Co., Philadelphia, (Proceedings of the Seventh National Cancer Conference, Los Angeles, September 27–29, 1972).

249. Sweet, W. H. Book Review of Neurological Surgery: A Comprehensive Reference Guide to the Diagnosis and Management of Neurosurgical Problems, 3 volumes, edited by J. R. Youmans, W. B. Saunders Co., Philadelphia, 1973. N. Engl. J. Med., *289:* 757–758, 1973.

250. Sweet, W. H. Pain. Ann. Roy. Coll. Phys. Surg. Can., *6:* 223–233, 1973.

251. Krayenbühl, H., Maspes, P., and Sweet, W. H. *In* Progress in Neurological Surgery, Editorial Preface, edited by H. Krayenbühl, P. Maspes and W. Sweet, Vol. 5, Basel (Switzerland), S. Karger, New York, 1973.

252. Sweet, W. H. Discussion of paper by Wassengar, W., and Tator, C. H. Glucose analogues as potential agents for brain tumour diagnosis and treatment. Trans. Am. Neurol. Assoc., *98:* 47–48, 1973.

253. Sweet, W. H. Discussion of paper by Cooper, I. S., Amin, T., and Gilman, S. Chronic cerebellar stimulation upon epilepsy in man. Trans. Am. Neurol. Assoc., *98:* 196, 1973.

254. Sweet, W. H., and Wepsic, J. G. Controlled thermocoagulation of trigeminal ganglion and rootlets for differential destruction of pain fibers. Part 1: Trigeminal neuralgia. J. Neurosurg., *40:* 143–156, 1974.

255. Sweet, W. H. Craniospinal surgery for pain. AVENS (Audiovisual Education Neurosurgery), Library of Congress Catalog number 73-701180, 1973.

256. Sweet, W. H., and Wepsic, J. G. Controlled thermocoagulation of trigeminal ganglion and rootlets for differential destruction of pain fibers. Part 1: Trigeminal neuralgia. *In* Advances in Neurology, Vol. 4, pp. 665–672, Raven Press, New York, 1974.

257. Sweet, W. H., and Wepsic, J. G. Stimulation of pain suppressor mechanisms: A critique of some current methods. *In* Advances in Neurology, Vol. 4, pp. 737–747,

Raven Press, New York, 1974.

258. Sweet, W. H. Book Review. Edited by M. Critchley, J. O'Leary, and B. Jennet, Scientific Foundations of Neurology. J. Neurosurg., *40:* 551–552, 1974.

259. Sweet, W. H., and Wepsic, J. G. Stimulation of the posterior columns of the spinal cord for pain control: Indications, technique, and results. Clin. Neurosurg., *21:* 278–310, 1974.

260. Mark, V. H. and Sweet, W. H. The role of limbic brain dysfunction in aggression. *In* Aggression, A. Res. Nerv. Ment. Dis., Proc., *52:* 186–200, 1974.

261. Sweet, W. H., and Wepsic, J. G. Controlled thermocoagulation of trigeminal ganglion and rootlets for differential destruction of pain fibers. Part 1: Trigeminal neuralgia. (Abstract) Hemicrania, *6:* 5, 1974.

262. Sweet, W. H., and Wepsic, J. G. Controllet thermocoagulation of trigeminal ganglion and rootlets for differential destruction of pain fibers. Part 1: Trigeminal neuralgia. Pain, *1:* 93, 1975.

263. Crowell, R. M., DeGirolami, U., and Sweet, W. H. Arteriovenous malformation and oligodendroglioma. Case Report. J. Neurosurg., *43:* 108–111, 1975.

264. Sweet, W. H., and Wepsic, J. G. Controlled thermocoagulation of trigeminal ganglion and rootlets. *In* Treatment of Pain, edited by H. C. Voris and W. W. Whisler, pp. 83–87. Charles C Thomas, Springfield, Ill., 1975.

265. Sweet, W. H. and Wepsic, J. G. Stimulation of the posterior columns of the spinal cord for pain control. Surg. Neurol., *4:* 133, 1975.

266. Sweet, W. H. (For the editors) *In* Progress in Neurological Surgery, Vol. 6, Editorial Preface, edited by H. Krayenbühl, P. Maspes, W. Sweet, Basel (Switzerland), S. Karger, New York, 1975.

267. Hoop, B., Ames, A., Ojemann, R. G., Sweet, W. H., and Ackerman, R. H. A technique for the assessment of cerebral circulation for diagnosis of cerebral death. *In* Cerebral Circulation and Metabolism, edited by T. Langfitt, L. McHenry, M. Reivich and H. Wollman, pp. 210–213. Springer-Verlag, New York, 1975.

268. Sweet, W. H. "Phantom" sensations following intraspinal injury. Neurochirurgia, *18:* 139–154, 1975.

269. Fields, W. S., and Sweet, W. H., Editors. Neural Bases of Violence and Aggression, 551 pp. Warren H. Green, Inc., St. Louis, 1975.

270. Fields, W. S., and Sweet, W. H. Neural Bases of Violence and Aggression, pp. vii–xvi. Warren H. Green, Inc., St. Louis, 1975.

271. Mark, V. H., Sweet, W. H. and Ervin, F. R. Deep temporal lobe stimulation and destructive lesions in episodically violent temporal lobe patients. *In* Neural Bases of Violence and Aggression, edited by W. S. Field and W. H. Sweet, pp. 379–391. Warren H. Green, Inc., St. Louis, 1975.

272. Sweet, W. H. Controlled thermocoagulation of trigeminal rootlets in man. Evidence that pain is related to nociception conducted only via unmyelinated and small myelinated fibers. *In* Controversies in Neurosurgery, edited by T. P. Morley. W. B. Saunders Co., Philadelphia, in press.

273. Sweet, W. H. Trigeminal neuralgias. *In* Facial Pain, edited by C. C. Alling, Lea & Febiger, Philadelphia, in press.

274. Sweet, W. H. Percutaneous differential thermal rhizotomy for management of facial pain. *In* Progress in Neurological Surgery, Vol. 7, edited by H. Krayenbühl, P. Maspes, W. Sweet, Basel (Switzerland), S. Karger, New York, in press.

275. Sweet, W. H. Percutaneous differential thermal rhizotomy for the management of facial pain. Advances in Neurosurgery, *3:* 274–286, 1975.

276. Sweet, W. H. Pain: Its mechanisms and treatment. *In* The Nervous System, Vol. 3, edited by D. B. Tower, Raven Press, New York, pp. 487–500, 1975.

277. Sweet, W. H. The difference between zero and one. Clin. Neurosurg., *23:* 32–51, 1976.

278. Sweet, W. H.: Radical surgical removal of craniopharyngioma. Clin. Neurosurg., *23:* 52–79, 1976.

279. Sweet, W. H. Recent observations pertinent to improving anterolateral cordotomy. Clin. Neurosurg., *23:* 80–95, 1976.

280. Sweet, W. H. Controlled thermocoagulation of trigeminal ganglion and rootlets for differential destruction of pain fibers. Part 2: Facial pain other than trigeminal neuralgia. Clin. Neurosurg., *23:* 96–102, 1976.

281. Sweet, W. H. Control of pain by direct electrical stimulation of peripheral nerves. Clin. Neurosurg., *23:* 103–111, 1976.

282. Sweet, W. H. What should the neurosurgeon do when faced with a malpractice suit? Clin. Neurosurg., *23:* 112–124, 1976.

283. Sweet, W. H., Editor. Neurosurgical Treatment in World Psychiatry. (Proc. V World Congress of Psychiatric Surgery, Madrid, 1975). University Park Press. Baltimore, in press.

284. Sweet, W. H. Central mechanisms of chronic pain. To be published.

285. Sweet, W. H. Pain after injuries in the spinal canal. To be published.

ACKNOWLEDGMENT

It is a pleasure to express appreciation to the Neuro-Research Foundation for the support of these studies.

CHAPTER

4

The Difference between Zero and One

WILLIAM SWEET, M.D., D.Sc.

This title would at first glance appear to be fruitless for extended analysis. The difference between zero and one is the same as that between one and two, namely one—end of analysis. Although the concept of zero as a number now seems obvious, the original systems of numeration did not include it. And it was not until the 11th century A.D. that the Hindu mathematician Bhāskara clearly stated that "if a number is multiplied by zero the product is zero only" (18).

The special quality of zero first appreciated by mathematicians becomes the more striking when placed alongside their concept of infinitesimal magnitudes whose use in the early 17th century led to the development in the middle of that century of the calculus (17). Clearly the latter notion has operational value. Zero, however, is less than something infinitely small, whereas one, though not infinitely great, is vastly more than an infinitely minute quantity. Two on the other hand is only twice as much as one. These reflections have little practical significance when we are thinking of concrete items like dollars. However when we move to the world of ideas we realize instantly that the first time a new and valid thought is conceived is the critical time. Having a massive number of identical ideas is fatuously monotonous; whereas having a massive number of identical dollars is a form of monotony to which most of us eagerly adapt. The significant step in the former case is the passage from no idea to one constructive idea.

The uncertainties and colossal number of variables inherent in the biological field make all of us working in the domain reluctant to publish an interpretation of a single observation, much less to construct an hypothesis unsupported by any observation. Indeed if the observation is strikingly unusual, we tend not to publish even that much but to wait hopefully for a similar event before we commit ourselves in print. We physicians and biologists are like the two Scotchmen in Figure 4.1. We prefer the avoidance of ridicule to the uphill struggle against skeptical colleagues fixed in the range of new ideas they are even willing to scrutinize. We would rather let someone else be the first to describe weird creatures in a flying saucer trying to land a Loch Ness monster.

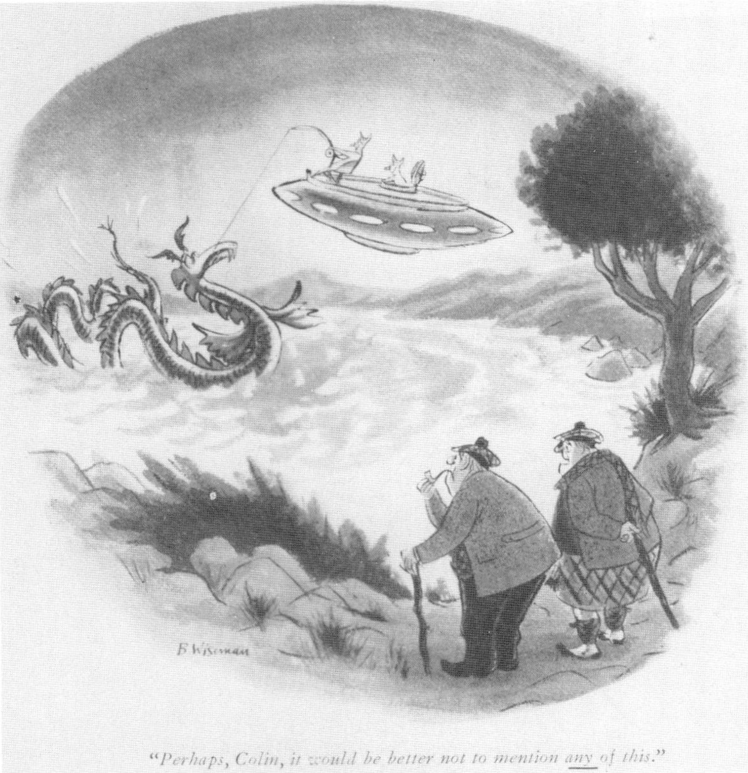
B. Wiseman
"Perhaps, Colin, it would be better not to mention any of this."

FIG. 4.1. Drawing by B. Wiseman; © 1956. The New Yorker Magazine Inc.

Not so our friends in such natural sciences as elementary particle physics. I grant that they are dealing with more precisely reproducible and to them more comprehensible phenomena. One example of many that could be cited will suffice to illustrate my point (Fig. 4.2). The theoretical physicist Murray Gell-Mann and colleagues (2) had predicted that a certain heavy fundamental particle should exist and, if found, might be the keystone to an orderly arrangement of the previously known particles. They called the particle omega, predicted it would have a negative charge, a mass of 1676 million electron volts, a hypercharge of −2, an isotopic spin of 0, etc.—never mind these details. In a search for this particle, about 1 million separate pictures were taken of events in the 80-inch liquid hydrogen bubble chamber in one of the target areas of the 33 billion electron volt proton accelerator at the Brookhaven National Laboratory (Fig. 4.3). The left-hand side of the figure is not the doodling of a schizophrenic draughtsman but an example of the series of tracks made by charged particles in a liquid hydrogen bubble chamber. This is

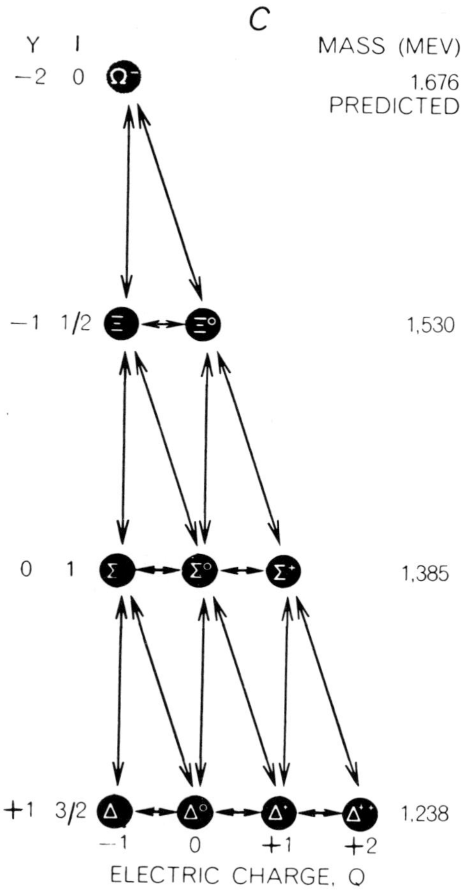

FIG. 4.2. From "Eightfold Way" Illustration C p. 88. Y = hypercharge I = isotopic spin. (From Chew, Gell-Mann and Rosenfeld. Scientific American *210:* 88, 1964.)

the discovery picture of the Omega minus particle, and the diagram on the right abstracts from the original picture relevant visible tracks of charged particles as well as the invisible tracks of the uncharged particles indicated by dotted lines. Upon these tracks precise measurements were made which revealed that a particle formed at a point just to the left of (3) where a K-meson smashed into a proton had to be the predicted Omega minus. It had among other features the expected life time of about one ten billionth of a second, the time for it to go the few millimeters until it decayed into a pi-meson and the uncharged baryon Xi° with the further complex decay scheme shown. The details are not relevant to the point I wish to make, *i.e.*, that a hypothesis could be

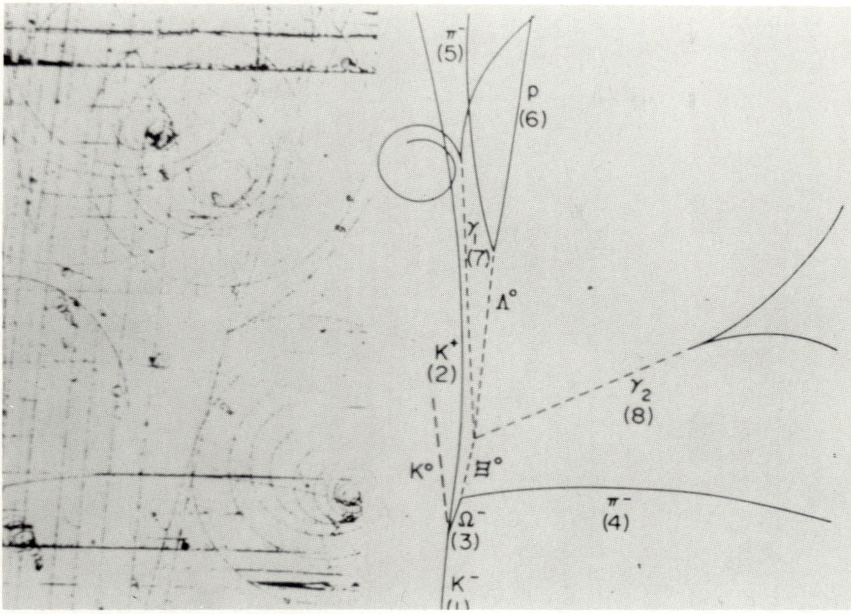

FIG. 4.3. Left half of figure; reproduction of portion of liquid hydrogen bubble chamber photograph depicting the event which was first objective demonstration of omega minus (Ω^-) particle. Right half of figure; diagram from the original indicating only those events related to the decay scheme of that particle. Collision of K-meson (1) and proton in the liquid hydrogen forms the Ω^- particle which decays in $\sim 10^{-10}$ seconds into a π^- meson (4) and a baryon Xi°. The latter decays into three other uncharged particles identifiable only because charged particles soon form related to each of them—from lambda° a π^- meson (5) and a proton (6) and from each of the 2 gamma rays (7) and (8) a charged particle. (Courtesy of Brookhaven National Laboratory and Associated Universities, Inc.)

devised and then confirmed by a *single* critically analyzable event among many millions. It is also worth commenting that the discovery picture did not come with an arrow labeled, "look this way for gold." But once that single segment of a much larger picture was spotted and then studied, the existence of the Omega minus particle was settled. In fact Dr. Gell-Mann soon became a Nobel laureate.

I think there is a lesson for us in such a sequence of facts and I should now like to describe three examples from early reports in which three neurosurgeons each failed to draw the logical conclusions from his observations of a single case. This led to a long unnecessary delay in the recognition of the syndrome of normal pressure hydrocephalus.

The first example is Case 6 in a 1956 publication of Foltz and Ward (7). In June, 1953 Dr. Foltz successfully clipped the neck of a left anterior cerebral aneurysm which had bled

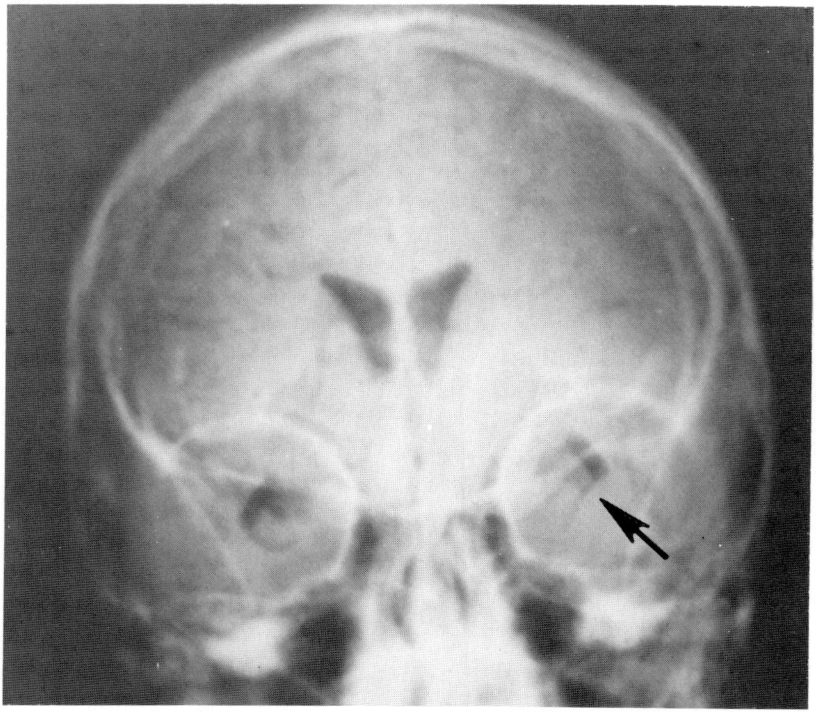

FIG. 4.4. Virginia C. Pneumonecephalogram. Elevation of left temporal horn by space-taking lesion (arrow).

twice in the preceding 3 weeks in a 28-year-old man. Slow steady improvement over the next 3 weeks was followed by reappearance of personality disturbances of the type which had preceded the first subarachnoid bleed. In 6 more weeks he began to have 2 weeks of headache, steady deterioration, and "catatonic-like" episodes lasting 10 to 18 hours. A new gross ventricular dilatation was depicted by the high arch of the supracallosal anterior cerebral arteries in an angiogram of September 11, 1953. However the normal spinal fluid was under a pressure of only 90 mm. of water. In a pneumoencephalogram (PEG) of October 29, 1953, the lateral ventricles were even larger and there was no supratentorial subarachnoid gas. The patient was now in a state like catatonia, totally disoriented with severe bilateral pyramidal and extrapyramidal signs and masklike facies. At right ventriculo-mastoidectomy on November 17, 1953, the intraventricular pressure was less than 50 mm. A startling recovery to an objectively normal state ensued within 4 days and was being maintained at follow-up 19½ months later. A PEG in January 1954 showed smaller ventricles. This remarkable case was published without special attention to it along with nine others under the title, hardly arresting, of "Communicating Hydrocephalus from Subarachnoid Bleeding."

My second example in chronological order is Case 2 in the doctoral thesis of S. Hakim (8) for his degree from Bogotá, Colombia. Gradual impairment of memory for 1 year in a 52-year-old musician had progressed through sluggishness of thought and action to apathy with urinary incontinence, stiffness of the legs, unsteady gait, slurring of speech and terminal tremor on finger-to-nose tests. Further steady deterioration is well documented in the report over the next 6½ weeks until late March 1958. Each of three times that a little spinal fluid was withdrawn at lumbar puncture, slight but definite improvement occurred, even though all three initial pressures were normal. At angiogram and air study, massive enlargement of all four ventricles was seen; there was no air in the cerebral sulci. Following a ventriculo-atrial shunt on March 30, 1958, there was again a dramatic recovery, largely complete within 7 days and maintained. When the thesis had its limited publication in 1964, it was included with two other case reports of hydrocephalus following head trauma with normal CSF pressure, but continuing deterioration.

My third example is my own Case 1 in a report by five of us with Dr. Raymond Adams as the first author (1). Gradual steady deterioration in mentation and gait in this previously vivacious 63-year-old lady during a 6½ month period had led to cessation of all social activity and occasional urinary incontinence. The CSF pressure was normal and, except for grossly unsteady gait, the neurological signs were normal. However, a PEG precipitated a state approaching akinetic mutism. By no maneuver could air be induced to enter the cerebral sulci at that study on April 21, 1959, or by a ventriculogram on May 25, 1959, but the ventricles were massively dilated. I did a ventriculo-atrial shunt on May 28, 1959. The improvement after this was so slow that the neurologists were inclined to ascribe it to spontaneous regression of an obscure disorder in the nadir of whose course I had happened to do this shunt. By 40 days after operation she was still forgetful, though talking, occasionally incontinent of urine, and so unsteady on her feet that with a person standing on either side of her she abruptly fell as she turned, fracturing the neck of the left femur. This event turned out to be a control experiment. Within 4 more days she had deteriorated to a state of unresponsiveness to commands and constant incontinence. I then noted a fluctuant mass over the McPherson valve assembly behind the right ear, and I discovered that when she fell, she also split the intervalvular tubing with an accumulation of CSF under the scalp. Upon my replacement of the tubing, the CSF pressure returned to low normal levels. Her mental and neurological status returned in a few days to that just before her fracture, and she went on to recover completely in all aspects, including to a "superior" verbal and nonverbal level in the WAIS. She remained totally well while we waited for two more somewht similar cases to come along, eventually reporting them in 1965 (1).

Each of the three cases was sufficiently decisive to warrant an individual report within a few months of the successful therapy. Each of us had made a virtually unassailable series of observations on his patient indicating that the simple treatment of a functional shunt was utterly and amazingly effective in restoring a derelict to normality in the presence of normal CSF pressure, given the unequivocal evidence of impaired flow of CSF provided by gross ventricular dilatation and no air in the cerebral sulci. The uniqueness of the case in the experience of each of us at that time should have spurred us on to report the unique event as such, not held us back or led us to mix it with less relevant cases. My sluggishness is particularly reprehensible in the face of the ultra-convincing episode related to shunt failure. In 1960 when an older member of Sir Geoffrey Jefferson's family was deteriorating mentally at a rapid pace, I described the foregoing case and suggested that his patient be studied to exclude the outside chance that a remediable impaired CSF flow was the cause of her trouble. Sir Geoffrey Jefferson was unconvinced by my account.

I believe we have become excessively imbued with the conviction that multiple consonant observations are necessary before even tentative conclusions can be drawn from biological phenomena, that a randomized statistically significant series is necessary for firm conclusions. It apparently suffices today to characterize a report as anecdotal to initiate its complete rejection. An anecdote is defined by the Oxford English Dictionary as "the narrative of one interesting or striking event." We need to establish faith in the capacity of the biologist to reach a valid novel conception on the basis of one single set of facts. There is a staggering difference between zero and one when the one is a good idea.

This is a protracted introduction to two anecdotes regarding unique totally unrelated observations I have made in two patients. Their nature makes unlikely an early attempt to repeat them.

Case 1. The first case is that of a 60-year-old woman with intractable pain associated with malignant tumor. Intending to do percutaneous cordotomy from the right side at C1-2, I introduced the electrode into the cord as indicated by a sense of increased resistance to the movement and demonstrated by a rise in the impedance from 280 to 600 ohms. I was proceeding to gentle electrical stimulation within the cord when, coincident with a little nod of her head, the patient suddenly declared with great agitation that both of her legs had become numb, were no longer lying on the table, but were floating about wildly and aimlessly in the air, both from side to side and up and down. This sensation was much worse in the right leg, soon disappearing in the left. She was not reassured by being able to see that the legs were, in fact, still lying quietly in the usual extended position. Although we took no film, a fluoroscopic lateral view showed the electrode tip behind the mid point of the anteroposterior diameter of the spinal canal. We withdrew the electrode at once, having made no electrical lesion and examined the patient continuously for about the next hour. She moved both lower limbs with excellent power at each joint exactly as commanded, but with her eyes closed she was uncertain that she was moving them as told. The "terrible feeling" of aimless floating movements was not dispelled by her strong voluntary movements in both legs. She said, "This must be the sensation the astronauts have when they are weightless." There was also some subjective "numbness" in the right hand. At this point, she localized touch on both upper limbs, throughout the torso, and on the left lower limb but could not feel or guess at the localization of touch or even of my hand stroking anywhere on the right lower limb. Proprioception at the left great toe was normal, but she felt no movement at the right great toe or ankle, and the sense of direction of passive movement was grossly diminished at the right knee. Despite her distraught state at her illusions of movement, she localized pin prick precisely throughout both lower extremities, feeling it as equally sharp on the two sides everywhere. This important point was repeatedly confirmed. Only at 19 minutes after the sensory illusions began could she for the first time localize a light stroking at one area in the right lower limb, the right sole. By 23 minutes later, gross movements of the right great toe were detected; at 27 minutes, light stroking was localized on the medial aspect of the right leg and ankle; and by 32 minutes, lesser movements of the right great toe were reported correctly. The illusion of aimless movements of the right lower limb virtually disappeared as soon as proprioception and touch returned to that structure. Although rapid improvement continued, she still retained by 2 weeks after the episode an exasperating numbness in both right limbs and the right torso. She could, however localize light touch throughout these areas and had normal proprioception at the right great toe, normal graphesthesia on the dorsum of the right foot and fully normal strength in dorsal and plantar flexion of that foot and in the rest of the lower limb. Occasionally, the right leg still had a sense of floating.

This relatively temporary lesion was presumably confined largely to the medial part of the right posterior column of white matter. The related findings help to resolve two, possibly three, uncertain points in the physiology of the cord.

The first has to do with the location of the pathways for tactile impulses. In addition to the long established ipsilateral ascending pathways in the posterior columns, a ventral (anterior) spinothalamic tract ascending contralaterally has long been described in the texts (4, 13, 21), and the mediation of the sense of touch has also been ascribed to it. May's (12) extensive review summarizes the varying and often contradictory accounts of animal and human studies in the 19th century on which this concept is based. The only histological evidence I know of in man for a separate ascending crossed ventral, presumably spinothalamic, pathway is that adduced by Kuru (11). Studying patients with islands of analgesia and thermanesthesia after cordotomies for pain, he was able in three of them to associate retrograde degeneration in the large cells within the nucleus proprius of the posterior horn with degeneration in a distinct ventral spinothalamic tract. However, Rose and Mountcastle (14) point out that the existence of a separate ventral spinothalamic tract as a tactile component of the spinothalamic system seems to be based mainly on suppositions. In the presence of intact posterior columns there is at most a minimal loss of tactile function after division of the anterior quadrant in man. Indeed this is ascertainable only by testing with calibrated hairs or the counting of touch-pressure points per square centimeter as shown first by Kroll (10), and confirmed by Foerster and Gagel (6) and by White, Sweet, Hawkins, and Nilges (22). Only on hairless analgesic areas did we find the threshold to light touch slightly increased from the ¼ to ½ gm. normal level in the majority of 20 patients studied. In several the threshold was unaltered; the greatest increase was only 6-fold, up to 3 gm. in one patient. In hairy analgesic areas the least contact was still felt. Dr. White has put the degree of this loss in its proper perspective, I think, by his statement to patients that they will be able to detect a mosquito landing on their cordotomized side but not feel the subsequent bite and itching.*

* Our observations have at times been misconstrued. Thus Ruch (Ref. 15, p. 335) has quoted us as stating that the threshold for light pressure is markedly reduced in man after the anterior quadrant has been divided.

The fact that our patient felt no touch at all at the height of her malfunction of the posterior column might be ascribable to a state of "neural shock" from which recovery had to take place before the ventral pathways for touch could function. Against this interpretation is the fact that the kinesthetic functions recovered in her *pari passu* with touch. Moreover, in the converse situation in which we eliminate pain and temperature sensation by thermal or incisional lesions in the anterior quadrant, there is no such shock despite the much more severe lesion. Excellent touch is always continuously preserved. Indeed, in testing the patient at once after we make such lesions, we must make it clear that his ability to tell us that we are stimulating at a given point is not the faculty we are trying to eliminate, but only the painful quality of that stimulus.

The only detailed study of sensation on patients in whom one posterior column was presumably all divided is that of Cook and Browder (3). In three patients they sought to cut all of one posterior column in the midthoracic region. Their incision to an estimated depth of 2½ mm. probably left intact some of the most ventral fibers in this column since the whole column occupies the posterior 60% of the 6.5 to 7.0-mm. anteroposterior diameter of the cord in this region (5). Such preservation would explain the merely temporary and questionable decreased appreciation of touch below the level of the cordotomy detected in only two of the patients. It does not, I think, controvert the significance of this observation. The temporary loss in my patient does not, of course, preclude the possibility that when the primary routes for touch in the posterior columns are lost, ventral pathways for touch may later develop clinically important function. In summary, I think this observation presents the first evidence that all of the usual clinically significant pathways for touch may lie in the posterior columns, and nowhere else.

However, an important case to remind us again of the variability from patient to patient is one reported by Head (Ref. 9, p. 357). His patient had the abrupt onset of temporary weakness of the left arm and leg. Although this gradually disappeared, the associated right-sided abolition of the sensations of light touch, steady pressure, pain and temperature from the costal margin on down persisted for years. The recognition of passive motion was always perfect throughout both lower limbs, so one must presume here that the pathways for touch travelled exclusively contralaterally along with those for pain and temperature.

My second point I can make briefly, namely that pin-pricks to the limb deprived of touch and kinesthesis were perceived at the same threshold, were as well localized, and had the same normal qualitative characteristics as those to the opposite limb. There was neither a latent period, a

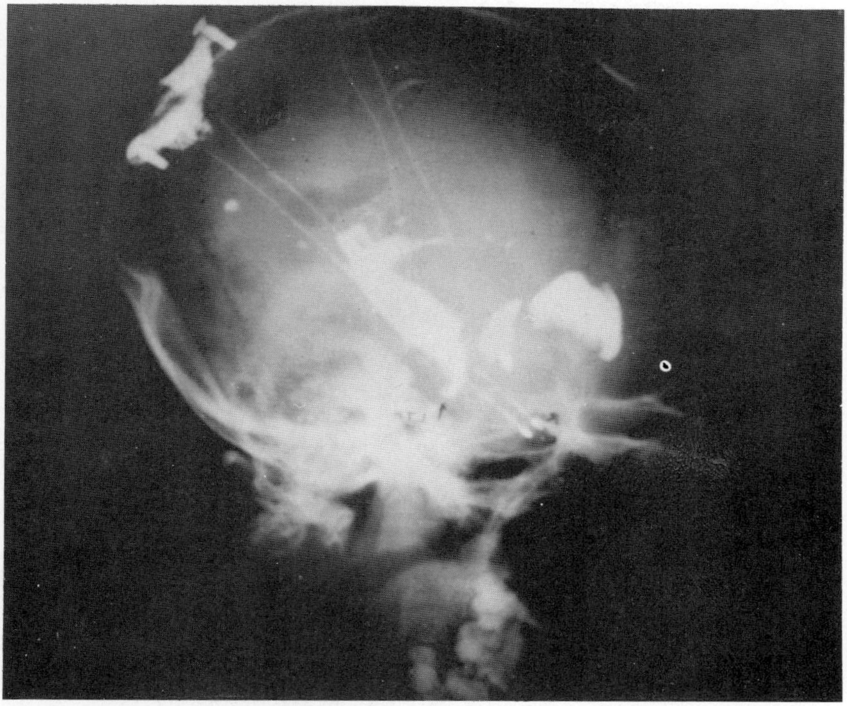

FIG. 4.5. Virginia C. Pantopaque ventriculogram showing positions of four electrode arrays. Lateral view. Pantopaque in frontal and temporal horns and anterior end of the third ventricle. Posteriorly external to skull plastic and screws hold firmly two tiny linear streamers of 20 electrodes each (numbered from front to back). These arrays inserted through posterior burr holes pass through the long axis of each hippocampus, into amygdala and temporal lobe white matter to the tip of the temporal lobe gray matter. A slight lateral tilt to the skull with the right side up permits both arrays to be seen, and on the original film the thin spot on the array marking each electrode site can be identified and counted back from the dense larger anterior tip of each array. Both arrays lie in the same horizontal plane. Two other arrays of electrodes each embedded in a thin plastic strip have been inserted on the floor of the middle cranial fossas extradurally in the coronal plane of the amygdalas. These structures lie just anterior to the tips of the temporal horns. Leads from these arrays extend upward and backward to the posterior parietal scalp.

peculiarly unpleasant quality, nor an after discharge of pain to pin-prick on the affected side. In other words, there was not discernable any descending pain suppressor mechanism in the posterior column whose activity was required to prevent pin-prick from being abnormally disagreeable, diffuse, or lasting. Nor was it necessary to have simultaneous large fiber impulses traversing the posterior columns induced by a pin-prick for this stimulus to be precisely localized.

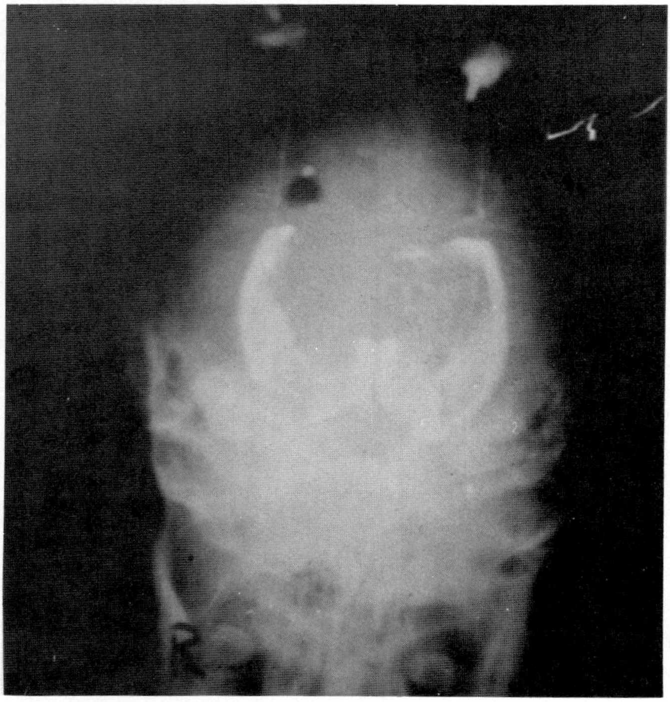

FIG. 4.6. Sagittal view with central x-ray entry above frontal eminences to show the lengths of the temporal lobes. The right longitudinal array extends 3 mm. further forward than the left one, but they pass through identical parts of the hippocampi and amygdalas.

My third point deals with the illusory or phantom sensations following spinal cord injury. In an extended discussion elsewhere (19), I refer to the phase of initial stimulation in which at once after injury, the patient may describe such sensations as that the legs were torn from the body, or flew up in the air remaining abducted or elevated, or that the legs seemed at first to be markedly flexed, floating, or suspended, or one patient who had a sensation, to him pleasant, of his having lost all weight and of flying high in the air. In three cases the whole body seemed catapaulted through the air. Two of these with cervical cord injury felt that only the head came back to earth! In five other patients recorded in the literature whose features I have summarized elsewhere, partial cord injuries indicated that it was loss of function in the posterior columns rather than in the anterolateral or anterior parts of the cord which was correlated with their illusory sensations of position and movement. This patient, the only one of the six with a lesion confined to the posterior column and

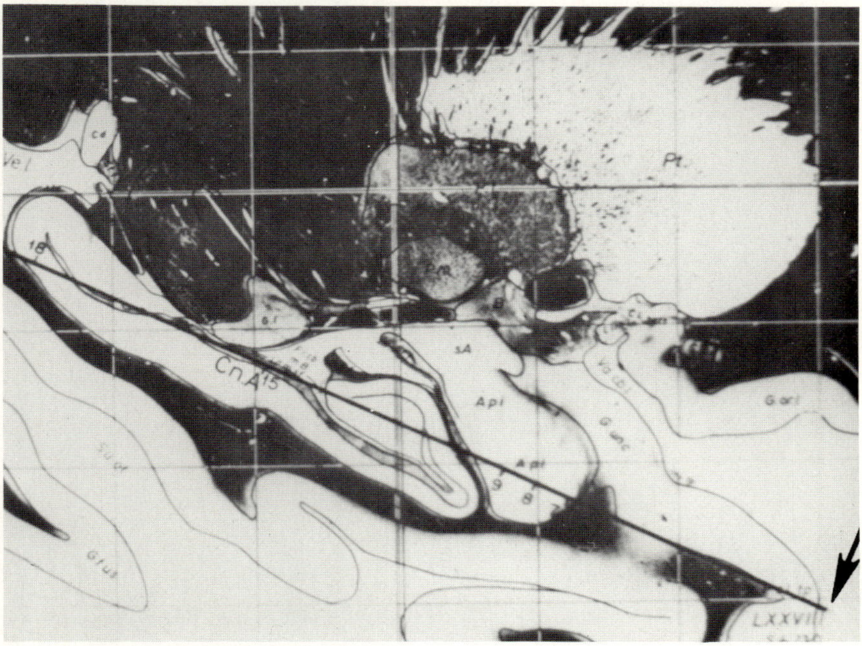

FIG. 4.7. Sagittal section 23 mm. lateral to midline taken from Schaltenbrand and Bailey Atlas (Plate LXXVIII). A long black line corresponding to the position of the right electrode array has been drawn on the original illustration. It extends backward and upward from the temporal tip (arrow) through the nucleus profundus lateralis of the amygdala (labelled Apl) into hippocampus (labelled Cn.A. = cornu ammonis). The numbers show the position of the specific numbered electrodes. The odd-numbered electrodes through 15 as well as numbers 16, 17 and 18 consist of coils of uninsulated wire extending for 3 mm. along the length of the array. They are separated by 3 mm. intervals of insulation. The even-numbered electrodes 2 through 14 are uninsulated points about 1 mm. in diameter lying in the insulated zone midway between the coils. Numbers 19 and 20 are similar points 5 mm. apart; number 20 lies 10 cm. behind the anterior tip of the array. The electrodes in the identical left array lie 3 mm. more posterior—*i.e.* numbers 6 through 8 instead of 7 through 9 lie in the amygdala.

not involving a posterolateral column, provides unequivocal confirmation that loss of posterior column function is the crucial factor in the development of phantom sensation after cord injury.

My second anecdote is longer but has much broader potential significance, in this instance, for our system of criminal justice.

Case 2. Patient Virginia C. had lived with attentive foster parents, her uncle and aunt, from the age of 1 month. Until December 1966 at age 13, they found her "the easiest child they had ever brought up." She then became moody and silent, spent the day in her room

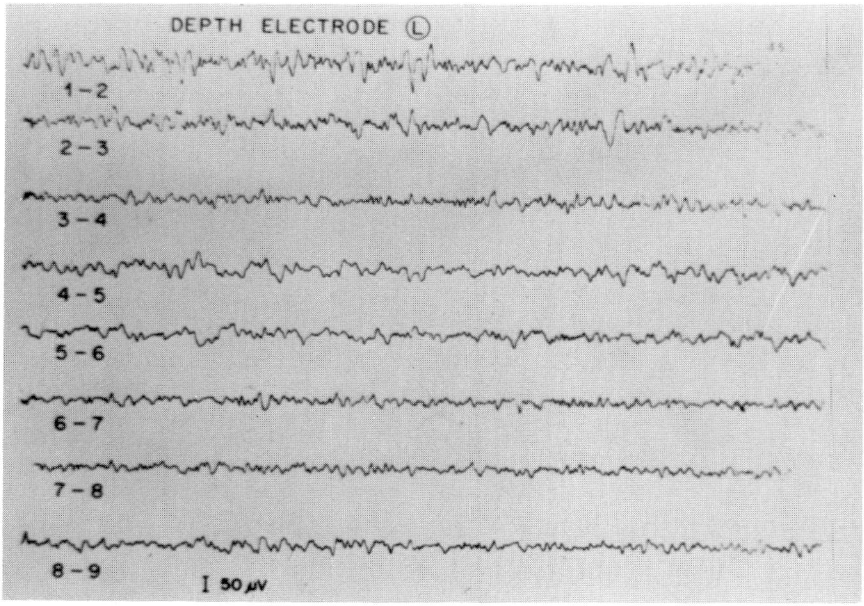

FIG. 4.8 through 4.11. Virginia C, age 14 years. Spontaneous resting potentials from longitudinal depth electrode arrays. Amplification 5 mm. = 50 microvolts.

FIG. 4.8. Anterior part of left array.

playing records. Asked on New Year's Eve 1966 to turn down the volume of the record player she flew into a rage and with an axe destroyed the contents, door, and floor of her room. The parents had to call the police to subdue her. For the next 4½ months there was no more destructive behavior. Then on May 11, 1967, she lost patience with a 21-month-old crying baby and suffocated it. Frightened at what she had done, she ran from her home. She was studied in several institutions during which she made several suicidal attempts and one more attack on a younger child. Professor Norman Geschwind suggested that her bursts of violence might be related to organic brain disease. The following examinations were normal, or virtually so: general physical, neurological, cerebrospinal fluid, EEG's asleep, awake, and after Metrazol activation, radiographs of the skull, a radioisotopic scan, and a left carotid angiogram. The last examination was done because a PEG (Fig. 4.4) showed a probably space-taking lesion inferolateral to the tip of the left temporal horn. Anticipating that we might be removing a lesion from the left medial temporal region, we sought to determine the degree of abnormality in both the temporal lobes lest the patient have a serious unsuspected lesion in the right hippocampus and we produce a catastrophic memory loss by removing much of the left hippocampus (Fig. 4.5). The two temporal lobes were studied further by installing in the coronal plane of the amygdalas two arrays of plate electrodes extradurally, one on each side in the floor of the middle cranial fossa, and a second pair of longitudinal arrays from back to front through Ammon's horn of the hippocampus, the amygdala and the white and gray matter at the tips of the two temporal lobes (Fig. 4.6). Aided by two projections of the pantopaque ventriculogram, Drs. Mark, Ervin, and I think we were able to plot within 1 to 2 mm. the positions of our two electrode arrays. Figure 4.7 shows the position of the right longitudinal array plotted on the

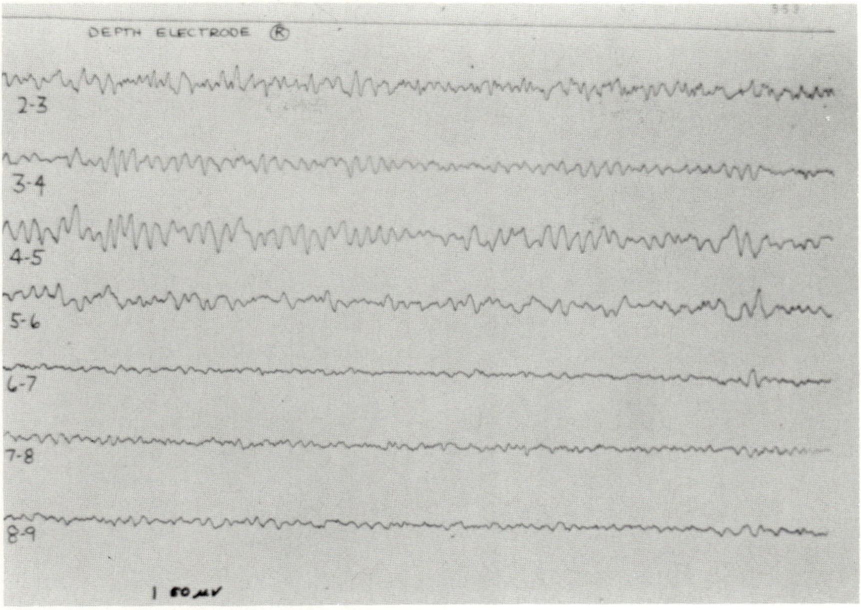

FIG. 4.9. Anterior part of right array. Relatively normal potentials throughout except for leads 1 and 2 at left temporal pole.

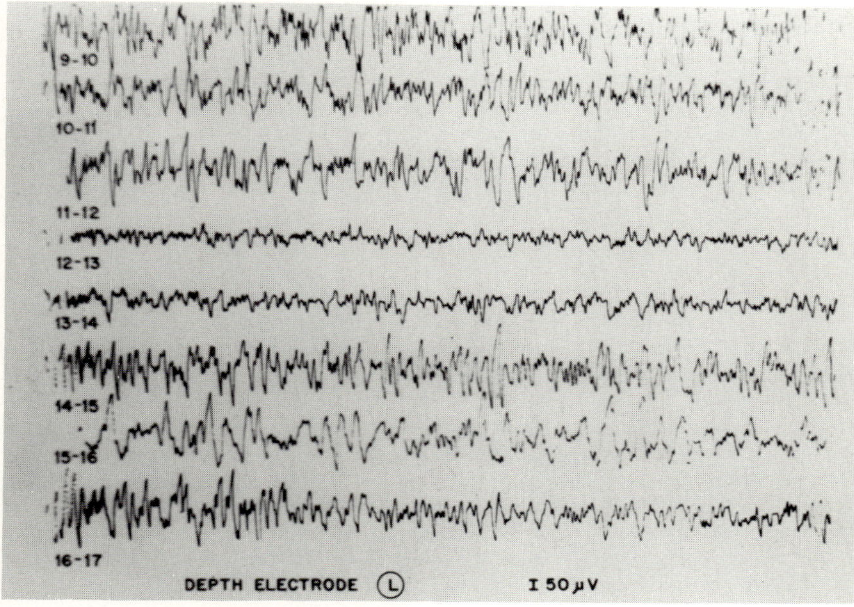

FIG. 4.10. Posterior part of left array—in hippocampus.

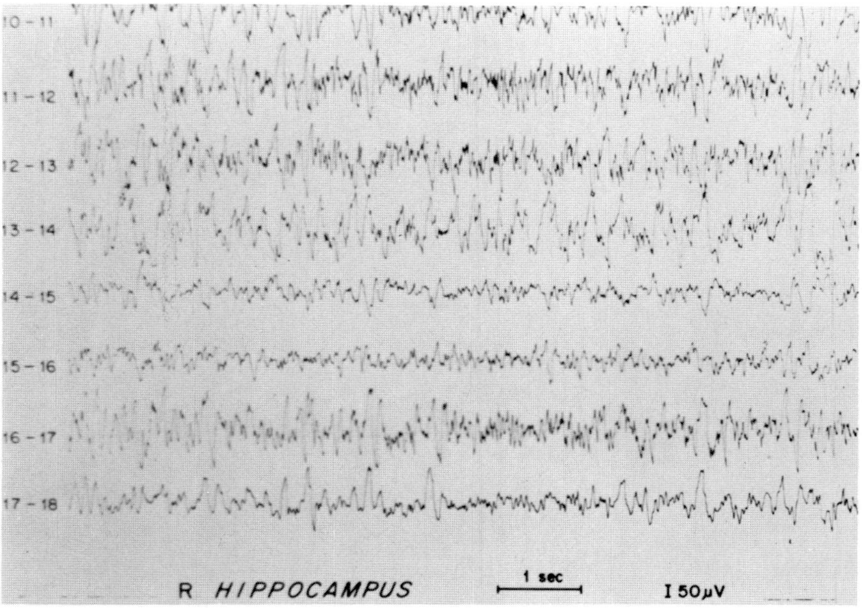

FIG. 4.11. Posterior part of right array in hippocampus. Continuous high voltage spikes and sharp waves worse left than right with only two relatively normal leads on the left. One of the most abnormal pairs on the right (13–14) corresponds in position to one of the normal pairs on the left (12–13). Hence the lesser right-sided abnormality probably does not represent merely mirror foci on the right of focal organic lesions on the left. The more normal pairs in both hippocampi serve to some extent as controls, indicating that the grosser deflections are not electrical features of a normally developing but still immature hippocampus. This degree of abnormality persisted through the final day's records 58 days after implantation. *Stimulation at hippocampal electrodes also evoked sensations of seeming to be at a distance from her environment characteristic of temporal lobe seizures. Once these had been evoked she described the occurrence of such mild seizures spontaneously.*

appropriate sagittal section of the Schaltenbrand-Bailey Atlas (16). Electrodes 7, 8, and 9 lie in the amygdala and 10 through 18 are in the hippocampus. The electrodes in the identical array on the left side lie 3 mm. more posterior so that 6 through 8 are in the amygdala and 9 through 17 in the hippocampus. The spontaneous potentials arising at the various electrodes were recorded from 7 to 58 days following implantation, and some were used for stimulation. The two arrays of eight electrodes each in the coronal plane beneath each temporal lobe dura revealed essentially normal traces (Ref. 20, p. 346) (Figs. 4.8 and 4.9). Likewise the anterior halves of the two arrays in anterior gray matter, white matter and amygdalas were nearly normal with the patient at rest (Fig. 4.10). But the leads from the hippocampi contrasted dramatically with extremely abnormal discharges present continually at rest in six of the eight pairs of leads both in the left and in the right Ammon's horn of the hippocampi. Only the pairs 11 through 13 on the left and 14 through 16 on the right failed to show incessant high voltage, spike-like potentials (Fig. 4.11). These brief excerpts are typical of all sections of the tracings from this patient lasting over scores of

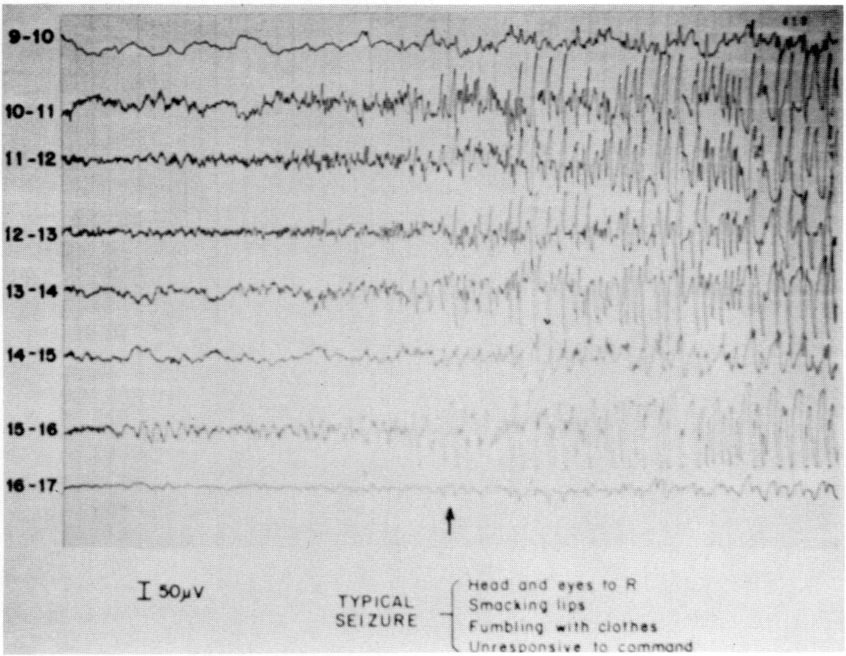

FIG. 4.12. Annette S. 24-year-old. Severe temporal lobe seizures. Longitudinal array placed as in previous patient. Left one-third of trace shows spontaneous resting potentials throughout hippocampus nearly normal in sharp contrast to the previous patient and to the high voltage discharges present in a typical seizure.

hours in the 41 days we recorded from her until the electrodes were removed. Because of the notable electrical lability of the hippocampus, one may ask what a normal human hippocampus in a teenage person would show. We cannot answer this, but Figure 4.12 is from a 24-year-old woman with severe temporal lobe seizures whose longitudinal electrode array was, we think, in essentially the same position. The left one-third of this record shows a hippocampal activity at rest much like that seen in the amygdalas of the previous patient. Not until just before the clinical insignia of a typical temporal lobe seizure were recognized did the depth electrodes record continuous high voltage spikelike deflections. Professor Herbert Jasper kindly spent 2 hours going over with me these tracings on the first patient and concluded that they unquestionably depict grossly abnormal bilateral hippocampal activity. In fact, the abnormality is not much less than that seen with many mild psychomotor seizures and suggests that this girl's brain is under a comparable but incessant abnormal bombardment.

In the course of our studies, the patient told us that actually another of her small siblings thought to have died of pneumonia had been suffocated by her when she became annoyed with the infant's crying. Hence it seemed logical to include the responses of the patient and her intratemporal potentials to such sounds. While she was chatting with the psychiatrist, Dr. John Lion, a tape recording of his own crying infant was started. Pre-amygdalar, hippocampal, and posthippocampal pairs of electrodes were recorded from simultaneously on the two sides. One of the least abnormal pairs in the right hippocampus was chosen for

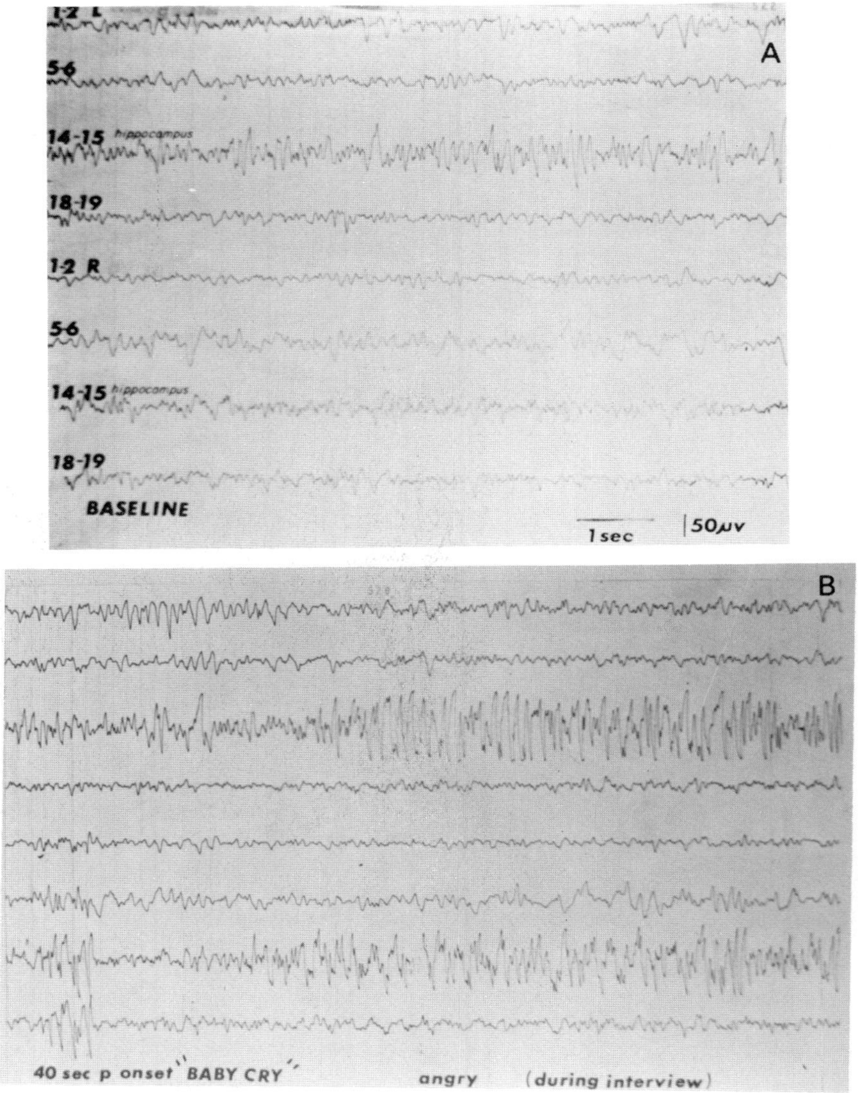

FIG. 4.13 (A–D). Virginia C. Tracings before, during, and after exposure of patient to a background tape recording of a crying infant. (A) Control period of quiet conversation with psychiatrist. (B) 40 seconds after start of tape-recording crying—striking increase in hippocampal abnormality both from the initially grossly abnormal left pair, 14–15, and the much less abnormal right pair 14–15. (C) 80 seconds after start of crying—both hippocampi still more abnormal with spread to posterior hippocampus on right leads 18–19. Electrodes 18 and 19 on left are posterior to hippocampus and show no high voltage spikes. (D) Two minutes after cessation of tape-recorded crying. Return to control levels.

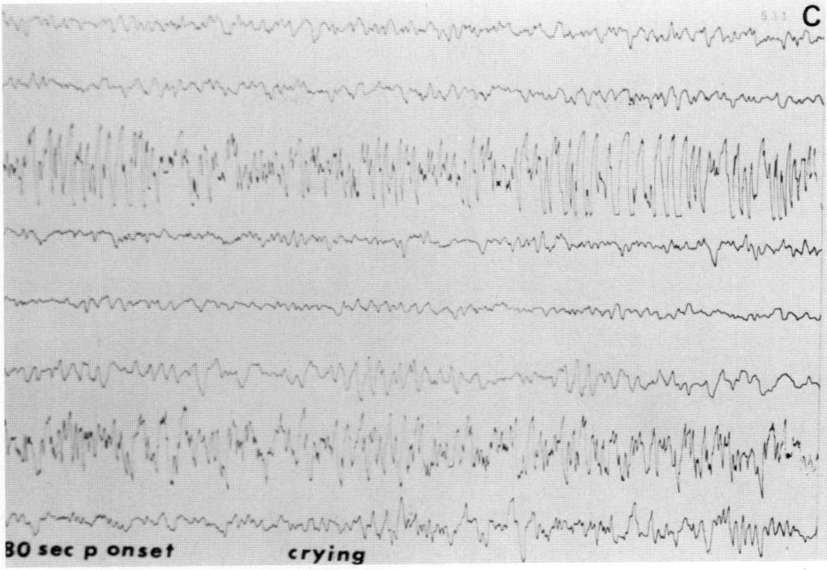

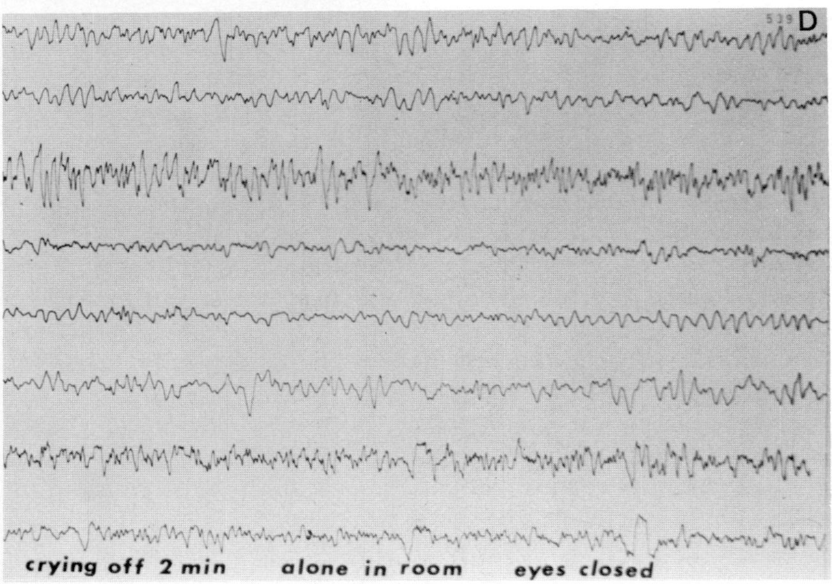

comparison with one of the six grossly abnormal pairs in the left hippocampus. Figure 4.13A in the immediately preceding control period is typical of the patient in quiet conversation. By 40 seconds after the onset of the tape-recorded crying, there is a striking increase in the abnormal spiking from both hippocampi (Fig. 4.13B). This is even worse at 80 seconds (Fig. 4.13C). The abnormal discharges did not spread to any of the other six pairs of leads in nearby structures. Figure 4.13D shows the prompt reversion to the original degree of abnormality after the tape was stopped. In four of five such sequences this same pattern of increased hippocampal activity occurred.

Of course I do not know what intrahippocampal electrodes would show in a normal person during an exasperating experience. However, we do know that the EEG may intimate the impending failure of anticonvulsant therapy, and we changed the regime of treatment to try to obviate a generalized seizure. Correspondingly, it is conceivable that such depth recordings, or even with luck, surface recordings may predict the efficacy of a therapeutic regime without subjecting society to a burst of the patient's assaultiveness. This tactic is perhaps the more likely to prove valid if environmental situations which have in the past provoked dangerous outbursts are duplicated or at least simulated. This patient had her electrodes removed because of the indignation of certain psychiatrists at this mode of study. She remained an involuntary inmate of institutions for 8 more years until 2 months ago when released for the present to the custody of her sister.

The principal interest in this congerie of facts however is that an impulsive murderess was proven to have gross focal abnormality in her brain only by sophisticated expensive diagnostic measures. How much more effort, if any, should be expended by society on what type of criminal conduct? We anticipated that any activity to extend this observation to other impulsive criminals, who destroy or assault for trivial reasons, might excite opposition from those who feel that more prompt, severe, and certain punishment is the proper solution for crimes of violence. They are sometimes referred to as the law and order group. They have not in fact been our problem. Instead it proves to be more the espousers of "liberal causes" who have been the greatest objectors to extension of these studies. If a "liberal" is defined as one who concentrates more on helping others than helping himself, I hope I may qualify and that efforts with patients such as the one just described are evidence in that direction. Robert Frost has a different definition for a "liberal," namely, a man who won't take his own side in a quarrel. I now understand what he means.

In summary, I hope you will wish to look thoughtfully at individual novel events in your experience, analyze them carefully, and decide whether or not they may contain the kernel of a new concept. My first anecdote has mainly confirmatory significance, but my second one may be a signpost toward a recognition of a new approach to grossly deviant actions of the special type deplored by the doer.

ACKNOWLEDGMENT

It is a pleasure to express appreciation to the Neuro-Research Foundation for the support of these studies.

REFERENCES

1. Adams, R. D., Fisher, C. M., Hakim, S., Ojemann, R. G., and Sweet, W. H. Symptomatic occult hydrocephalus with "normal" cerebrospinal fluid pressure. A treatable syndrome. N. Engl. J. Med., *273:* 117–126, 1965.

2. Chew, G. F., Gell-Mann, M., and Rosenfeld, A. H. Strongly interacting particles. Sci. Am., *210:* 74–93, 1964.
3. Cook, A. W., and Browder, E. J. Function of posterior columns in man. Arch. Neurol., *12:* 72–79, 1965.
4. Crosby, E. C., Humphrey, T., and Laver, E. W. Correlative Anatomy of the Nervous System, pp. 85–86. MacMillan Co., New York, 1962.
5. Elliott, H. C. Cross-sectional diameters and areas of the human spinal cord. Anat. Rec., *93:* 287–293, 1945.
6. Foerster, O., and Gagel, O. Die Vorderseitenstrangdurchschneidung bein Menschen. Eine-klinisch-patho-physiologisch-anatomische Studie. Neurol. Psychiatr., *138:* 1–92, 1932.
7. Foltz, E. L., and Ward, A. A., Jr. Communicating hydrocephalus from subarachnoid bleeding. J. Neurosurg., 13: 546–566, 1956.
8. Hakim, S. Some observations on CSF pressure hydrocephalic syndrome in adults with "normal" CSF pressure. Thesis #957, Javeriana University School of Medicine, Bogato, Colombia, S. A. March 10, 1964.
9. Head, H. Studies in Neurology, Volume II. Hodder & Stoughton, Ltd., London, 1920.
10. Kroll, F. W. Schwellenuntersuchungen bei Lasionen der afferenten Leitungsbahnen. Z. Neurah Psychiatr., *128:* 751–776 1930.
11. Kuru, M. Sensory Paths in the Spinal Cord and Brain Stem of Man, 39 pp. Sogensya, Tokyo and Osaka, 1949.
12. May, W. P. The afferent path. Brain, *29:* 742–803, 1906.
13. Ranson, S. W., and Clark, S. L. Anatomy of the Nervous System. Ed. 10, p. 190. W. B. Saunders Co., Philadelphia, 1959.
14. Rose, J. E., and Mountcastle, V. B. Touch and Kinesthesis. Handbook of Physiology. Sect. I: Neurophysiology, Vol. 1, Chap. 17. American Physiological Society, Washington, D.C., 1959.
15. Ruch, T. C., Patton, H. D., Woodbury, J. W. and Towe, A. L., Eds. Neurophysiology. 521 pp. W. B. Saunders Co., Philadelphia, 1961.
16. Schaltenbrand, G. Introduction to Stereotaxis with an Atlas of the Human Brain. Georg Thieme Verlag, Stuttgart, 1959.
17. Smith, D. E. History of Mathematics, Vol. II. Special Topics of Elementary Mathematics, p. 676. Ginn and Company, Boston, 1925.
18. Smith, D. E. History of Mathematics, Vol. I. General Survey, p. 274. Ginn and Company, Boston, 1925.
19. Sweet, W. H. "Phantom" sensations following intraspinal injury. Neurochirurgia, *18:* 139–154, 1975.
20. Sweet, W. H., Ervin, F., and Mark, V. H. The relationship of violent behaviour to focal cerebral disease. *In* Aggressive Behavior, edited by S. Garattini and E. B. Sigg, pp. 336–352. Excerpta Medica Foundation, Amsterdam, 1969.
21. Truex, R. C., and Carpenter, M. B. Human Neuroanatomy, pp. 263–265. Williams & Wilkins, Baltimore, 1969.
22. White, J. C., Sweet, W. H., Hawkins, R., and Nilges, R. G. Anterolateral cordotomy: results, complications and causes of failure. Brain, *73:* 346–367, 1950.

CHAPTER

5

Radical Surgical Treatment of Craniopharyngioma

WILLIAM H. SWEET, M.D., D.Sc.

INTRODUCTION

There is a striking divergence of opinion on the management of craniopharyngioma. It was hoped in the early fifties that with the availability of cortisone and other hormones related to pituitary function many of these tumors could be totally removed. However, in the past 12 years there has been a major trend toward a minor or even minimal role of extirpative surgery. This statement will be documented in the later discussion. Matson and I appear to be the only neurosurgeons to have maintained for many years a program of radical, hopefully total removal for the great majority of these patients. Matson, noting a zero long term survival in their patients treated by less than total removal, operated radically on nearly all of the 51 children with this tumor he saw after 1950, once good hormonal replacement therapy became available (18). Katz' late followup of these patients treated during the last 18 years of Matson's professional life (1950 to 1968) reveals that a primary operation with presumed total excision was carried out in 34 cases without a single postoperative death—a record not yet equalled (13). Unhappily his own death prevented him from completing the operative atlas he started to tell us how he did it.

ANALYSIS OF PERSONAL CASES

This will be divided into 4 parts: (1) Evidence for the extent of tumor which can be totally removed, (2) role of special glial reaction provoked by craniopharyngioma cells, (3) suggestions regarding operative management, and (4) results.

Evidence for the Extent of Tumor which can be Totally Removed

My own encouragement toward radical surgery of this tumor came from a distinguished experienced neurologist who referred to me a patient especially important to him with the proviso that I carry out a total removal even if, as I was so doing, I estimated a mortality as high as

90%. He was led to this attitude, he said, by the relentlessly downhill course and unsatisfactory life of those surviving less aggressive measures. Since that time, 1954, I have sought to remove these tumors radically in all 30 patients in whom I was doing the primary therapeutic procedure and in six of the seven in whom my effort was at a second or later operation.

The first three cases illustrate the major extent of some of the tumors removed.

Case 1. John G., aged 7 years, showed before my first operation on him a relatively small tumor encroaching on the anterior part of the 3rd ventricle (Fig. 5.1A. The fluid and soft tissue part of this were readily removed, but his preoperative ataxia, to our surprise, became progressively worse. An air study 6 weeks later (Figs. 5.1B and C) revealed extreme displacement of the aqueduct and the 4th ventricle posteriorly and to the right. At suboccipital craniectomy, his giant craniopharyngiomatous cyst presented at the foramen magnum. After 56 cc. of fluid had been aspirated, one could see to the left and in front of the displaced brain stem right up to the top of the dorsum sellae. The cyst wall was everywhere so thin as to be almost transparent. It seemed reasonable to leave in the shreds of cyst attached firmly to cranial nerve VII, in a few places to the brain stem, and engulfing a large vein at the Vth cranial nerve. Within 8 months the cyst wall had been reconstituted and massively refilled. The suboccipital approach was repeated and all identifiable cyst removed with an ensuing paralysis of cranial nerves V and VII. The patient died 8 months later after a 4-month effort to treat subacute bacterial endocarditis. Postmortem showed no recurrent soft tissue or cystic neoplasm.

Case 2. Joseph P., aged eight, had a huge bilateral subfrontal lesion rising straight up from the sella as shown in Figures 5.2A and B. Aspiration trans-sphenoidally by Dr. Hamlin with injection of air revealed (Fig. 5.2C) that there was so much solid tumor the cyst would not collapse completely. At my subfrontal operation this tumor separated with great ease from the frontal lobes but required a critical dissection from its attachment to the visual pathways. He is well 13 years later, but his preoperative mental retardation has not improved and he remains unemployable.

Case 3. Evan D., aged 6 years, was legally blind when admitted for study. After the radiographs illustrated in Figures 5.3A and B revealing extremely dilated lateral ventricles and marked lateral displacement of the narrow posterior crescent of the 3rd ventricle unoccupied by tumor, he was totally blind. He has recovered only light perception after presumed total removal of his tumor, but now 11 years later he will be graduating from the Perkins School for the Blind.

Role of Glial Reaction Provoked by Craniopharyngiomatous Epithelium

My attention was forcefully drawn to this phenomenon by the following experience. Having removed the typical content and much of the capsule of this tumor lying within the 3rd ventricle (Fig. 5.4), I brought out finally as the last of the presumed capsule the tissue shown in Figure 5.5A. I was aghast at this spectacle and wondered how many hypothalamic nuclei were included in it. However, the H&E stain (Fig. 5.5B) showed only astroglia with Rosenthal fibers and occasional epithelial neoplastic nests. The densely fibrous character of the glia is

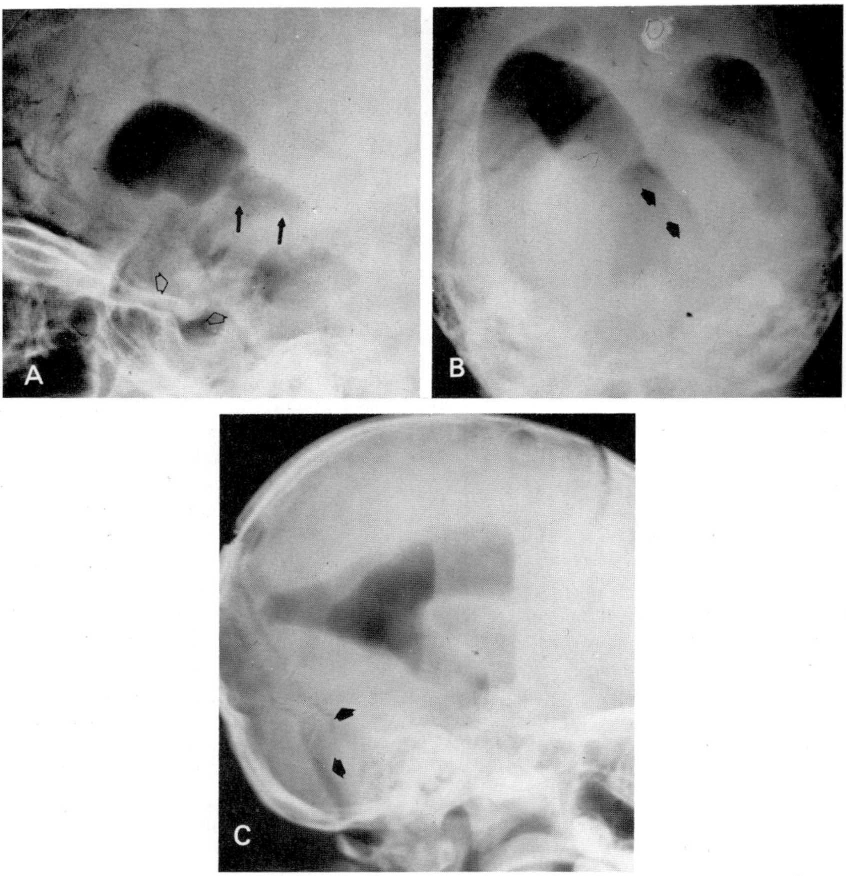

FIG. 5.1. (A) John G. First lateral fractional pneumoencephalogram (PEG) showing moderate sized indentation into anterior floor of 3rd ventricle (closed arrows), rising above extensive supra- and retrosellar calcification (open arrows). (B and C) John G. Second PEG 6 weeks later. Lateral ventricles more dilated, 4th ventricle and aqueduct deviated to the extreme right and posteriorly (closed arrows).

shown in the phosphotungstic acid hematoxylin stain in Figure 5.6. No neurones are to be seen.

As far back as 1939, Bailey, Buchanan and Bucy (2) had noted that the epithelial cells of these tumors are imbedded in a dense gliosis surrounding the tumor and into which papillae of tumor extend. In their case 90, for example, the outer wall of the cyst was a dense mass of neuroglia with Rosenthal fibers, which "pulled free from brain tissue at postmortem." In only one of their five cases was there no dense gliosis; here the cyst wall was "comprised of epithelium with a small amount of

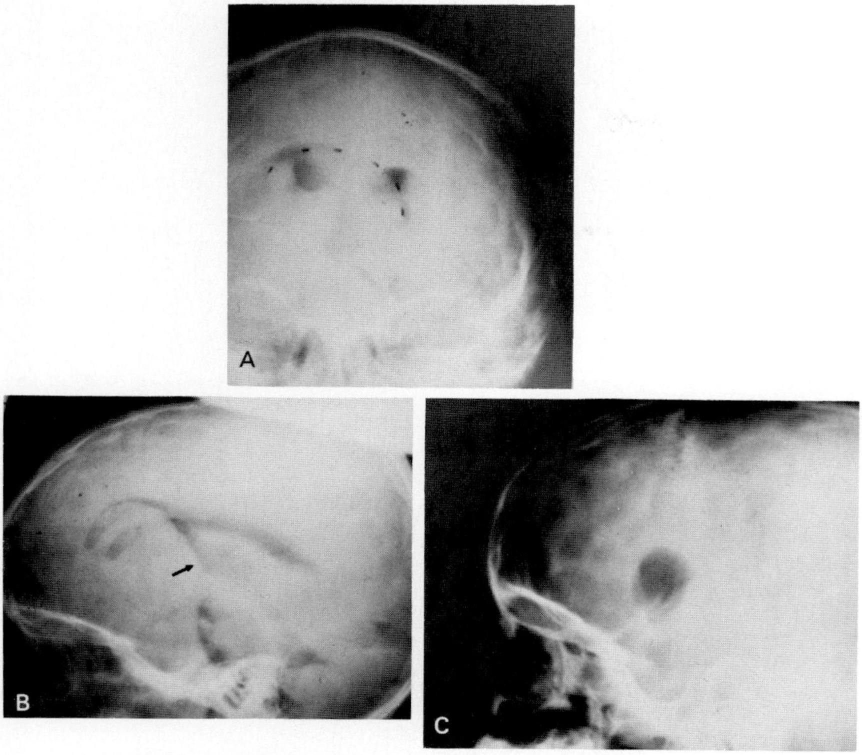

FIG. 5.2 (A and B) Joseph P. Sagittal and lateral projections showing extreme upward displacement of anterior parts of lateral ventricles right greater than left, black dashes mark upper surface dome of tumor; filling defect anterior 3rd ventricle (arrow). No filling any basal cisterns in front of cisterna interpeduncularis. (C) Joseph P. Lateral view after trans-sphenoidal aspiration of cyst by Dr. H. Hamlin and injection of air into it showing cyst far from completely collapsed. Separation of coronal suture and increased convultional markings.

supporting connective tissue.'' This observation of a fibrillary gliosis including abundant Rosenthal fibers at the contiguous hypothalamus in association with these tumors has been repeatedly confirmed among others by Grcevic *et al.* (7), Zülch (28), van der Bergh (27), and Ghatak *et al* (6). Timperley (26) has pointed out that this marked eosinophilia of the glial fibers, often expanded to form tadpole-shaped ''Rosenthal'' bodies characterizes craniopharyngiomas, whereas, an epidermoid cyst is enclosed by ''an unremarkable gliosis.'' Incidentally, his four craniopharyngiomas and an ameloblastoma of the jaw had a high activity of alkaline phosphatase. Normal squamous epithelium from six sites and epithelium from three epidermoid cysts did not show this high activity.

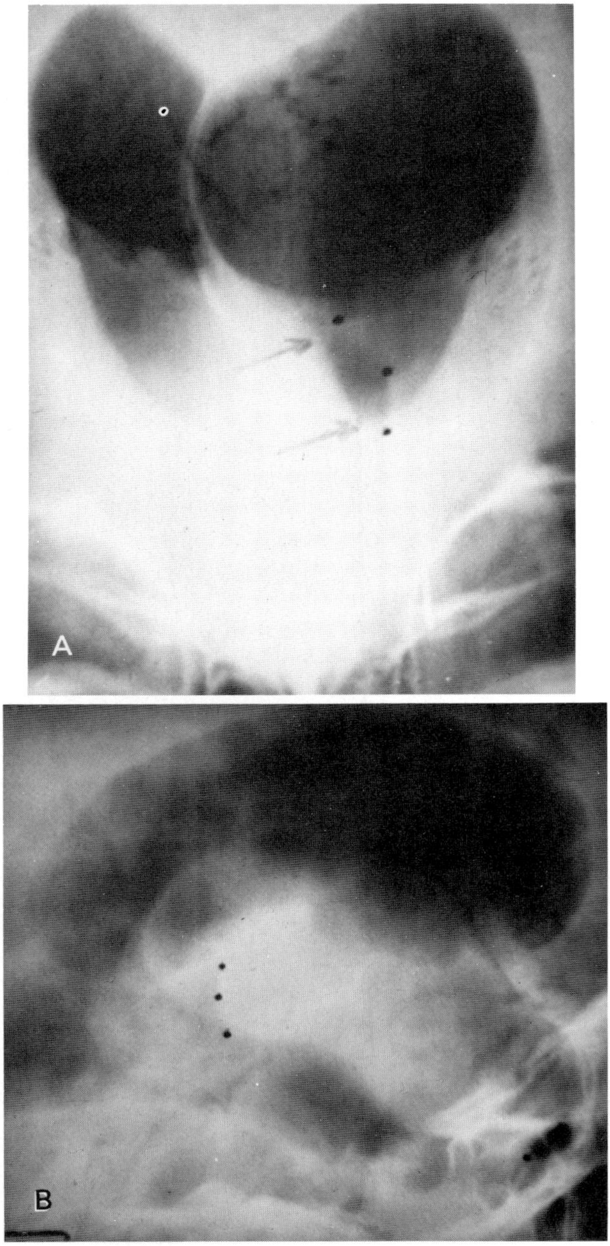

FIG. 5.3. Evan D. Ventriculogram. (A) Sagittal view showing extreme displacement of 3rd ventricle to the left (3 black dots mark its convex left border; arrows its straight right border). (B) Lateral view showing 3rd ventricle as a tiny posterior crescent (3 black dots mark its anterior boundary).

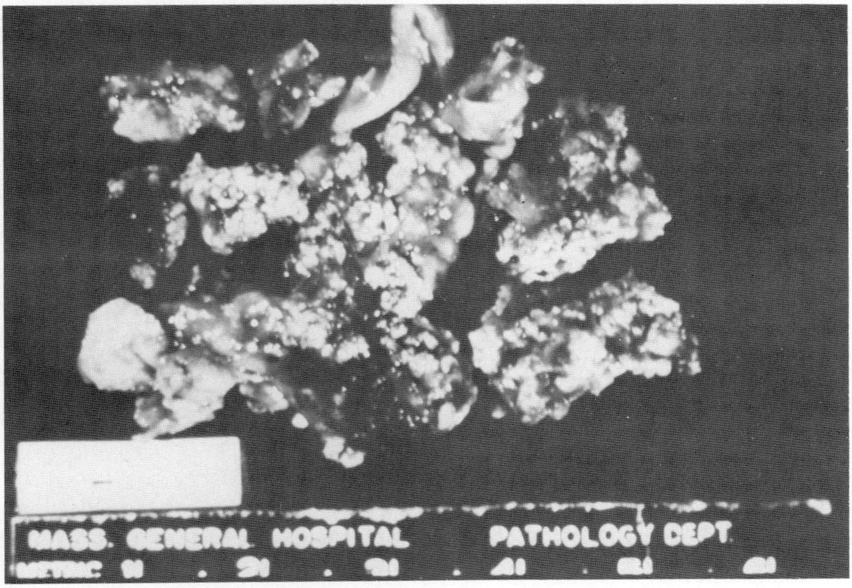

FIG. 5.4. Nancy C. Typical gross appearance of craniopharyngioma fragments.

"This intimate mixture of nests of tumor cells and severely altered brain tissue" to quote Ghatak and associates (6) has been generally regarded as a major obstacle to total surgical removal of craniopharyngiomas impinging on brain tissue, the assumption being that the reactive glia adheres to the normal neural structures. My experience has led me to regard the reverse point of view as the more tenable, namely, that this glial reaction may well constitute a margin of safety between the proliferating epithelial cells we seek to remove and the functioning neurones we wish to leave behind. Happily my gentle traction on this densely gliotic tissue has nearly always yielded a trophy free of neurones. Figure 5.7A from another case illustrates this point. Figure 5.7B from the same patient shows that at other points the capsule may be much more tenuous.

One is concerned that some gliotic tissue with epithelial tongues in it may be left behind. Thus the tissue shown in Figure 5.8 was taken from the posterior edge of the chiasm 11 years ago. It looked, under the operating microscope at that time, indistinguishable from the rest of the chiasm, so I stopped. The tissue removed, as you see, contained some epithelial clumps but no nerve fibers and the patient recovered with no visual field defect. However, 10 years later his tumor recurred. He is now well 1 year after its second nearly total removal.

The intense glial reaction can at times dominate the picture the

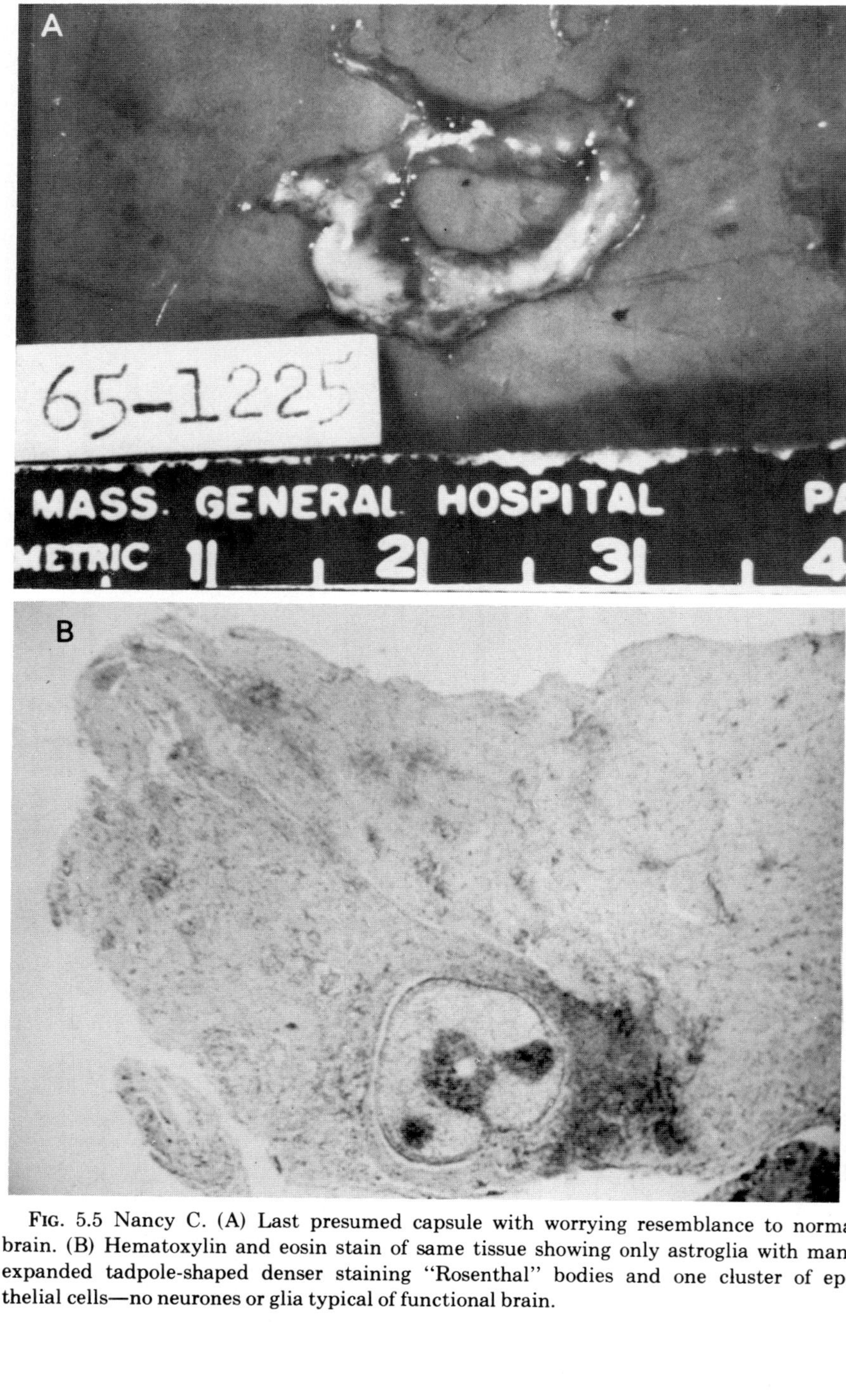

FIG. 5.5 Nancy C. (A) Last presumed capsule with worrying resemblance to normal brain. (B) Hematoxylin and eosin stain of same tissue showing only astroglia with many expanded tadpole-shaped denser staining "Rosenthal" bodies and one cluster of epithelial cells—no neurones or glia typical of functional brain.

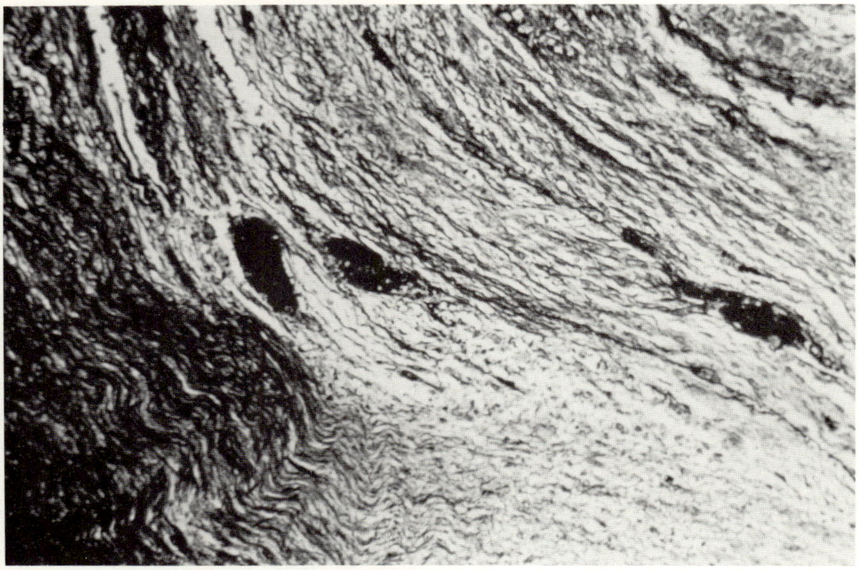

FIG. 5.6. Nancy C. Same Specimen as Figure 5.5 (A). Phosphotungstic acid hematoxylin stain showing densely fibrous nature of glia.

surgeon first sees. In two of my cases the chiasm, the apparently grossly swollen optic tracts and lamina terminalis seemed to be expanded by a glioma of the visual pathways or hypothalamus. In the first case the radiographs had shown no intracranial calcification; I could find no cleavage plane between a presumed medial border of optic tract and tumor, and no cyst fluid could be aspirated (Fig. 5.9). My several biopsies taken from zones halfway between the lateral borders of the 2 optic tracts were reported as glial tissue with a few chronic inflammatory cells. I sadly closed the wound, but Dr. E. P. Richardson sent over word as I was taking the last scalp stitches that he had seen one epithelial cluster characteristic of craniopharyngioma. I reopened the wound, decided the best place to find tumor surface would be in the midline where it was abutting on the cavity of the 3rd ventricle. Once a clearcut posterosuperior end of tumor was felt, its center was removed and the cleavage plane followed by easing wall of tumor toward the midline from all the way around. Her three quadrant defects in the visual field of each eye and her visual acuity promptly returned to normal. She has had no evidence of recurrence 12 years later. In a second patient, the pathologist was promptly able to diagnose a craniopharyngioma from a small biopsy and the cleavage plane was found in the same way.

I have shown, however, to my entire dissatisfaction that it is possible to

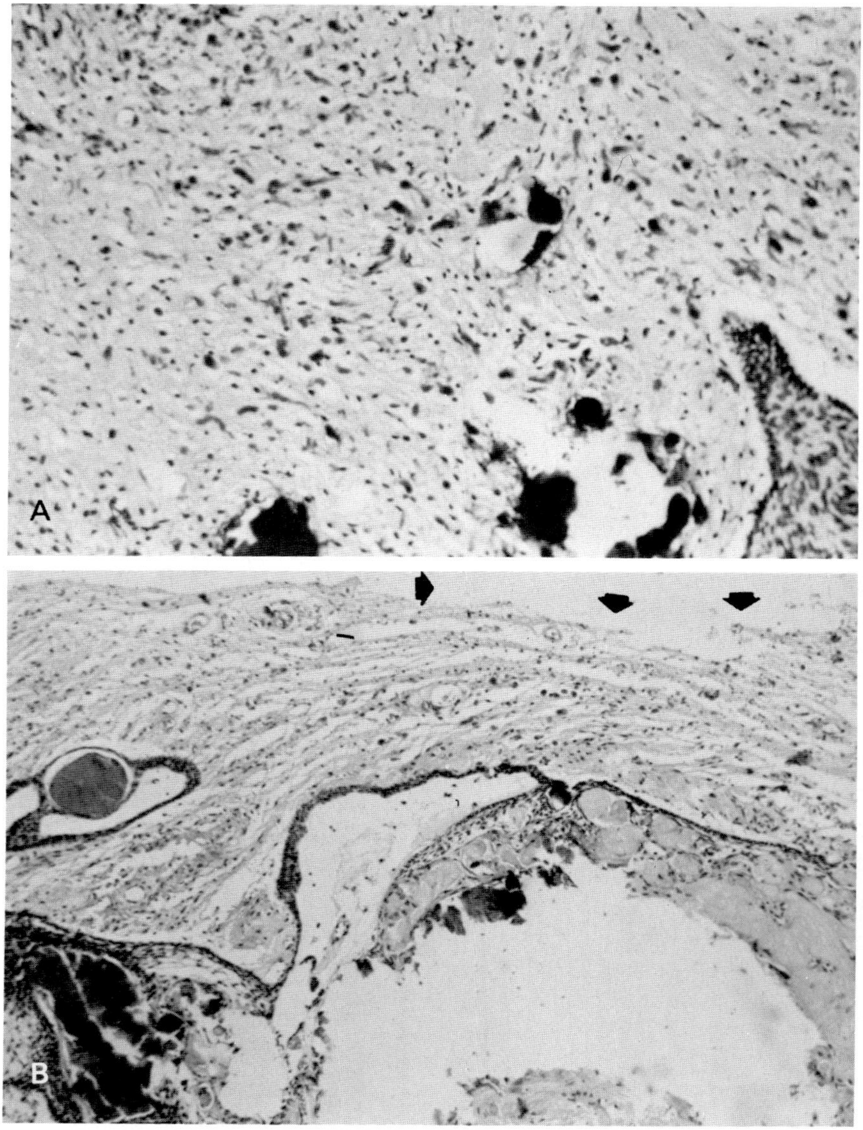

FIG. 5.7. Frederick N. Histology of tumor capsule. (A) One area with dense astroglia, many Rosenthal bodies, one epithelial tongue, and bits of calcification (dense black blobs). (B) Another area within thin, much less densely fibrous capsule (arrows).

remove some hypothalamus along with the gliotic tumor boundary. Figure 5.10 shows this in a patient's biopsy (James D.) taken at a second operation 14 years after the first one and 9 years after we had known of his tumor recurrence. The patient had abandoned both medical and

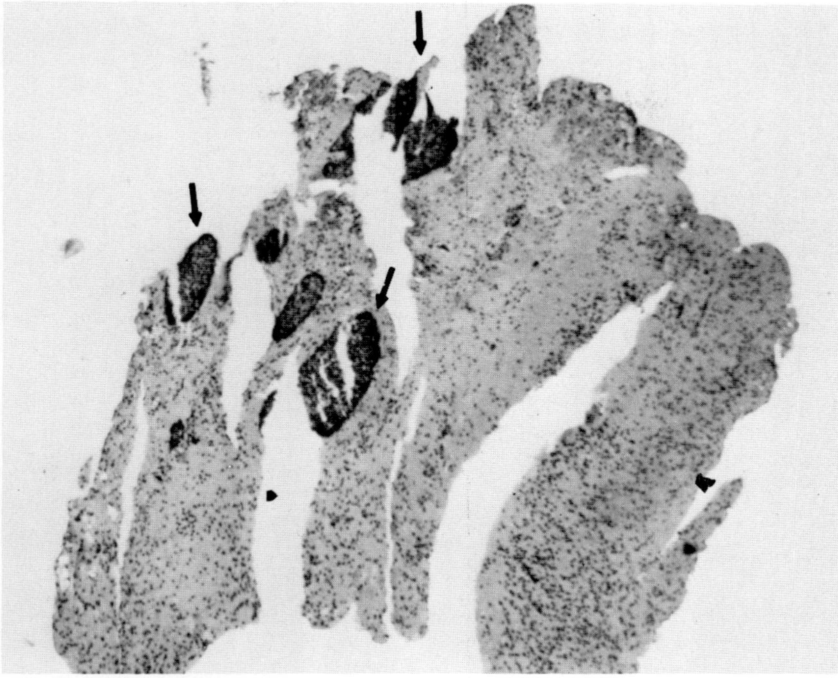

FIG. 5.8. Nicholas D. Histology of tissue from posterior edge of chiasm grossly indistinguishable from remainder of chiasm. H&E stain—only astrocytes with small epithelial nests (arrows).

further surgical treatment until his condition became desperate. At reoperation, the boundary tissue between tumor and hypothalamus was obviously more tenacious than anything I had ever encountered before. Because of a wound infection the patient did not survive the postoperative period, but the hypothalamic trauma may well have played a role in the fatal outcome. Van der Bergh and Brucher (27) have made several observations of both types; *i.e.*, in their Case 1 at postmortem they noted in several places a plane of cleavage between the perineoplastic spongioblastic gliosis and the actual hypothalamic nervous tissue. Contrariwise, in their Case 5 at postmortem, the dense spongioblastic gliosis with tumor tongues contained as well some normal looking neurons and some atrophic ones with vacuolar degeneration.

Another patient in whom the tumor grew for many years and became firmly adherent to adjoining brain was a patient (Anna M.) who was treated with 3000 rads of radiation to her presumed 3rd ventricular pinealoma in 1949. She did well until 1972 when her increasing mental confusion was treated by ventriculoatrial shunt of her grossly dilated lateral ventricles. Finally, over a year later when she was in a state of

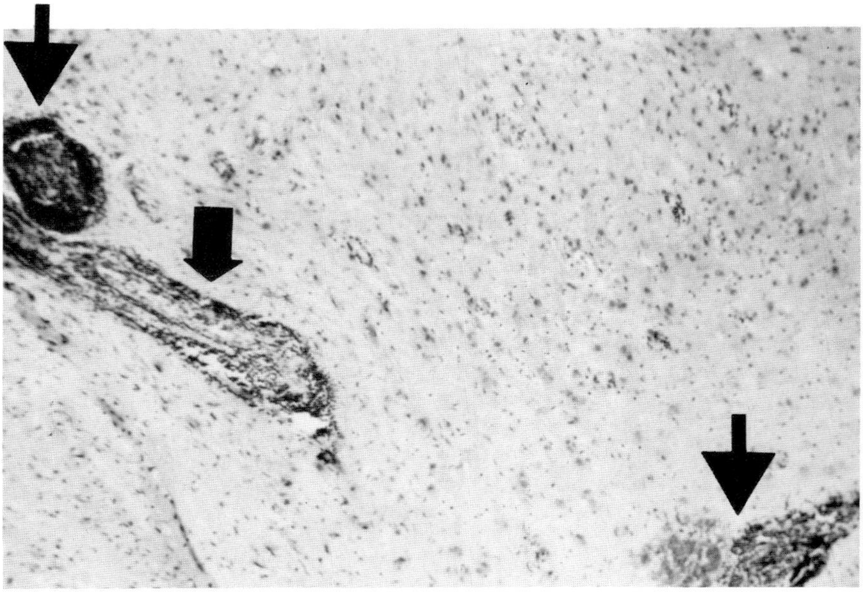

FIG. 5.9. Jean P. Histology of tumor biopsy originally in frozen section erroneously diagnosed as optic nerve glioma because only astroglia with a few clusters of chronic inflammatory cells (arrows) are seen.

useless dementia and the center of her brain was a mass of solid tumor, I made a forlorn effort to remove her craniopharyngioma. The central part of the lesion came away fairly readily, leaving a tenacious glial rind whose separation from brain I had to abandon. The operation served no useful purpose.

However, in all 22 of my other patients in whom tumor could apparently be eased away essentially totally from the surrounding 3rd ventricular wall, the operative specimen shows only gliosis with or without epithelial nests and without neurones. In particular, in 10 of these 22 patients in whose operative specimens I directed Dr. Richardson's attention to a worrying gross appearance to some of the tissue, he saw nothing containing neurones. However, the gliosis elicited by these tumors appears to be an increscence into ventricle, not a part of functional brain, and largely separable from it by gentle dissection. I have no evidence that gliomas of the visual pathways, ectopic pinealomas or any other anterior 3rd ventricular tumor excite this specific, apparently surgically helpful, form of gliosis.

Suggestions Regarding Operative Management

Matson and I independently concluded that these tumors should all be approached *via* the subfrontal route. Their most tenacious attachments in my experience are to the chiasm and adjoining optic tracts, pituitary stalk, and neighboring hypothalamus, or to the medial aspects of the internal carotid, posterior communicating, or anterior choroidal arteries. Only the subfrontal route permits a good view of all of these areas. In particular, since the neoplasm and much of its accompanying special gliosis can almost always be safely drawn downward and forward out of the 3rd ventricle, the 2 superior approaches *via corpus callosum* or lateral ventricle lose their special advantage of a good view of the walls of the 3rd ventricle. However, these tumors may send a tongue down into the cerebellopontine angle oftener than I had realized 2 decades ago. As already pointed out, such extension may require a suboccipital craniectomy, or if the tongue is less extensive, a supratentorial lateral approach.

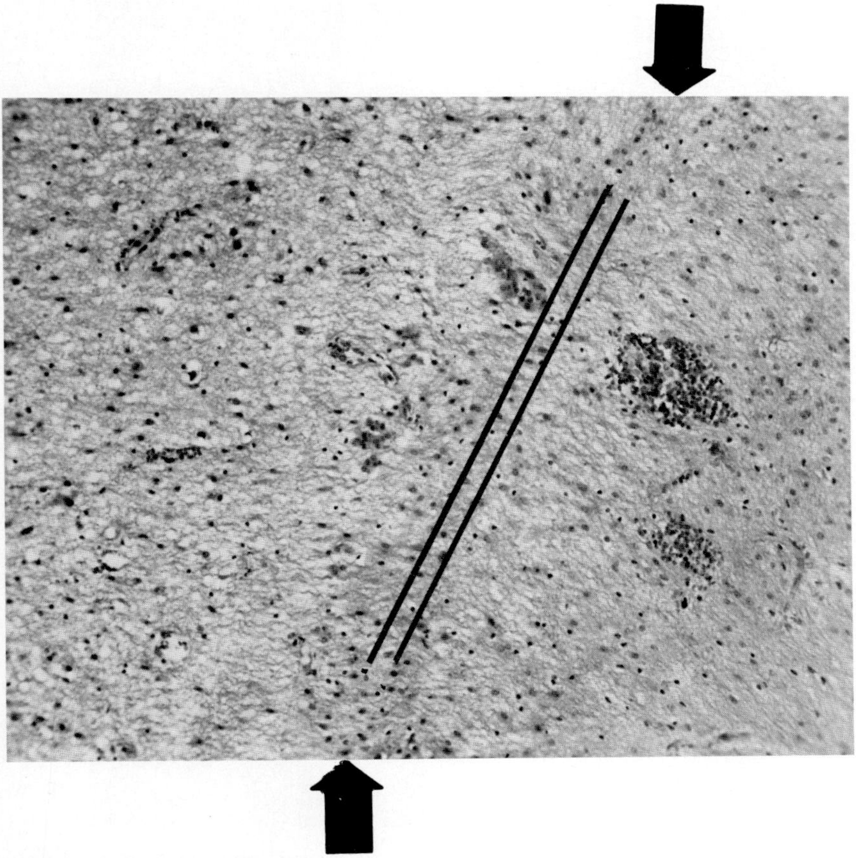

FIG. 5.10. James D. Histology of tissue biopsy × 130. Hypothalamus is present along with glial reaction in this tenaciously adherent recurrent tumor of long standing. To the left of the lines joining the arrows is hypothalamus; to the right of that line lies dense astroglia.

Either elevation of the temporal lobe or division of arachnoid at the horizontal limb of the Sylvian fissure and depression of temporal lobe may achieve the necessary exposure. Malis (17) has presented an excellent description of this exposure.

It is important to select the appropriate side from which to work. I favor working from the side of the worse vision and the larger mass of tumor. Figure 5.11 illustrates a little larger tumor to the left of the midline in the CT scan in a patient whose vision was down to finger counting and that only in the upper nasal quadrant of the right eye. As Figure 5.12 shows, this tumor had to be approached from the left since it lay mainly lateral to the left optic nerve displacing it over against the

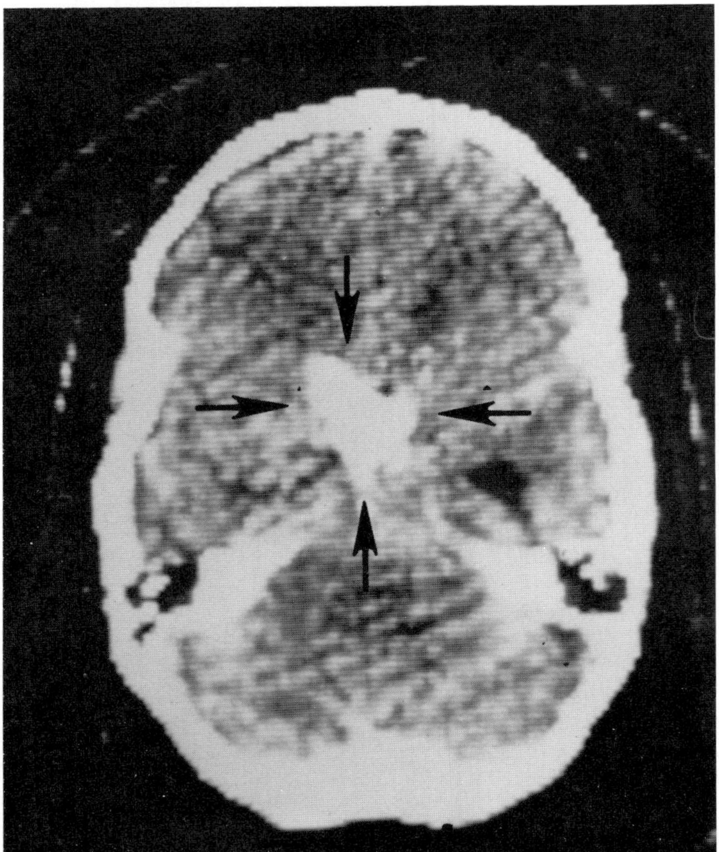

FIG. 5.11. Charles W. CT (EMI) scan. Low horizontal cut shows abnormal parasellar dense calcification of tumor (arrows) not much more to left than to right of midline.

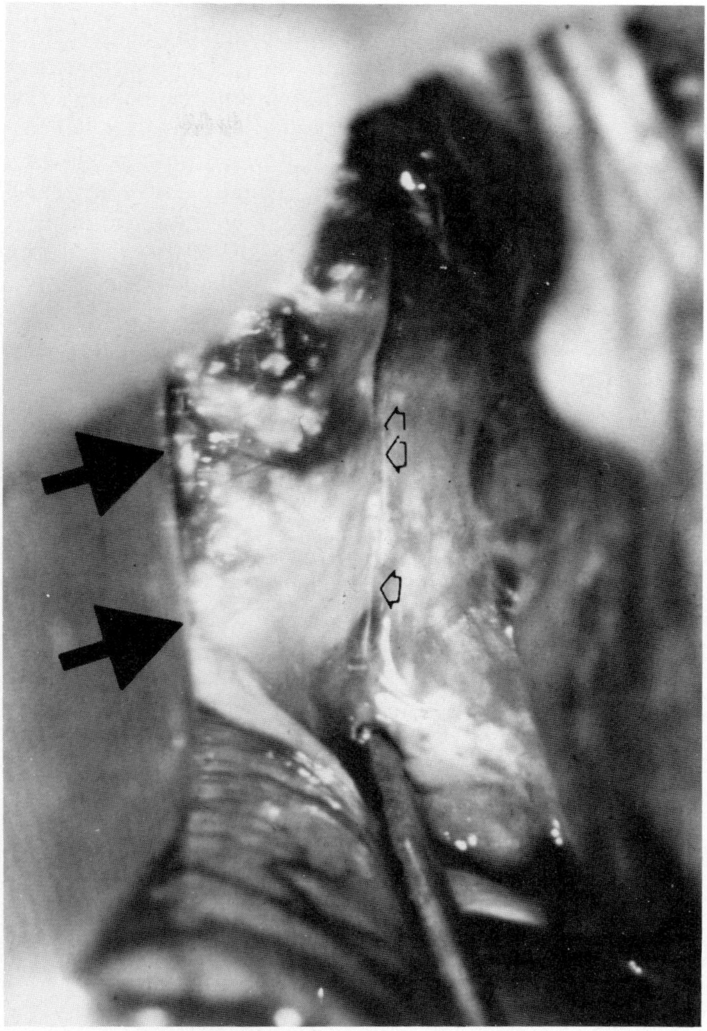

FIG. 5.12. Charles W. Operative photograph. After elevation of left frontal lobe to expose left optic nerve and tumor. Suction tip points to lateral edge of posterior part of grossly elongated left optic nerve. Extreme displacement to right of left optic nerve by tumor (open arrows indicate lateral edge of nerve). Retraction on medial edge of temporal lobe exposes tumor beyond tips of closed arrows.

right optic nerve and pushing the internal carotid downward. The dislocation of the usual normal structures and the frequent presence of unusual arteries require unrelenting maintenance of orientation. After the tumor was removed largely *via* the space lateral to optic nerve and chiasm, the pituitary stalk appears to run diagonally behind the dorsum sellae with the right posterior communicating artery just to its right (Fig. 5.13). One tongue of the tumor was drawn anterosuperiorly out of the cerebellopontine angle. A sizable unnamed artery lies ventral to the anterior end of the left internal carotid. From it came one of the main feeding arteries to the tumor capsule, an unusually long one. One seeks to find nutrient arteries to the inferior surface of the optic nerves and to save them separate from tumor capsule. In this patient, the tumor was located superior to the left anterior and middle cerebral arteries pushing their perforating branches posteriorly. The tumor, although adherent to these vessels, could be slowly freed from them with no oozing from any of them. The extreme zigzag course of the left optic tract is probably cor-

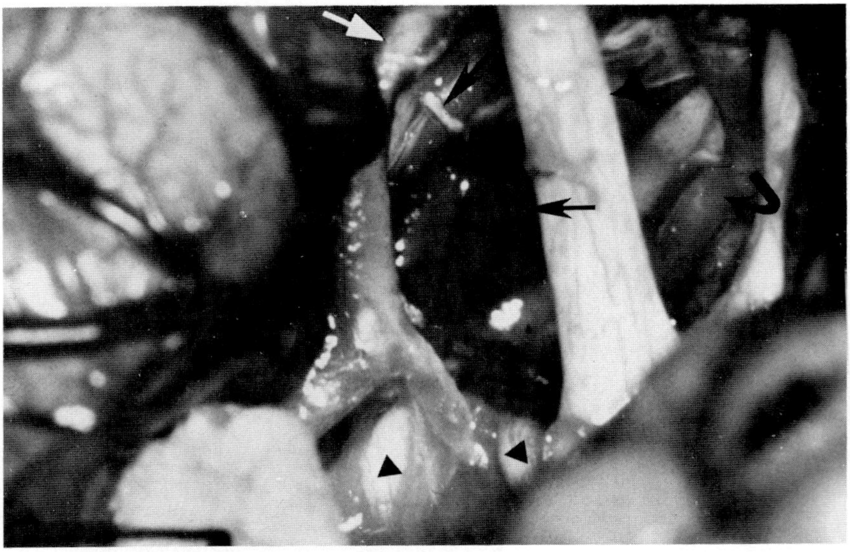

FIG. 5.13. Charles W. Same view as Figure 5.12 after removal of tumor which extended inferoposteriorly into left cerebellopontine angle (arrow on left optic nerve points to black void of the empty angle). Proceeding clockwise from this arrow, ➤ to right of left optic nerve points to intact pituitary stalk; curving arrow on right optic nerve points to origin of right posterior communicating and anterior choroidal arteries from right internal carotid. Closed triangles lie on zigzag left optic tract which had been displaced by tumor, so as to move straight lateral to the chiasm about 1 cm, then angle sharply backward. The right closed triangle lies just to the right of left anterior cerebral artery crossing the optic tract. The left closed triangle lies between perforating branches running backward from anterior and middle cerebral arteries. The largest arrow at top left points to anterior end of left internal carotid artery. The smaller arrow below and to the right of this points to the largest feeding artery to the capsule electrocoagulated and divided several mm from its origin from a large anomalous artery running inferomedial and parallel to the anterior end of the left internal carotid. The shaft of the arrow lies on that anomalous artery.

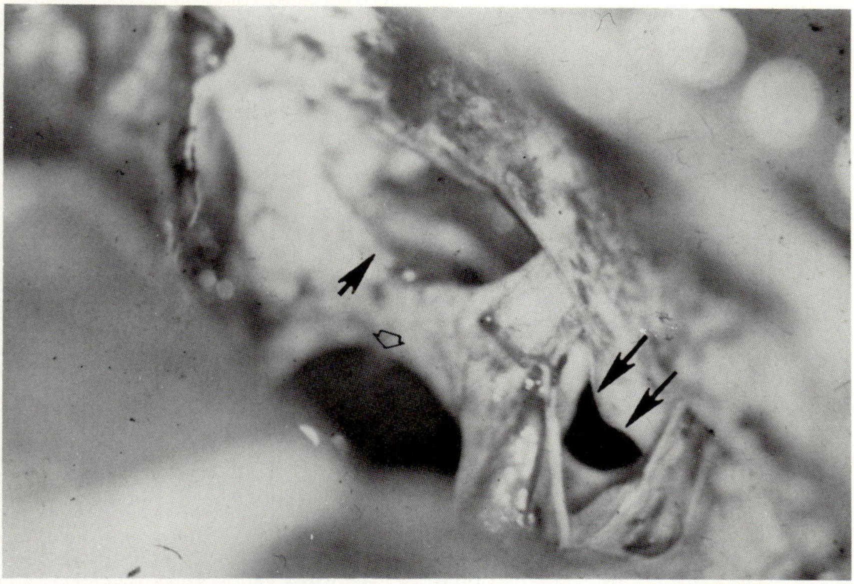

FIG. 5.14. Nancy C. Operative photo after tumor removal *via* subfrontal approach to show empty spaces anterior to the chiasm (left solid arrow) and lateral to right optic tract and right internal carotid artery (double solid arrows) beneath which tumor was pushed for removal behind the chiasm and between the two optic tracts (open arrow).

related with no recovery of vision related to it despite the resumption of a nearly normal appearance of the optic nerves once the tumor was out.

The tumors in 23 of my 37 patients lay mainly in the 3rd ventricle and in them removal was from between the two optic tracts through the lamina terminalis. Often they pushed the chiasm forward almost to the tuberculum sellae. Especially in the three completely solid tumors, there was initially almost no space to work between the anterior cerebral artery behind and the posterior edge of the chiasm in front. This space gradually increased as the center of the tumor was removed. I sought to avoid piecemeal removal of any of the capsule. This may become tenuous, and it is important to have as much of it as possible on which to exert gentle traction as one seeks to bring tumor downward and forward out of the back of the 3rd ventricle. Use of the double binocular microscope affording a chance for a second surgeon to bring at least one of his hands into play has been an advance in technique, as Dr. Kjellberg and I demonstrated to our satisfaction in this situation several years ago. Those tumors largely in the 3rd ventricle often erode through its anterior and/or anterolateral floor, and I have found it advantageous to push them backward from the suprasellar area under the chiasm or from

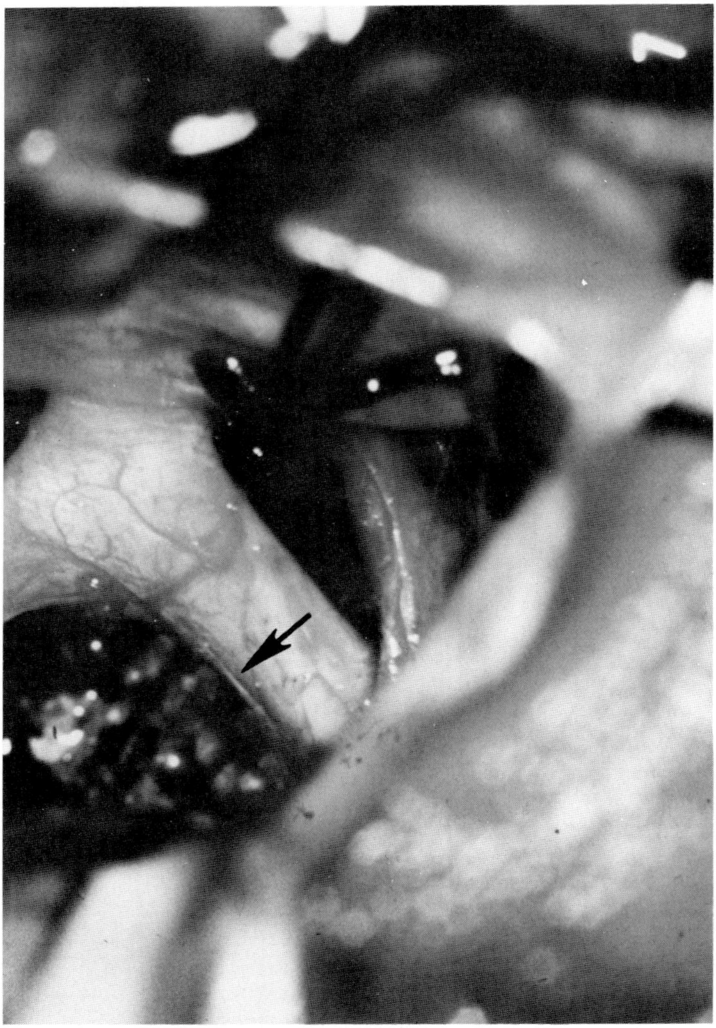

FIG. 5.15. Scott S. Operative photo. Similar general view as for Figure 5.14; glistening tumor remnants in 3rd ventricle behind chiasm and to left of right optic tract on which arrow lies pointing to tumor. To right of right optic tract lies empty space medial to right internal carotid previously occupied by lateral wall of hypothalamus plus tumor. *By pushing this medially, the lateral wall of hypothalamus was kept intact and tumor all removed medial to tract, via the safest opening available for an intra-third ventricular tumor—i.e. that provided by removal of ultra-thin, functionless lamina terminalis.*

medial to the carotid artery under the optic tract as shown in Figures 5.14 in one patient and Figure 5.15 in another. In the latter patient, the bloodstained hypothalamic floor seen after the tumor was out proved consistent with useful hypothalamic function. Via the hole in the anterior 3rd ventricular floor made by tumor in such a case, one sees after its removal the basilar artery and its main upper branches through the intact arachnoid over the prepontine and cerebellopontine angle cisterns. The same vessels may be seen from in front of the chiasm when this has been pushed far back by tumor. The arachnoid appears to form a barrier preventing adherence of tumor to the important structures near to it in these cisterns and permitting its forward withdrawal with relative impunity.

Unusual directions of growth were taken by one tumor (Fig. 5.16) which engulfed the right internal carotid and proximal anterior, middle, and posterior cerebral arteries, following the latter two vessels out into the Sylvian fissure and back around the cerebral peduncle. Those vessels were lying free in air after Dr. John Tew and I spent the day picking out

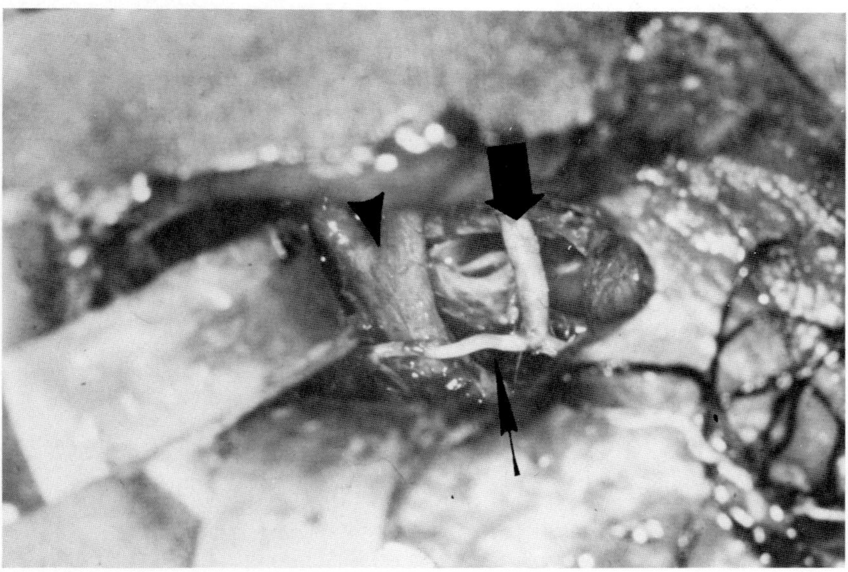

FIG. 5.16. Kevin A. Operative photo after right subfrontal removal of tumor which had engulfed right internal carotid and proximal anterior, middle and posterior cerebral and posterior communicating arteries. Right internal carotid displaced markedly to right (upper right arrow); horizontal part of anterior cerebral remarkably free of any branches (lower right arrow), apparently because of early embryonic development of congenital nests around it; visual pathways enclosed in unusually thick arachnoid (upper left arrow between right and left optic nerves).

neoplasm, birdseed bites at a time. An atypical slight arachnoidal thickening enclosed the optic nerve, chiasm, and proximal optic tracts in this patient.

The pink posterior communicating and anterior choroidal arteries may make little ridges in the pink wall of the capsule and obviously should not be grasped. Indeed every effort is made to avoid starting up any arterial bleeding of even minimal degree. In two patients, I started bleeding which was readily controlled by application of Oxycel. In one of them, a whole succession of tiny holes in one anterior cerebral artery and the opposite internal carotid were made because the adherent tumor capsule was apparently supplied directly therefrom. In the other patient, I placed divergent retractors in such fashion as to cause a slight tear at the angle of origin of anterior cerebral from internal carotid, obviously a maneuver to avoid. The ease of stopping the bleeding led me to push on with extirpation. Both patients, at first doing well after operation, died of spreading thrombosis in the basal arteries. In three later patients in whom such bleeding occurred, the operation was stopped forthwith to allow time for endothelium to cover the opening. In two, the operation was successfully completed at a second stage some weeks later, but the third died postoperatively from hemorrhage at the operative site. An additional abrupt death occurred from a tiny hemorrhage into the hypothalamic floor on the 14th postoperative day. A premonitory moderate subarachnoid hemorrhage had occurred in her on the 4th postoperative day, from which she was recovering, and which led to determination of normal blood coagulation mechanisms. Doing well, she suddenly expired without another subarachnoid hemorrhage. No tumor was identified in the hypothalamus, but if I left behind tissue of the type seen in part of the operative specimen from another patient, showing many blood vessels in the midst of the gliosis, it might have caused the tiny fatal bleed. The result has led me to ease out all I dare of the periphery of tumor.

In only six patients, was I able to keep the pituitary stalk intact; in several I had to cut it as it splayed out into tumor; in others, I did not see it either because it was presumably engulfed in tumor lying in front of and within the 3rd ventricle or lying beneath a broad fixed chiasm. In one patient, a huge stalk proved to be invaded by a central cord of neoplasm and was excised.

An important point already stressed by many surgeons is the need to line the working area with cottonoid so that irritative fluid and solid debris in the cyst will not set up a chemical meningitis. Patrick's case (22) of a spontaneous rupture of such a cyst is especially instructive. At the height of the reaction, the CSF total protein was 7.5 g/100 ml., the white cell count 23,700/cu. mm., and the pressure > 300 mm. H_2O. Everytime a new locule of cyst is entered, its contents should be thoroughly sucked and irrigated out before one works on the solid tumor again. The mica-like crystals come to the top of the fluid and irrigation should continue until not a one is visible. Inadequate attention to this may have led to the need for a postoperative ventriculoatrial shunt after 5 of my 44 operations. (The cottonoid strips were removed to facilitate orientation in the operative photographs).

All of these tumors were removed with the aid of magnifying loupes, the operating microscope, or both. As special instruments I have found long, tiny shafted delicate alligator type scissors, toothed and smooth forceps, and tiny cup rongeurs useful, especially when three hands are manipulating them in the small field. The surgeon must learn to use reflections from a mirror to look and work beneath the chiasm, hypothalamic floor, and *tuberculum sellae* for tumor remnants.

POSTOPERATIVE MANAGEMENT

The need for assiduous attention to water and electrolyte balance and to hormonal requirements has received full discussion elsewhere and need not be repeated. Rapid deterioration in the patient's condition may be associated either with hyperosmolarity usually with hypernatremia, or hypo-osmolarity and hyponatremia. A similar clinical picture is present in each type of disorder. Clearly the treatment differs in the two situations. It is imperative that the neurosurgeon have skilled associates, neurosurgical or otherwise, who are constantly on call to manage such problems if he himself is not promptly available.

An avoidable cause of death after one of our reoperations deserves mention. Four hours after the wound was closed, the patient's systolic blood pressure rose from 140 to 220 mm. Hg, remained at 230 to 190 levels for 13 hours and then spontaneously subsided to its preoperative 150/90 level. But probably during this period, oozing began intradurally at his craniotomy site. By his 2nd postoperative day, increasing stupor led to evacuation of the hematoma but this 63-year-old man did not survive the two operations. Now with constant monitoring of the blood pressure, as soon as this rises to 160 to 170 mm. Hg, a slow intravenous infusion of sodium nitroprusside is started to maintain the pressure in the normotensive range while active investigation of the cause of that rise proceeds.

It is not superfluous to repeat that for the majority of these patients with varying degrees of hypothalamo-hypophyseal deficits they and their relatives must be aware of their particular vulnerabilities. They must themselves increase their doses of glucocorticosteroid upon any added stress of mild illness or injury, and they must have a physician skilled in the management of their deficits whom they consult at once on minimal provocation.

In our patients the most common annoying postoperative problem is their need to wage an even more relentless battle against the tendency to gain weight than the average overnourished American. I describe to them in vivid terms two patients who lost this battle to the extent of requirement of jejunoileostomy in one and extreme corpulence contributing eventually to death in the other. A Danish drug, a resin, containing as the active agent the sympathomimetic drug, phentermine, and marketed in this country as Ionamin has proven helpful to decreasing the incessant appetite for food. A 30-mg. capsule each morning usually suffices for an adult. One highly intelligent patient has pointed out to me that when she is very thirsty and needing another dose of pitressin she may combine unnecessary eating with the necessary drinking of fluids. I pass on to other patients the word that they must satisfy thirst only with water or other noncaloric fluids.

The capacity of some of the tumors to recur even after radical or presumed total excision makes it advisable to restudy the patients at one-to-two year intervals for this possibility by CT scanning and polytomograms of the sellar region. The former study has higher sensitivity for tiny bits of calcification in the suprasellar and retrosellar area than do tomograms. However, Figure 5.17 illustrates the special value of sellar polytomography for calcification within the sella near its bony borders. The CT scan could not distinguish the craniopharyngioma calcification from the bony shadows of the anterior clinoid process in Figure 5.17(A) and from the sellar floor in Figure 5.17(B).

Results

MORTALITY OF VIRTUALLY TOTAL REMOVAL

Radical operations were done in those 37 of my patients who had a reasonable chance for a productive life; there were 19 children 16 years or under and 18 adults. The lone exception was the deteriorated dement with a known tumor for 30 years mentioned earlier. I did the initial radical operation in 30 of these patients with a postoperative death in two. I thought I had left definite tumor remnants behind in five of the 28 survivors. On four of the five I have operated for recurrences: after 8 months (John G. already described), 2½, years, 10 years, and 14 years. Only one of these four is still living. The fifth died of a myocradial infarct 21 years later. A more conservative operation will not necessarily suffice in the older age group. A tiny remnant beneath the chiasm in a 61-year-old man had regrown to cause near blindness by 2½ years; my colleague, Dr. Ojemann, had the same state develop within 7 weeks in a 69-year-old

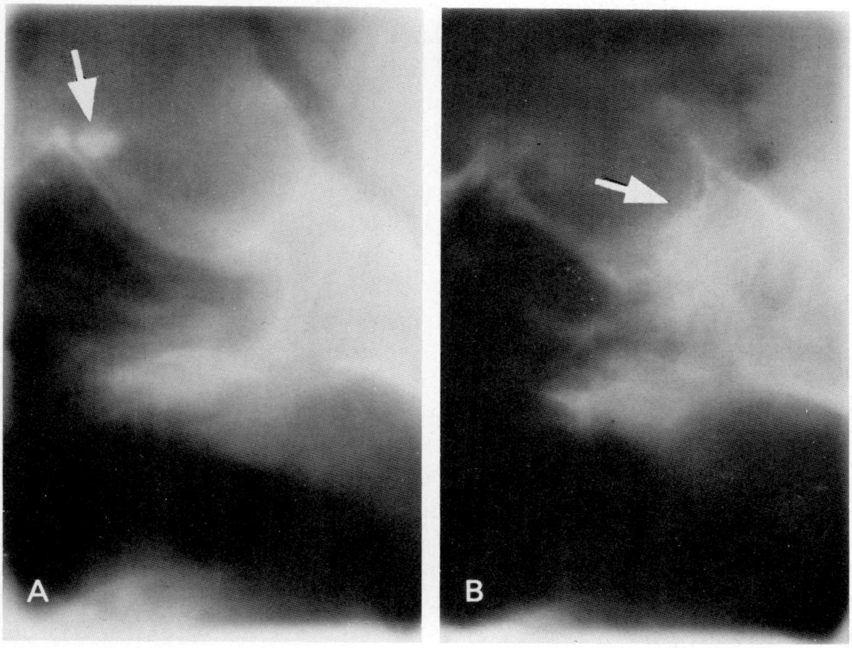

FIG. 5.17. Roger Q. (A) Tomographic cut to right of midline shows spheroidal calcification independent of normal bony structures (arrow). (B) Tomographic cut to left of midline shows an additional shell of calcification in tumor lying above the line of the sellar floor (arrow).

woman after he had emptied her cyst and removed a generous portion of its wall. In four other patients, I suspect I may have left tumor at one point under chiasm or in 3rd ventricle. None of these has clinical, CT scan, or polytomographic evidence of recurrence 8, 10, and 11 years later in the three children and 8 years later in the adult. However, two children in whom I thought my removal was total have required reoperation 4 and 6 years later; both have died, one in the postoperative period and one from the late effects of hypothalamic injury.

Of the seven patients in whom I did a secondary radical operation, four are living and two died postoperatively. The seventh in this group is lost to follow-up.

QUALITY OF SURVIVAL AND CAUSES OF DEATH

The status of the 26 known to be living is on the whole encouraging. I have used the same classification as Katz (13) did for evaluating the quality of survival in Matson's patients. "Excellent": normal independent functioning; "Good": functioning well despite deficiency; "Fair":

functional but dependent; "Poor": nonfunctional. As in Katz' series, our endocrine consultants, Drs. Crawford, Fields, and Kliman, have with the exception of one patient been able to manage the endocrine and metabolic problems so that the quality of survival has been determined by the neurological, primarily the general mental status. Thus we have classified a patient who has dropped from "A–B" student to the "C–D" level as "good." The one metabolic exception is a lad whose hyperphagia could be managed only by jejunoileostomy, but who has in addition now developed Huntington's chorea (Table 5.1).

Results in the two series are summarized in the two tables. The quality of survival as shown in Table 5.1 is remarkably similar. In Table 5.2, the causes of mortality are compared. Matson's total early postoperative mortality is much lower, 10%, compared with my 17%. However nine of his patients have died later of hypothalamo-hypophyseal dysfunction compared with one of mine. In particular, persistent hyperosmolarity, usually with hypernatremia, was present in all nine. Katz also notes elevated intracranial pressure in some of their five later deaths—a problem we handled by ventriculoatrial shunt. Although nine of his radical primary excisions have been operated for recurrence to only five of mine, his series terminated in 1968 and I have done nine of my 30 such patients since that time so the recurrence rates are not validly comparable. The major point evident in both series is the much better chance of long survival after primary than after secondary radical excision (Table 5.2).

None of the patients in either of these two series has been treated by radiation after our radical removal. The subsequent section will summarize the views of others on these topics.

DISCUSSION

Objections to Aggressive Surgery

Olivecrona reported in 1967 (21) that in his 107 personal cases only 46% of 25 cases had a "useful survival" after radical removal and 21% of 53 cases had a "useful survival" after partial removal. Hence he favored giving radiation therapy a trial—either by an external source or by stereotactic puncture of and instillation into the cyst of a β-emitting isotope or both. However, study of the detailed tables of Svolos (25) on the same series of cases reveals that the follow-up was carried out in January, 1961, that the last operation was in December, 1958, and that only 32 of the patients were operated on after 1951. Hence, about three-fourths of the series was carried out in the precortisone days.

However, other discouraging reports on the advisability of radical removal in the postcortisone era include: (1) Kerr (14)—seven postopera-

TABLE 5.1
Comparison between Results in the Matson (Ma) and Sweet (Sw) Series of Those Still Alive after Surgical Removal

	Primary total excision		No. patients Reoperative, presumed total excision		Partial excision	
	Ma	Sw	Ma	Sw	Ma	Sw
Excellent	9	16	1		2	
Good	6	4	1	1	2	1*
Fair	7	1	1	2	1	
Poor			1			
Totals	22	21	4	3	5	1

* At reoperation.

TABLE 5.2
Operative and Postoperative Mortality, Matson (Ma) and Sweet (Sw) Series

	Radical primary excision			Reoperation	
	Ma	Sw		Ma	Sw
Total No. of patients	34	30		24	12
Postoperative death	0	2		6	5
Later death from hypothalamic, hypophyseal dysfunction	3	0		9	1
Later death from nonneural or nonmetabolic cause	0	2*		2	1
Reoperated for recurrence	9	5			
Still living without recurrence	22	21	Still living	7	4
			Lost to followup		1

* Myocardial infarct after 21 years in an adult; pneumonia after 3 years in a child.

tive deaths after radical removals in 16 of 17 patients. Of the nine survivors, the tumor was thought to be completely removed in seven. (2) Bartlett (3)—only six radical removals carried out in 72 patients since about 1948; two of these died 2 decades later of proven recurrence. Of the whole group, only 43% are still alive or survived more than 10 years. He concluded that the problems created by these tumors and attempts at radical excision are so formidable that they should be treated at a few special centers. (3) Hoff and Patterson (9)—a radical removal of tumor at first operation in four and at a second operation in only two more patients out of a total of 51 during the last 35 years. (4) Kahn *et al.* (12)—"As a result of our experience over the years we have become less radical in our operations upon children." The long term survival rate in his 28 children was only 50% and, more importantly, only 21% could be classified as having a good to excellent result. "Eventually severe seizure disorders or organic brain syndrome, total blindness, obesity, marked endocrine dysfunction and lack of general physical and mental maturation" featured the poor quality of survival. This longer follow-up has led Kahn (11) to modify his earlier optimism regarding radical surgery. (5) Rougerie after a personal experience of 100 craniopharyngiomas has sentiments similar to those of Kahn. (6) Nakagawa and Tsuru (20) did total removals in 5 cases and subtotal removals in 18 of 26 cases after 1958 with an operative and hospital mortality of 27% and 46% respectively. (7) A tentative attitude toward radical surgery in the postcortisone era is that of Michelsen *et al.* (19). Their mortality after primary procedures is only 7%. However, the surgeon thought he had achieved total removal in only 11 (34%) of 32 children and 12 (23%) of 52 adults. Moreover, five of the 11 children have since shown recurrent or remaining tumor. These authors recommend radical removal "when the operative conditions are ideal."

Evidence Regarding Radiation Therapy

Pari passu with waning enthusiasm for radical surgery has appeared an increasing intimation of the efficacy of radiation therapy. Leddy and Marshall (16), among the first to draw attention to this, gave convincing details of 10 patients who were benefited by tumor doses usually in the range of 1000 to 2500 rads by the then available dosimetry. A greater percentage of their patients were still living more than five years after operation if they had received roentgen therapy in addition (five of six such patients), than if they had had operation only (16 of 35 patients). Microscopic examinations months or years after these modest doses revealed no radiation effect on the tumor in cases in whom obvious clinical improvement had occurred. The authors agree with Carpenter and colleagues (5) who had suggested as the basis for the improvement in their four cases that the radiation inhibited the formation of cystic fluid.

Kramer *et al.* (15) have the first intensively treated series with the longest follow-up to date. They used large doses of 2 million volt x-ray or ^{60}Co photons. Of 12 children treated with 5500 rads in 6 weeks, two died with tumor, and of 14 adults treated with 7000 rads in 7 weeks, one died with tumor and one with radiation necrosis. In two patients who died of causes unrelated to radiation, none of the tumor left behind at the original operation was visible at postmortem. The other 20 were alive and "reasonably well" up to 15 years after treatment. Bloom and Harmer (4) agree with Kramer *et al.* in favoring a combination of a conservative cyst evacuation and biopsy only, followed by radical irradiation. They are assessing results of treatment in a series of 100 patients of all ages with primary or recurrent craniopharyngioma. The 5- and 10-year survival rates for cases treated as they recommend were 85% and 72%, respectively. Over 90% of the patients were in good general health with no serious neurological or mental disability at 2 years; vision was at least useful in 82%. Of 12 patients treated on a 6 mev. linear accelerator over 5 years ago, 11 were still alive and well.

Hoff and Patterson (9) have also presented evidence that partial removal of the tumor with radiation therapy is better than the same type of operation alone. Ten-year follow-ups revealed a 63% recurrence rate in the 24 patients in whom radiation was added, whereas 85% of 17 patients who were not radiated had shown recurrence. However, Matson and Crigler (18) comment that all but one of the 11 patients sent to them for recurrence after an operation elsewhere had also had radiation therapy. The crucial data regarding the detailed parameters of that therapy are given in neither of the last two publications.

Sharma *et al.* (24) have treated 21 patients by "limited surgery" and 5000 to 5500 rads over *circa* 1 month from a Theratron-60 unit. In a follow-up on 18 patients—from 2 to 7 years later in 11 of them—none had yet shown brain damage or other clinical deterioration and all are alive and well (the remaining three patients were lost to follow-up).

In a little contrast to these encouraging reports, Backlund (1) cites five publications which describe radiation necrosis disasters at the "radical" dose levels. He and Leksell have for nearly 10 years been developing a regime of a more localized radiation involving the stereotaxic injection of colloidal, β-emitting ^{90}Y into the cystic part of the tumor and stereotaxicly directed focused multiportal gamma-irradiation from ^{60}Co to the solid parts of the tumor. A personal communication from Dr. Backlund, dated October 8, 1975, summarizes his highly gratifying data from a follow-up just completed in 34 primary cases treated in the last 10 years; there were only two deaths and two "partially disabled." It will be instructive to compare the long term results of this logical approach as well as those of less focused radiation with those of radical surgery. These encouraging results from radiation are consonant with the observations of Rubin and Casanett (23) of the "fairly high" radiosensitivity of skin and oropharyngeal epithelium.

Rarely the tumors have or develop so vicious an invasive tendency that at that point no therapy can succeed. Thus, in Iyer's (10) 3-month old baby, the tumor had critically invaded and replaced not only hypothalamic but also midbrain tegmental structures. Grover and Rorke's (8) patient had "a 95% removal" of his solid tumor at age 5 followed by 6100 rads of ^{60}Co radiation at age 12. When he died at age 17, there was almost no residual normal structure in the left caudate nucleus, thalamus, midbrain, or pons. These areas and the basal subarachnoid space were filled with tumor.

SUMMARY AND CONCLUSIONS

There is evidence from this publication and those of Matson and colleagues that a determined effort at total excision of these tumors as the initial therapy is a tenable course of action. The main bases for this concept are: (1) that the dense gliosis characteristically intervening between these epithelial tumors and normal brain constitutes a margin of safety for the surgeon at least for the first several years such tumors are growing in the 3rd ventricle; (2) improved early diagnosis and better operative instruments, magnification, lighting, and technique are decreasing operative morbidity and mortality; and (3) new knowledge and new replacement therapy are reducing the burden of the metabolic and endocrine defects.

Competing with this is the concept that rotationally delivered or even more precisely focused high energy photons and intracavitary β-radiation have lower morbidity and mortality. The detailed and long term data on which to draw conclusions are not yet available. My medical colleagues and I are preparing case-by-case tables with all of the relevant facts to supply one component of the total picture.

ACKNOWLEDGMENT

It is a pleasure to express appreciation to the Neuro-Research Foundation for the support of these studies.

REFERENCES

1. Backlund, E. O. Studies on craniopharyngiomas III. Stereotactic treatment with intracystic Yttrium-90. Acta Chir. Scand., *139:* 237–247, 1973.
2. Bailey, P., Buchanan, D. N., and Bucy, P. C. Intracranial Tumors of Infancy and Childhood, 598 pp. The University of Chicago Press, Chicago, Ill., 1939.
3. Bartlett, J. R. Craniopharyngiomas–a summary of 85 cases. J. Neurol. Neurosurg. Psychiatry, *34:* 37–41, 1971.
4. Bloom, H. J. G., and Harmer, C. L. Craniopharyngiomas. Br. Med. J., *2:* 288–289, 1972.
5. Carpenter, R. C., Chamberlin, G. W., and Frazier, C. H. The treatment of hypophysial stalk tumors by evacuation and irradiation. Am. J. Roentgenol. Radium Ther. Nucl. Med., *38:* 162–177, 1937.
6. Ghatak, N. R., Hirano, A., and Zimmerman, H. M. Ultrastructure of a craniopharyngioma. Cancer, *27:* 1465–1475, 1971.
7. Grcevic, N., and Yates, P. O. Rosenthal fibers in tumors of the central nervous system. J. Pathol., *73:* 467–472, 1957.
8. Grover, W. D., and Rorke, L. B. Invasive craniopharyngioma. J. Neurol. Neurosurg. Psychiatry, *31:* 580–582, 1968.

9. Hoff, J. T., and Patterson, R. H. Craniopharyngiomas in children and adults. J. Neurosurg., *36:* 299–302, 1972.
10. Iyer, C. G. S. Case report of an adamantinoma present at birth. J. Neurosurg., *9:* 221–228, 1952.
11. Kahn, E. A. Some physiologic implications of craniopharyngiomas. Neurology (Minneap.), *9:* 82–90, 1959.
12. Kahn, E. A., Gosch, H. H., Seegar, J. F., and Hicks, S. P. Forty-five years experience with the craniopharyngiomas. Surg. Neurol., *1:* 5–12, 1973.
13. Katz, E. L. Late results of radical excision of craniopharyngiomas in children. J. Neurosurg., *42:* 86–90, 1975.
14. Kerr, A. S. Craniopharyngiomata. J. Neurol. Neurosurg. Psychiatry, *31:* 646, 1968.
15. Kramer, S., Southard, M., and Mansfield, C. M. Radiotherapy in the management of craniopharyngioma: further experiences and late results. Am. J. Roentgenol. Radium Ther. Nucl. Med., *103:* 44–52, 1968.
16. Leddy, E. T., and Marshall, T. M. Roentgen therapy of pituitary adamantinomas (craniopharyngiomas). Radiology, *56:* 384–393, 1951.
17. Malis, L. I. The transnasal and transpterional approach to lesions of the clivus. Presented at Congress of Neurological Surgeons Meeting, Atlanta, Ga. October, 1975.
18. Matson, D. D., and Crigler, J. F., Jr. Management of craniopharyngiomas in childhood. J. Neurosurg., *30:* 377–390, 1969.
19. Michelsen, W. J., Mount, L. A., and Renaudin, J. Craniopharyngioma. A thirty-nine year survey. Acta Neurol. Lat. Am., *18:* 100–106, 1972.
20. Nakagawa, Y., and Tsuru, M. Post-operative course of craniopharyngioma. Brain Nerve (Tokyo), *23:* 993–1002, 1971.
21. Olivecrona, H. The craniopharyngiomas. *In* Hanbuch der Neurochirurgie. Vol. IV, Part IV. Edited by H. Olivecrona and W. Tonnis, pp. 269–279. Springer, Berlin, 1967.
22. Patrick, B. S., Smith, R. R., and Bailey, T. O. Aseptic meningitis due to spontaneous rupture of craniopharyngioma cyst. Case report. J. Neurosurg., *41:* 387–390, 1974.
23. Rubin, P., and Casanett, G. W. Clinical Radiation Pathology, Vol. I and II. 1057 pp. W. B. Saunders, Philadelphia, 1968.
24. Sharma, U., Tandon, P. N., Saxene, K. K., Singhal, R. M., and Baruah, J. D. Craniopharyngiomas treated by a combination of surgery and radiotherapy. Clin. Radiol., *25:* 13–17, 1974.
25. Svolos, D. G. Craniopharyngiomas. A study based on 108 verified cases (of Olivecrona). Acta Chir. Scand. (Suppl.), *403:* 1–44, 1969.
26. Timperley, W. R. Histochemistry of Rathke pouch tumours. J. Neurol. Neurosurg. Psychiatry, *31:* 589–595, 1968.
27. van der Bergh, R., and Brucher, J. M. L'abord transventriculaire dans les craniopharyngiomes du troisième ventricule. Neurochirurgie, *16:* 51–65, 1970.
28. Zülch, K. J. Brain Tumors. Their Biology and Pathology. 2nd American Edition. 326 pp. Springer, New York, pp 228–233, 1965.

CHAPTER

6

Recent Observations Pertinent to Improving Anterolateral Cordotomy

WILLIAM H. SWEET, M.S., D.Sc.

The unreliability of external landmarks on the cord for determining the proper site of an incision to destroy pain pathways has already been reported.

However, in view of the frequency with which the origin of the dentate ligament from the cord is used as the basic landmark to guide the incision, I shall draw your attention to the disaster which can ensue if the case in which this origin is well posterior to the equator of the cord is not

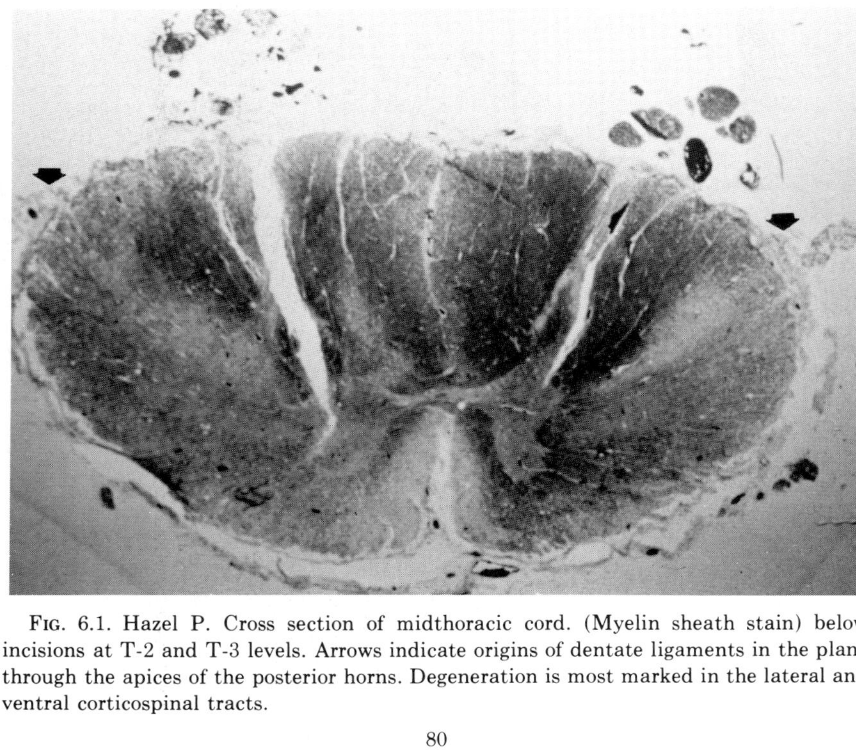

FIG. 6.1. Hazel P. Cross section of midthoracic cord. (Myelin sheath stain) below incisions at T-2 and T-3 levels. Arrows indicate origins of dentate ligaments in the plane through the apices of the posterior horns. Degeneration is most marked in the lateral and ventral corticospinal tracts.

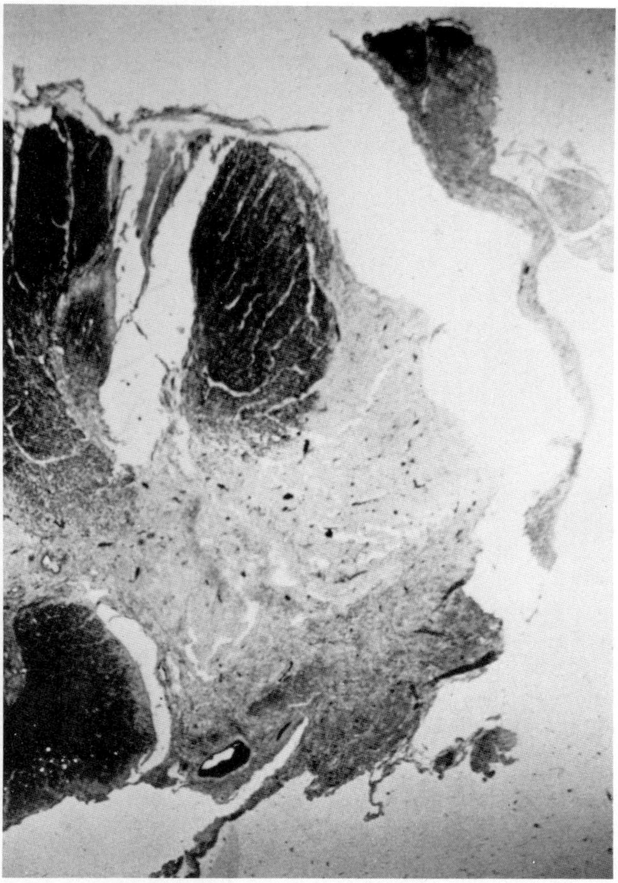

FIG. 6.2. Hazel P. Cross section at level of the right incision showing major encroachment into posterolateral white matter. (The broad vertical cleft in the right posterior column is an artefact).

recognized. Figure 6.1 caudal to the actual incision in this patient shows the origin of the ligaments in the plane through the apices of the posterior horns and the descending degeneration in the lateral corticospinal tracts following their section by an incision ventral to the dentate origins. Figure 6.2 shows one of my two huge incisions. Although they produced only temporary paraplegia and the patient recovered the ability to walk, she gradually developed the most devastating postcordotomy painful dysesthesia I have ever seen. Figure 6.3A shows the posteriorly misplaced incision in another patient whose dentate ligament arose far dorsally and who had a large motor rootlet going straight lateral to the ven-

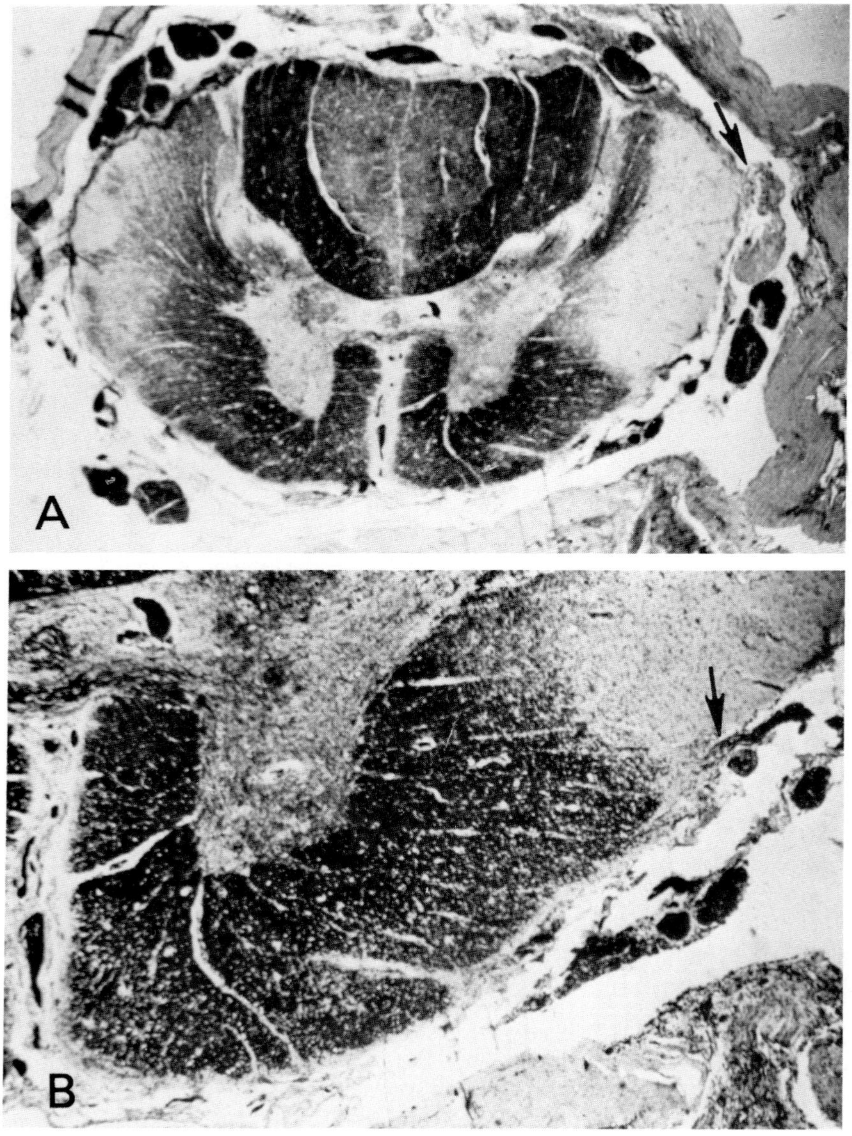

FIG. 6.3. (A) Cross section of midthoracic cord. Myelin sheath stain. The upper thoracic incisions on each side were placed too far posteriorly not only because of a posterior displacement of the origin of the dentate ligament (arrow on right) but also because a conspicuous anterior rootlet emerged from the cord straight lateral to the anterior horn. (B) Closeup of right anterior quadrant of the cord at the level of (A). Arrow indicates the large anterior rootlet whose emergence led to sparing of most of the anterolateral white matter.

tral horn. Figure 6.3B is a closeup of this showing that rootlet at which the surgeon stopped his incision with resultant sparing of most of the anterolateral white matter.

These are relatively easy problems to correct. Much more serious is the accumulating evidence that the entire anterior quadrant of the cord may be neither as safe nor as successful a target as many of us have thought. Frazier (6) first recommended an incision in this quadrant only 2.5 mm. deep, extending ventrally to the anterior root. A swelling chorus of voices later pointed out that such an incision is likely to be inadequate. In 1937 Kahn and Barney (10) reported that persistent high levels of analgesia are more likely if the incision is carried 1 to 2 mm. anterior to the anterior nerve root. Hyndman and van Epps (9) soon recorded agreement as did Voris (23). Dr. White and I have repeatedly emphasized our opinion that extensive incisions in the anterior quadrant are needed to give the greatest chance of sustained relief of pain (Ref. 25, pp. 213–217; Ref. 26,

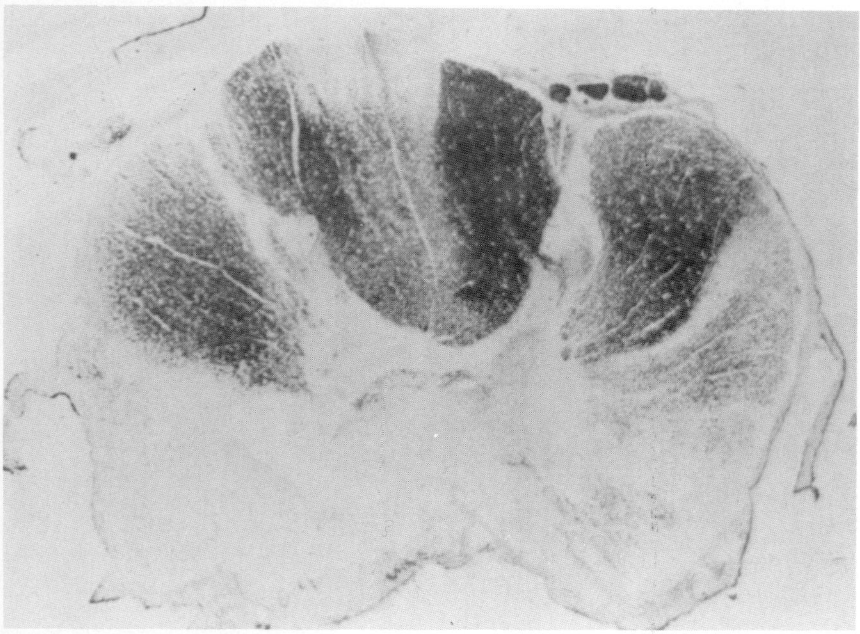

FIG. 6.4. Foerster and Gagel's Figure 29 (Ref. 5). Cross section of cord at T-5 level indicating extent of bilateral incisions into anterior quadrants at same horizontal level. Today we would always stagger the two sides of such incisions at least 1 cord segment apart, making the lower incision no lower than T-3. The surgical lesion produced analgesia of skin from T-6 segment down but the senses of pressure, pain, and temperature were not lost and the patient's spontaneous gastric crises continued.

pp. 753–758). Although Foerster's hypothetical diagrams (Ref. 4, p. 345) depict a zone in the medial part of the ventral quadrant assigned exclusively to touch, he made his incisions under local anesthesia, steadily deepening them until the contralateral analgesic level was within a single dermatome of the incision. Figure 6.4 shows one of his pairs of incisions at the T-5 segment (5). Even this total wipeout of the anterior quadrants at the same level on both sides of the cord did not abolish pressure pain, temperature sense, or the painful gastric crises of *tabes dorsalis*, although there was the expected cutaneous analgesia. Such observations led Dr. White and me (26) to conclude that delayed crossing of some of the pain fibers in the cord might account for some of our failures. For example, Figure 6.5 shows one of our patients whose destruction of one whole anterior quadrant at T-3 achieved contralateral analgesia only to T-10.

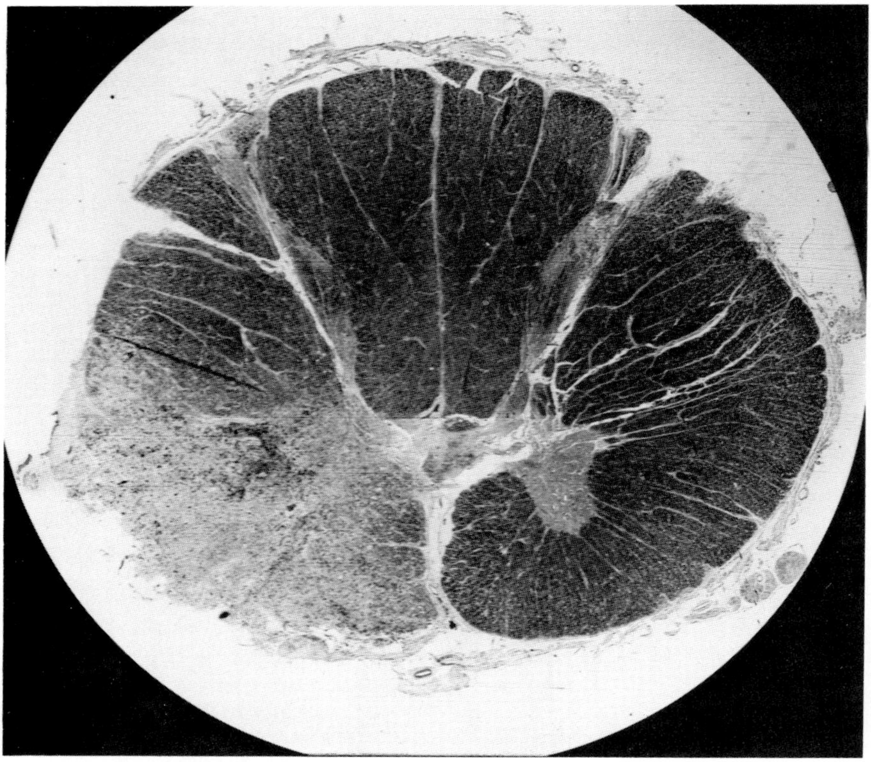

FIG. 6.5. Patient M. B. Cross section of cord at T-3 level of incisions. Despite destruction of one entire anterior quadrant, contralateral analgesia only to T-10 indicating delayed crossing of fibers and need for making cord incision well above highest segmental level of pain (Fig. 68, White and Sweet, 1955).

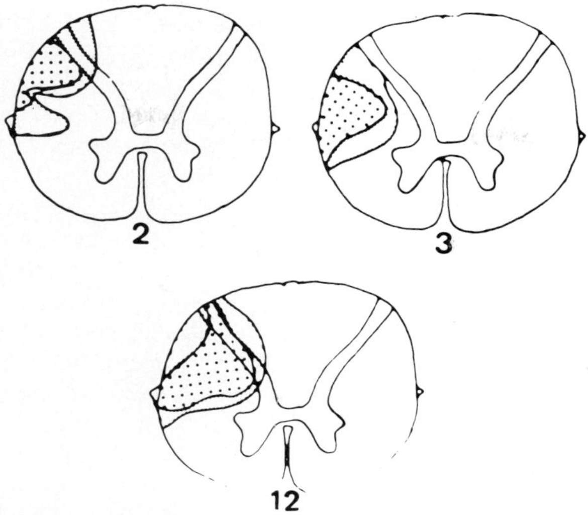

FIG. 6.6. Diagram of postmortem demonstration of cord lesions made at C1-2. All three of these patients had "an analgesic level to pin" and relief of pain of unstated duration with no hemiparesis even though the lesion was confined to the posterolateral sector of the cord. (Courtesy of Moossy and Rosomoff, AVENS.)

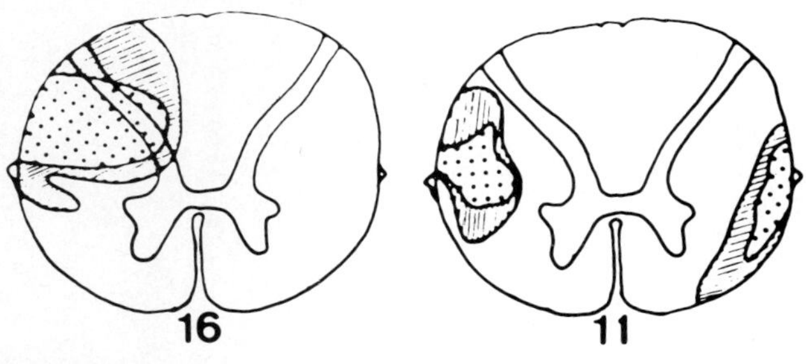

FIG. 6.7. Diagram of postmortem demonstration of cord lesions at C1-2. Similar lesions (as noted in Fig. 6.6) in these two patients did not give pain relief but they did not cause hemiparesis. (Courtesy of Moossy and Rosomoff, AVENS.)

Through the fifties and sixties a number of us were describing patients with atypical disposition of the pain fibers: (1) only partial crossover requiring bilateral cordotomy for one-sided pain (two cases by White *et al.* (24), others by French, Chou and Story (7)); (2) no crossover at all (French and Peyton (8), Voris (22) each one case); and (3) at 187 individual electrical stimulations in the anterior half of the cord in man the sensation was referred ipsilaterally in 11% and bilaterally in 6% (20); (4) reversal of the usual topography with the sacral dermatomes lying far ventrally, three cases of Schwartz (17). However, it is worth commenting that despite all of our detailed directions to each other about how to do these procedures, we all note an exasperating percentage of failures to achieve the desired analgesia.

With the important advent of percutaneous cordotomy (13), the grossly inaccurate electrode placements possible thereat plus the excellent responses to testing usually given during this procedure have given rise to some startling findings at postmortem. Thus, Mooney and Rosomoff cited by Sweet (19) show cords of three patients whose posterolateral C1-2 lesions yielded an analgesic level to pin prick and pain relief of unstated duration unaccompanied by ipsilateral motor weakness (Fig. 6.6). Kurze (11) reported to me a similar experience in which such surprising lesions were seen bilaterally at postmortem. In two other of the Moossy-Rosomoff patients with similar lesions there was no hemiparesis; neither was there pain relief (Fig. 6.7). In addition to these indications of aberrant placement of the motor pathways, I was finding motor responses on single shock stimulation within the cord at unexpected sites. For example, muscle jerks occurred in one patient in the contralateral forearm or hand within 2 to 3 mm. of the surface of the ventral quadrant

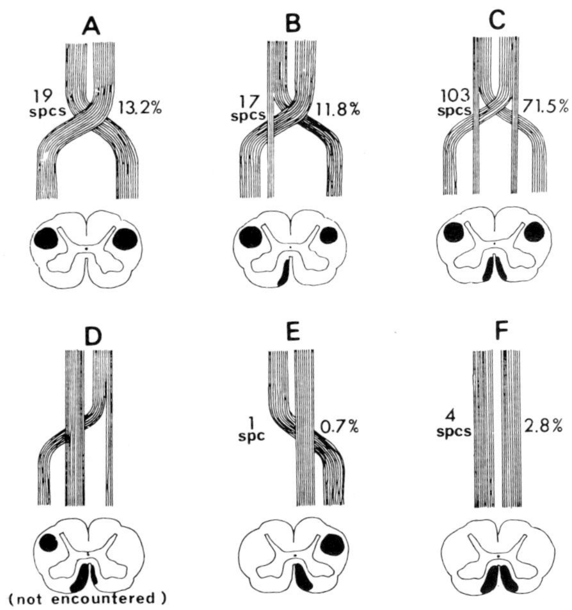

FIG. 6.8. Diagram of disposition of pyramidal tracts in cords of 144 specimens of human fetal or neonatal spinal cords and/or brain stem. Although pattern C is shown in the diagram as bilaterally symmetrical, the pyramidal tracts were "patently unequal" in 81 of these 103 specimens.

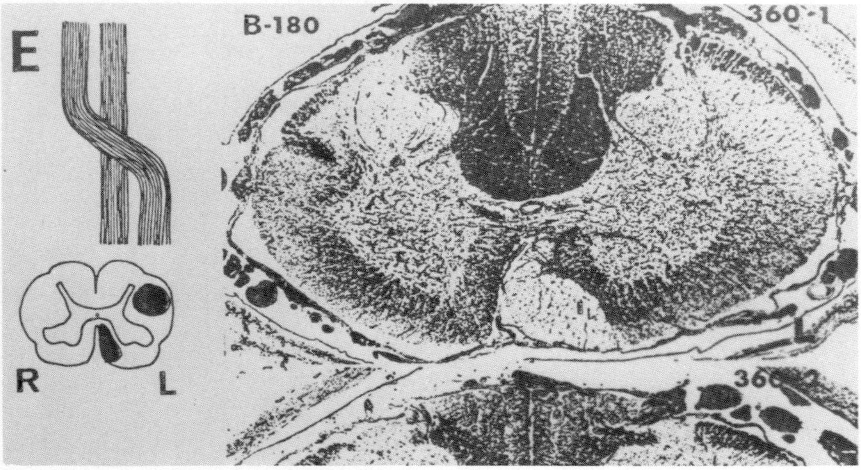

FIG. 6.9. Pattern E. All pyramidal tract fibers lie on one side of the cord.

of the cord—much too superficial for the ventral corticospinal tract. Even more striking to me were evidences that the pain pathways may in some patients be far more concentrated than we have thought in the past few decades. Either the initial few second bursts of heating at 55°C. or some later small fragment of heating may abruptly produce an extensive zone of analgesia.

When I complained of these anatomical uncertainties to my neuroscience colleagues, Dr. R. Sidman advised me to consult with Dr. P. Rakic. This basic neuroscientist and Dr. P. Yakovlev completed in 1967 an extensive manuscript based on a study of serial sections of 144 specimens of human fetal and neonatal cords and/or brain stems, 94 specimens of medullas with spinal cords, and 50 of spinal cords only. The pyramidal tracts are the last to undergo myelination and in this age group are almost totally unmyelinated. Hence they stand out clearly in cross sections with myelin sheath stains. Figure 6.8 summarizes Yakovlev and Rakic's findings (16). They didn't seem important enough to the program committee of the American Neurological Association to justify presentation at its annual meeting (27). Hence Yakovlev and Rakic have not yet sent them off for full publication but are kindly allowing me to draw them to your attention. I classify these as of crucial importance to those doing or having cordotomies for pain; especially at the C1-2 level. Their patterns A and B with bilateral or unilateral absence of the uncrossed corticospinal tract were seen in 36 or 25% of the specimens. The material studied is not dominated by congenital lesions. In only one of these 36 was the presence of malformations described in the obstetrical

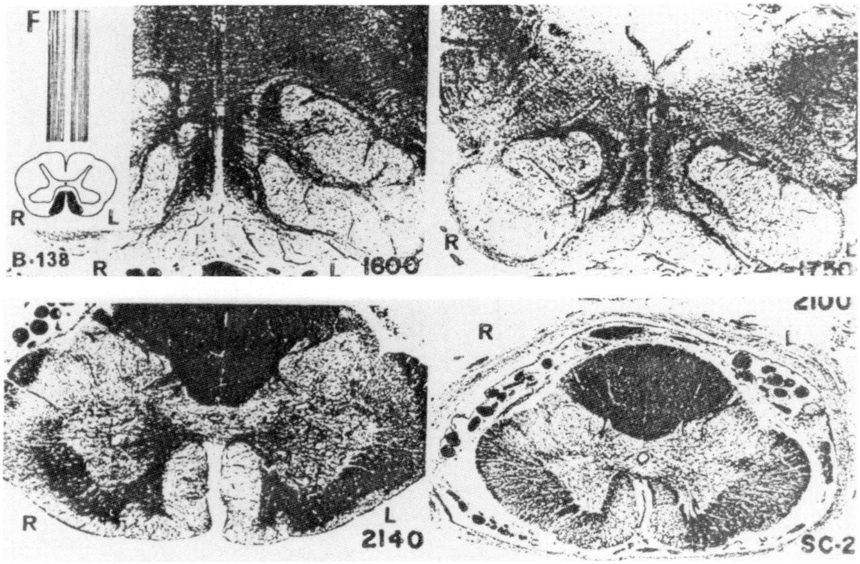

FIG. 6.10. Pattern F. All pyramidal tract fibers lie ventro-medially. (Sections 2140 and Sc-2 Courtesy of Rakic and Yakovlev, unpublished data.)

and autopsy record; these were visceral not neural. Of even more importance statistically is the fact that in their standard pattern C, although all four pyramidal tracts are present, they vary widely in size from specimen to specimen having by no means the symmetry shown in the diagram. They found the pyramidal tracts "patently unequal" in 81 specimens (79%). In 82% of those 81 the tracts were largely on the right side. Of the 66 specimens showing pattern C in whom there were medullas and matching spinal cords, the pyramid which began its decussation more rostrally came nearer crossing completely than the other one in 94% of the cases. Figures 6.9 and 6.10 show how clear these anomalous distributions are in the myelin stain; Figure 6.9 with the pyramidal tracts all on the left side and Figure 6.10 with them all ventral. Although earlier accounts describe gross asymmetries in the pyramidal tracts (1) (p. 563) (Figure 6.11), their significance for neurosurgeons has been proven only by Rakic's determination of their great frequency.

For neurosurgeons the lesson is clear that unusually disposed motor pathways probably push sensory pathways into unusual positions and that these may well vary as much or more than their motor counterparts. The conclusion is obvious that in every patient we must try to determine where the pain fibers are in him and tailor the lesion to his anatomy. Schwartz (17) has already presented evidence that a smaller and more lateral percentage of the anterior quadrant requires transection at the high cervical than at the high thoracic level. The importance of the patient's protracted effective cooperation is evident. Generous use of the neuroleptic agents such as fentanyl and droperidol (Innovar, McNeil Laboratories, Fort Washington, Pa.) helps on this score. Because of the far less consistent and less explicable responses of the patient to stimulation in the cord, than in *e.g.*, the trigeminal posterior rootlets, guidance from this is far from decisive at this juncture, at least for me.

Current discrepancies in experience are highlighted by statements last month of Tasker (21) and Mazars (12). The former, after 240 percutaneous cordotomies, sought to elicit a contralateral warm or cool tingle; he found that 94% of his patients who developed satisfactory analgesia had this prelesional response. Mazars, on the other hand, said he characteristically elicited no response to stimulation at sites wherein a lesion produces analgesia. My own experience is intermediate between these two contradictory generalizations and leans more toward Tasker's formulation.

Because the motor fibers show a more consistent and lower visible threshold of activity which is elicited by single shocks, we may have to

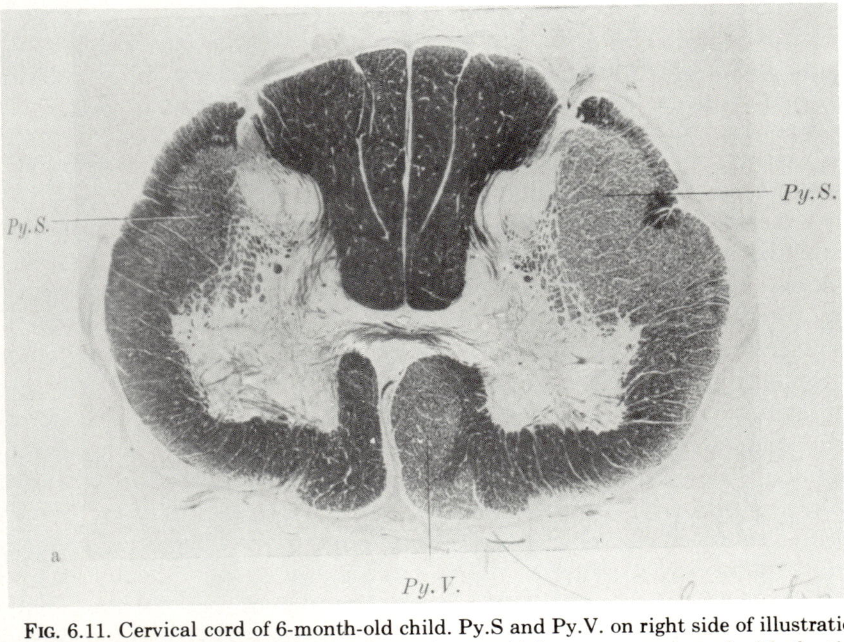

FIG. 6.11. Cervical cord of 6-month-old child. Py.S and Py.V. on right side of illustration shows gross enlargement of the unmyelinated pyramidal tracts as compared with the tiny unmyelinated lateral pyramidal tract and no ventral pyramidal tract on left.

learn how better to be guided by these responses. Unfortunately, details of the anatomy of the human ventral and lateral pyramidal tracts important to us are not presently known (3). Descending fibers in the ventral pyramidal tract may end anywhere from the highest thoracic to the midthoracic cord (15, 2). In very rare instances, the tract extends into the upper lumbar segments. However, the fibers leaving the tract in the upper cord segments are not necessarily all destined for the upper limb or torso; there is some evidence that as they descend in the cord they gradually pass to the lateral pyramidal bundle before they terminate (2). Nor can we be sure that a contralateral motor response in limb or torso will be obtained from stimulation of the ipsilateral ventral pyramidal tract. The anatomists are not certain how many ventral pyramidal fibers fail to cross over just before they terminate at a ventral horn cell. Further complicating features include the description by Barnes (1), Swank (18), and other writers of a "ventrolateral pyramidal tract." This aberrant bundle moves laterally away from the pyramid at the level of the XIIth cranial nerve lying on the surface of the medulla just external to the inferior olive. The descending part of this tract has been seen by both these observers to extend in some cases as low as the lumbar region. What sort of motor function it has is unknown. Moreover, Nathan and Smith (14) have assembled their own evidence and that of others for spinocortical fibers in man intermingled in the upper cervical cord with the main motor lateral corticospinal fibers. Whether electrical stimulation of these spinocortical fibers gives rise to any subjective sensation in man is likewise unknown. All of these fine features in human anatomy we neurosurgeons need to ascertain from our own observations in order to improve our results of cordotomy for pain.

A recent operative protocol brings out a number of these points which explain my uncertainty on the subject. Figure 6.12 illustrates a case in which I think there may have been an unusually large lateral corticospinal tract. Figure 6.12A shows the position of the cordotomy electrode tip 3 mm. anterior to the unusually clear line of pantopaque on the dentate ligament. (The tip measures 4 mm. ventrally on the film.) At three different depths 1 mm. apart within the cord as judged by the impedance, and along the same horizontal line, there were only ipsilateral *i.e.*, left, sternomastoid contractions at 0.5V single shocks and no other sensation on continuous stimulation at 50/cps. Assuming I had to be in the anterior horn or near an intramedullary motor rootlet or ventral to it, I made six progressively longer and hotter lesions, the last at 60°C for 30 seconds. No sensation was evoked during any interlesion stimulation. At this juncture he complained of numbness and virtual paralysis in his ipsilateral (left) upper limb, (the lower was already paralyzed from his primary disease). He still had no analgesia. I decided I was probably too

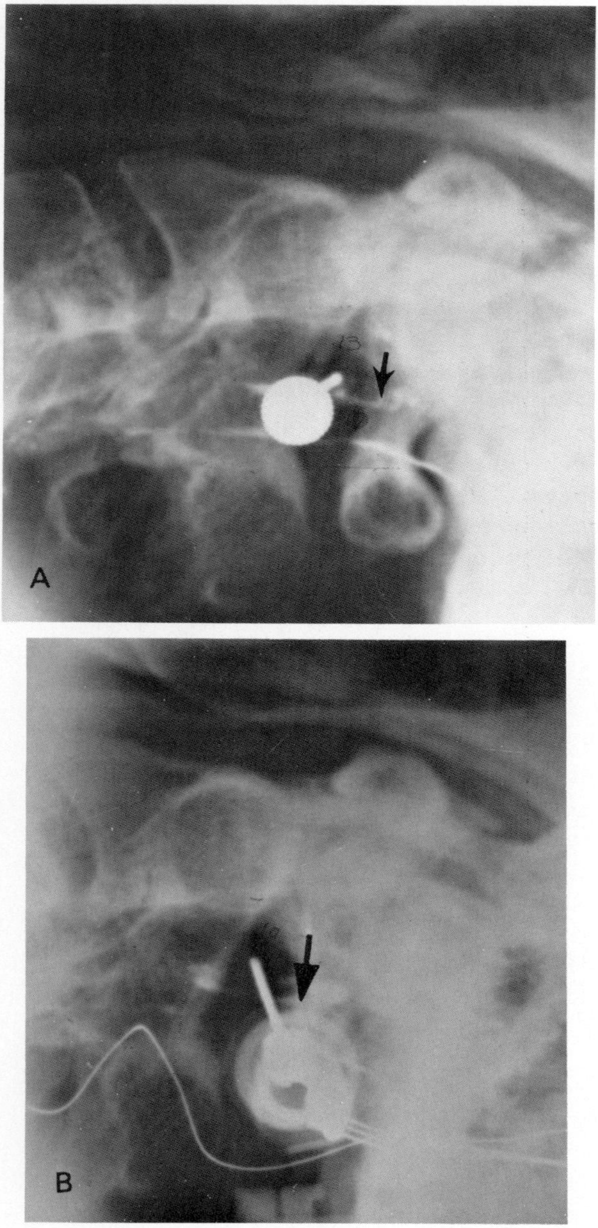

FIG. 6.12. Edward T. Lateral views upper cervical spine, patient supine, after injection through electrode sheath of one-half cc. pantopaque and one-half cc. 1% lidocaine emulsified with 3 cc. csf and 10 cc. air. (A) electrode tip 3 mm. ventral to line of pantopaque lying ventral to dentate ligament (arrow). In this position the electrode produced paralysis of the ipsilateral arm. (B) electrode tip 5.5 mm. ventral to same line of pantopaque (arrow). In this position the electrode heated to 55° V for 5 seconds produced complete analgesia of the contralateral lower limb.

dorsal, that were I in the ventral pyramidal tract, the weakness would presumably have been in the right arm. The electrode was replaced 3 mm. more ventrally in the film (2.5 mm. *in vivo*) almost at the ventral surface of the cord as judged by the pulsating air shadows and shown in Figure 6.12B. Here at the threshold sensation of 1.2 volts at 50/cps., there was a pressure sensation in the left ipsilateral leg, later stimulation caused a pulsing sensation there. Despite no evident change in the position of the electrode on a second radiograph the response changed to a cold tingle in the right forearm at 0.3V. An initial lesion at only 55°C for only 5 seconds yielded complete analgesia of the entire right lower limb. Obviously the pain fibers from that limb were densely concentrated in that immediate vicinity, even though the responses to stimulation certainly did not suggest this. The lesion was gradually increased in size during a total of 8 steps; only 65°C for 15 seconds was required to produce analgesia on the right from C-4 to S-5. During this lesion-making sequence, analgesia gradually increased from below upward, although the interlesion stimulations never evoked any sensation outside the right shoulder and right upper limb. In the next patient our objective was to relieve left midthoracic cancer pain. In him a warm tingle over the precordium was consistently evoked by stimulation from the very start, yet many lesions of increasing size at that site yielded only patchy analgesia from C-2 on down to the groin.

I think our most unequivocal gross anatomical landmark at percutaneous C1-2 cordotomy is the location of the ventral surface of the cord, and I favor delineating this both with pantopaque layered on that surface and with air. Figure 6.13A shows a minimal concavity in the ventral aspect of the cord at the rostrocaudal level of the needle insertion. Figure 6.13B taken at the end of the lesion-making sequence shows that the angle of the electrode shaft in the dorsoventral plane had changed slightly but that the interval between electrode tip and ventral surface of the cord is the same.

I am so convinced that we must maximize our effort to make a small lesion in the proper place that I am seeking to extend the tactic of flexible search to include open upper thoracic cordotomy. Figure 6.14A shows a right angle bipolar electrode insulated except at the tip (held by the Dott self-retaining retractor assembly) which can be thrust a measurable and precisely held distance into the cord. When the dentate ligament is allowed to fall back, Figure 6.14B, the electrode does not move in the cord as the patient moves about. This procedure I am now using when a cordotomy is required on the second side. The ventral percutaneous approach through the intact disc gives inadequate leeway for search. I present these thoughts on technique on a tentative basis.

In summary: I think there is good evidence that we should change our

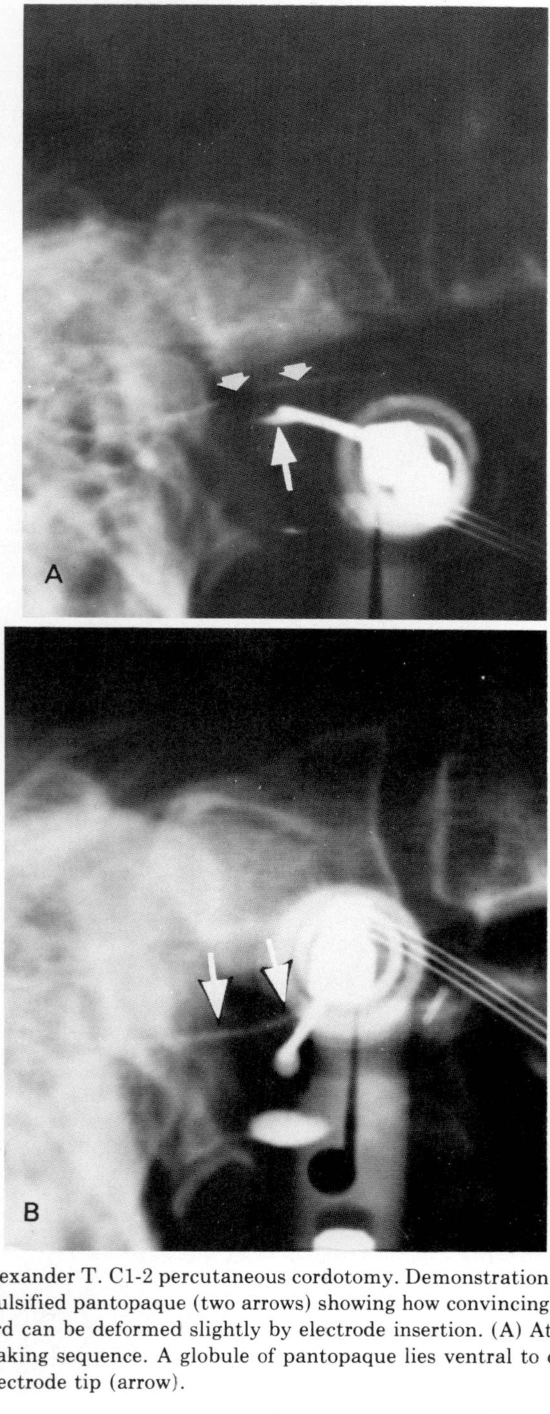

FIG. 6.13. Alexander T. C1-2 percutaneous cordotomy. Demonstration of ventral aspect of cord with emulsified pantopaque (two arrows) showing how convincing this landmark is and how the cord can be deformed slightly by electrode insertion. (A) At start and (B) at end of lesion-making sequence. A globule of pantopaque lies ventral to dentate ligament and dorsal to electrode tip (arrow).

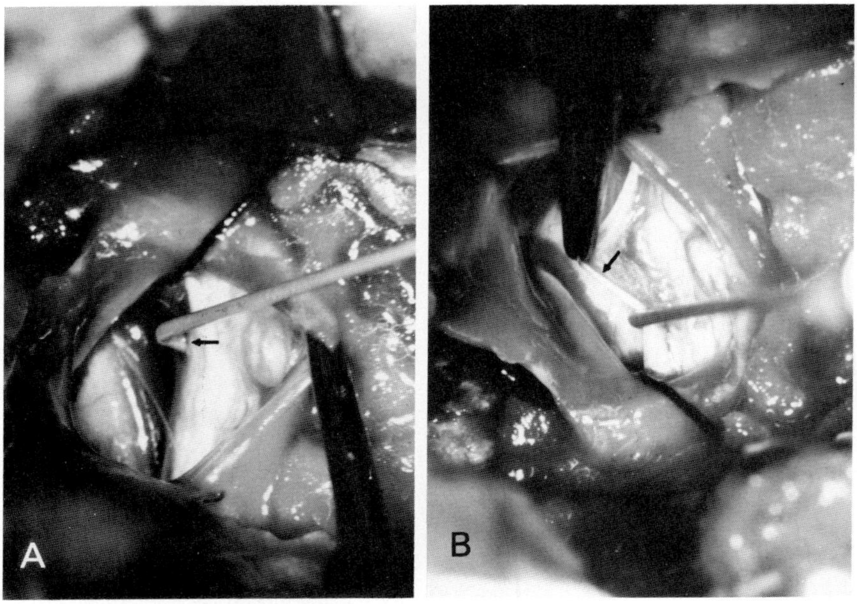

FIG. 6.14. Irvin F. Exposure left side of cord at T-2 level. (A) Bipolar electrode held firmly in Dott retractor clamps and tip inserted 2 mm. ventral to origin of dentate ligament. (B) Cord rotated back into normal position by drawing dentate ligament laterally during stimulation and lesion making.

fundamental objective in cordotomy to one of minimizing and placing precisely the lesion to produce extensive dense analgesia, hopefully with fewer complications. There have to be better ways of doing this than the one I am using.

ACKNOWLEDGMENT

It is a pleasure to express appreciation to the Neuro-Research Foundation for the support of these studies.

REFERENCES

1. Barnes, S. Degeneration in hemiplegia: With special reference to a ventro-lateral pyramidal tract, the accessory fillet and Pick's bundle. Brain, *24:* 463–501, 1901.
2. Bok, S. T. Das Rückenmark. *In* Handbuch der Mikroscopischen Anatomie des Menschen, Nervensystem, edited by W. von Möllendorf, Vol. 4, pp. 562–567, Springer, Berlin, 1928.
3. Bucy, P. C., Keplinger, J. E., and Siqueira, E. B. Destruction of the "pyramidal tract" in man. J. Neurosurg., *21:* 385–398, 1964.
4. Foerster, O. Die Vorderseitenstrangleitung. *In* Handbuch der Neurologie, edited by O. Bumke and O. Foerster, Vol. 5, pp. 320–340, Springer, Berlin, 1936.
5. Foerster, O., and Gagel, O. Die Vorderseitestrangdurchschneidung beim Menschen. Eine klinisch-patho-physiologisch-anatomische Studie. Zrschr. f. d. ges. Neurol. Psychiat., *138:* 1–92, 1932.

6. Frazier, C. H. Section of the anterolateral columns of the spinal cord for the relief of of pain. A report of six cases. Arch. Neurol. Psychiatry, *4:* 137–147, 1920.
7. French, L. A., Chou, S. N., and Story, J. L. Cervical tractotomy: Technique and clinical usefulness. *In* Pain, edited by R. S. Knighton and P. R. Dumke, pp. 311–319. Little, Brown & Co., Boston, 1966.
8. French, L. A., and Peyton, W. T. Ipsilateral sensory loss following cordotomy. J. Neurosurg., *5:* 403–404, 1948.
9. Hyndman, O. R., and van Epps, C. Possibility of differential section of the spinothalamic tract. A clinical and histologic study. Arch. Surg., *38:* 1036–1053, 1939.
10. Kahn, E. A., and Barney, B. F. Anterolateral chordotomy for intractable pain of *tabes dorsalis*. Arch. Neurol. Psychiatry, *38:* 467–472, 1937.
11. Kurze, T. Personal communication, June, 1975.
12. Mazars, G. J. Discussion of Tasker *et al.*, September, 1975.
13. Mullan, S., Harper, P. V., Hekmatpanah, J., Torres, H., and Dobbin, G. Percutaneous interruption of spinal-pain tracts by means of a strontium^{90} needle. J. Neurosurg., *20:* 931–939, 1963.
14. Nathan, P. W., and Smith, M. C. Spino-cortical fibres in man. J. Neurol. Neurosurg. Psychiatry, *18:* 181–190, 1955.
15. Nyberg-Hansen, R., and Rinvik, E. Some comments on the pyramidal tract with special reference to its individual variations in man. Acta Neurol. Scand., *39:* 1–30, 1963.
16. Rakic, P., and Yakovlev, P. I. The right-of-way in the decussation of bulbar pyramids, the patterns of decussation and the torque in the distribution of the pyramidal tracts on the two sides of the cord. To be published.
17. Schwartz, H. G. High cervical cordotomy: Technique and results Clin. Neurosurg., *8:* 282–293, 1962.
18. Swank, R. L. The relationship between the circumoliary pyramidal fascicles and the pontobulbar body in man. J. Comp. Neurol., *60:* 309–317, 1934.
19. Sweet, W. H. Craniospinal surgery for pain. *In* Audiovisual Education in Neurosurgery (AVENS), 1973.
20. Sweet, W. H., White, J. C., Selverstone, B., and Nilges, R. Sensory responses from anterior roots and from surface and interior of spinal cord in man. Trans. Am. Neurol. Assoc., *74:* 165–169, 1950.
21. Tasker, R. R., Organ, L. W., Rowe, I. J., and Hawreylshyn, P. The human spinothalamic tract. Stimulation-mapping in the spinal cord and brain stem. Presented at First World Congress on Pain, Florence, Italy, September 5–8, 1975.
22. Voris, H. C. Ipsilateral sensory loss following chordotomy: Report of a case. Arch. Neurol. Psychiatry, *65:* 95–96, 1951.
23. Voris, H. C. Variations in the spinothalamic tract in man. J. Neurosurg., *14:* 55–60, 1957.
24. White, J. C., Richardson, E. P., Jr., and Sweet, W. H. Upper thoracic cordotomy for relief of pain. Postmortem correlation of spinal incision with analgesic levels in 18 cases. Ann. Surg., *144:* 407–420, 1956.
25. White, J. C., and Sweet, W. H. Pain: Its Mechanisms and Neurosurgical Control, 736 pp. Charles C Thomas, Springfield, Ill., 1955.
26. White, J. C., and Sweet, W. H. Pain and the Neurosurgeon. A Forty Year Experience, 1000 pp. Charles C Thomas, Springfield, Ill., 1969.
27. Yakovlev, P. I., and Rakic, P.: Patterns of decussation of bulbar pyramids and distribution of pyramidal tracts on two sides of the spinal cord. Trans. Am. Neurol. Assoc. *91:* 366–370, 1966.

CHAPTER

7

Controlled Thermocoagulation of Trigeminal Ganglion and Rootlets for Differential Destruction of Pain Fibers: Facial Pain other than Trigeminal Neuralgia

WILLIAM H. SWEET, M.D., D.Sc.

In five previous publications I have concentrated mainly on describing the technique and results of this procedure in the treatment of trigeminal neuralgia both of the typical and atypical varieties including that seen with multiple sclerosis (6–9, 14). In my most recent paper a detailed account of the method including its pitfalls is given. All other reports on the procedure likewise emphasize its use in trigeminal neuralgia (2–4, 11–13).

This paper deals with the much smaller number of patients in other diagnostic categories of facial pain on whom trigeminal thermal rhizotomy has been performed. Table 7.1 includes the types of disorder and the results of the operation in each group.

I use the term atypical trigeminal neuralgia about as Taarnhøj (10) does, *i.e.*, for patients whose paroxysmal pains occur on a background of a variable aching or burning or who have other features less typical such as inconsistent provokability of the pain or spontaneous hypesthesias ascertained by standard clinical testing. Wilfred Harris (1) gave the first good delineation of the disorder he called "periodic migrainous neuralgia." This is described under many other labels, *e.g.*, autonomic faciocephalgia, histamine headache, petrosal neuralgia, cluster headache, etc. Only in those few patients in whom medical management fails and the attacks are no longer confined to clusters is neurosurgical treatment in order. "Trigeminal neuropathy" is used for those with objective trigeminal deficits and at times facial pain in whom no focal cause such as multiple sclerosis, vascular lesion, or tumor can be found. "Atypical facial neuralgia" is essentially a waste basket diagnosis for those with constant pain of unidentifiable cause usually not worse on local stimulation, and with no objective neurological deficit. The "post-traumatic facial neuralgias" have been separated out of the clinically similar atypical facial pain group on the basis of a history of local injury or infection antedating the pain. This feature appears to improve the likelihood of success of trigeminal denervation (14).

With the possible exception of the cancer patients, these individuals have a higher incidence of postoperative unacceptable paresthesias than do those with the trigeminal neuralgias as above defined. I have tried to reduce this incidence by: (1) retrogasserian differential lidocaine block (applied rarely to those with trigeminal neuralgia) and (2) appraisal with the patient of his own reaction to his sensory loss after each addition to the lesion during the operation. I have described elsewhere (6) the easy technique of differential lidocaine block to produce analgesia to pin but not anesthesia to touch. No lesion was made in any patient unless he was satisfied with the pain relief as well as with the new sensations which replaced it after this differential type of anesthetic block.

Table 7.2A depicts the results in four categories of patients in whom the tactic appears tentatively to have positive merit. Only three of the atypical trigeminal neuralgias were sufficiently worrying as to general personality or specific symptoms so that I did not proceed at once to a lesion. In two of them the lidocaine block has yielded continuing relief for longer than 1 year. The post-traumatic neuralgias had done so poorly with only two of 13 successes in our first group that we tried lidocaine initially in the last four cases. Of the three who were satisfied with the

Table 7.1
Differential Thermal Rhizotomy

Diagnosis	No. Patients	No. Procedures	Total Relief
Cancer	20	23	4
Postherpetic neuralgia	3	3	1 of 2
Periodic migrainous neuralgia	8	9	4
Trigeminal neuropathy	3	3	3
Central pain	2	2	1
Post-traumatic neuralgia	16	17	5
Atypical facial neuralgia	18	27	1
Total	70	84	19

Table 7.2A
Lidocaine Block V Rootlets

Pain Diagnosis	No. Cases	Acceptable Relief with Block	Needed no Lesion	Relief with Lesion
Atypical trigeminal	3	2	2	
Post-traumatic	4	3	1	2
Periodic migrainous	7	3	2	0
Acromegaly	1	1		1

block, this alone has continued to relieve one and the other two have been relieved by a differential lesion. Of the seven periodic migrainous neuralgias, only three accepted the numbness but in one of these three the relief has persisted for 17 months after the block alone. However, another of the three failed to get relief from a technically excellent lesion which gave him complete analgesia without any anesthesia. The lone acromegalic with 12 years of constant facial pain followed up relief from a block with relief from two lesions sustained now at 15 months.

In the next four categories (Table 7.2B) most of the patients were unrelieved by the block. In the one postherpetic who was relieved, we could not get the electrode into the rootlets of the second division, the site of her pain. We were encouraged by her temporary relief and have made it long lasting by implantation of stimulating electrodes to the second division behind the foramen rotundum. The atypical facial neuralgias have remained our major bête noir. In our first series of 274 patients, not one of the 14 patients in this intransigent group was relieved. We have submitted another 19 to preliminary lidocaine block. Only six of them were clearcut in describing relief; we made lesions in four of these. Only one of the four is a success. She isn't totally atypical, since her pain had begun 8 years before apparently as typical tic douloureux, but had soon changed over to a continuous, unprovokable pain present in most of her waking hours for over 5 years. One of the three failures expressed tearful gratitude for the removal of her shroud of pain upon hospital discharge after my lesion producing analgesia, and only two months later she wrote as follows: "Dear Dr. Sweet, I have just received your bill. It is outrageous that you should be charging me for the terrible operation you did on me. You have made my first awful pain ten times worse and added a lot of new pains. You are the one who should be paying me, etc." In the 18 cases selected for radiofrequency lesions, I have sought, of course, to exclude psychogenic regional pain. However, my hope that preservation of touch fibers in these patients would not only decrease denervation dysesthesias but preserve some mechanisms

TABLE 7.2B
Lidocaine Block V Rootlets

Pain Diagnosis	No. Cases	Acceptable Relief with Block	Needed no Lesion	Relief with Lesion
Postherpetic	4	1		V2 lesion not achieved
Atypical facial	19	6	2 No lesion yet	1
Trigeminal neuropathy	3	0		
Hyp- or analgesia dolorosa	2	0		

successful in suppressing pain and travelling in the large myelinated fibers has *not* been realized. Siegfried (5) has made a lesion in eight patients with atypical facial neuralgia, reporting short term success in three.

I do not subscribe to the view that all of these patients have some form of neurosis. Inasmuch as the extremely severe pains of trigeminal neuralgia are so consistently relieved by trigeminal operations, one has a tendency to be skeptical of a focal organic cause when facial pain is not so relieved. However, when I become impatient with these people for failing to respond to my best efforts, I remind myself that the deep facial structures are very difficult to denervate and that there is a high failure rate to relieve cancer pain in these areas even by drastic high rostral bubar tractotomies or multiple rhizotomies. I fear that there may be elusive organic factors in some of these patients we have yet to identify. In the final two categories, the patients were unrelieved by differential block and no lesions were made. The block has been helpful not only in most instances with temporary relief but also in an important way in those who have found unacceptable the sensations accompanying analgesia or severe hypalgesia—namely, it has discouraged them from badgering surgeons to operate on their trigeminal nerve.

The second tactic I now use on all of the patients in all diagnostic categories during the procedure. I ask them after each increment to the lesion how annoying the sensations are which accompany the sensory loss. Many are emphatic about preferring much more numbness in the hope of permanent elimination of their intense pains. Others, though, are wary about the new sensations and, especially if neither of us can provoke a bout of pain, they prefer to settle for hypalgesia. Asking the patient to participate in the decision regarding the extent of his lesion leads to less dissatisfaction if the pain returns and less grumbling at least to me about dysesthesias. Of course, the sensations during either a differential block or a lesion do not cover the range of those possibly occurring later. Happily we can assure patients that subsequent operations are no more difficult to complete than the original one. This makes them less uneasy about stopping with hypalgesia. Table 7.3 shows the extent of our experience and that of Thiry (12) with multiple operations.

The results of the differential thermal lesions will now be described in each diagnostic group. They include those treated before as well as after the tactic of differential lidocaine block was begun.

CANCER

In two of our 20 patients, trigeminal sensory loss was not achieved—in one because the area of the foramen ovale was invaded by neo-

TABLE 7.3
Multiple Operations

No. Patients	No. Operations
Sweet	
1	6
2	5
1	4
6	3
Thiry	
4	5
10	4
12	3

plasm and could not be entered. We sought to produce anesthesia as well as analgesia in those patients and succeeded in 16 of the 18. One of the two patients with analgesia only, as well as three others, never had useful relief. Two of them said the pain lay deep to the denervated skin. Another four patients were completely relieved until death from 3 weeks to 3 months later. The remainder, after varying short periods of partial or total relief, had renewed pain on the same or the opposite side as the lesion spread.

POST-HERPETIC NEURALGIA

One of the three patients has been relieved of his first division pain for 4½ years by a lesion producing only analgesia of that division. One soon lost his relief from a lesion producing sustained second division analgesia—the zone of the pain. The third patient's deteriorating mental status precluded evaluation.

PERIODIC MIGRAINOUS NEURALGIA

Four of the eight patients have had no more attacks for follow-up periods from 7 months to 7 years. All four have analgesia of at least the first division. One of them has complete trigeminal anesthesia and analgesia and is worse than before the lesion because of an anesthesia dolorosa. Another with analgesia and severe hypesthesia of all 3 divisions remains at 3½ years unhappy about the "numbness like novocain." His unhappiness is tempered by the total absence of pain now during spectacular daily or twice daily autonomic attacks of profuse ipsilateral lacrimation and watery rhinorrhea, ipsilateral flaming red face and eyeball, miosis, and ptosis. These last for 2 to 3 hours and are accompained by nausea, generalized weakness, and bilateral facial sweating.

Preoperatively, such manifestations were associated with totally disabling pain. I have seen the converse after superficial petrosal neurectomy, namely, continuing absence of lacrimation and rhinorrhea as the attacks of pain recurred. One of the eight patients with trigeminal analgesia is incompletely relieved by operation alone but now remains attack free at 4½ years on doses of propranolol he can tolerate. However two patients with technically excellent lesions providing total trigeminal analgesia and only mild hypesthesia had no relief of their attacks even though the pain is referred exclusively to the trigeminal zone as in the successes. Clearly, the afferent pathways in this disorder vary from patient to patient. The 8th case is too recent to evaluate.

ACROMEGALY

The one patient in this group has been given sustained relief.

TRIGEMINAL NEUROPATHY

These three patients are all relieved of their original pain by appropriately placed production of analgesia; unfortunately, one with total first division sensory loss has anesthesia dolorosa. These complicated patients deserve a fuller account elsewhere. Three other such patients unrelieved by differential lidocaine block had no lesion made.

CENTRAL PAIN

We shall also describe elsewhere our two patients with posterior fossa lesions. One has remained relieved of his original pain; the other soon lost his early relief, although he maintains analgesia in his painful eyeball and forehead.

POST-TRAUMATIC NEURALGIA

Only five of these 16 patients in whom a lesion was made have had lasting relief of the original pain and one of these has anesthesia dolorosa.

ATYPICAL FACIAL NEURALGIA

Our only totally successful lesion in this group of 18 patients was in a woman whose pain had begun as a series of provokable paroxysms. One other has had a degree of relief for which she is grateful.

SUMMARY

I describe the results of retrogasserian differential lidocaine block to aid in the selection of patients for a differential thermal lesion in the trigeminal ganglion and rootlets. This procedure temporarily duplicates the state of analgesia without anesthesia one seeks to make permanent with the radiofrequency heating. The results of this heating procedure are described in the treatment of 71 patients with facial pain of cancer, postherpetic, periodic migrainous neuralgia, acromegaly, trigeminal neuropathy, central pain, post-traumatic facial neuralgia, and atypical facial neuralgia.

ACKNOWLEDGMENT

It is a pleasure to express appreciation to the Neuro-Research Foundation for the support of these studies.

REFERENCES

1. Harris, W. Migrainous neuralgias and periodic migrainous neuralgia. *In* Neuritis and Neuralgia, edited by W. Harris, pp. 295–306. Oxford University Press, London, 1926.
2. Nugent, G. R., and Berry, B. Trigeminal neuralgia treated with percutaneous radiofrequency lesions. J. Neurosurg., *40:* 517–523, 1974.
3. Onofrio, B. M. Radiofrequency percutaneous Gasserian ganglion lesions. Results in 140 patients with trigeminal pain. J. Neurosurg., *42:* 132–139, 1975.
4. Schürmann, K., Butz, M., and Brock, M. Temporal retrogasserian resection of trigeminal root versus controlled elective percutaneous electrocoagulation of the ganglion of Gasser in the treatment of trigeminal neuralgia. Report on a series of 531 cases. Acta Neurochir. (Wien), *26:* 33–35, 1972.
5. Siegfried, J. Results of percutaneous controlled thermocoagulation of the Gasserian ganglion in 300 cases of trigeminal pain. Advances in Neurosurgery, *3:* 287–295, 1975.
6. Sweet, W. H. Percutaneous differential thermal trigeminal rhizotomy for the management of facial pain. Advances in Neurosurgery, *3:* 274–286, 1975.
7. Sweet, W. H. Trigeminal neuralgias. *In* Facial Pain, edited by C. C. Alling III, pp. 100–101. Lea & Febiger, Philadelphia, 1968.
8. Sweet, W. H., and Wepsic, J. G. Controlled thermocoagulation of trigeminal ganglion and rootlets for differential destruction of pain fibers. Part 1: Trigeminal neuralgias. J. Neurosurg., *40:* 143–156, 1974.
9. Sweet, W. H., and Wepsic, J. G. Controlled thermocoagulation of trigeminal ganglion and rootlets. *In* Treatment of Pain, edited by H. C. Voris and W. W. Whisler, pp. 83–87. Charles C Thomas, Springfield, Ill., 1975.
10. Taarnhøj, P. Decompression of the trigeminal root. J. Neurosurg., *11:* 299–305, 1954.
11. Tew, J., and Mayfield, F. Trigeminal neuralgia: A new surgical approach. (Percutaneous electrocoagulation of the trigeminal nerve.) Laryngoscope, *83:* 1096–1101, 1973.
12. Thiry, S., and Hotermans, J. M. Traitement de la névralgie essentielle du trijumeau par stéreotaxie et electrocoagulation partielle sélective du ganglion de Gasser. Expérience portant sur 365 cas traités entre 1950 et 1970. Neurochirurgie, *20:* 55–60, 1974.
13. Turnbull, I. Percutaneous rhizotomy for trigeminal neuralgia. Surg. Neurol., *2:* 385–392, 1974.
14. White, J. C., and Sweet, W. H. *In:* Pain and the Neurosurgeon. A Forty Year Experience, edited by J. C. White and W. H. Sweet, pp. 196–197. Charles C Thomas, Springfield, Ill., 1969.

CHAPTER

8

Control of Pain by Direct Electrical Stimulation of Peripheral Nerves

WILLIAM H. SWEET, M.D., D.Sc.

Wall and I (6) noted about 10 years ago that temporary low threshold stimulation *via* subcutaneous electrodes at peripheral nerves in five patients and *cauda equina* rootlets in three others relieved their clinical pain. In the peripheral nerve group, 2 to 5 minutes of stimulation gave longer lasting relief usually for more than ½ hour after the cessation of stimulation. In the summer of 1965, we had a patient (Doris S.) whose constant burning pain with superimposed sharp stabs in her medial three left fingers had not been helped by posterior rhizotomies C-6 through T-2, even though these had produced anesthesia and analgesia in her medial two and one-half fingers. The fact that she was relieved only by rubbing her first two lateral sentient fingers against cloth all day long led Wall and me to make her, in October, 1965, the first patient in whom we tried for long term relief by stimulation of the large myelinated low threshold fibers. Electrodes implanted around the median nerve provoked a pleasant tingle in her lateral three fingers and corresponding hand and stopped the pain and tenderness in the medial three fingers and hand. Details of her encouraging first 2 years of stimulation and of a number of other such peripheral nerve patients were described long ago (1968) (5, 8). Since then my unrelenting mystification as to what is happening here has rendered me virtually mute on this topic, but at least a brief account is in order of the experiences Dr. Wepsic and I have had in 69 such patients in whom electrodes were placed around 74 nerves.

The history of Doris S. from 1968 illustrates some of the problems. Her after effect of continuing relief upon stimulation by a mechanical vibrator to the thenar eminence or electrically to the skin over the median nerve gradually disappeared over a 2½ year period. The electrodes originally placed around the median nerve in 1965 had been removed 2 weeks later when stimulation to the skin over the median nerve proved so effective. But in May, 1968, reimplantation and activating of the electrodes gave no relief at all so they were removed 2½ months later. In late 1969, a Brown-Séquard type of lesion related to the right side of the lower cervical cord gradually became apparent with leg weakness, increased tendon jerks, and a positive Babinski on that side, and analgesia with higher hypalgesia up to T-2 on the opposite side. This slightly expanding cord lesion associated with arachnoidal adhesions was seen at operation but not biopsied. It has advanced only slightly in the last 6 years. Her pain in an anesthetic zone seems almost certainly due to an intramedullary lesion. None of our maneuvers to decrease it is quite as effective as her own incessant rubbing of a soft cloth with her first two left nonpainful sentient fingers. She remains an active housewife.

Our 69 patients selected for implantation had had a variety of medical, physiotherapeutic, and surgical procedures for pain of clearcut focal organic etiology except for the four patients with atypical facial neuralgia (Table 8.1). In these latter patients, the pain was referred only to one of the three trigeminal divisions, but not one of them had sustained relief from the electrodes. The pain followed trauma, surgical or accidental, in 68% of the total group; it was almost always to a single nerve; even four of the six amputation stumps were of a finger. The miscellaneous category consists of neuropathies—two diabetic and one each tabetic, ischemic, and toxic—one rhizopathy after accidental vertebral injury, and two myelopathies. The principal criterion for selection for the operation in addition to chronicity and organicity of the pain was reference to a limited zone of the body, preferably that of one nerve. We checked this point by a lidocaine block where it was in the least doubt, as well as in many in whom reference of pain and/or injury to a single nerve root was unequivocal (Table 8.2). Such blocks were carried out in 52 patients.

TABLE 8.1

Peripheral Nerve Implants, Diagnoses

Neuropathy, after accidental trauma	31
Neuropathy, after accidental trauma with amputation stump and/or phantom pain	6
Neuropathy, after surgical trauma	10
Postherpetic neuralgia	5
Spinal rhizopathy and disc removal	5
Atypical facial neuralgia	4
Miscellaneous	8
Total	69

TABLE 8.2

Result Nerve Block Correlated with Result Stimulation

No relief block with no relief stimulation	5
No relief block but relief stimulation	1
Relief block with temporary relief stimulation	8
Relief block with sustained relief stimulation	13
Relief block but no relief stimulation	25
Total	52

Often the same nerve was blocked two or three times or adjoining nerves, roots, or the sympathetic trunk were blocked. Most of these procedures were carried out by or under the aegis of Dr. Donald Todd with whom Dr. White and I have been working on pain problems for over 25 years. The injection as carried out by a man of his experience involves a fairly standard amount of additional pain for the patient. The degree to which the patient complains has proven of value in determining his general threshold for protesting about pain. A block giving pain relief was achieved in nearly 90% of the patients. In only one of the six who had no relief from the block have the implanted electrodes given relief. Herewith a vignette of that case.

F. D., aged 79 years, had been complaining for two decades of suprapubic pain after a transurethral prostatectomy and bilateral herniorrhaphy. Suprapubic prostatectomy and division of the right ilioinguinal nerve 9 years previously had not helped. Innumerable blocks of all the relevant peripheral nerves at other clinics as well as ours had given no relief. A differential spinal anesthetic progressing to a full anesthesia with a motor and sensory paralysis to T-1 worsened the pain. This led to a diagnosis of psychogenic regional pain at the institution. Dr. Todd's paravertebral block of the left T-12 nerve produced anesthesia over the iliac crest and into the area of pain without relief. The following day I placed temporary electrodes on the left 12th intercostal nerve at open operation. For 2 days there was no suggestion of relief; then enough developed so that I put in a permanent system on the 14th postoperative day. According to the patient, the vibrating soothing effect at 13 to 16 cps and 5 volts dissipated the pain. He gradually stopped all medication and had longer and longer relief with short periods of stimulation. He has needed neither the stimulator nor any medication since 16 months after operation, and remains vigorously active 4½ years later.

I remain dumbfounded at this sequence of events. The remainder of Table 8.2 makes it clear that relief with a lidocaine block is not a predictor of relief upon simulation.

The results nerve by nerve are given in Tables 8.3A–8.3D. The outcome has been far better with the superficial radial implants than with any other nerve. All eight had either surgical or accidental trauma; seven have had temporary or sustained relief; the eighth is lost to follow-up. This nerve differs from all the others implanted in its purely sensory function (Table 8.3A). The first patient in the median nerve group is our very first patient whom I have already described. The remainder in this group with any degree of success all had their pain related to some form of local trauma (Table 8.3B). In the ulnar group, the 66-year-old patient with postherpetic neuralgic pain had his hyperpathia and spontaneous pain relieved in his hypalgesic fourth and fifth fingers both times the ulnar nerve was blocked with lidocaine, an unusually favorable response in this disorder. Relief from appropriate

TABLE 8.3A
Results with Each Nerve

	Total No. Cases	Temporary Relief for	Sustained Relief at	Diagnosis
Trigeminal	8		15 mos	Postherpetic neuralgia
Superficial radial	8	4 wks		Post-traumatic neuropathy
		5 mos		Post-traumatic neuropathy
			68 mos	Post-traumatic neuropathy
		4 mos		Amputation stump and phantom
			49 mos	Amputation stump and phantom
			>3 yrs	Postsurgical neuropathy
			3 yrs	Postsurgical neuropathy

TABLE 8.3B
Results with Each Nerve

	Total No. Cases	Temporary Relief for	Sustained Relief at	Diagnosis
Median	14	See text		Myelopathy & arachnoiditis
		Few weeks		Post-traumatic neuropathy
		1 mo		Amputation stump and phantom
		2 mos		Amputation stump and phantom
			17 mos	Post-traumatic neuropathy
			2 yrs	Postsurgical neuropathy
			40 mos	Postsurgical neuropathy

trigeminal blocks had also occurred in the patient with second division postherpetic neuralgia. Both of them have sustained their excellent benefit from the implanted electrodes. Of the other three with postherpetic pain who are failures, in one we did not achieve total relief with the lidocaine, and in the other two we did not try it. None of the five patients had a major loss of touch sensation in their zone of pain; these may represent a fruitful group for further studies.

We devoted much effort to the nine individuals with sciatic lesions, using multiple pairs of electrodes and leads but with no really good lasting result in any of them (Table 8.3C). In the tibial and common peroneal nerve group we were a bit better (Table 8.3D). The success rate in the superficial radial group and the annoyance to the patient when motor fibers are stimulated too near the low threshold sensory fibers has led me to try to separate out predominantly sensory bundles in the larger mixed nerves. Figure 8.1 shows the electrode around the one of the three fascicles of the common peroneal nerve which gave predominantly sensory responses. The other two fascicles into which the nerve was readily divided were mainly motor. Stimulation in this patient continues to give him almost instantaneous relief of the pain in his leg and pedal dorsum even though sensation is evoked only in the former zone. I am now leaning toward almost invariable use of local or wakeup anesthesia in order to carry out this fractionation maneuver if it is feasible; however, this type of anesthesia was used in only 24 of our 69 patients. None of our five spinal rhizopathies after disc removal were helped.

The technical problems with operation and the equipment are relatively minor. It is so easy to remove the electrodes that we usually do so if they don't help and in 37 patients they are now out. The receiver buttons are usually placed under the skin of the torso especially if the large size, delivering a symmetrical biphasic signal, is used. On the limbs they are subject to much minor trauma often with a tight skin over them. It is easy to regard the operation as so trivial that scrupulous aseptic technique and minimally traumatic dissection may not be maintained. We had eight wound infections, usually late in onset. Two of the patients were getting such good relief that I reimplanted the electrodes and sustained relief was reachieved.

TABLE 8.3C
Results with Each Nerve

	Total No. Cases	Temporary Relief for	Sustained Relief at	Diagnosis
Ulnar	9	8 mos		Postsurgical rhizopathy
			>1 yr	Postherpetic neuralgia
			15 mos	Post-traumatic neuropathy
			32 mos	Post-traumatic neuropathy
Intercostal nerves	2			
	T8 and 9	8 wks		Post-traumatic neuropathy
	T12		55 mos	Postsurgical neuropathy
Sciatic	9	5 mos		Post-traumatic neuropathy
			Partial	Amputation stump and phantom
			5 yrs	

TABLE 8.3D
Results with Each Nerve

	Total No. Cases	Temporary Relief for	Sustained Relief at	Diagnosis
Tibial	10	9 mos		Postsurgical neuropathy
			9 mos	Post-traumatic neuropathy
			2 yrs	Post-traumatic neuropathy
Common peroneal	9	13 mos		Post-traumatic neuropathy
		14 mos		Diabetic neuropathy
			2 yrs	Post-traumatic neuropathy
			10 mos	Post-traumatic neuropathy
			37 mos	Post-traumatic neuropathy

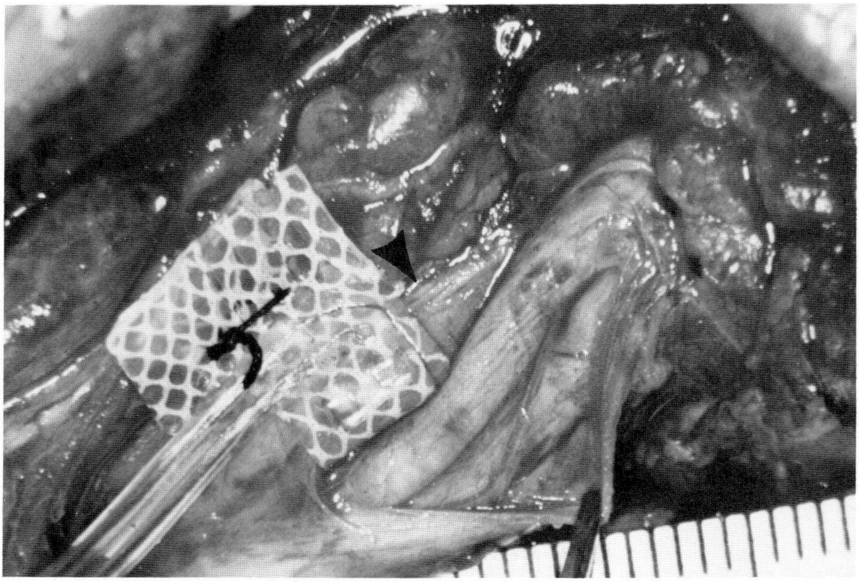

FIG. 8.1 Vernon H. Exposure of common peroneal nerve in popliteal fossa. Sheath enclosing entire nerve has been opened longitudinally and one leaf of it is held down against mm. scale by forceps. The main nerve was readily separable into 3 fascicles. Electrical stimulation elicited largely sensory responses from the highest one of the three (arrow) around which a silastic cuff containing two platinum electrodes is visible; one of the two electrodes is on the other side of the nerve. From the two lower fascicles in the field the responses were mainly motor.

Late scarring around the nerve does not seem to be the problem it may be in the spinal canal. For example, in a recent patient electrodes were removed from the superficial radial after 3⅓ years, revealing a nerve which looked normal even though stimulation had been for many hours per day.

Most tantalizing is our lack of understanding of how to recoup a good result once it fades. The patient just referred to suggests one answer. His sensations from a constant electrical signal had become erratic, varying from abrupt sharp stabs of pain through an acceptable range to no sensation at all. Some of his pain had spread from the back of the lateral hand and thumb around to the volar aspect. Shift of the electrode to the median nerve yielded by far the best result he has had. Even though the stimulus tingle is exclusively volar and most of his pain is dorsal, at 14 months after the second operation he is down to 0 to 15 minutes of stimulation per day, after working a 16-hour day. In general, the lower the signal strength and the less frequent the usage, the more likely is the patient able to wean himself off the device entirely. One alert individual noted that his pain abruptly stopped shortly before the threshold voltage for any positive sensation. Such experiences make me think a more flexible attitude toward this therapy with a sturdier determination to try to make it work may improve the gloomy results I have shown.

As a consequence of the reports of others (see discussion), we have resumed transcutaneous stimulation prior to implantation, with the results shown in Table 8.4. These certainly suggest that we should pursue this tactic further.

DISCUSSION

There are numerous features of the patients in whom we must try in continuing studies to arrive at more definitive statements. These include the correlation with the clinical result of any changes during stimulation in the various modalities of sensation. A complicating feature of many in this group is the presence of litigation or workman's compensation factors. We need a more objective means of assessing the patient's total personality, the effect of it on the pain, and *vice versa*.

Probably the most detailed and thoughtful account of the results of stimulation for control of pain *via* electrodes implanted around peripheral nerves is that of Picaza and his colleagues (4) who by the spring of 1974 had treated 50 patients in this way. They implanted no patient who had not had consistent benefit from transcutaneous stimulation and in whom other therapy short of narcotics has been tried for less than 1 year. They have made a thorough effort to appraise the patient's pain and its influence on his life by semiquantitative parameters. At a follow-up after 6 to 12 months in 15 patients and after 14 to 20 months in eight others, only five were on drugs with a "high or moderate abuse potential", *i.e.*, substances listed in schedule II or III respectively of the Bureau of Narcotics and Dangerous Drugs. Moreover, only eight patients described their pain as worse than mild, and only nine had their pain 50% or more of the time during the day. These results are strikingly better than those I have just described and have been obtained in a much wider assortment of pathological disorders than we have treated in this way. The major difference in management has been their insistence on a sustained response to transcutaneous stimulation before they would install electrodes. As in our series, constant attention and follow-up by the

Table 8.4
Transcutaneous Stimulation (TCT) Correlated with Implantation Stimulation (IMP)

Relief TCT	Relief IMP	No. of Patients
Decreasing	None	1
Partial	Temporary	1
Complete	Sustained	2
5 mos then failed	Sustained	1
None	None	2

neurosurgeon were essential as reoperations for a variety of reasons were needed.

There are two much shorter reports in the same Pain Symposium number of *Surgical Neurology*. Cauthen and Renner (2) placed electrodes around one sciatic and two ulnar nerves in patients with painful injuries of these nerves. Relief remained effective at 4, 6, and 8 months, respectively. Clark (1) at first had "excellent" results in four of five patients following sciatic nerve implants. By a year later pain had returned completely in one of the four. One patient with both median and ulnar electrodes continued to have pain in her palm and ulnar three fingers—areas to which no stimulus-evoked sensation was felt; by 1 year later she was getting no relief at all.

Long (3) gives excellent detailed reports on 10 patients in whom pain associated with injury of nerve trunks was treated by implantation of electrodes around the relevant nerve. He selected only patients in whom stimulation needles percutaneously placed near the nerve predicted relief. Pain from injuries of the ulnar nerve in four patients and to the brachial plexus in two others has been satisfactorily treated for periods of up to 32 months. In the four other patients whose electrodes were placed around the sciatic nerve in three and around this and the femoral nerve in the fourth, the results were unconvincing or poor. This is consonant with our bad batting average with this nerve. Weinstein and Sacks (7) comment briefly on the failure of transcutaneous stimulation to give relief which was then achieved in three of their cases of peripheral nerve injury by percutaneously placed needles. Electrodes implanted in these three have given "good results". They note a positive correlation between relief of pain and reference of stimulus-evoked sensation to the painful area.

SUMMARY AND CONCLUSIONS

Our results after implanting electrodes around peripheral nerves in 69 patients over a 10 year period are only fair with but 17 individuals maintaining relief until death or until the present time. Thirteen others had weeks or months of temporary relief. A continuing use of transcutaneous and better still of percutaneous electrodes to guide the decision regarding implantation is almost certainly advisable. Intensive efforts in laboratory animal studies with models of chronic pain are needed to improve our understanding of exactly what we should be doing. Empirical sustained work with the individual patient is likely to improve the figures we have presented, even in our present state of ignorance.

ACKNOWLEDGMENT

It is a pleasure to express appreciation to the Neuro-Research Foundation for the support of these studies.

REFERENCES

1. Clark, K. Electrical stimulation of the nervous system for control of pain: University of Texas Southwestern Medical School experience. Surg. Neurol., *4:* 164–166, 1975.
2. Cauthen, J. C., and Renner, E. J. Transcutaneous and peripheral nerve stimulation for chronic pain states. Surg. Neurol., *4:* 102–104, 1975.
3. Long, D. M. Electrical stimulation for relief of pain from chronic nerve injury. J. Neurosurg., *39:* 718–722, 1973.
4. Picaza, J. A., Canon, B. W., Hunter, S. E., Boyd, A. S., Gruma, J., and Maurer, D. Pain suppression by peripheral nerve stimulation. Part II. Observations with implanted devices. Surg. Neurol., *4:* 115–124, 1975.
5. Sweet, W. H. Lessons on pain control from electrical stimulation. Trans. Coll. Physicians Phila., *35:* 171–184, 1968.
6. Wall, P. D., and Sweet, W. H. Temporary abolition of pain in man on stimulation of large diameter cutaneous afferent fibers. Science, *155:* 108–109, 1967.
7. Weinstein, P. R., and Sacks, L. B. Transcutaneous stimulation for the evaluation and treatment of post-traumatic neuralgia, p. 183. Abstracts First World Congress on Pain, Florence, Italy, Sept. 5–8, 1975.
8. White, J. C., and Sweet, W. H. Control of pain by activation of inhibitory mechanisms. *In* Pain and the Neurosurgeon. A Forty Year Experience, edited by J. C. White and W. H. Sweet, pp. 888–904. Charles C Thomas, Springfield, Ill., 1969.

ADDENDUM

The most recent report of Picaza and associates presents a less optimistic account of their results than their earlier report (4). The later report describes follow-ups of less than 12 months in 22 patients and after 1 to 4 years in 37 others. About one-half of their patients in both groups reported 50% or more relief of pain; this they designated as "significant relief." Our classification of "relief" was more rigorous; we required that the patient: 1) be off all but mild analgesic medication, and 2) have resumed productive activity, in order to place him in this category. This would correspond roughly to the 75 to 100% relief group of Picaza and associates. Thirty percent of their 37 patients followed for over 1 year were benefited to this degree—only a bit better than our results. Of 30 patients they selected for implantation who responded well to transcutaneous stimulation, only half of them maintained significant relief after implantation. Likewise three of seven implanted patients who did not respond to transcutaneous stimulation were also in the success group. Thus the result of transcutaneous stimulation was not a reliable predictor of the response to operation. We are grateful to Picaza and his colleagues for their frank appraisal of their earlier conclusions.

REFERENCE

Picaza, J.A., Hunter, S.E., and Cannon, B.W. Pain suppression by peripheral nerve stimulation. Part IV. Chronic effects by implanted devices. Presented to the American Association of Neurological Surgeons, San Francisco, April 1976.

CHAPTER

9

What Should the Neurosurgeon Do When Faced with a Malpractice Suit?

WILLIAM H. SWEET, M.D., D.Sc.

Many articles on the subject of professional negligence suits are written from the vantage point of medicolegal experts, plaintiff's or defendant's attorneys, public officials, sociologists, etc. Having had a worm's eye view of the scene twice as the defendant myself and having had four more court appearances testifying in defense of colleagues, I have a keen awareness of the reason so few doctors write of their experiences. These are so unpleasant and the physician finds his role so ignominious and so distastefully time consuming that once the performance is over and he is again beginning to get a decent night's sleep, he prefers to expunge the memories from consciousness.

In my two cases in 1963 and 1967, the contest was carried through to the end of a jury trial with victory for me both times, but the neurosurgical defendant won in only two of the other four cases, in which I have testified, although I state categorically, there was no professional negligence in any of them. In still another two instances, after a careful study of the facts, I urged both defendant neurosurgeons to fight their cases in court and offered to testify in their behalf. They elected, however, to settle before trial for handsome sums; both were soon faced by other malpractice suits. On the basis of these experiences, I am going to venture some practical suggestions for the avoidance of such suits and for increasing the chance of winning them once they are instituted.

I should lead off, however, by making it crystal clear that if the doctor has in our view been guilty of malpractice, my colleagues and I say so without reservation. In the lone instance of this type which I have studied, all the several neurosurgeons consulted by the insurance company reached such a conclusion. The expected out-of-court settlement for a colossal sum took place. Since in my experience an overwhelming percentage of physicians are honest, it is futile for the negligent defendant to expect his colleagues to rally to his defense with a view to keeping down their own malpractice insurance premiums or out of professional loyalty.

A more difficult situation is posed by the neurosurgeon some of whose practices are making his colleagues uneasy. At the present time, we tend to confine our active expression of discontent to refusing to testify in his behalf if a malpractice suit is brought against him. I could cite two specific instances of well known neurosurgeons in my area who, in the actual cases in question, were in my view not in the least guilty of professional negligence, and I urged them to fight the suit. But they and their attorneys, discouraged by their rebuffs from other neurosurgeons, elected to settle out of court for scores of thousands of dollars—sums to which all of us, of course, contribute. If there is any more idiotic way for us to discipline our possibly wayward confreres, I don't happen to be able to think of it. A more logical though distasteful *modus operandi* is for a group of us to make a conscientious survey of the cases of a neurosurgeon whose conduct is called in question and develop written recommendations. In fact, we are now doing this in Boston in exactly that situation.

But the occasional occurrence of negligence does not, I think, justify the generalized current use of our courts repeatedly to achieve flagrant piracy. While I view many plaintiff's attorneys in malpractice suits against physicians as buccaneers, I gather that these characters tend to view themselves as modern Robin Hoods riding forth to redress the wrongs of their poor defenseless clients at the hands of the robber barons of medicine and, especially, surgery. I may point out that these lawyers enjoy one advantage Robin Hood never had, namely, the Sheriff of Nottinghamshire and all the rest of the sheriffs are on their side if they win in court. (Nor in fact do many of these lawyers find it necessary to rough it in the forest of Arden.)

We surgeons must be able to present convincing evidence to the public that we are constantly on the lookout to prevent overcharging for our services. At the Massachusetts General Hospital and Massachusetts Eye and Ear Infirmary, we have not come fully to grips with this problem. Evidence for this, in my view, is that the charge for intradiscal injections of chymopapain at our hospital, prior to the recent FDA restrictions on this procedure, was $750, in accord with the custom in several states. The charge made by Dr. Ian McNab who, as one of the most thoughtful students of this procedure, addressed this society on the subject in 1973, is $50 for one disc; $75 for two. The retired minister of my church was recently charged $440 at the Massachusetts Eye and Ear Infirmary for the removal of a benign nodule a few millimeters in diameter from one eyelid. The operation under local anesthesia required about 1/2 hour. Should these examples of questionable charges be examined by an ongoing peer review mechanism? Although the published surgical fee schedules for Blue Shield and other insurance plans have gone most of the way to eliminate charge abuses, it is worth pointing out that the charges within any specialty are set by the members thereof. A more broadly representative review group would, I think, check any specialist groups who may have become habitually overgenerous to themselves.

Another contention of the plaintiff's attorneys is that there is a conspiracy of silence among doctors not to testify against each other in court on malpractice suits. In the above cited cases in which I have been concerned, there has not only been no such conspiracy detectable, the testimony given in behalf of the plaintiff by physicians was, in my opinion, patently ridiculous in three of the cases.

A neuroradiologist friend of mine was in 1969 told by a plaintiff's attorney that "it could mean in the neighborhood of $50,000 for her if she were willing to testify against our Chief of Neuroradiology and a former neurosurgical resident in a pending court case involving a patient who became quadriplegic after a catheter angiogram. She refused, but a pathologist, working at the time in a local hospital, appeared on the witness stand in her stead, presenting himself as a neuroradiological expert. His testimony apparently failed to convince the jury because the plaintiff lost the case.

But once the statement under oath of that physician and of the two in the other two cases were given in court, no further questioning of the validity of the statements took place by any medical or any other group as far as I know. I suggest that the opportunity to explicate the basis for their testimony be made available to such ladies and gentlemen. I am happy to inform you that the American Association of Neurological Surgeons is arranging for such opportunities. If a proposal currently before the AANS becomes operative, any sworn testimony of a neurosurgical expert witness may be reviewed by the Professional Liability Committee of the AANS upon request thereto, with appropriate procedures thereafter to secure a fair hearing for all concerned. These will include publication and distribution of the full and unabridged testimony.

I may point out that our malpractice suits in the field of neurological disease in the Boston area took a giant leap forward in frequency when one of our most respected neurosurgeons settled out of court for a handsome sum an action pending against him. The patient, with a modest degree of visual impairment and a suspected parasellar mass, had a bilateral carotid angiogram under general anesthesia. The man awoke blind and remained so. In the neurosurgeon's letter to the referring physician, he indicated that it had not been good judgment to do the angiogram on the second side without testing the patient's vision after the first side had been studied. This statement cost a bit less than $100,000.

One of the first lessons I needed to learn was that it is imperative to take seriously the threat of legal action no matter how ill founded the allegation of professional negligence may in fact be. I was under the mistaken impression that, if the medical facts clearly disproved negligence, an unfavorable jury verdict could be appealed with expectation of reversal. This is not necessarily so.

When an untoward result occurs, it is, of course, vitally important to devote protracted intensive effort to help the patient. The more belligerent and contentious he or his relatives are, the more important it is to maintain a calm, sustained friendly, cooperative attitude—and the harder it is to do.

The standard ploy used by a plaintiff in my own two cases was for him to testify that I had acknowledged that a mistake had been made; I then testified that no such admission was made by me. The plaintiff's statement has two advantages from his standpoint: (1) it would constitute evidence of negligence which an appeal court might be unwilling to overrule, and (2) it prevents the original trial judge from withholding the case from a jury decision in the first place because of inadequate evidence of negligence. My admission of negligence as alleged by the plaintiff constitutes important evidence that it had occurred; my own denial of such admission represents a dispute on a relevant fact. It is the province of the jury to decide which witness is telling the truth, so the whole case is decided by the jury. The plaintiff and his attorney count on the defendant's plight to elicit a favorable verdict regardless of the evidence of any negligence. In one instance, my admission of guilt was said to have been made before one other family member in addition to the patient—so it became the words of two against me. In my two cases, the jury apparently decided to believe me, but I would prefer to come into court with more recorded evidence on my side and suggest the following procedure in the case of those patients who have a major adverse sequel to one's efforts. One arranges a conference with the patient and/or responsible relative to discuss and explain the unhappy turn of events. At this conference there just happens to be present a resident or assistant and a nurse. At the completion of this conference, one makes a note in the record as to precisely how one has accounted for the major complication, states that this is the definitive and complete discussion of the problem with the family, and writes down the names of the other doctor, the nurse, and any others who were present at the time. This is part of the permanent record available to the plaintiff and the court. It will constitute, hopefully, a major deterrent to the plaintiff's attorney bringing suit with the automatic expectation that his client's standard falsehood regarding acknowledgment of guilt will get the case to a sympathetic jury.

Plaintiffs are also often contending that they have not been adequately informed as to the risks of the procedure; certainly, patients or other doctors who have had or seen superb results from an operation may oversell its advantages to others similarly afflicted. Of course, the surgeon years later when the case comes to court may not recall exactly how he described the procedure to the patient. In one of the cases in which I could enthusiastically testify that the patient's neurosurgical care had been exemplary, the defendant neurosurgeon honestly stated that he did not remember the details of how he had described to the patient his retrogasserian operation for first and second division pain. The patient insisted that he had said these rootlets would be sectioned. Largely on the basis of this "lack of informed consent" a judge—not a jury—awarded the plaintiff $18,000.

For many months I have provided patients a three-page detailed account of the procedure and risks of a percutaneous differential thermal retrogasserian rhizotomy. There is a terminal line for his signature, indicating he has read and understood and agreed to the operation. A copy of this statement and one I have written for cordotomy may be obtained on request. The descriptions of these two procedures, which involve active patient cooperation during them, are intended primarily to help the patient aid the surgeon, but secondarily they are proof of informed consent.

Another type of activity I commend to all of us is the cooperative analysis of the management of specific problems by 10 or 20 prominent groups of neurosurgeons. For example, at the last meeting of the German Society for Neurosurgery in Heidelberg the host, Professor Penzholz, described the outcome with a detailed description of all the complications seen after each of the various forms of injection and surgical treatment used in a total of 1946 cases of trigeminal neuralgia in the 17 clinics participating in the study. No one clinic, much less one surgeon, was identifiable in the figures given. The numbers and types of all the complications were substantially greater than those published by any single group, reflecting the natural tendency of all of us to describe our best series in the literature. Incidentally, this article will appear in the next volume of *Advances in Neurosurgery* (1). However, such cooperatively obtained data are not only valuable in a defense against alleged negligence, they should probably be used by all of us with a small personal experience of a specific procedure to indicate to patients the risks thereof.

Another suggestion is that the doctor make a careful word for word study of the entire record of any patients in whom he suspects a suit for professional negligence may be in the offing. One surgeon of my acquaintance was aghast to discover, after the record had been seen by the plaintiff's attorney, that he had dashed off his signature to an operative note dictated by a resident which had described one small component of the operation erroneously and in a way grossly damaging to the surgeon. This probably was a critical factor in the verdict against him by the jury, despite his statement on the witness stand correcting the written error.

A further suggestion is that the surgeon promptly make a copy of any record in which a suit for professional negligence may be threatened. He would do well to keep this under lock and key in his own files. This recommendation is based on the following sequence of events in the third case in my own experience. There was a crucial admission note containing the detailed description of the risks of a vertebral arteriogram and noting that these risks had been accepted by the patient. The event stood out clearly in the memories both of the resident and intern who had made the note because they wished to make it so clear they had secured fully informed consent that the note was written in red ink. It happens to be a Massachusetts General Hospital rule that only operative procedures are to be described in red ink, and the nurse in charge took the men to task for this infraction of the rules. Some years later when the patient brought suit because she alleged she had not been informed of the risks of the study, this critical red ink component of the record was missing.

A further thought relates to the need of securing one's own personal legal counsel in the event that the suit exceeds one's insurance coverage. Some years ago when I had written to my own insurance carrier suggesting that my $100,000 coverage for a single case be increased, the carrier wrote back stating that this was a poor idea since it only served to encourage law suits for exorbitant amounts. So I didn't increase my coverage. In 1967 I faced a suit for $1,000,000 in damages in a man who had a peculiarly catastrophic outcome following my bilateral anterior rhizotomy of the three uppermost cervical roots along with the spinal portion of the spinal accessory nerves for the relief of torticollis. He was left with a bilateral total atrophic and areflexic paralysis of both upper limbs. Although he had no other motor and no sensory loss, his plight was utterly pathetic and any verdict against the defendant would probably have been for more than my $100,000 insurance coverage. Hence, close friends in the legal profession advised me to secure my own attorney to protect my own financial interests regarding any verdict over and above the sum the insurance company would have to pay. The securing of such additional counsel proved to entail what then seemed a memorable expense. My personal attorney had no overt role during the trial. The insurance company routinely insists that its attorney control every aspect of the defense. Moreover, that attorney uttered every syllable heard by the court from any defense counsel. As far as I could see, my own attorney was privileged during the trial to do no more than pass sweet tidbits of advice to the king man, the insurance company's attorney. However, if he were to be a real value he had to prepare for the trial, allotting just as much time as his colleague employed by the insurance company. So, even though during the trial he seemed to play less of a role than the first assistant at a surgical operation, his professional fee for me came to $5,617. It is cheaper in the long run to be covered for at least $1,000,000 per law suit and in some jurisdictions for even more. Don't let your insurance carrier talk you out of it—great help though it may be to reducing unemployment in the legal profession if there are two law firms involved in the defense of every physician.

Now to return to the medicolegal problems posed by the gloomy facts about my patient with the eventual atrophic paralysis of both arms. When I did my operation of bilateral C-1, C-2, and C-3 anterior rhizotomy, I thought I had preserved any significant vessels on these roots, but when he awoke after operation he was paralyzed in all voluntary muscles below the neck except the diaphragm. Some sensation was preserved. Re-exploration of the wound disclosed only a slightly swollen spinal cord and no hematoma. The explanation seemed to be an ischemic myelopathy consequent upon need for some of the cut arterial supply accompanying those cut rootlets. After a stormy course he recovered bowel, bladder, and all sensory and motor functions except for a remarkable areflexic atrophic total paralysis of every muscle in the upper limbs. There was at that time no report in the literature of any such remotely similar disaster following this operation. The lower motor neuron quality of the paralysis in the arms meant that the anterior horn cells in the brachial plexus enlargement of the cord opposite C-5, C-6, C-7, and T-1 vertebrae were the only totally ischemic structures—an extraordinary phenomemon in view of the fact that my operation had exposed the cord only at the Cl-2 level (Fig. 9.1). Normally the brachial plexus enlargement of the cord receives the most generous portion of main arterial feeders of any portion of the cord. There are usually three or four as shown in this simplified diagram taken from a publication by Lazorthes. The most tenable explanation of the peculiar disaster in this patient was that he had none of these main feeders; had been relying upon tiny much higher vessels coming in over the uppermost anterior roots.

Although chagrined at the catastrophic sequel of my operation I thought that from the medicolegal standpoint of defending myself in a malpractice suit, I was lucky. It seemed to me that there was no conceivable manipulation anyone could have carried out on the cord in

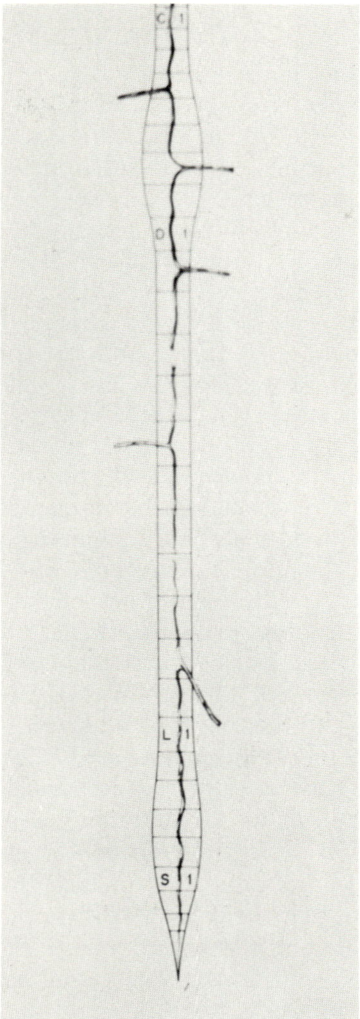

FIG. 9.1. Main arterial supply to spinal cord, illustrating that of the five principal arterial trunks three of them usually go to the brachial plexus enlargement of the cervical cord. (From G Lazorthes: Rev. Neurol., *106:* 552, 1962; Masson & Cie, Paris.)

my operative field—no matter how clumsy or inadvertent it was—which could have produced the findings in this man. These required that the lesion be confined to the anterior column of grey matter of C-5 to T-1 segments—all well below my operative field. I was at first placid in the blithe feeling of assurance that my position was unassailable because of the peculiar congeries of the facts described. I was dumbfounded when the insurance company attorney with decades of experience in malpractice suits insisted that despite all his experience at understanding medical facts, my explanation of this situation was incomprehensible even to him and hence utterly worthless in terms of persuading a jury. He strongly urged me to think of some other defense because this was useless!! These disputes with my council convinced me of the imperative necessity of adjusting myself to a mode of intellectual operation previously foreign to me. It gradually filtered into my consciousness that I would have have to prepare myself for an entirely new profession. The modes of thought and action of the court room are so alien to those of the practicing physician or surgeon that if he is to defend himself effectively he does well to spend literally scores of hours schooling himself in order to respond effectively to every conceivable court room contingency. The attitude that no such intense preparation is necessary should, I think, be abandoned because I think one sound way for the medical profession to cope with the meteroric rise in suits for professional negligence against us is to learn ourselves how to present a convincing defense in court.

In my case one of the first requirements was for me to change my mental orientation to the problem from one of a feeling of injured martyrdom that such a thing was happening to me to an attitude that I was now engaging in a fascinating intellectual experience of an entirely new ilk. Trial attorneys may seek deliberately to infuriate opposition witnesses and attorneys in order to befuddle their capacity for orderly thought. Attorneys tell me they must develop tactics to calm themselves when they feel anger supervening. One must avoid global activation of the autonomic nervous system and adrenal glands in favor of a highly selective outpouring of neurotransmitters in the cerebral areas for cognition. Gradually I was able to convince the insurance company attorney that the best defense was to present the facts in a simple graphic way so that they would not only be comprehensible to the jury but would carry with that comprehension the firm conviction inherent to them. I think the clincher in presenting the case to the jury was a repeatedly practiced description of the medical reasoning employing absolutely no technical terms and accompanied by simple slides projected on a screen in the court room. The first figure in that series you have already seen. The next four figures are operative photographs in the field of another patient who was having the same operation (Fig. 9.2). The first figure shows the typical appearance of the posterior roots seen in this picture. Figure 9.3 with a millimeter rule giving the scale of magnification enabled the jury to appreciate the superior view one has of these tiny structures. The blood vessel was saved on the right C-2 anterior root

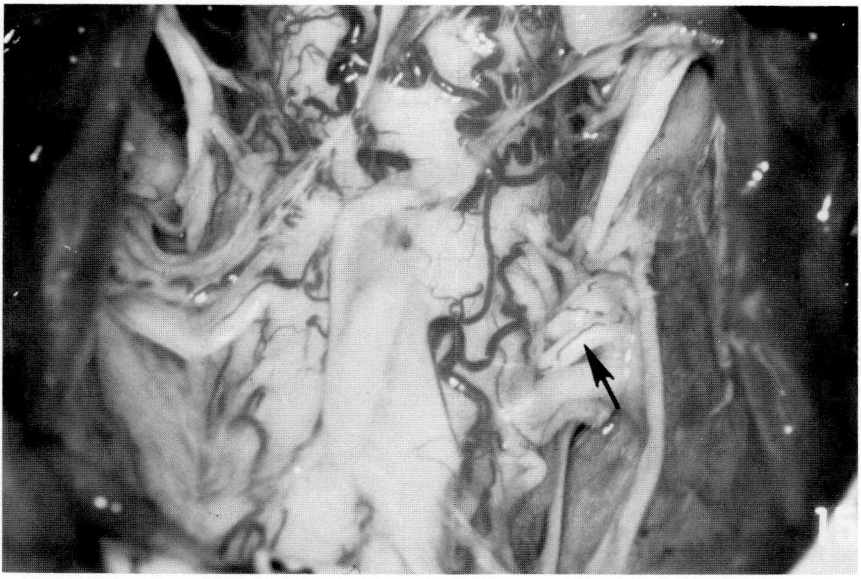

FIG. 9.2. Appearance of normal cervical cord after dural opening at C-1 and C-2 levels showing tiny arteries on C-2 posterior rootlets (arrow).

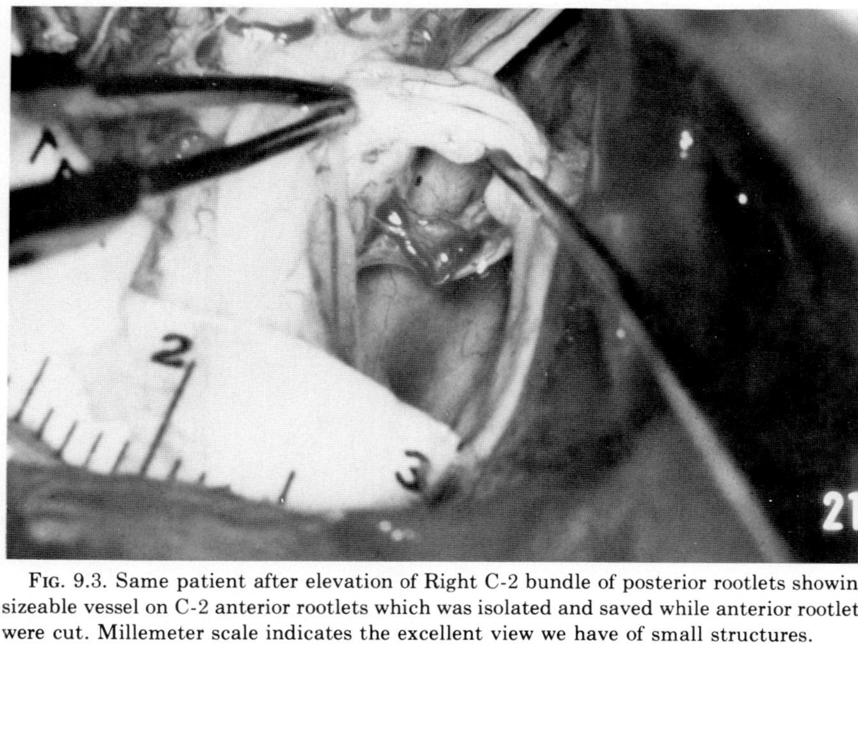

FIG. 9.3. Same patient after elevation of Right C-2 bundle of posterior rootlets showing sizeable vessel on C-2 anterior rootlets which was isolated and saved while anterior rootlets were cut. Millemeter scale indicates the excellent view we have of small structures.

which has come into view as the posterior root is not elevated. Figure 9.4 shows a smaller vessel on the right C-1 anterior rootlets which we also saved while cutting the root. In Figure 9.5 there was a larger vessel with the left C-1 anterior rootlet on the left side which was again saved. However, on the left, one also sees the anterior lateral end of the C-2 anterior root on which is a tinier vessel of the size that we are never able to save. My point to the jury was that this is the typical view we have at operation and the control of our dissection we are able to achieve under magnified vision. We and the jury witnessed the tragic fact of a young man who had none of these vessels of modest size on his uppermost anterior rootlets, much less the normal complex of three huge arteries nourishing the brachial plexus enlargement of the cord. Before I went on the witness stand, the two lawyers for my defense made it clear to me that the burden rested squarely on my shoulders and that if I could not persuade the jurors, if I could not give an effective tutorial to the jury on this set of medical facts, my case was lost. The plaintiff's attorney rested his case by dramatically demonstrating the pathetic figure stripped to the waist with a pair of spindly flail arms unable to take care of even his needs at toilet.

The evening after this dramatic scene my own personal council

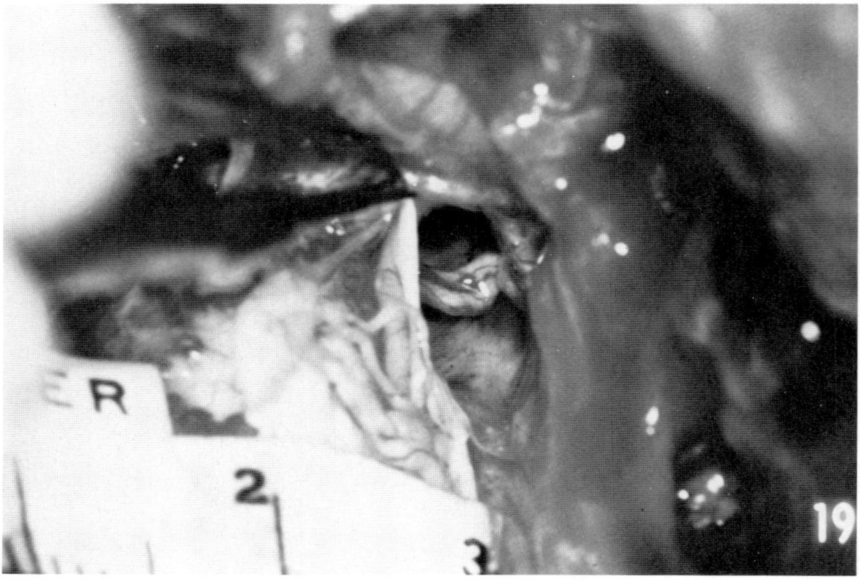

FIG. 9.4. Same patient after elevation of Right C-1 small posterior rootlet bundle on dentate ligament showing a smaller vessel on C-1 anterior rootlets which could also be saved while the rootlets were cut.

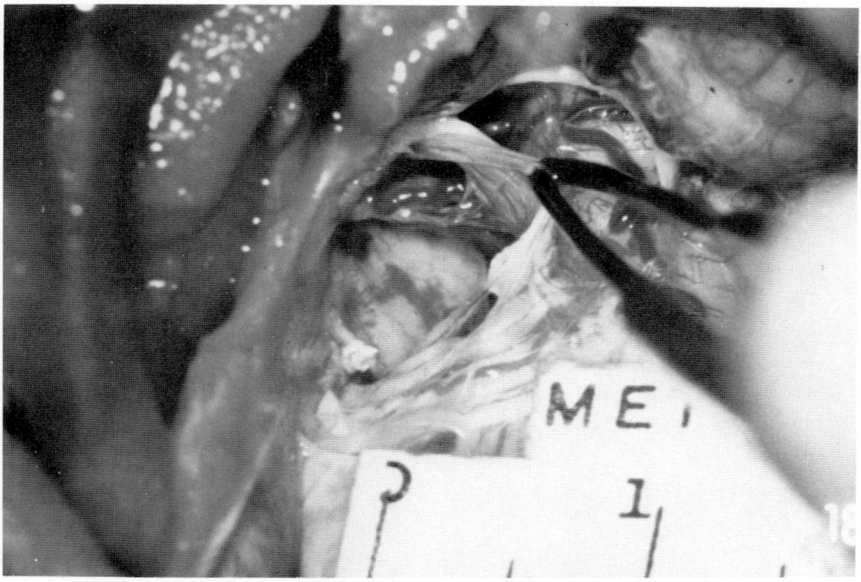

FIG. 9.5. Same patient after elevation of Left C-1 posterior rootlet bundle showing a large vessel on C-1 anterior rootlets; this too was saved while the rootlets were cut.

strongly urged me to settle the case without further trial for up to $140,000. I refused to accept his advice. The trial was completed and the verdict was for the defense. In 1967 the net financial result of this was that my annual malpractice insurance premium dropped to some hundreds of dollars from the thousands of dollars to which it had risen when my original insurance company cancelled my coverage while this case was pending against me.

With the present annual premiums at tens of thousands of dollars for neurosurgeons, I doubt that there is going to be a useful substitute for winning the case at the showdown. Although my colleagues and I are under no illusions that we have any special skills in defending ourselves in the court room, we are convinced that we must undertake such defense after tremendous preparation and with the determination to grapple with this problem by meeting it head on. Settling out of court or during the trial in an action in which there was no professional negligence only invites a massive proliferation of such suits.

ACKNOWLEDGMENT

It is a pleasure to acknowledge the generosity of the Congress of Neurological Surgeons in allowing me such a full opportunity to amplify my thoughts in print on all 6 of my subjects as contrasted with the more limited spoken presentations.

I have a special debt to Mrs. Deborah Norton whose intensive assiduous follow-up of the patients and unflagging energy in retyping the multiple drafts of these 6 manuscripts have finally yielded results fairly satisfactory to both of us.

This work was supported in part by the Neuro-Research Foundation.

REFERENCE

1. Penzholz, H., Menzel, J., and Hagenlocher, H. J.: Results of surgical treatment of idiopathic trigeminal neuralgia using different operative techniques (a cooperative study). Adv. Neurosurg., *3:* 320–327, 1975.

CHAPTER

10

Hematological and Vascular Concepts in Relation to Stroke*

Paul Didisheim, M.D, and **Valentin Fuster, M.D.**

INTRODUCTION

Stroke may be defined as a permanent or protracted loss or impairment of neurological function resulting from ischemia of a portion of the brain. Ischemia from extrinsic conditions such as occlusion of an artery by pressure from an extravascular mass is extremely rare. We will consider in this review only the causes of stroke related to intrinsic abnormalities in the blood or blood vessels.

In the mid-1800's Virchow described a triad of changes which predispose to thrombosis. These are changes in the blood, changes in the vessel wall, and stasis. Virchow's triad is still a useful point of departure in considering the mechanisms of *thromboembolism*. Recently acquired knowledge has allowed us to be more specific regarding each component of the triad. Changes in the blood may now be subdivided into coagulation, fibrinolytic, and platelet abnormalities. Changes in the vessel wall may be congenital, proliferative, or ulcerative. Stasis now encompasses turbulence, vortex formation, and the rheological properties of blood and its components. Abnormalities in these mechanisms may result not only in thrombosis but also in hemorrhage.

Hemostasis depends upon a triad as well. Hemostasis is the complex set of mechanisms which operate to prevent bleeding; it is dependent upon the integrity of the vasculature, the normal function of the plasma coagulation system, and the presence of platelets in normal numbers and functions. Following a vascular injury, interaction of these processes leads to the formation of the hemostatic plug. The hemostatic plug is merely a thrombus which seals a vascular leak rather than occluding or stenosing a vascular lumen. The structure and mechanisms of formation of a hemostatic plug and of a thrombus are similar.

Thrombi may be classified into three types according to their distribution: arterial, venous, and disseminated. Fibrin deposition is common to all three, serving as a consolidating meshwork holding the

* Supported by National Institutes of Health Grants NS 6663 and HL 17443

cellular elements together. However, in arterial thromboembolism platelets occupy a prominent role, resulting in a "white thrombus," whereas in venous thrombosis, occurring in a comparatively slow flow system, the blood elements are distributed according to their occurrence in flowing blood, producing a "red thrombus." In disseminated intravascular coagulation (DIC), platelet-fibrin thrombi are scattered in multiple sites but are usually primarily limited to the microvasculature.

Atherosclerosis is influenced in its genesis by local stresses (fluid, mechanical, or chemical), permeability, the lipids in plasma, and perhaps factors in platelets.

FACTORS INFLUENCING THE GROWTH AND FATE OF THROMBI

We will now review the elements of Virchow's triad in modern terms. These will be considered under the headings of blood rheology and flow, blood coagulation, fibrinolysis, the role of platelets, and interaction of factors.

Blood Rheology and Flow

Blood is a non-Newtonian fluid: unlike water, the viscosity of blood increases as its flow velocity decreases. The practical implication of this fact is clear: failure to maintain high flow velocity will result in increased viscosity, thereby enhancing the risk of stasis and coagulation. Red cells contribute more than plasma to the viscosity of blood. The relation of hematocrit to viscosity is continuous over the hematocrit range of 0 to 70 but is not linear: viscosity increases at an accelerated rate especially above a hematocrit of 50 (50). Elevated blood viscosity has been observed in some patients with stroke (36). Whether such an abnormality is a significant risk factor influencing either the incidence or natural history of stroke is not clear. Red cell deformability affects viscosity. The high frequency of vascular occlusion in patients with spherocytosis or sickle cell anemia is attributable to the reduced deformability of the red cells in these conditions. Abnormalities of plasma proteins (macroglobulinemia, multiple myeloma) can contribute to elevated viscosity of whole blood and to the so-called "hyperviscosity syndromes" (29), which can be relieved rapidly by plasmapheresis.

As already stated, arterial thrombi contain more platelets than do venous thrombi. Histologically, venous thrombi resemble blood which has been allowed to clot in a test tube. This difference is probably due to a physical effect of red blood cells (RBC). Under conditions of high shear rate (as in arteries), the complex motions of RBC increase the frequency of collision of platelets with the vessel wall where they then interact with surface abnormalities, adhere, and aggregate, and thus participate in thrombogenesis. In veins where the shear rate is lower, these forces are not so prominent. By contrast, high shear rates oppose RBC deposition on vessel walls, accounting for the relative paucity of RBC in arterial thrombi as compared with venous thrombi.

As blood flows past a stenotic area and enters a dilated segment, vortices form, resulting in the rotary motion of cells in a restricted area for prolonged periods of time. Perhaps such conditions lead to the injury of cells or the accumulation of "activation" products which then contribute to thrombogenesis in such locations. In any event, thrombosis on normal endothelial surfaces is commonly seen in venous valve pockets (47), perhaps as a consequence of this kind of flow pattern.

Shear stress can injure cells (5). Injured platelets release various components which include serotonin and nucleotides such as ADP. ADP may then induce the platelet aggregation that is observed following exposure to shear stress. The stresses required to produce ADP release from platelets can exist in patients with prosthetic cardiovascular devices. It may be that a similar mechanism is responsible for the formation of platelet-fibrin thrombi embolizing from an ulcerated atherosclerotic plaque in a carotid artery. The kinetics of certain plasma coagulation factor reactions are also influenced by fluid shear (48).

It is of interest that the sites of maximal turbulence in the systemic arterial circulation are the sites of predilection for atherosclerosis. This relationship will be discussed in further detail in the section on Etiologies of Atherogenesis.

Blood Coagulation

The final product of the reactions comprising the blood coagulation mechanism is fibrin. Fibrin is an essential component of all thrombi. It follows that if fibrin formation can be completely prevented, thrombosis cannot occur. This is the rationale for the use of anticoagulants. Heparin, once thought to interfere only with thrombin's action on fibrinogen, now appears to have multiple actions on the coagulation mechanism. It activates normally present antithrombin, which neutralizes thrombin by forming a thrombin-antithrombin complex. It also accelerates the neutralization by antithrombin of several activated coagulation factors in the coagulation sequence. These include factors IXa, Xa, XIa, and perhaps all the other serine proteases of the clotting mechanism as well (41). Coumarin-like oral anticoagulants inhibit blood coagulation by blocking hepatic synthesis of four coagulation factors: prothrombin (II) and factors VII (stable), IX (Christmas; plasma thromboplastin component), and X (Stuart). Recent evidence suggests that these drugs may lead to the production by the liver of abnormal protein molecules which are immunologically related to the above four clotting factors, but which lack their coagulant activities (26).

The classical blood coagulation theory of Morawitz, published in 1905, contained only two steps: (1) prothrombin, the plasma precursor of thrombin, is converted to thrombin by thromboplastin (tissue extract) in the presence of ionized calcium; and (2) fibrinogen, the plasma precursor of fibrin, is converted to fibrin by thrombin. An over-simplified description of blood coagulation today is that it involves the sequential activation of at least ten inactive plasma protein precursors into biologically active coagulation factors. The sequence is believed to be as follows: XII (Hageman), XI (plasma thromboplastin antecedent), IX, VIII (antihemophilic), X, V (labile), prothrombin, fibrinogen, and XIII (fibrin stabilizing). Calcium ions are required for a number of these steps; phospholipid (platelets serve as a source) plays a role at several stages. Factor VII occupies a unique role: it is not required for the "intrinsic" coagulation of blood (without addition of factors not normally present in blood), but is essential in the "extrinsic" coagulation mechanism (in the presence of tissue thromboplastin, as in the performance of the prothrombin time). Factor XIII is required for cross linkage of fibrin molecules; in its absence, fibrin is formed but is unstable. Evidently each of these coagulation factors (except XII) is essential for normal hemostasis, since patients deficient in any one of them (except XII) are prone to bleed excessively when subjected to significant injury or surgery.

Whether "hypercoagulability" plays a role in stroke is not clear. Several reports (40, 51) indicate that a spectrum of coagulation abnormalities exists in the blood of patients with thrombotic stroke. These include shortened activated partial thromboplastin test (APTT) and glass and silicone-clotting times, elevations of platelet count, fibrinogen and soluble fibrin, accelerated thromboplastin generation, and reductions in plasminogen activator and heparin tolerance. Since these measurements were made on the blood of patients with completed thrombotic stroke, the relevance of these observations to the etiology of stroke is not certain. Whether these abnormalities are correlated with survival or with recurrence of stroke also is not clear.

Fibrinolysis

Normal blood contains a fibrinolytic mechanism which, like the coagulation mechanism, is normally quiescent but is activated by various stimuli. Normal plasma contains an inactive protein precursor of the fibrinolytic enzyme called plasminogen or profibrinolysin. Plasminogen is converted to active plasmin (fibrinolysin) by activators in bacteria (such as streptokinase), tissues (particularly vessel walls), and urine (urokinase). Plasmin splits fibrinogen (or fibrin) into a series of fibrinopeptides which exert varying inhibitory effects on coagulation and platelet functions. Plasma also contains at least two inhibitors of plasmin (antiplasmins). The heightened fibrinolytic activity of the blood which is seen with emotional stress or surgery is usually short lived and of no clinical consequence. The normal fibrinolytic mechanism may contribute to the dissolution of certain types of clinical thromboemboli. Fibrinolytic activity may become clinically significant and contribute to major hemorrhage when it is associated with disseminated intravascular coagulation (DIC). We have named this clinical-laboratory constellation the intravascular coagulation-fibrinolysis (ICF) syndrome (37). It may be acute or chronic and may be associated with surgery, obstetrical complications, malignancies, infections, and a group of miscellaneous disorders. The fibrinolytic component of the syndrome is probably in response to the DIC. Clinically significant primary fibrinolysis is extremely rare. For these reasons, it seems unwise to administer inhibitors of plasminogen activation such as epsilon aminocaproic acid (EACA, Amicar, Lederle Laboratories, Pearl River, N.Y.) to bleeding patients who have enhanced fibrinolytic activity. Occasionally, such treatment has been followed by acceleration of DIC with dire thromboembolic consequences. Fibrinolysis associated with DIC should be regarded as a protective response the interruption of which may allow the underlying DIC to proceed unchecked. The benefits and risks of EACA treatment of subarachnoid hemorrhage are the subject of current investigations.

Thrombolytic therapy of thrombotic stroke or other thromboembolic events with a fibrinolytic activator such as streptokinase or urokinase (14) is theoretically appealing, but it has a number of real and potential limitations: (1) Such treatment is unlikely to be of benefit unless it can be instituted within a few hours after the onset of the thrombotic episode; after that, fibrin becomes increasingly resistant to lysis. (2) Induction of a systemic fibrinolytic state entails an increased risk of bleeding. (3) Discontinuation of fibrinolytic therapy may be associated with recurrence of the underlying predisposition to thrombosis. (4) Streptokinase or urokinase is effective only intravenously and must be administered continuously or repeatedly every day. (5) Frequent laboratory monitoring of the patient's plasma fibrinolytic activity during therapy is advisable; but this requires specialized tests which are not widely available. (6) Finally, the use of streptokinase or urokinase as thrombolytic agents in the United States is currently limited to investigational protocols.

The Role of Platelets

Platelets, the smallest cells in the blood, occupy a vital role in the genesis of thrombosis and perhaps atherosclerosis as well, as will be discussed in the following sections. Platelets serve an essential role in preventing bleeding from small vessels: a reduction of platelet count to less than 20% of normal levels is commonly associated with bleeding. It has been suggested that platelets are continually utilized in a process of maintenance of vascular integrity. This hypothesis would explain the occurrence of petechiae in thrombocytopenic patients who deny any known trauma.

Platelets are discoid, 2 to 3 μ in diameter and about 0.5 μ thick. Immediately upon contact of platelets with glass or most other nonbiological surfaces, platelets undergo a dramatic sequence of responses which include change in shape from discoid to spheroid and the extension of pseudopods which attach to the surface. Elements in the vessel wall to which platelets adhere are collagen, noncollagenous microfibrils of elastic tissue (but not elastin itself), and, in small blood vessels, basement membrane. Certain surfaces such as collagen fibers and antigen-antibody complexes and certain compounds such as ADP, epinephrine, thrombin, arachidonic acid, and prostaglandin G_2 induce additional responses in the platelet which include complex changes in ultrastructure and a secretory process called the "release" reaction during which serotonin, ADP, ATP, and other constituents are released from platelets. The released ADP in turn causes platelets to aggregate to one another. Such aggregates form the nidus of a thrombus.

The precise mechanisms of this sequence of events are not clear. Prostaglandin metabolism has been implicated in the regulation of release and aggregation. Reaction of platelets with collagen, thrombin,or ADP leads to hydrolysis of arachidonic acid from platelet membrane phospholipid; arachidonic acid is then converted by a cyclo-oxygenase to a labile cyclic endoperoxide, which is a precursor of prostaglandins E_2 and $F_{2\alpha}$. This endoperoxide can directly induce release of ADP and serotonin from platelets. Aspirin inhibits the synthesis of this endoperoxide. This action is believed to be the mechanism by which aspirin inhibits ADP release and the platelet aggregation that follows release. Cyclic adenosine monophosphate (cAMP) may also play some regulatory role in release and aggregation. Elevation of platelet cAMP levels is associated with inhibition of platelet aggregation. Conversely, a fall in platelet cAMP is commonly observed as platelets aggregate. Comprehensive reviews of platelet physiology and pharmacology have appeared recently (34, 52).

Interaction of Factors

From the above discussion it can been seen that a number of forces interact in the pathogenesis of thrombosis. Factors in the circulating *blood* include elevated levels of coagulation factors or the presence of activated products, increased numbers of platelets (paradoxically, bleeding may occur in essential thrombocythemia), and an imbalance in the fibrinolytic system with reduced plasminogen or activator or raised levels of inhibitors. Properties of blood which influence thrombogenesis due to altered *flow* are high hematocrit, presence of abnormal proteins or increased fibrinogen (contributing to increased blood viscosity), reduced red cell deformability, and slow flow and eddy formation which may contribute to accumulation of activated coagulation products. *Vascular* factors include any conditions resulting in interruption of the nonthrombogenic endothelial layer, permitting contact of circulating blood elements with subendothelial components, principally collagen.

It is commonly stated as a corollary to Virchow's triad that no one of these factors alone suffices to cause thrombotic occlusion of a major vessel. This is not strictly true. Experimentally, increased concentrations of coagulation factors, inhibition of fibrinolysis, or even induction of stasis will not by itself cause the formation of a thrombus. However, vascular injury to a localized region of the vessel wall alone suffices to initiate the thrombotic process. At the site of injury, cellular elements accumulate. These are mostly platelets; little fibrin is deposited (11). If a larger vascular surface is denuded of endothelium (*e.g.*, in endarterectomy of cat carotid arteries), thrombotic occlusion regularly occurs (39). Whether a vessel occludes following vascular injury depends upon such factors as the extent of endothelial surface area which has been altered, the nature and severity of the endothelial abnormality (*e.g.*, ulcerated atherosclerotic plaque vs. fatty streak), the effect of the abnormality on the pattern of blood flow (*e.g.*, local eddies or high rate of shear), the diameter of the vascular lumen, and the blood flow rate.

By considering all of these factors together, one may arrive at the following concept of the mechanism of transient ischemic attacks (TIA's). At a site of vascular irregularity such as an ulcerated atherosclerotic plaque in a carotid artery, a number of conditions may exist which favor the formation of platelet-fibrin thrombi. High local rates of shear, turbulent flow, and access of blood to subendothelial collagen, tissue thromboplastin, and plaque lipids provide the environment in which platelet adhesion, release, aggregation, and fibrin formation can all occur. Flow forces cause the resulting thrombi to embolize periodically, briefly interrupting cerebral blood flow locally, giving rise to the symptoms observed. The transient nature of the attacks may be due to the fragmentation of the thrombotic mass in the small intracerebral arteries in which they lodge by processes which include fibrinolysis and platelet disaggregation. It is of interest that platelet aggregates, perhaps remnants of the platelet-fibrin thrombi, have been observed in the circulating blood of patients with TIA's (55).

ETIOLOGIES OF ATHEROGENESIS

Despite widespread recognition of the importance of atherosclerosis, relatively little is known about the cellular mechanisms associated with its production. Most studies have concentrated upon the importance of extracellular factors such as plasma lipids, elevated blood pressure, and smoking habits, all of which tend to be associated with increased incidence of atherosclerosis and hence are thought to influence the development of the disease (2). One of the most critical areas in atherosclerosis is the nature of the interaction of the arterial wall with blood elements, particularly platelets, and lipoproteins, in the early steps of atherosclerotic plaque formation.

Smooth Muscle Proliferation

The sequential ultrastructural changes in spontaneous atherosclerosis, particularly of the early lesions, have recently been clarified by the groups of Haust and More (24), McGill (30), Knierem and Wissler (28), and the group in Albany (8) who by light and electron microscopy and different histochemical techniques studied the atherosclerotic lesions in patients dying at various ages. It is now widely accepted that the earliest microscopically detectable lesion of atherosclerosis is an intimal proliferation of smooth muscle cells mainly at branch points in arteries (3). Initially these cells proliferate when no free fat is demonstrable in the cells or in the intercellular tissues (25). With advance of the lesion, free fat frequently appears in intimal cells and later in the intercellular space (25) while the "fatty streak" becomes macroscopically apparent. The further progress of the lesion is characterized by abundant intimal fibrous tissue or "fibrous plaque" which can progress into "complicated lesions" when ulceration, hemorrhage, thrombosis or calcification develops (31).

Because of the recent accepted concept that proliferation of smooth muscle cells mainly at branch points in arteries is associated with the genesis of the early atherosclerotic lesions, investigations in recent years have placed major emphasis on studying the causes of this local smooth muscle proliferative response, its relation to the properties of the endothelial cells and hemodynamic stress at the branch points, to the lipid deposition and to the interaction of the arterial wall and blood elements.

Lipid Deposition

Recent evidence from *in vivo* (45) and *in vitro* (42) studies suggests that the smooth muscle cell is responsible for the synthesis of collagen and elastic fiber proteins. However, the origin of the lipid material in the lesion is unclear. Morphological studies of spontaneous atherosclerosis in humans (21) and in atherosclerosis induced by injury (32) suggest that both smooth muscle cells and macrophages are the precursors of the foam cells which contain most of the lipid material in atherosclerotic plaques. Various blood cells have been implicated as sources of macrophagic elements, but direct evidence is lacking. Studies of the composition of lipids in atherosclerotic lesions have shown a striking similarity between spontaneous atherosclerosis in humans (9) and animals (46) and atherosclerosis induced by injury (4).

Endothelial Cells and Hemodynamic Stress

The aortic branch points and other areas where atherosclerotic plaques usually develop have been shown to be sites of increased endothelial damage. Packham and associates (38) and Jørgensen and associates (27), using ^{131}I albumin and Evans blue in young rabbits and pigs, demonstrated an increased passage of proteins into those areas before the atherosclerotic lesions develop. In the same arterial sites, Bjorkerud and Bonjers (4), by supravital dye exclusion, demonstrated that the endothelial cells were devitalized, Wright (54) found increased mitotic activity, and Caplan and Schwartz (6) showed increased endothelial cell turnover. These observations indicate that there may be increased endothelial injury and continuous replacement at those sites where atherosclerotic lesions develop. Furthermore, studies by transmission and scanning electron microscopy in these arterial sites showed endothelial cell shape changes and gaps between the endothelial cells suggestive of damage (6).

There is now increasing evidence that hemodynamic and rheological mechanisms are the primary factors in causing a focal and continuous vascular injury (15). Wesolowski and associates (53), from experiments using hydraulic models of various flow patterns, predicted by the site of maximal turbulence the areas of predilection for the occurrence of atherosclerosis within the human arterial tree. The concept that atherosclerosis is a local response to continuous endothelial injury has recently received further support since experimental intimal injury, without disruption of the internal elastica lamina, which imitates the physiological mechanical injury due to hemodynamic factors, reproduces the full spectrum of early atherosclerotic lesions (49). In such experiments one of the first structural changes, as in spontaneous atherosclerosis, is an intimal proliferation of smooth muscle cells which presumably derive from the media of the artery (43).

Platelet Interaction with the Arterial Wall

In the development of atherosclerosis, hemodynamic factors with endothelial injury and smooth muscle cell proliferation appear to play an important role in the development of the disease. Recently, studies suggest that platelets, by interaction with the arterial wall, may be involved in such early stages of the disease. Examination of the endothelial surface of aortas of pigs, rabbits and mice, and young humans who died suddenly (27) showed clumps of formed elements, mainly platelets and leukocytes, on the surface of the endothelium about those sites where atherosclerosis develops.

In experimental atherosclerosis induced by chronic endothelial injury, one of the first morphological events is the appearance of platelets undergoing intracytoplasmic degranulation and adhering to the endothelial surface and subendothelial denuded areas. This precedes the migration and proliferation of smooth muscle cells (49).

A recent important finding by Ross and associates (44) was that a substance derived from platelets was necessary for the proliferation of smooth muscle cells in culture. Serum derived from platelet poor plasma did not support smooth muscle cell growth in culture. When isolated platelets were incubated in the presence of thrombin, a heat stable dialyzable substance was derived which, when added to plasma, would substitute for whole platelets in the process of initiating smooth muscle cell growth in culture. Some of the known physicochemical characteristics of this substance indicate that it may be platelet factor 4, a platelet-heat-stable protein with antiheparin activity which is released into the plasma when platelet aggregation or destruction occurs and is therefore present in high concentration in normal serum (18).

A possible role of platelet factor 4 in the development of atherosclerosis has been recently suggested by the reports of O'Brien and associates (35). Furthermore, Fuster and associates have done extensive studies on the kinetics of platelet factor 4 (17, 18, 20) which they have recently measured (19) in White Carneau atherosclerotic pigeons in collaboration with B. A. Kottke. This species is known to develop spontaneous aortic atherosclerotic lesions similar to those observed in humans. The first lesions appear grossly when the birds are 1 year old, all of the birds having lesions by age 3 (7). Sequential studies in these birds showed a progressive elevation of platelet factor 4-like activity in serum after the age of 6 months, with elevated levels persisting at 3 years of age. In the Show Racer species of pigeons which do not develop spontaneous atherosclerotic lesions (7), serum platelet factor 4-like activity fell progressively from the age of 6 months, persisting at a low level at 3 years. These studies suggest that platelet factor 4 may be involved in the pathogenesis of atherosclerosis.

Insight into the significance of the role played by platelets in the initiation of atherosclerosis would be gained by a biological approach, investigating whether experimental animals or humans with inhibited platelet function are resistant to the development of atherosclerosis. For several years a colony of pigs with all the characteristics of human von Willebrand's disease have been maintained in Rochester at Mayo Institute Hills farm. In order to evaluate whether such von Willebrand pigs with impaired platelet function are less prone to the development of spontaneous atherosclerosis than normal control pigs, in collaboration with E. J. W. Bowie, Fuster initiated a detailed pathological study (16) of the aortas from normal pigs and the pigs with von Willebrand's disease. Both groups of pigs were 1 to 3 years of age, were of the same breed, and were rigidly matched by heart weight. Of the 11 normal pigs, six showed multiple arteriosclerotic plaques. In contrast, none of the von Willebrand pigs had multiple plaques.

PLATELET INHIBITORS AND STROKE

Platelet adhesion and aggregation are not prevented by heparin, or by warfarin, or related oral anticoagulants given in therapeutic doses. The partial protective effect exerted by these drugs in patients with arterial thromboembolic disease is probably due to prevention of the formation of fibrin that maintains the stability of the thrombus. Recent studies in experimental animals have shown that aspirin does not prevent platelet adherence to a damaged endothelial surface but does prevent the subsequent platelet aggregation. The mechanisms whereby dipyridamole and sulfinpyrazone exert their beneficial effect in the treatment of arterial thromboembolism are not clearly understood.

Harrison and colleagues (23), over a five-month study of a patient with multiple TIA's, reported a significant reduction in the number of attacks during treatment with aspirin, 600 mg. 4 times daily. Mundall and associates (33) reported a patient with recurrent episodes of transient monocular blindness associated with increased platelet aggregability and thrombocytosis (740,000 platelets/μl). The patient's platelets in anticoagulated blood aggregated spontaneously without the addition of any aggregating agent. During two episodes of left monocular blindness, multiple dull yellow emboli were observed moving along the left retinal arterioles. While receiving aspirin, 600 mg. by mouth every 6 hours, the episodes ceased and platelet aggregation returned to normal. On aspirin, she remained symptom free for a 5-month follow-up period.

Further support for the beneficial effect of aspirin in patients with TIA's is found in the retrospective study reported by Dyken and associates in 1973 (12). They reported 26 patients with TIA's; 15 were treated with aspirin, 600 mg. daily, and 11 were not. Only 13% of those treated with aspirin had an additional attack compared to 82% of those who had no aspirin.

Evans in 1972 (13) carried out a double-blind crossover study in which each of 20 patients with TIA's in the form of transient blindness or amaurosis fugax received either sulfinpyrazone, 200 mg. 4 times daily, or an identical appearing placebo. At 6 weeks both groups of patients were crossed over to the alternate therapy for a further 6 weeks. There was a marked reduction in the number of attacks in the patients during the sulfinpyrazone treatment period when compared with the placebo or control pretrial period.

The beneficial effect reported for aspirin and sulfinpyrazone on the natural history of transient cerebral ischemia has now led to the design of two large multicenter trials, one in Canada (22) and another in the United States, with the objective to determine whether aspirin, sulfinpyrazone, or both drugs together are effective in reducing the number of subsequent cerebral ischemic attacks, in preventing strokes, and in increasing survival. In these two large trials, dipyridamole is not being investigated, presumably because in a well controlled study reported by Acheson in 1969 (1) this drug when used alone did not affect the natural history of cerebrovascular disease. However, it would seem reasonable to test the effectiveness of a combination of dipyridamole and aspirin on the incidence of stroke and on survival in patients with transient cerebral ischemia.

The rationale and results of therapeutic trials with inhibitors of platelet functions in the management of various thromboembolic disorders have been recently reviewed (10).

SUMMARY

This review has highlighted some of the factors which influence the formation and fate of thrombi. Rheology and flow, the coagulation mechanism, the fibrinolytic enzyme system, and the properties of platelets to adhere and aggregate all play a significant role. Of paramount importance to neurosurgeons is the role of the vascular wall in thrombogenesis. The ulcerated atherosclerotic plaque demonstrates this point. Factors contributing to thromboembolism in this setting include stenosis and reduced flow, turbulence, and the elements in the lesion with which blood interacts. These are principally collagen, ADP, fatty acids, and the thromboplastic activity of vascular subendothelial tissue.

Current concepts of the etiologies of atherosclerosis were discussed. Along with other predisposing factors, platelets may play a significant role in the initiation of the process. The current status of clinical trials with inhibitors of platelet function in the treatment of cerebrovascular disorders was reviewed.

In vascular reconstructive surgery, the principles which underlie good technique are those which best insure against thrombosis. The briefest possible period of stasis during surgery should be maintained. The reconstruction should result in a smooth blood flow pattern with rapid runoff and minimal stenosis or gaps between apposed endothelial surfaces.

ACKNOWLEDGEMENTS

V. F. Fairbanks, E. F. Grabowski, F. J. Kazmier, E. R. Laws and T. M. Sundt, Jr. made valuable suggestions in the preparation of this manuscript.

REFERENCES

1. Acheson, J., Danta, G., and Hutchinson, E. C. Controlled trial of dipyridamole in cerebral vascular disease. Br. Med. J., *1:* 614–615, 1969.
2. Atherosclerosis and epidemiology study groups. Primary prevention of the atherosclerotic diseases. Circulation, *42:* A55–A95, 1970.
3. Atherosclerosis. Publication No. 72-219. National Heart and Lung Institute Task Force on Arteriosclerosis. Department of Health, Education and Welfare, Washington, D.C., 1971.
4. Bjorkerud, S., and Bondjers, G. Endothelial integrity and viability in the aorta of the normal rabbit and rat as evaluated with dye exclusion tests and interference contrast microscopy. Atheroscerosis *15:* 285–300, 1972.
5. Brown, III, C. H., Leverett, L. B., Lewis, C. W., Alfrey, C. P., and Hellums, J. C. Morphological, biochemical and functional changes of human platelets subjected to shear stress. J. Lab. Clin. Med., *86:* 462–471, 1975.
6. Caplan, B. A., and Schwartz, C. J. Increased endothelial cell turnover in areas of *in vivo* Evans Blue uptake in the pig aorta. Atherosclerosis, *17:* 401–417, 1973.
7. Clarkson, T. B., Prichard, R. W., Netsky, M. G., and Lofland, H. B. Atherosclerosis in pigeons. Its occurrence and resemblance to human atherosclerosis. Arch. Pathol., *68:* 143–147, 1959.
8. Daoud, A., Jarmolych, J., Zumbo, A., Fani K., and Florentin, R. "Preatheroma" phase of coronary atherosclerosis in man. Exp. Mol. Pathol., *3:* 475–484, 1964.
9. Day, A. J. Lipid metabolism by macrophages and its relationship to atherosclerosis. Adv. Lipid Res., *5:* 185–207, 1968.
10. Didisheim, P., Kazmier, F. J., and Fuster, V. Platelet inhibition in the management of thrombosis. Thromb. Diath. Haemorrh., *32:* 21–34, 1974.
11. Duval, D. L., Didisheim, P., Titus, J. L., Spittell, Jr., J. A. and Owen, Jr., C. A. Experimental arterial thrombosis: description of a method. Mayo Clin. Proc., *45:* 388–395, 1970.
12. Dyken, M. L., Kolar, O. J., and Jones, F. H. Differences in the occurrence of carotid transient ischemic attacks associated with antiplatelet aggregation therapy. Stroke, *4:* 732–736, 1973.

13. Evans G. Effect of platelet-suppressive agents on the incidence of amaurosis fugax and transient cerebral ischemia. *In* Cerebral Vascular Diseases: Transactions of the Eighth Conference, edited by F. H. McDowell and R. W. Brennan, pp. 297–299. Grune and Stratton, New York, 1973.
14. Fletcher, A. P. Current status of thrombolytic agents in acute cerebrovascular disease. J. Clin. Pathol., *25:* 649–650, 1972.
15. Fry, D. L. Certain chemorheologic considerations regarding the blood vascular interface with particular reference to coronary artery disease. Circulation *39-40* (Suppl. IV): 38–59, 1969.
16. Fuster, V., Bowie, E. J. W., and Brown, A. L. Spontaneous arterial lesions in normal pigs and pigs with Von Willebrand's disease. Proceedings of International Workshop–Conference on Atherosclerosis. London, Ontario, Canada, in press, 1976.
17. Fuster, V., Bowie, E. J. W., Kazmier, F. J., and Owen, Jr., C. A. Platelet factor 4-like activity reflecting rate of platelet consumption in chronically induced intravascular coagulation in dogs. Thromb. Res., *4:* 247–260, 1974.
18. Fuster, V., Kazmier, F. J., Cash, J. D., Bowie, E. J. W., and Owen, Jr., C. A. Assay of Platelet factor 4 in plasma. Mayo Clin. Proc., *48:* 103–106, 1973.
19. Fuster, V., Kottke, B. A., Ruiz, C. E., Lewis, J. C., and Bowie, E. J. W. Increase in platelet factor 4-like activity in the initial stages of atherosclerosis in pigeons. Proceedings of International Workshop–Conference on Atherosclerosis. London, Ontario, Canada, in press, 1976.
20. Fuster, V., Owen, Jr., C. A., and Pintado, T. Platelet kinetics and the effect of aspirin in chronically induced intravascular coagulation in dogs. Thromb. Diath. Haemorrh. (Suppl.), *60:* 371–376, 1974.
21. Geer, J. C. Fine structure of human aortic intimal thickening and fatty streaks. Lab. Invest., *14:* 1764–1783, 1965.
22. Gent, M. Platelet inhibitor therapy in cerebrovascular disease. Thromb. Diath. Haemorrh. (Suppl.), *60:* 509–516, 1974.
23. Harrison, M. J. G., Marshall, J., Meadows, J. C., and Russell, R. W. R. Effect of aspirin in amaurosis fugax. Lancet, *2:* 743–744, 1971.
24. Haust, M. D. The morphogenesis and fate of potential and early atherosclerotic lesion in man. Hum. Pathol., *2:* 1–29, 1971.
25. Haust, M. D., and Moore, R. H. Significance of the smooth muscle cell in atherogenesis. *In* Evolution of the Atherosclerotic Plaque, edited by R. J. Jones, pp. of blood clotting enzymes. III. Demonstration of an inhibitor of prothrombin 51–63. The University of Chicago Press, Chicago, 1963.
26. Hemker, H. C., Veltkamp, J. J., and Loeliger, E. A. Kinetic aspects of the interaction of blood clotting enzymes. III. Demonstration of an inhibitor of prothrombin conversion in vitamin K deficiency. Thromb. Diath. Haemorrh., *19:* 346–363, 1968.
27. Jørgensen, L., Packham, M. A., Rowsell, H. C., and Mustard, J. F. Deposition of formed elements of blood on the intima and signs of initial injury in the aorta of rabbit, pig and man. Lab. Invest., *27:* 341–350, 1972.
28. Knierem, H. J., Kao, V. C. Y., and Wissler, R. W. Demonstration of smooth muscle cells in bovine arteriosclerosis. J. Athero. Res., *8:* 125–136, 1968.
29. MacKenzie, M. R., and Babcock, J. Studies of the hyperviscosity syndrome. II. Macroglobulinemia. J. Lab. Clin. Med., *85:* 227–234, 1975.
30. McGill, H. C., and Geer, J. C. The human lesion, fine structure. *In* Evolution of the Atherosclerotic Plaque, edited by R. J. Jones, pp. 65–67. The University of Chicago Press, Chicago, 1963.
31. Mitchell, J. R. A., and Schwartz, C. J. Arterial Disease 411 pp. F. A. Davis Co., Philadelphia, 1965.
32. Moore, S. Thromboatherosclerosis in normolipemic rabbits. A result of continued

endothelial damage. Lab. Invest., *29:* 478–487, 1973.

33. Mundall, J., Quintero, P., von Kaulla, K., Harman, R., and Austin, J. Transient monocular blindness and increased platelet aggregability treated with aspirin–a case report. Neurology, *22:* 280–285, 1972.
34. Mustard, J. F., and Packham, M. A.: Platelets, thrombosis and drugs. Drugs, *9:* 19–76, 1975.
35. O'Brien, J. R., Etherington, M., Jamieson, S., and Lawford, P. Heparin thrombin clotting-time and platelet factor 4. Lancet, *2:* 656–657, 1974.
36. Ott, E. O., Lechner, H., and Aranibar, A. High blood viscosity syndrome in cerebral infarction. Stroke, *5:* 330–333, 1974.
37. Owen, Jr., C. A., Bowie, E. J. W., Didisheim, P., and Thompson, Jr., J. H. The Diagnosis of Bleeding Disorders, 300 pp. Little, Brown, Boston, 1969.
38. Packham, M. A., Rowsell, H. C., Jørgensen, L., and Mustard, J. F. Localized protein accumulation in the wall of the aorta. Exp. Mol. Pathol., *7:* 214–232, 1967.
39. Piepgras, D. G., Sundt, T. M., and Didisheim, P. Effect of anticoagulants and inhibitors of platelet aggregation on thrombotic occlusion of endarterectomized cat carotid arteries. Stroke, in press, 1976.
40. Pilgeram, L. O., Chee, A. N., and von dem Bussche, G. Evidence for abnormalities in clotting and thrombolysis as a risk factor for stroke. Stroke, *4:* 643–657, 1973.
41. Rosenberg, R. D. Heparin action (Editorial). Circulation, *49:* 603–605, 1974.
42. Ross, R. The smooth muscle cell. II. Growth of smooth muscle in culture and formation of elastic fibers. J. Cell Biol., *50:* 172–186, 1971.
43. Ross, R., and Glomset, J. Atherosclerosis and the arterial smooth muscle cell. Science, *180* 1332–1339, 1973.
44. Ross, R., Glomset, J., Kariya, B., and Harker, L. A. A platelet dependent serum factor that stimulates the proliferation of arterial smooth muscle cells *in vitro*. Proc. Natl. Acad. Sci., *71:* 1207–1210, 1974.
45. Ross, R., and Klebanoff, S. J. The smooth muscle cell. I. *In vivo* synthesis of connective tissue proteins. J. Cell Biol., *50:* 159–171, 1971.
46. St. Clair, R. W., Lofland, H. B., and Clarkson, T. B. Influence of atherosclerosis on the composition, synthesis and esterification of lipid in aortas of squirrel monkeys (Saimiri Scimrius). J. Atheroscler. Res., *10:* 193–206, 1969.
47. Sevitt, S. Pathology and pathogenesis of deep vein thrombosis. *In* Recent Advances in Thrombosis, edited by L. Poller, pp. 17–38. Churchill Livingstone, Edinburgh and London, 1973.
48. Spaeth, E. E., Roberts, G. W., Yadwadkar, S. R., Ng, P. K., and Jackson, C. M. The influence of fluid shear on the kinetics of blood coagulation reactions. Trans. Am. Soc. Artif. Intern. Organs, *19:* 179–187, 1973.
49. Stemerman, M. B., and Ross, R. Experimental arteriosclerosis. I. Fibrous plaque formation in primates, an electron microscope study. J. Exp. Med., *136:* 796–789, 1972.
50. Talbot, L., and Berger, S. A. Fluid-mechanical aspects of the human circulation Am. Sci., *62:* 671–682, 1974.
51. Todd, M., McDevitt, E., and McDowell, F. Stroke and blood coagulation. Stroke, *4:* 400–405, 1973.
52. Weiss, H. J. Platelet physiology and abnormalities of platelet function. N. Engl. J. Med., *293:* 531–541 and 580–588, 1975.
53. Wesolowski, S. A., Fries, C. C., Sabini, A. M., and Sawyer, P. N. The significance of turbulence in hemic systems and in the distribution of the atherosclerotic lesion. Surgery, *57:* 155–162, 1965.
54. Wright, H. P. Mitosis patterns in aortic endothelium. Atherosclerosis, *15:* 93–100, 1972.
55. Wu, K. K., and Hoak, J. C. Increased platelet aggregates in patients with transient ischemic attacks. Stroke, *6:* 521–524, 1975.

CHAPTER

11

Host—Dose—Time: A Concept for Atherosclerosis

JAMES C. ROBERTS, JR., M.D.

In the past 25 years, many facts have entered our medical knowledge of arteriosclerosis. First among these is the indisputable fact that there is some degree of atherosclerosis present in all Americans over the age of 16. The observations identifying this fact were first made by pathologists in the field such as Enos, Holmes and Beyer (6) in Korea. Their observations were complemented, extended, and correlated by academic pathology groups such as ours in Pittsburgh; (16, 18, 24) and they are now firmly supported by angiography (14). Every day thousands of angiograms in living, often asymptomatic, people, demonstrate significant lesions of atherosclerosis.

This endemic atherosclerosis starts at some unknown time in the artery in the intima and inner media in as yet unknown cells, cells which are probably related to smooth muscle cells. These first changes are invisible to the unaided eye and are reversible, as are many of the visible lesions which we will discuss. Some time after these changes, one may see small atheromata composed of plump, lipid rich cells which convert into fibrofatty, and then fibrous, plaques. Since we are active biological organisms, not merely slides in my laboratory, this process may repeat itself numerous times, appearing as a layered plaque with the microscopy ranging from the early changes, often only histochemically identifiable, through to a more advanced, visible lesion. This kind of plaque is a common occurrence. Subsequent to these continuing dynamic developments, changes which we call complications occur. Areas of hypoxia in the plaque lead to necrosis. This necrosis may lead to disruption of the delicate endothelium over the plaques. A hemorrhage may appear in the plaques. A thrombus may attach itself to the plaques. The plaque may excavate and embolize. The wall of the artery may be so weakened that it expands and an aneurysm appears. Every one of these changes may occur without clinical symptoms (16, 17).

There is a predictable pattern and a predictable timetable to the occurrence, localization, and focalization of these visible lesions (16, 18, 24). The first are in the heart and aorta and are observed in the teens and

20's. There is then a centrifugal spread so that by the 30's and 40's in North Americans some lesions are visible in all vessels including the cerebral and visceral arteries. This baseline atherosclerosis is the same atherosclerosis which causes disease. There is a time lag of about 20 years from pathologist observing to clinician talking with relatives. Not only do we see intracerebral atherosclerosis later than we see myocardial atherosclerosis (11), but we have some indirect proof from the halls of learning in Boston as is witnessed by the inclusion of a 45-year-old lady with cerebral atherosclerosis in the renowned "Stamp Collection" of the Cabot Clinical Pathological Conferences in the *New England Journal of Medicine* (20). This is indirect evidence because myocardial infarcts at the age of 45 are so common that the selectors of these Cabot cases ignore them.

While the pathologists were observing vessels, clinicians and epidemiologists were organizing and examining humans for prospective studies in the hope of discovering differences between those who would and those who would not demonstrate clinical evidence of atherosclerotic disease. The pioneering studies of Keys and his group on the middle-aged business and professional men in the upper Midwest were expanded to include entire towns, such as Framingham, Massachusetts and Tecumseh, Michigan; and finally counties, such as Evans County in Georgia (9).

From these clinical studies came recognition and appreciation of what are now known as "risk factors" for arteriosclerotic disease (9). These factors are, however, only factors, not necessarily cause or effect. The primary risk factors are hypercholesterolemia of over 250 mg./100 ml.; resting diastolic blood pressure of 90 mm. of mercury or more, and cigarettes (9). Other factors have also been introduced, but these three are the primary factors with which age studies are combined (23). If a group of men aged 30 to 40 have all three of these factors, in 10 years, this group will have 8 times the atherosclerotic catastrophes than a group of men similarly aged and socio-economically classed, without these factors (9). However, these data cannot be applied to any one patient. A recent report in the *British Heart Journal* collected 240 young men, under the age of 40, from around the world, with documented myocardial infarctions (5). Eleven per cent of these men had no risk factors. Unfortunately, their coronary arteries did not know this. At this time, a 50-year-old white male is in the cardiac care unit of the hospital with which I am associated with a documented myocardial infarct. He is of normal weight for his height; his triglycerides are low-normal (80 mg./100 ml.); his cholesterol is 180 mg./100 ml.; he does not smoke, and his blood pressure is 106/76!

These risk factors are also difficult to modify in this era. Aronow, in conjunction with the Long Beach Heart Association, reported that 11 months of intensive education changed the risk factors in 1800 men very little (3). However, the factors are of remarkable value in studying large groups of patients, and from them, we are learning.

When a physician makes an observation, two or more physicians shall develop a theory. This dictum must be engraved somewhere, and atherosclerosis is no exception. Over the past 25 years, we have had many theories advanced to explain the above and other observations (1, 2, 8–10, 12, 17, 22).

Among the theories which have been engendered, espoused, championed and/or shrilled about in the past 25 years are DIET: including too much sugar; too much refined sugar; too much fat; too much saturated fat; too much protein; too much animal protein; too much soft drinking water; too little unsaturated fat; too little vitamin C; too little vitamin D, and too little vitamin E; or the wrong kinds of any of the above. CIVILIZATION's indictments include usually too much of the following: carbon monoxide, smoking, nicotine, radiation, micro-organisms and their toxins, urban living, changing from rural to urban living, lack of physical activity, trace elements, such as chromium, manganese, cadmium, or not enough zinc and too much copper; and stress.

STRESS had been subdivided into reaction to stress; the kinds of stress such as the kind managers receive *vs.* the kind subordinates receive; and personality differences in handling the differing kinds of stress. Endogenous theories include race, genes (whatever that means), aging or senescence, thrombogenic changes including sludged blood, mechanical and hydraulic and gravitational factors, sex and anoxemia. Other theories include homocysteine and hyperhistidemia. As yet, no convincing evidence has been presented incriminating the low residue diet.

For every one of the above theories, reasonably intelligent human beings have reported apparently convincing (to them, at least) epidemiological, experimental, or clinical observations. "Each was partly in the right, and all of them were wrong (19)."

The Blind Men and the Elephant
It was six men of Indostan
To learning much inclined,
Who went to see the elephant
Tho' all of them were blind.
That each by observation
Could satisfy his mind.

The first approached the elephant
And happening to fall

Against his broad and sturdy side
At once began to bawl:
"God bless me, but the elephant
is nothing but a wall. "

The second, feeling of the tusk,
Cried: "Ho, what have we here?
So very round and smooth and sharp
To me 'tis mighty clear;
This wonder of an elephant
Is very like a spear."

The third approached the animal
And happening to take
The squirming trunk within his hands
Thus boldly up and spake:
"I see," quoth he,
"This elephant is very like a snake."

The fourth reached out his eager hand
And felt around the knee
"What this wondrous beast is like
Is mighty plain," quoth he:
"Tis clear enough the elephant,
Is very like a tree."

The fifth, who chanced to touch the ear.
Said, "Even the blindest man can tell
What this resembles most:
Deny the facts who can:
This marvel of an elephant
Is very like a fan."

The sixth no sooner had begun
About the beast to grope
Than seizing on the swinging tail
That fell within his scope,
"I see," quoth he,
"The elephant is very like a rope."

And so these men of Indostan
Disputed loud and long,
Each in his own opinion
Exceeding stiff and strong,
Though each was partly in the right
And all were in the wrong.

—John Godfrey Saxe (1875).

On the other hand, therapeutic generalities can be obtained from these theories. A reasonable diet; moderation in such enjoyable habits as cigarettes, whiskey, and wild women; physical fitness; and attempting to *enjoy* stress. Subsequent to symptoms, we should think of the anatomy of the arteries, the effects of hydraulics in this low pressure, pulsatile system, and search for obstructive lesions with a logical *modus operandi*.

At this time, I would like to introduce a concept, rather than a theory; a concept which attempts to incorporate the many theories, and which will degrade none of them. This concept is based on three variables: the HOST, the DOSE, and TIME.

The HOST is born with anatomic, biochemical, and neurological pathways. The HOST has variable ability to develop anatomic, biochemical, and neurological pathways. The DOSE is the factor or factors to which the HOST is exposed over TIME.

The HOST is a dynamic, biological, multidimensional organism; the DOSE is variable in quality and quantity; TIME is the element which allows HOST to react to DOSE.

In the anatomy of the HOST there may be small vessels, larger vessels, many vessels, fewer vessels. These vessels in the brain may appear or develop into tortuous or coiled arteries (7). In these vessels are hydraulic and mechanical factors. The biochemical parts of the HOST include appetite, ingestion, absorption, metabolism, storage, and excretion.

All exogenous factors may apply in the DOSE. Radiation, carbon monoxide, fats, carbohydrates, proteins, vitamins, vitamin inhibitors, chemicals, cigarettes, whiskey, and wild, wild women. Ethnic and demographic influences are pertinent through this portal, with special emphasis on diet. A significant part of our immoderate diet in this modern age of less needed physical activity is the old rural American diet of large meals for heavy workers. Exogenous calorie consumption is far greater than the usual caloric demand to perform a day's work.

I have used TIME instead of aging or senescence. I consider TIME as a lateral, passive constant, rather than as a vertical implication of degeneration.

Emphasis on the *host* may be credited to Sir William Osler, who said in 1892 (15):

> To a majority of men, death comes primarily or secondarily through this portal (of arteriosclerosis) . . . The onset of what may be called physiological arteriosclerosis depends in the first place upon the quality of arterial tissue (vital rubber) which the individual has inherited, and secondarily, upon the amount of wear and tear to which he has subjected it.

This concept can be used to skeptically analyze observations on etiology and treatment. This concept is also intended to appreciate therapy: the reaction of the HOST to DOSE over TIME.

Very exciting observations are emanating from Bassler (4) and the

American Medical Joggers Association, who have nearly 100,000-man years obtained from middle-aged males; those considered top risks for atherosclerotic catastrophes (23). They have yet to observe a fatal atherosclerotic catastrophe in anyone who has finished a marathon in under 6 hours. This observation may be sorted into the HOST, with elements of masochism; and the DOSE, since training for a marathon involved almost total redirection of life style: more and earlier sleep, fewer and lighter meals, fewer cigarettes, and less whiskey. I am advised that wild, wild women need not be eliminated.

Effective therapy for atherosclerosis over the past 25 years has been primarily a surgical bypass (21) or replacement of obstructed arteries (14). Pioneered by neurological and vascular surgeons, these efforts involve the HOST. Nonsurgical therapy involves the DOSE.

In the next 25 years, I hope that earlier detection and treatment of high risk people (13), without induction of hysteria, will be achieved. For this hope, more studies of intracranial atherosclerosis and correlation with DOSE and HOST are needed.

SUMMARY

Advances in knowledge about atherosclerosis in the past 25 years were discussed. Areas of disagreement and agreement were identified.

A concept of HOST-DOSE-TIME was introduced for the skeptical analysis of past, present, and future observation and treatment of atherosclerosis.

ACKNOWLEDGMENTS

Elizabeth Roberts, Catherine Roberts, John H. Bridge, and Joan Copeland helped in the generation of these thoughts.

REFERENCES

1. Altschul, R. Selected Studies on Atherosclerosis, 182 pp. Charles C Thomas, Springfield, Ill., 1950.
2. Altschule, M. D., Editor of Symposium on Atherosclerosis. Med. Clin. North Am., *58:* 243–462, 1974.
3. Aronow, W. S., Allen, W. H., De Cristofaro, D., and Ungermann, S. Follow-up of mass screening for coronary risk factors in 1817 adults. Circulation, *51:* 1038–1045, 1975.
4. Bassler, T. J. Personal communication. 1970, 1971, 1972, 1973; 1974, 1975.
5. Dolder, M. A., and Oliver, M. F. Myocardial infarction in young men: study of risk factors in nine countries. Br. Heart J., *37:* 493–503, 1975.
6. Enos, W. F., Beyer, J. C., and Holmes, R. H. Pathogenesis of coronary disease in American soldiers killed in Korea. J.A.M.A., *158:* 912, 1955.
7. Fields, W. Aortocranial occlusive vascular disease (Stroke), Clin. Symp. (CIBA), *26(4):* 3–31, 1974.
8. Jain, R. C., Onion and garlic in experimental atherosclerosis. Lancet, *1:* 1240, 1975.
9. Keys, A., Coronary heart disease—The global picture. Atherosclerosis, *22(2):* 149–192, 1975.

10. McCully, K. S., and Wilson, R. B., Homocysteine theory of arteriosclerosis. Atherosclerosis, *22(2):* 215–227, 1975.
11. McMillan, G. C., The pathology of cerebral arteriosclerosis, *In* Biological Basis of Medicine, edited by E. E. Bittar and N. Bittar, vol. 6, pp. 235–255, Academic Press, J. A. Constable Ltd., Edinburgh, 1969.
12. Moses, C. Atherosclerosis: Mechanisms as a Guide to Prevention, 239 pp. Lea and Febiger, Philadelphia, 1963.
13. Mulcahy, R., Hickey, N., Graham, I., McKenzie, G. Factors influencing long-term prognosis in male patients surviving a first coronary attack. Br. Heart J., *37:* 158–165, 1975.
14. Mundth, E. D. and Austen, W. G., Surgical measures for coronary heart disease (third of three parts). N. Engl. J. Med., *293:* 124–130, 1975.
15. Osler, W., Principles and Practice of Medicine, 1079 pp. Appleton and Co., New York, 1892.
16. Roberts, J. C., Jr., Moses, C., and Wilkins, R. H. Autopsy studies in atherosclerosis. I. Distribution and severity of atherosclerosis in patients dying without morphologic evidence of atherosclerotic catastrophe. Circulation, *20:* 511, 1959.
17. Roberts, J. C., Jr., and Straus, R., eds. Comparative Atherosclerosis, 426 pp. Harper and Row, New York, 1965.
18. Roberts, J. C., Jr., Wilkins, R. H., and Moses, C. Autopsy studies in atherosclerosis. II. Distribution and severity of atherosclerosis in patients dying with morphologic evidence of atherosclerotic catastrophe. Circulation, *20:* 520, 1959.
19. Roberts, J. C., Jr. Closing Address in Some Recent Developments in Comparative Medicine. Symposia of the Zoological Society of London, Edited by R.N. T-W-Fiennes, No. 17, p. 423. Academic Press, London, 1966.
20. Scully, R. E. and McNeely, B. U., eds. Case Records of the Massachusetts General Hospital. N. Engl. J. Med., *291:* 966–973, 1974.
21. Starzl, T. E., Chase, H. P., Putnam, C. W., and Nora, J. J. Follow-up of patient with portacaval shunt for the treatment of hyperlipidemia. Lancet, *2:* 714–715, 1974.
22. Stehbens, W. E., Pathology of the Cerebral Blood Vessels, 661 pp. C. V. Mosby Co., St. Louis, 1972.
23. Wilder, Charles, Prevalence of Chronic Circulatory Conditions, U.S. Department of Health, Education, and Welfare, Public Health Service, Health Resources Administration, Series 10: 94. 55 pp., 1972.
24. Wilkins, R. H., Roberts, J. C., Jr., and Moses, C. Autopsy studies in atherosclerosis. III. Distribution and severity of atherosclerosis in the presence of obesity, hypertension, nephrosclerosis, and rheumatic heart disease. Circulation, *20:* 527, 1959.

CHAPTER

12

Pathophysiology of Cerebral Infarction*

ARTHUR G. WALTZ, M.D.

Doctors Didisheim and Roberts have described for you many of the events that can occur in the major blood vessels and in the blood itself and that can be associated with cerebral infarction. They also have discussed certain aspects of the prevention of cerebral infarcts in patients who may or may not have had premonitory symptoms or a specific earlier event. However, it is quite likely that there always will be a number of persons, productive and effective, who will have acute ischemic strokes, regardless of the results of preventive measures. Therapeutic measures must be developed and used to minimize neurological disability and maximize functional capacity in such patients.

It is probable that surgical procedures will be among the most effective measures for treating cerebral infarcts; thus, I plan to discuss three aspects of cerebral infarction that have a direct bearing on the therapeutic effectiveness of surgical procedures: the responses of neurons to ischemia; reperfusion of ischemic regions; and brain swelling from ischemic cerebral edema. The discussion will include results and conclusions of studies carried out in the Cerebrovascular Clinical Research Center of the Department of Neurology, University of Minnesota, from 1971 through 1974, and earlier in the Cerebrovascular Clinical Research Center of the Department of Neurology, Mayo Clinic.

RESPONSES OF NEURONS TO ISCHEMIA

Functional Activity of Individual Neurons

The key to the minimization of neurological disability resulting from acute focal cerebral ischemia is the preservation or restoration of function of individual neurons. The functional behavior of individual neurons can be inferred from observations of neurological deficits, measurements of electroencephalographic and electrocorticographic activity, or detection of cortical potentials evoked by such peripheral

* Partial support for the studies reported here was provided by United States Public Health Service Research Grants NS 3364, NS 6663, and RR 5566.

stimuli as repetitive flashes of light, sounds, and tactile pressure. Studies of the relationships between cerebral blood flow (CBF) and electroencephalographic activity in humans undergoing carotid endarterectomy and between CBF and evoked cortical potentials in baboons undergoing occlusion of one middle cerebral artery (MCA) have shown a remarkable consistency: changes or disappearance of the electrical activity occur with decreases of regional CBF to approximately 17 to 20 ml/100 gm./min., with recovery of the electrical activity if CBF increases after a relatively short time (4, 32, 35). Moreover, the structural integrity of brain tissue appears to be affected only if CBF is less than about 20 for an extended period (34).

Direct measurement of the function of individual neurons requires detection of depolarization with intracellular or extracellular microelectrodes. Doctors W-D Heiss, T. Hayakawa, and I have recorded the action potentials of 162 individual cortical neurons in seven cats, using extracellular glass electrodes, before and up to 7 hours after occlusion of the left MCA by a device implanted transorbitally 4 to 8 days earlier (13). CBF was measured at the same times and in the same locations by recording polarographically the rate of clearance of inhaled hydrogen gas with platinized platinum-iridium electrodes 125 microns in diameter (15, 29). Immediately after MCA occlusion, abnormal patterns of neuronal activity included bursts; prolonged, high frequency repetitive discharges, or seizures; increases of frequency; decreases of frequency; and cessation of activity. Subsequently, neuronal activity was related to the corresponding CBF. No activity was detected in regions with calculated CBF values of less than 18 ml./100 gm./min.; activity was present in regions with greater CBF values, although frequently the patterns of activity were abnormal. Initial marked decreases of CBF to values less than 18 ml./100 gm./min. could be followed by spontaneous increases of CBF to higher values; a spontaneous increase after an initial decrease could be accompanied by resumption of the activity of individual neurons even though the region studied was still ischemic, with CBF less than before MCA occlusion (16).

Thus, the evidence available at present indicates that in normal brain there is a considerable reserve of CBF, in that neuronal function does not cease until a relatively low value for CBF is reached, although activity may be abnormal at higher values of CBF. Moreover, neurons that cease functioning at CBF less than about 20 may resume functioning when CBF is greater than 20, although still less than normal (16). However, the patterns of neuronal activity after resumption of function may be abnormal, and it is possible that neurological deficits would not be appreciably lessened or modified. It is of particular interest that the critical value for both neuronal function and structural integrity has been found to be roughly the same in three species: humans, baboons, and cats.

Neurological Deficits: Prevention and Recovery

Studies of electrical activity related to neuronal function have not as yet provided information about the maximum duration of a period of ischemia from which a neuron can recover. In the studies mentioned earlier, increases of CBF occurred within minutes of the impairment of electrical activity. However, other studies in which neuronal function has been inferred from observations of neurological deficits have indicated that recovery of function may be possible many hours after the onset of acute ischemia.

In an experimental model, acute focal cerebral ischemia can be induced inside an intact cranium containing cerebrospinal fluid (CSF) under normal pressure in a conscious, comfortable, and normally functioning animal (13). When the model is used in cats, regional CBF (measured by the hydrogen method) may decrease to very low values within seconds, at times becoming too low to calculate (15). Neurological deficits likewise begin within seconds to minutes and include forced deviations and circling movements as well as weakness of limbs. In certain situations, however, the exact characteristics of which are unknown, spontaneous lessening of the neurological deficits may begin within several hours of MCA occlusion and continue to the point that no neurological deficit is detectable several days after the onset of ischemia (13). Moreover, in anesthetized rhesus monkeys an occluding device can be removed from one MCA many hours after occlusion with no resultant neurological deficit (8). In some monkeys, ischemia persisting as long as 24 hours has not produced a deficit.

These experimental models are not precisely comparable to an acute stroke in humans; the influences of differing collateral circulation, effects of anesthesia, and other experimental maneuvers are not known with certainty. Nonetheless, even in humans there is indirect evidence that nonfunctioning regions of brain can remain viable for up to several hours (17). Thus, functional impairment of neuronal activity due to ischemia may be reversible, and neurons may resume functioning after restoration of the flow of blood. It is obvious that focal cerebral ischemia from the occlusion of a major or minor vessel supplying the brain is not the same as total cerebral ischemia (as from cardiac arrest or clamping all major thoracic vessels) or anoxia (as from respiratory arrest) in which recovery of cerebral function may not occur after as short a time as 5 minutes of ischemia. In focal ischemia, although the flow of blood in a central zone may be undetectable, at least some flow is maintained in surrounding zones through collateral channels, and the anatomic, enzymatic, and chemical integrity of neurons may be preserved during periods of impaired function (4, 11, 15, 25, 34, 37).

REPERFUSION OF ISCHEMIC REGIONS

There is, then, accumulating evidence that neurons can remain in a state of "functional paralysis" for a period of time after the onset of ischemia, during which restoration of the flow of blood may lead to recovery of function. However, there is still some concern about whether or not it is possible to restore normal perfusion in an ischemic region. With total cerebral ischemia, as from clamping the major thoracic arteries, there may be no reflow of blood into the brain after as short a time as 5 minutes to 1 hour, perhaps because of intravascular aggregation of blood elements or swelling of endothelial and perivascular tissue (1, 7, 37). However, just as with neuronal function, the situation is not the same for focal cerebral ischemia in which some flow of blood is preserved through collateral channels. There is abundant evidence from studies of experimental models that relatively normal perfusion can be restored to ischemic regions of the brain up to 24 hours after the onset of ischemia (8, 10, 12, 21, 22, 31, 33, 36).

Thus, there appears to be a period of time after an acute ischemic stroke during which blood flow can be restored to the ischemic regions and impaired neuronal function can be reversed. The implication of these findings is that appropriate neurovascular surgical procedures could prevent or minimize a developing neurological disability. In practice, however, immediate surgical procedures for ischemic strokes have not met with unqualified success. Consideration must also be given to ischemic cerebral edema.

BRAIN SWELLING FROM ISCHEMIC CEREBRAL EDEMA

Edema occurring in response to ischemia may be a major factor in the processes involved in the development of cerebral infarcts and neurological deficits. Although there is some information available about the characteristics of ischemic cerebral edema, conclusions about modification by therapeutic measures are largely speculative.

In experimental models of acute cerebral ischemia in animals, increases of the water content of perivascular glial cells begin to develop within minutes of the onset of ischemia (2, 19). Within hours, as the water content of cerebral tissue increases and focal swelling of the brain occurs, edema can be demonstrated both intracellularly and extracellularly and in both gray matter and white matter (23, 28). Edema is maximal 1 to 3 days after the onset of ischemia (28). At this time, swelling of the brain can produce intracranial pressure gradients which may cause shifts of midline structures, transtentorial herniation, worsening of neurological deficits, or death (6, 14, 27). Lesser degrees of swelling from focal cerebral edema may be adequate to produce focal increases of vascular resistance causing decreases of blood flow in regions with impaired vascular reactivity and contributing to neurological deficits (2, 6, 14). Edema is greatest in areas of cell death and necrosis, but it also develops in regions of brain that are ischemic but not infarcted (18, 28). In studies in animals, if ischemia is severe and infarcted regions are large, edema may develop in remote, nonischemic parts of the brain, even in the opposite hemisphere (19, 28). The mechanisms involved in the development of remote edema are unknown.

If an animal survives acute induced focal cerebral ischemia, edema resolves within 3 to 5 days, regardless of the resulting neurological deficit. The time course of ischemic cerebral edema—quick development to a maximum at 1 to 3 days and resolution within a few more days—is different from the time course of the transendothelial distribution of other molecules, such as sodium pertechnetate containing technetium-99m, labeled albumin, dyes, and other protein tracers (26). Thus the mechanisms that underlie ischemic cerebral edema are different from those involved in the development of necrosis and the production of a positive brain scan. The transendothelial distribution of water may take place across cellular membranes by diffusion or mass transport; the transendothelial distribution of other substances may occur through intercellular clefts, or pores, which are not normally present in the cerebral endothelium but which may be caused to "open" by ischemic or other changes in endothelial cells (5, 24, 30). Ischemic cerebral edema cannot be characterized as "cytotoxic" or "vasogenic;" ischemic cerebral edema has many, but not all, of the characteristics of both these types of edema (23, 28).

Ischemic cerebral edema may be worsened by anything that worsens the ischemia, such as systemic hypotension or hypoxia (28, 36, 37). However, induced hypertension or spontaneous reactive hyperemia also may worsen ischemic cerebral edema and cause extension of a cerebral infarct if the hyperemia develops within several hours of the onset of ischemia (15). Presumably, the hypertension or hyperemia causes increased transudation of water through damaged endothelial cells in response to an increase of intracapillary and intravascular pressure. In an experimental model of acute focal cerebral ischemia in cats, spontaneous hyperemia occurring within 4 to 6 hours of MCA occlusion may cause severe brain swelling with tentorial herniation and death within 12 hours, accompanied by a characteristic Cushing response of hypertension and bradycardia associated with a massive increase of intracranial pressure (14). However, hyperemia occurring later, 2 to 3 days after occlusion, does not produce a catastrophic reaction of massive edema and brain swelling (15).

Restoration of the flow of blood to an ischemic zone of the brain, perhaps by an appropriate neurovascular surgical procedure, may be followed by the restoration or preservation of function of neurons and the minimization of neurological disability. Alternatively, it may lead to worsening of ischemic cerebral edema with a resultant increase of neurological disability. For neurovascular surgical procedures to be effective, it appears that they must be undertaken relatively shortly after the onset of ischemia, and that worsening of edema must be prevented. Unfortunately, corticosteroids and osmotic agents are not as useful for the treatment of ischemic cerebral edema as for edema associated with cerebral tumors and head injuries (2, 3, 9, 18, 20). The resolution of this paradox awaits further study of the treatment of ischemic cerebral edema.

I have not mentioned as yet the possibility of converting an ischemic infarct to a hemorrhagic infarct by increasing perfusion pressure in an ischemic zone because in experimental models in animals this has not been a problem (8, 31, 33). In humans, early surgical experience with acute cerebral infarcts included the development of hemorrhagic infarcts and left many surgeons abandoning early intervention. I understand from my surgical colleagues, however, that recent experience with vascular procedures has been different; I will leave a discussion of this aspect of surgical therapy to those with appropriate experience.

SUMMARY

Evidence available at present from animal studies indicates that the flow of blood can be restored to ischemic zones in the brain as long as 24 hours after the onset of ischemia, and that such reperfusion could result in the restoration of function of neurons that have not been functioning during the period of ischemia. However, reperfusion also can cause worsening of ischemic cerebral edema resulting in increased neurological disability or death. Adequate measures for control of cerebral edema will be necessary if surgical intervention is to become an effective therapy for acute ischemic cerebral infarcts.

REFERENCES

1. Ames, A., III, Wright, R. L., Kowada, M., Thurston, J. M., and Majno, G. Cerebral ischemia. II. The no-reflow phenomenon. Am. J. Pathol., *52:* 437–453, 1968.
2. Bartko, D., Reulen, H. J., Koch, H., and Schürmann, K. Effect of dexamethasone on the early edema following occlusion of the middle cerebral artery in cats. *In* Steroids and Brain Edema, edited by H. J. Reulen, and K. Schürmann, pp. 127–137. Springer-Verlag, New York, 1972.

3. Bauer, R. B., and Tellez, H. Dexamethasone as treatment in cerebrovascular disease. 2. A controlled study in acute cerebral infarction. Stroke, *4:* 547–555, 1973.
4. Branston, N. M., Symon, L., Crockard, H. A., and Pasztor, E. Relationship between the cortical evoked potential and local cortical blood flow following acute middle cerebral artery occlusion in the baboon. Exp. Neurol., *45:* 195–208, 1974.
5. Brightman, M. E., Hori, M., Rapoport, S. I., Reese, T. S., and Westergaard, E. Osmotic opening of tight junctions in cerebral endothelium. J. Comp. Neurol., *152:* 317–326, 1973.
6. Brock, M., Beck, J., Markakis, E., and Dietz, H. Intracranial pressure gradients associated with experimental cerebral embolism. Stroke, *3:* 123–130, 1972.
7. Chiang, J., Kowada, M., Ames, A., III, Wright, R. L., and Majno, G. Cerebral ischemia. III. Vascular changes. Am. J. Pathol., *52:* 455–476, 1968.
8. Crowell, R. M., Olsson, Y., Klatzo, I., and Ommaya, A. Temporary occlusion of the middle cerebral artery in the monkey: clinical and pathological observations. Stroke, *1:* 439–448, 1970.
9. Donley, R. F., and Sundt, T. M., Jr. The effect of dexamethasone on the edema of focal cerebral ischemia. Stroke, *4:* 148–155, 1973.
10. Garcia, J. H., Cox, J. V., and Hudgins, W. R. Ultrastructure of the microvasculature in experimental cerebral infarction. Acta Neuropathol., *18:* 273–285, 1971.
11. Garcia, J. H., and Kamijyo, Y. Cerebral infarction: evolution of histopathological changes after occlusion of a middle cerebral artery in primates. J. Neuropathol. Exp. Neurol., *33:* 408–421, 1974.
12. Harrington, T., and DiChiro, G. Effect of hypocarbia and hypercarbia on experimental brain infarction: a microangiographic study in the monkey. Neurology, *23:* 294–299, 1973.
13. Hayakawa, T., and Waltz, A. G. Immediate effects of cerebral ischemia: evolution and resolution of neurological deficits after experimental occlusion of one middle cerebral artery in conscious cats. Stroke, *6:* 321–327, 1975.
14. Hayakawa, T., and Waltz, A. G. Intracranial pressure, blood pressure, and pulse rate after occlusion of a middle cerebral artery in cats. J. Neurosurg., *43:* 399–407, 1975.
15. Heiss, W-D., Hayakawa, T., and Waltz, A. G. Unpublished observations, 1974a.
16. Heiss, W-D., Hayakawa, T., and Waltz, A. G. Unpublished observations, 1974b.
17. Heyman, A., Saltzman, H. A., and Whalen, R. E. The use of hyperbaric oxygen in the treatment of cerebral ischemia and infarction. Circulation, *33* (Suppl. II): 20–27, 1966.
18. Hoppe, W. E., Waltz, A. G., Jordan, M. M., and Jacobson, R. L. Effects of dexamethasone on distributions of water and pertechnetate in brains of cats after middle cerebral artery occlusion. Stroke, *5:* 617–622, 1974.
19. Kogure, K., Busto, R., Scheinberg, P., and Reinmuth, O. M. Energy metabolites and water content in rat brain during the early stage of development of cerebral infarction. Brain, *97:* 103–114, 1974.
20. Lee, M. C., Mastri, A. R., Waltz, A. G., and Loewenson, R. B. Ineffectiveness of dexamethasone for treatment of experimental cerebral infarction. Stroke, *5:* 216–218, 1974.
21. Levy, D. E., Brierly, J. B., Silverman, D. G., and Plum, F. Brief hypoxia-ischemia initially damages cerebral neurons. Arch. Neurol., *32:* 450–456, 1975.
22. Little, J. R., Kerr, F. W. L., and Sundt, T. M., Jr. Microcirculatory obstruction in focal cerebral ischemia: relationship to neuronal alterations. Mayo Clin. Proc., *50:* 264–270, 1975.
23. Little, J. R., Sundt, T. M., Jr., and Kerr, F. W. L. Neuronal alterations in developing

cortical infarction: an experimental study in monkeys. J. Neurosurg., *40:* 186–198, 1974.
24. Lorenzo, A. V., Shirahige, I., Liang, M., and Barlow, C. F. Temporary alteration of cerebrovascular permeability to plasma protein during drug-induced seizures. Am. J. Physiol., *223:* 268–277, 1972.
25. MacDonald, V. D., Sundt, T. M., Jr., and Winkelmann, R. D. Histochemical studies in the zone of ischemia following middle cerebral artery occlusion in cats. J. Neurosurg., *37:* 45–54, 1972.
26. O'Brien, M. D., Jordan, M. M., and Waltz, A. G. Ischemic cerebral edema and the blood-brain barrier: distributions of pertechnetate, albumin, sodium, and antipyrine in brains of cats after occlusion of middle cerebral artery. Arch. Neurol., *30:* 461–465, 1974.
27. O'Brien, M. D., and Waltz, A. G. Intracranial pressure gradients caused by experimental cerebral ischemia and edema. Stroke, *4:* 694–698, 1973.
28. O'Brien, M. D., Waltz, A. G., and Jordan, M. M. Ischemic cerebral edema: distribution of water in brains of cats after occlusion of middle cerebral artery. Arch. Neurol., *30:* 456–460, 1974.
29. Pasztor, E., Symon, L., Dorsch, N. W. C., and Branston, N. M. The hydrogen clearance method in assessment of blood flow in cortex, white matter and deep nuclei of baboons. Stroke, *4:* 556–567, 1973.
30. Rapoport, S. I., Hori, M., and Klatzo, I. Testing of a hypothesis for osmotic opening of the blood-brain barrier. Am. J. Physiol., *223:* 323–331, 1972.
31. Sundt, T. M., Jr., Grant, W. C., and Garcia, J. H. Restoration of middle cerebral artery flow in experimental infarction. J. Neurosurg., *31:* 311–322, 1969.
32. Sundt, T. M., Jr., Sharbrough, F. W., Anderson, R. E., and Michenfelder, J. D. Cerebral blood flow measurements and electroencephalograms during carotid endarterectomy. J. Neurosurg., *41:* 310–320, 1974.
33. Sundt, T. M., Jr., and Waltz, A. G. Cerebral ischemia and reactive hyperemia: studies of cortical blood flow and microcirculation before, during, and after temporary occlusion of middle cerebral artery of squirrel monkeys. Circ. Res., *28:* 426–433, 1971.
34. Symon, L., Crockard, H. A., Dorsch, N. W. C., Branston, N. M., and Juhasz, J. Local cerebral blood flow and vascular reactivity in a chronic stable stroke in baboons. Stroke, *6:* 482–492, 1975.
35. Trojaborg, W., and Boysen, G. Relation between EEG, regional cerebral blood flow and internal carotid artery pressure during carotid endarterectomy. Electroencephalogr. Clin. Neurophysiol., *34:* 61–69, 1973.
36. Waltz, A. G. Pathophysiology of cerebral ischemia. *In* Cerebral Vascular Diseases: Transactions of the Eighth Conference, edited by F. H. McDowell, and R. W. Brennan, pp. 119–126. Grune & Stratton, New York, 1973.
37. Waltz, A. G., and Sundt, T. M., Jr. The microvasculature and microcirculation of the cerebral cortex after arterial occlusion. Brain. *90:* 681–696, 1967.

CHAPTER

13

Neurosurgical Consideration of some Features of the Cerebral Dural Sinuses and their Tributaries

HARRY A. KAPLAN, M.D. and JEFFERSON BROWDER, M.D.

The major venous sinuses of the cerebral dura mater have been categorized in most anatomical textbooks as the superior and inferior sagittal, the straight, the lateral or transverse, the cavernous, the sphenoid, the superior and inferior petrosal, the occipital, and marginal sinuses. Basic components of these venous pathways are for the most part present in all individuals; however, developmental alterations lead to a great variation in their final configuration which in some has surgical significance.

Nine hundred and forty-eight specimens of cerebral dura mater and their enclosed sinuses have been obtained at autopsy. These have been processed, described, probed, diagrammed, and in approximately one-half, segments of the sinuses injected with vinylite and subsequently corroded. The resultant casts showed the details of the sinuses and their joining veins. From this material we have drawn conclusions of surgical import which are herein presented in brief.

EMBRYONIC DEVELOPMENT OF THE CEREBRAL DURAL SINUSES

Early in the course of this study it became evident that a working knowledge of the development of the cerebral dural sinuses would be an asset. Available information concerning the embryology of the cerebral dural sinus has been repeatedly reviewed, and the Mall collection of human embryos, which is at present housed in Sacramento, California, has been studied. The present account is drawn for the most part from Streeter's (1915) report of the development of the venous sinuses of the dura mater in the human (15).

Our knowledge of the earliest phases of growth of the embryo stems from the studies of Evans (8) and Sabin (14) in the chick and pig. A chain of angioblasts along the border of the hindbrain sprouts into a capillary mesh to cover this structure. A similar type mesh sprouts from the aortic arch to cover the fore and midbrain. These two meshes combine to cover the brain with a primary head plexus. This vascular mesh then divides into a deeper primary head plexus, the forerunner of the blood vessels of the brain and a second or more superficial portion, the vascular channels of the dura mater. The superficial dural plexus begins at the ventral aspect of the cephalic neural tube by forming large venous lakes. As the superficial dural plexus develops dorsally, small intermediate connecting channels unite the two layers. As the meningeal layers grow dorsally, these connecting channels are obliterated except at the dorsal midline where they form a confluence which persists throughout life. Surgeons of experience are aware of the occasional connections between the dural and cerebral circulations.

In the early phase of the formation of the superficial dural venous plexus, the ventrally placed channels coalesce to form the primary head vein of Evans. The rostral part of this vein forms between the diencephalon and optic bulb and continues caudomedially just ventral to the trigeminal ganglion. This rostral segment will ultimately become the cavernous sinus in the adult. The middle segment of the primary head vein develops from the superficial dural plexus overlying the hindbrain. It will ultimately become segmental and give rise to both the superior and inferior petrosal sinuses. The anterior cardinal vein forms the caudal segment of the primary head vein and remains as the jugular vein of the adult.

The vein of Evans is the first true drainage channel of the head. Dorsal tributaries join this vein in three groups. The anterior dural group or plexus, draining venous blood from the fore and midbrain, joins the primary head vein in front of the semilunar ganglion; the middle dural plexus draining the region of the cerebellum joins between the semilunar and the acousticofacial ganglia; and the posterior plexus from the medullary region empties into the primary head vein caudal to the otic capsule.

In the 12-mm. crown-rump(C-R) length embryo, the ventral portions of the dural plexuses as described are more or less completely separated from the deeper lying plexus or capillary sheet. The vascular mesh of the dorsum of the anterior and middle dural plexuses advance toward the mid-dorsal part of the telencephalon to form a sagittal plexus. It is in this sagittal plexus dipping between the cerebral hemispheres that the superior and inferior sagittal sinuses arise. The superior sagittal sinus forms asymmetrically with a tendency to drain more freely to one side, usually to the right.

In the 18-mm. C-R embryo, the middle section of the primary head vein becomes smaller and ultimately fades away leaving segments for the formation of the petrosal sinuses. The blood from the anterior and middle dural plexuses is now shunted caudalward through their dorsally placed channels. This represents the first stage in the development of the transverse sinus.

In the 20-mm. C-R embryo, the veins are intermediate between the embryonic and the fetal types. Venous drainage from the anterior, middle, and posterior dural plexuses is now through the newly forming dorsal channel, the transverse sinus, into the jugular vein. The dural area lying between the caudal aspects of the cerebral hemispheres and the dorsum of the cerebellum will combine to form the tentorium cerebelli. In the loose tissue of the tentorium are the meshes of the tentorial plexus. With the growth of the cerebrum and cerebellum, the tentorial mesh becomes compressed. In the midline of the mesh, the straight sinus is formed and in its lateral aspects, the transverse sinuses. The junction of all the sinuses, superior sagittal, straight, and lateral sinuses gives rise to the confluence of sinuses or torcula herophili.

In the 40-mm. C-R embryo, beginning of the fetal stage, morphological features of the adult are appearing. Although the primitive transverse sinus is well outlined in the tentorial plexus, the only definitive segment is the sigmoid segment.

In the 50-mm. C-R embryo, the channels for venous drainage of the head correspond fairly well to those found in the adult. The external or veins of the integument, the dural veins, and the cerebral veins represent three separate systems. The external venous plexus of the scalp has a few connections with the dural system especially at the superior midline. The rostral portion of the superior sagittal sinus in most instances lacks only a connective tissue investment to make it an adult type of sinus while the caudal part remains plexiform. A plexiform arrangement caudally not infrequently persists throughout life.

In the 80-mm. C-R stage, the sinuses approach the adult appearance. In some instances the development of the adult type occipital sinus is not completed until infancy.

An understanding of the many phases in the development of the cerebral dural sinuses during embryonic, fetal, and neonatal periods as above set forth serves as a basis for an interpretation of the aberrancies of the cerebral venous system encountered in the adult. We are here concerned with the so-called anomalies that are to be recognized by clinical neurosurgeons. For sake of clarity and facility of presentation, they are categorized, and each is drawn from the list and discussed from the viewpoint of their clinical import.

ITEMS FOR CONSIDERATION

A. Vascular channels of the scalp, skull, dura mater, and brain
B. Vascular spaces in the mid-dorsal dura mater

C. Superior sagittal sinus and the confluence of sinuses
D. Transverse sinuses
E. Occipital sinus
F. Straight sinus
G. Vascular channels in the tentorium cerebelli
H. Vascular connections of the cavernous sinuses
I. Tumors in the dural sinuses

VENOUS CHANNELS OF THE SCALP, SKULL, DURA MATER, AND BRAIN

As stated, there are three venous systems for the head (3): (a) the superficial which serves as drainage pathways from the scalp, the fronto-occipital muscles and their tendons, the galea aponeurotica; (b) the intermediate for drainage of the skull, diploe, and the dura mater; and (c) the deep system which drains the brain. The confluence of these, which persist throughout adult life, is located for the most part along the sagittal plane of the head. Connections between the superficial and intermediate are few, irregularly located, and mostly of small caliber. They are found along the midline of the head and a few along the superior temporal line of the skull. Connections between the diploe and the dural vessels are generous as would be expected since these in aggregate constitute the intermediate venous system of the head. The large cortical veins that connect with the major dural sinuses represent the deep venous system. Our studies strongly support these anatomical conclusions.

Clinical observations have not helped appreciably in an attempted estimation of blood flow from scalp to skull and/or skull to scalp. Occasionally, one encounters a patient with a vascular malformation implicating the veins of the scalp and has vascular pathways through multiple foramina of a segment of the skull which unite with the dural venous system. In other words, complete cleavage between the superficial and dural venous systems did not occur at the site of malformation during embryonal development. Experienced neurosurgeons have no doubt encountered an occasional vein crossing the subdural space of the cerebral convexity, which unites the dural and cerebral venous systems. Ray and associates (13) observed dilatation of the scalp veins in association with obstruction of the superior sagittal sinus. Kalbag and Woolf (10) discussed dilatation of the veins of the scalp associated with inflammatory implication of the cerebral dural sinuses. A determination of the extent of thrombosis of dural sinuses is difficult to make at autopsy. Such an estimation is even less accurate when made at surgery. In the examples of occlusion of the superior sagittal sinus in its posterior part by a meningioma appears to lend support to the notion that the venous pathways draining the scalp and those subserving the skull are in close proximity but not connected. The zone of hyperostosis that usually caps a meningioma involving the underlying dura mater is frequently very vascular; however, enlargement of the regional vessels of the scalp has not been observed. In the instances in which a meningioma invades the epicranium and the deep part of the scalp, veins of the scalp are strikingly enlarged. Elsberg and Schwartz (7) described enlargement of the diploic channels of the skull in the area of a meningioma attached to the dura mater but did not mention dilatation of the veins of the overlying scalp. We are convinced that the anatomical arrangement of the veins of the head conform to that established during embryonic and fetal life and that this persists in the vast majority throughout adult life.

VASCULAR SPACES IN THE MID-DORSAL DURA MATER

During the development of some of the great dural sinuses from an embryonal mesh, the superior sagittal and the straight sinus in particular, remnants of this vascular network persist. These are found in the adult within the dorsal wall of the superior sagittal sinus, within the walls of the straight sinus and the adjacent part of the tentorium cerebelli, in the dorsal leaflet of the confluence of sinuses, and rarely within the dorsal walls of the proximal transverse sinuses. Most of the remnants consist of a spongy vascular network, however, the pads that project into the lumen of the proximal parts of a transverse sinus frequently have a substantial fibrocollagenous component. Baló (1) studied these vascular networks and assigned a functional capacity to them, namely, a mechanism for regulation of blood flowing from the intracranial cavity. This appears untenable since in the majority of instances the lumen of a sinus is not encroached upon by the network. Furthermore, this mesh is not present at all in some specimens.

We have observed two areas where the lumen of a sinus may be mildly to moderately narrowed; the dorsal wall of the middle third of a superior sagittal sinus may be 2 to 3 mm. thick over a 2- to 4-cm. segment and the thickened part sag into the lumen of this sinus; and two, a wedge-shaped pad of vascular mesh mixed with strands of fibrocollagenous tissue may, mildly to almost completely, occlude a proximal transverse sinus (Fig. 13.1). The former situation is not clinically important since the sag of the dorsal leaf has not been found sufficient to compromise the lumen of the sinus. The latter, however, should receive consideration since at times it may be of surgical significance. Frequently, the transverse sinus implicated is small; consequently, under these circumstances the major part of blood flow from the superior sagittal sinus passes into the unobstructed larger transverse sinus. In some instances the straight sinus also joins this large transverse sinus; therefore, a substantial amount of the total outflow of venous blood from the brain exits through one internal

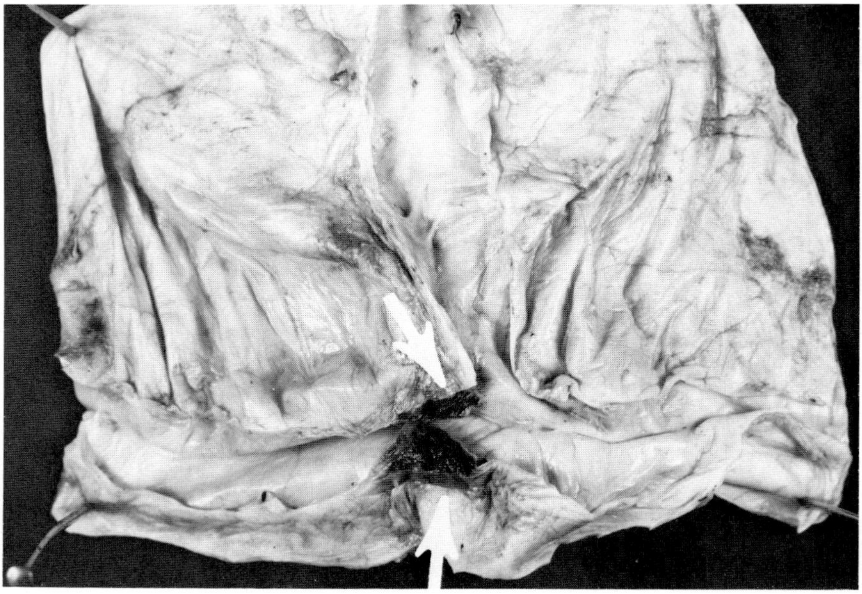

FIG. 13.1. The superior sagittal sinus and both transverse sinuses have been opened through their dorsal leaves. Just to left of confluence of sinuses is located a wedge-shaped vascular mesh (arrows) which almost occludes the lumen of the proximal left transverse sinus. The size of the lumen of the right transverse sinus is the same as the superior sagittal sinus.

jugular vein. Pathophysiological dysfunctions resulting from ablation of this major channel in the neck would be approximately the same as bilateral occlusion of both internal jugular veins.

SUPERIOR SAGITTAL SINUS AND THE CONFLUENCE OF SINUSES

This sinus has been accorded more consideration by anatomists, pathologists, experimentalists, and clinicians than all other cerebral dural sinuses combined. The neurosurgeon has followed in the footsteps of his predecessors and perforce has become knowledgeable regarding its size, course, and major tributaries. Some surgeons have not given thought to the embryonal development that results in aberrations in both the rostral and caudal ends of the superior sagittal sinus. This deficit in knowledge is related to a lack of understanding of the significance of the various patterns of cortical veins of the frontal lobes and the multitude of so-called anomalies involving the confluence of sinuses. In addition, the neurosurgeon should have insight into the arrangement of the maze of venous channels located in the parasagittal regions.

The most intriguing of the developmental departures from average or normal of this sinus are those located in its rostral part. Reference to the embryology as described in the first section of this presentation will help clarify the manner of formation of the superior sagittal sinus from the embryonal mesh that dips between the two cerebral hemispheres, *i.e.*, the sagittal plexus. The lumen of the most rostral end of the sinus is not formed by a vein passing through the foramen caecum of the frontal bone. In a few, the sinus begins at the intracranial level of this foramen by confluence of small veins of the frontal poles. In the vast majority, a cordlike fibrocollagenous structure extends for variable distances caudally along the course usually occupied by the sinus. This cord or atretic sinus ranges in length from a few millimeters to 9 cm., the maximal found in our studies (11). In most instances, cortical veins of various configurations course caudomedially over the frontal lobe and unite in the midline to establish the lumen of the sinus at a level representing the caudal end of the atretic segment (Fig. 13.2). A phlebographic x-ray film in a lateral projection with the vessels opacified with contrast medium simulates a depression of the superior sagittal sinus. In the anteroposterior projection the real anatomical position of the opacified vein becomes evident, that is, coursing caudomedially in the parasagittal region to

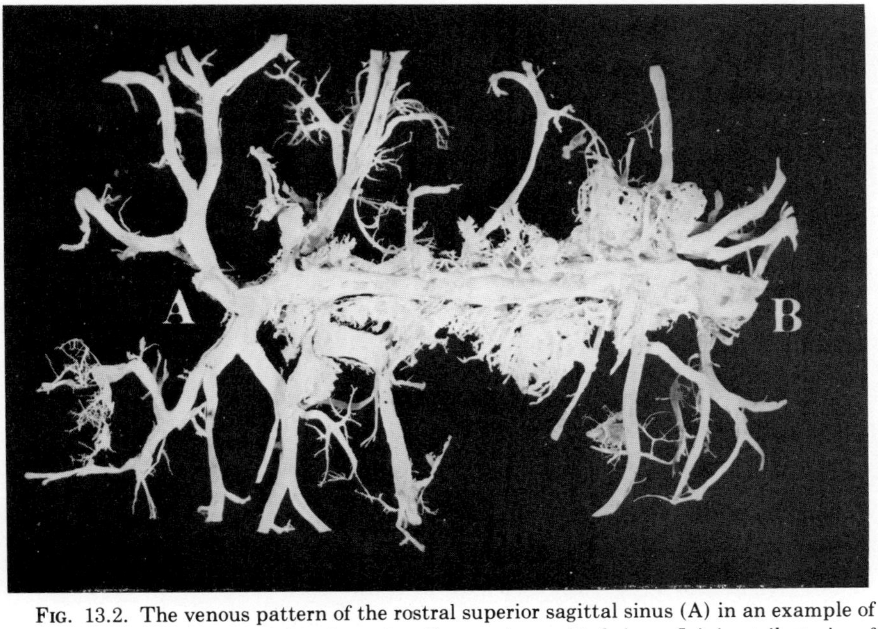

FIG. 13.2. The venous pattern of the rostral superior sagittal sinus (A) in an example of atresia of the rostal 5 cm. of this sinus. A to B, superior sagittal sinus. Joining tributaries of the sinus and the lateral lacunae are shown.

produce with its joining fellow of the opposite side a midline sinus. Also a segment of atresia of the rostral superior sagittal sinus, 8 to 9 cm. in length, may be mistaken for an inflammatory occlusion of the sinus. The histological appearance of these atretic cords of embryonal origin is not that of a chronic inflammatory process. Both arteries and venous channels are found in this fibrocollagenous atretic segment, the veins represented by ramifying pathways without proper wall but with endothelial lining that course through the dura-like matrix. When the rostral 5 to 6 cm. of an average superior sagittal sinus is isolated by ligature and the isolated segment injected with contrast medium, the preferential avenue of outflow is over the frontal veins, into the superficial Sylvian veins, and thence through the veins of Labbé to the transverse sinuses. Only minimal flow is "around" the site of occlusion to more caudally placed cortical veins and then into the superior sagittal sinus (4). It would appear that the collaterals formed bilaterally subsequent to the surgical resection of the rostral part of this sinus is by way of the frontal veins, superficial Sylvian veins, and veins of Labbé to the transverse sinuses. As aforementioned, a substantial segment of the rostral superior sagittal sinus may not be present. Surgical resection of a cordlike segment of sinus with preservation of the cortical veins that course dorsomedially over the frontal lobes leaves the venous system of the frontal lobe intact. Consequently, the postoperative course is not complicated by dysfunctions due to cerebral edema.

Passing caudally with the lumen laid open by a longitudinal incision through the dorsal leaf of the sinus there are brought into view numerous orifices, bands, bridges, and tunnels located in the lateral walls, in the aggregate, chordae willisii. In the zones just lateral to the sinus, *i.e.*, parasagittal areas, are located the lateral lacunae which contain about four/fifths of all Pacchionian granulations found in the venous channels of the dura mater. The superior cerebral veins pass beneath the lacunae and most of them course in a rostral direction within the lateral wall of the sinus before entering it (Fig. 13.3). This channel within the wall may be as much as a centimeter in length. This represents an important anatomical arrangement if the sinus is to be resected at the junction of its anterior and middle thirds or more caudally for the cure of a meningioma. Dividing the sinus a few millimeters rostral to the junction of the superior cerebral vein and the sinus may occlude the orifice of the vein. Passing further caudally, the last of the large superior cerebral veins is represented by a collecting channel draining the dorsomedial part of the posterior parietal lobe and a comparable cortical part of the entire occipital lobe. This vein enters the superior sagittal sinus in a rostral course in the wall of the sinus as described for the more rostrally

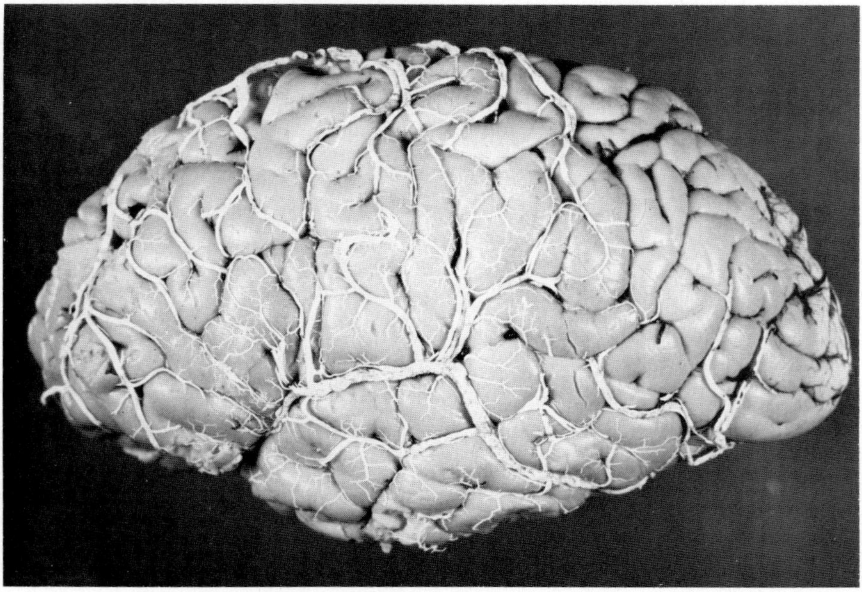

FIG. 13.3. Lateral view of left cerebral hemisphere. At the vertex of the brain the rostral courses of the superior cerebral veins are shown. This specimen had atresia of the rostral superior sagittal sinus 4½ cm. in length. The substitute vein for the atretic sinus courses over the anterior pole of the brain.

positioned superior cerebral veins. Occlusion of the trunk of this vein just parasagittally in the performance of occipital lobectomy should not be carried out since postoperative edema commonly follows this type of ablation.

Consideration of the great variety of venous patterns that are to be found at the confluence of sinuses will not be presented here. Suffice it to say that the head and neck surgeon should have accurate knowledge of the pattern of veins and sinuses of this region in each patient who is a candidate for internal jugular ablation in the eradication of cancer of the nasopharynx and neck. The development of a technique for complete and detailed phlebographic demonstration is sorely needed in order to appraise the surgeon preoperatively of the configuration of intracranial channels with which he will be concerned and to give him a clear notion of the jugular vein carrying the major outflow of blood from the brain.

TRANSVERSE SINUSES

During the preantibiotic era, the relatively common implication of a transverse sinus by inflammatory disease secondary to infection of a contiguous ear and/or mastoid cells prompted many reports dealing with thrombotic lesions in this sinus. A deficit in knowledge of the connections of the venous channels involved initiated several important studies of the fundamental anatomy of these sinuses within the posterior part of the head. Some of these have served as milestones and their accuracy and importance are attested by the frequency of reference to them at the present time. The attention of neurosurgeons was attracted by complications of the infected ear-mastoid cell lateral sinus complex that extended into the intracranial cavity, in the main, cerebellar abscesses. Since the development of antibiotic therapies, most of these problems have vanished. The head and neck surgeons have assumed the responsibility of assessing and further investigating the patterns of venous outflow from the brain into the jugular systems. There remains, however, an occasional circumstance which requires the surgical division of a transverse sinus for total removal of a bilobed meningioma occupying the occipito-cerebellar region. It is not a difficult task to uncover both transverse sinuses by enlarging the bony opening of a bilateral suboccipital craniectomy and exposing these sinuses to direct vision. Decision regarding the advisability of dividing the sinus homolateral to the tumor can be made on the basis of comparative size of the sinuses. Ablation of a large transverse sinus which represents a continuation of the superior sagittal sinus and a small transverse sinus of the other side receiving blood almost exclusively from the straight sinus is followed by uncontrollable swelling of the brain.

OCCIPITAL SINUS

In the vast majority of patients requiring bilateral suboccipital craniectomy, the occipital sinus presents no technical problem. This sinus is usually small, courses in the dorsal aspect of the cerebellar falx, and extends from the proximal part of a transverse sinus, or the caudal limits of the confluence of sinuses to the marginal sinuses and/or the upper reaches of the vertebral plexus. Transverse division of the occipital sinus in its midpart produces no recognizable dysfunctions. In less than one per cent of adults, the occipital sinus is large, courses in the midline, and serves as a conduit for blood from the straight sinus. In fact in most of these, the occipital sinus represents a continuation of the straight sinus. The authors have not had surgical experiences with patients having this configuration of sinuses. *A priori*, occlusion of the occipital sinus under these circumstances should produce some congestion of blood in the Galenic venous system. More rarely a superior sagittal sinus continues within the dura mater covering a cerebellar hemisphere as a large parasagittal occipital sinus. Such a channel is occasionally double barreled, a channel coursing in the dura mater parasagittally over the midpart of each cerebellar lobe. A midline occipital sinus is not present in these circumstances. Ablation of these large channels, which may represent the major outflow pathways of venous blood from the head, produces vascular congestion and swelling of the brain.

The most unusual configuration of the occipital sinus or sinuses within the dura covering the dorsal cerebellum is found in infants. In 25% of patients in this age group, there are variable sized venous channels in the sagittal and parasagittal dura mater covering the dorsal cerebellum (Fig. 13.4). These lakes or coarse network of venous channels usually extend into the falx cerebelli. They may implicate about half of the dorsal dura of the posterior cranial fossa. Their presence is not associated with an alteration in the size of the transverse sinus. The walls of this venous plexus are thin and their interior consists of a reticular-like formation (5). A neurosurgeon who has encountered such a venous aberration is well aware of the technical difficulties that may be encountered when surgically exposing the cerebellum. That these venous plexuses dwindle or otherwise disappear is attested by their absence after adolescence. Here again complete preoperative phlebograms would alert the neurosur-

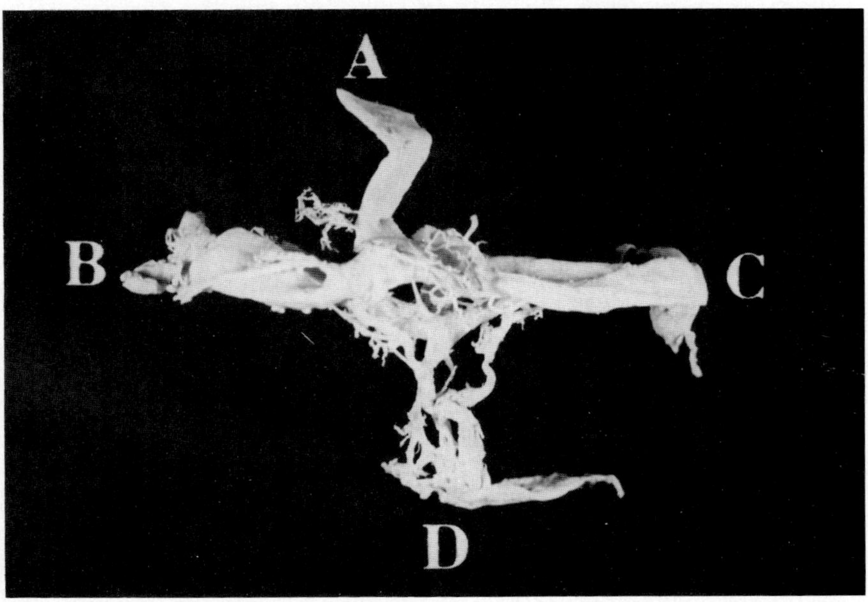

FIG. 13.4. Posterior view of a cast showing multiple connecting channels representing the occipital sinus. (A) Stub of superior sagittal sinus, (B) left transverse sinus, (C) double right transverse sinus, and (D) site of junction of multichannelled occipital sinus and marginal sinuses. This specimen was obtained from a child aged 2½ years.

geon regarding the extent of such an anomaly in an infant requiring bilateral suboccipital craniectomy.

STRAIGHT SINUS AND THE VEIN OF GALEN

Some of the essential anatomical features of the straight sinus and its tributaries have been recently reviewed and reported. In all specimens this sinus is the major pathway for drainage of venous blood from the inner structures of the brain and those at its base. Its principal tributaries are the vein of Galen, the inferior sagittal sinus, and an occasional channel in the caudal falx cerebri coursing rostroventrally to connect the superior sagittal with the rostral straight sinus. The straight sinus courses in the ridge of the cerebellar tent to join the confluence of sinuses, one of the transverse sinuses, rarely the occipital sinus, and still more uncommonly the distal superior sagittal sinus. In its course through the apex of the tentorium cerebelli, segments of the sinus may be doubled or more rarely tripled.

The paucity of reported cases in whom the straight sinus and/or the great vein of Galen have been ablated for the cure of a tumor indicates that neurosurgeons believe that such a procedure is extremely hazardous. This is probably true; however, this should not be since generous potential collateral channels exist which should be sufficient to accommodate reverse flow of venous blood of the inner brain and this not associated with vascular congestion of significance. Relatively recent experiments show that occlusion of the vein of Galen in the primate is not followed by recognizable dysfunction of the brain (9). Scanty evidence suggests that this does not hold in the human.

VASCULAR CHANNELS IN THE TENTORIUM CEREBELLI

If one reviews the embryonic development of the tentorium cerebelli, it comes as no surprise that numerous venous channels exist between the leaflets of this structure (6) (Fig. 13.5). These are most numerous and larger in the posterior half of this tent. They join with and seemingly drain into regional dural sinuses; namely, transverse, straight, and superior petrosal sinuses. They may join one of these sinuses with another.

The surgical import is related to incision through the tentorium to expose the anterior cerebellum and/or the pontile region of the brain stem. It is to be recognized that this fold of dura mater is not a bloodless partition but contains sizable venous channels without constant patterns.

VASCULAR CONNECTIONS OF THE CAVERNOUS SINUSES

The cavernous sinuses are reticular structures situated in the medial aspect of the middle cranial fossae and having rather generous connec-

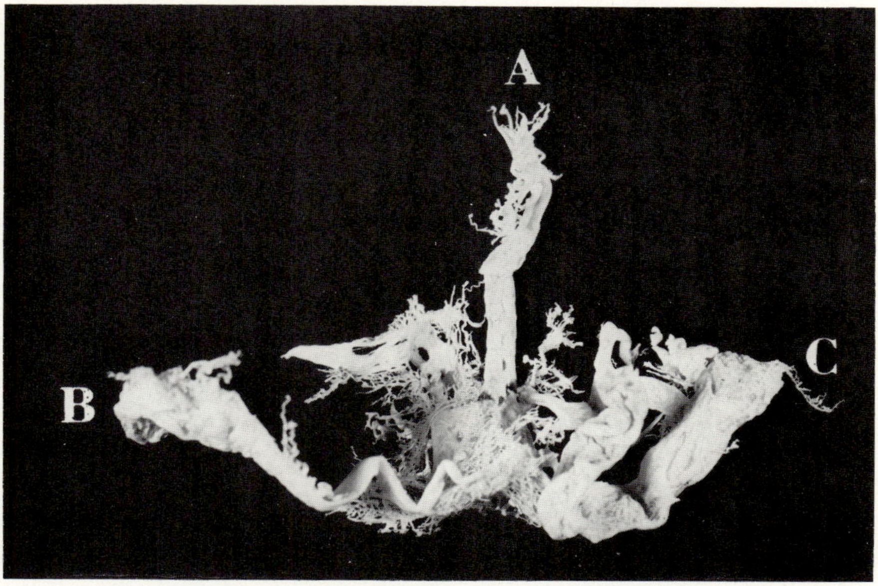

FIG. 13.5. Dorsal view of a cast of the straight and both transverse sinuses, confluence of sinuses, and the complex of venous channels within the posterior half of the tentorium cerebelli. (A) Straight sinus, (B) left transverse sinus, and (C) right transverse sinus.

tions by channels crossing the midline. These intercavernous connections comprise the basilar venous plexus lying over the upper clivus, the posterior arm of the superior circular sinus, the anterior arm of the circular sinus, and the network of channels within the dura mater lining the hypophyseal fossa (Fig. 13.6). The channels crossing the cavity of the hypophyseal fossa were called the inferior circular sinus by Winslow (16); however, they are in no way comparable to the configuration of the superior circular sinus. In some specimens of the series, they represented the largest of all intercavernous connections.

Three of the structures comprising the cavernous sinus and its connections merit consideration from a surgical viewpoint. Firstly, the transcavernous sinus approach for cure of a carotid artery cavernous sinus fistula as reported by Parkinson (12). We have had no experience with this operation, consequently, refer the reader to the publications of Parkinson. Secondly, division of the anterior arm of the circular sinus when incising the diaphragma sellae in its rostral midline for exposure of the pituitary by the transfrontal route. In the presence of a hypophyseal tumor, this channel is attenuated and seldom offers technical difficulties subsequent to its division. It is to be remembered that a circular avascular zone approximately 3 mm. in width is present around the central opening of the diaphragma sellae through which the pituitary

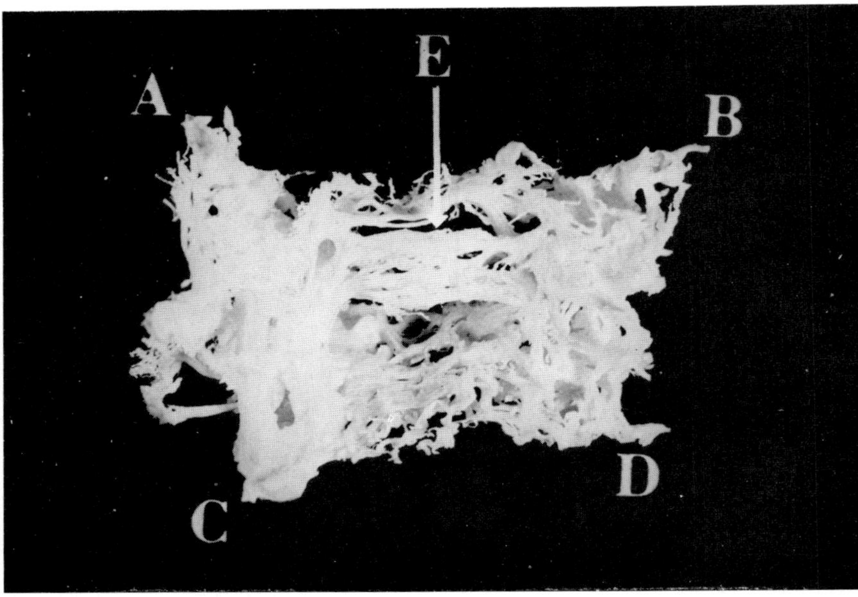

FIG. 13.6. Vinylite case of cavernous sinuses and their connections. (A) Left ophthalmic vein, (B) right ophthalmic vein, (C) left superior petrosal sinus, (D) right superior petrosal sinus, and (E) arrow pointing to the relatively large venous connection which crosses from one sinus to the other in the dura mater of the hypophyseal fossa. Crossing the midline just rostral to the arrowhead is the multichannelled anterior arm of the circular sinus.

stalk passes. Thirdly, the crossing venous channels of the base of the hypophyseal fossa may be relatively large and the source of troublesome bleeding when divided in the midline during a trans-sphenoidal approach to the pituitary gland.

TUMORS OF THE CEREBRAL DURAL SINUSES

Some 4 years ago shortly after embarking on a study of the "Venous sinuses of the cerebral dura mater and their tributaries," we encountered a roundish, pale gray, pedunculated tumor attached to a lateral wall of the superior sagittal sinus in its distal third. The lumen of the sinus was mildly dilated at the level of the lesion but not so rostral to it. Subsequently, two additional tumors of comparable size were found, one in the distal superior sagittal sinus, approximately the same location as the first, and the other at the knee of the left transverse sinus (2). In addition, 67 small tumors with histological findings suggesting that they arose from Pacchionian granulations have been found. Essential details of these small masses, which we have termed hypertrophic Pacchionian granulations, has been recorded (3).

It appears possible, if not probable, that some of the larger growths may compromise the lumen of a sinus and initiate a series of clinical events comparable to the syndrome of so-called pseudo tumor cerebri. This brief discussion of tumors located solely within the lumen of a large cerebral dural sinus has been included here to indicate that such a lesion exists and to urge neuroradiologists and neuropathologists to be on the alert regarding their possible presence.

REFERENCES

1. Balo, J. The dural venous sinuses. Anat. Rec., *106:* 319–325, 1950.
2. Browder, J., Browder, A., and Kaplan, H. A. Benign tumors of the cerebral dural sinuses. J. Neurosurg., *37:* 576–579, 1972.
3. Browder, J., Kaplan, H. A., and Howard, E. M. Hyperplasia of pacchionian granulations. Arch. Pathol., *95:* 315–316, 1973.
4. Browder, J., and Kaplan, H. A. Venous drainage following ablation or occlusive isolation of the rostral superior sagittal sinus. Surg. Neurol., *1:* 249–251, 1973.
5. Browder, J., Kaplan, H. A., and Krieger, A. J. Venous lakes in the suboccipital dura mater and falx cerebelli of infants: surgical significance. Surg. Neurol., *4:* 53–55, 1975.
6. Browder, J., Kaplan, H. A., and Krieger, A. J. Venous channels in the tentorium cerebelli: surgical significance. Surg. Neurol., *3:* 37–39, 1975.
7. Eisberg, C. A., and Schwartz, C. W. Increased cranial vascularity in its relation to intracranial disease (with special reference to enlargement of the veins of the diploe and its relation to the endotheliomas). Arch. Neurol. Psych., *11:* 292–307, 1924.
8. Evans, H. M. Development of the vascular system. *In* Manual of Human Embryology, edited by F. Keibel and F. P. Mall, Vol. 2, Ch. 18, pp. 570–709. J. B. Lippincott Co., Philadelphia, 1910–1912.
9. Hammock, M. K., Milhorat, T. H., Earle, K., and DiChiro, G. Vein of Galen ligation in the primate. J. Neurosurg., *34:* 77–83, 1971.
10. Kalbag, R. M., and Woolf, A. L. Cerebral Venous Thrombosis. Oxford University Press, London, 1967.
11. Kaplan, H. A., Browder, A., and Browder, J. Nasal venous drainage and the foramen caecum. Laryngoscope, *83:* 327–329, 1973.
12. Parkinson, D. Collateral circulation of cavernous carotid artery: anatomy. Can. J. Surg., *7:* 251–268, 1964.
13. Ray, B. S., Dunbar, H. S., and Dotter, C. T. Dural sinus venography as an aid to diagnosis in intracranial disease. J. Neurosurg., *8:* 23–37, 1951.
14. Sabin, F. R. Origin and development of the primitive vessels of the chick and of the pig. Contr. Embry. Carneg. Inst., *6:* 61–124, 1917.
15. Streeter, G. L. The development of the venous sinuses of the dura mater in the human embryo. Am. J. Anat., *18:* 145–178, 1915.
16. Winslow, J. B. An Anatomical Exposition of the Structures of the Human Body, G. Douglas (Trans.), Ed. 5, Vol. 2. J. F. Rivington and others, London, 1776.

CHAPTER

14

Cardiogenic Factors in the Stroke Syndrome*

CHARLES E. RACKLEY, M.D.

INTRODUCTION

Since vascular and circulatory disturbances are involved in the production of the stroke syndrome, an analysis of cardiogenic factors will often elucidate the mechanism for the alterations in cerebral blood flow. Pathophysiological mechanisms for the stroke syndrome include intrinsic cerebrovascular disease, arterial emboli, reductions in the cardiac output and localized disturbances in cerebral circulation. This review will examine the underlying circulatory diseases which may be involved in the production of cerebral emboli, the abnormalities imposed by arteriosclerosis and hypertension on cranial and extracranial vessels, the role of cardiac arrhythmias, current complications of cardiac resuscitation, and abnormal alterations in cardiac output. Currently available forms of therapy for each of these disorders will be discussed and the potential role of metabolic support for combined cardiovascular and cerebral vascular disorders.

EMBOLIC PHENOMENA

Clinically, the most common underlying diseases in patients with cerebral emboli are rheumatic heart disease, coronary artery disease, and bacterial endocarditis (Table 14.1). Patients under the age of 50 years presenting with cerebral emboli often reveal underlying rheumatic heart disease involving stenosis of the mitral valve. Left atrial enlargement and atrial fibrillation further predispose to the development of thrombus formation in the left atrium. Patients over the age of 50 years frequently present with complications of coronary artery disease which may be due to a recent myocardial infarction and mural thrombus or the subsequent development of a ventricular aneurysm. Patients with congenital heart disease, cyanosis and a large right to left intracardiac shunt present

* Supported in part by Specialized Center of Research for Ischemic Heart Disease, Contract #1P17HL1767-01, Cardiovascular Research and Training Center, Program Project Grant #HL,310 (Division of Heart and Vascular Diseases, National Heart and Lung Institute), NIH Grant #T01LM00154, National Institutes of Health.

TABLE 14.1
Sources of Cerebral Emboli

1. Rheumatic heart disease
2. Coronary artery disease
3. Congenital heart disease
4. Bacterial endocarditis
5. Cardiac and vascular surgery

occasionally cerebral emboli. Despite the availability of effective antimicrobial agents, bacterial endocarditis continues to be a frequent cause of cerebral emboli. In the early developmental and technical period, cardiac surgery was occasionally associated with interruptions in cerebral blood flow due to technical complications, but advances have greatly reduced the frequency of this complication. Rarely emboli can originate from intracardiac tumors or sterile thrombotic material that has developed on valve leaflet margins. Therefore, any patient presenting with a stroke syndrome should have careful consideration of these potential underlying cardiac conditions.

ATHEROSCLEROSIS

A major vascular factor underlying the pathophysiology of cerebrovascular disease is atherosclerosis of the intracranial and extracranial arteries (Table 14.2). This occlusive process can disturb cerebral blood flow in the carotid arteries or the basilar artery system. Extracranial arterial involvement often develops at the bifurcation of the arteries at the junction of the common carotid artery and the internal and external carotid branches. In addition to the intimal accumulation and stenotic process of the atheromatous disease, extracranial arteries may further produce emboli to the cerebral circulation which originate from ulcerated areas of the sclerotic plaques. Such emboli may consist of fibrin, platelet aggregations, or cholestrol. The cholestrol emboli may sometimes be visualized in the retinal circulation as highly refractile areas at the bifurcation of retinal arteries.

Hypertension also plays a prominent role in the production and acceleration of atherosclerotic disease in the intracranial and extracranial vessels. The elevated arterial pressure may lead to disruption of the intracranial vessel with hemorrhagic strokes. Hypertension remains a contributory factor in the development of berry aneurysms at the bifurcation of cerebral vessels from the internal carotid. Hypertension is one of the most common cardiovascular disorders and is estimated to affect twenty-three million Americans. Therefore, atherosclerosis and hypertension are common factors in the pathophysiology of the stroke syndrome.

TABLE 14.2
Atherosclerosis

1. Cerebral arteries
2. Extra cranial arteries
3. Ulcerated plaques
4. Hypertension

CARDIAC ARRHYTHMIAS

Intermittent or sustained reductions in cardiac output can result from a variety of rhythm disturbances of the heart (Table 14.3). Electrocardiographic monitoring in coronary care units and intensive care units has significantly improved the recognition of rhythm disturbances which may produce transient cerebral ischemic episodes and potential strokes. Disease of the sinus node which is located in the right atrium may produce a clinical syndrome of intermittent bradycardia which can be further complicated by escape ectopic beats or tachycardia. Disturbances in sinus node impulse formation develop when the sinus node is diseased. When impulse formation is reduced, other pacemaking centers assume the role of the sinus node. Whenever the frequency of impulse generation falls below a critical level, ectopic rhythm disturbances develop in other areas of the atrium, the junctional areas between the right atrium and ventricle, or in the ventricle. These escape rhythms may produce significant tachycardias which can severely reduce the cardiac output. Either the bradycardia or the escape tachycardia can result in sufficient reduction of the cardiac output to impair cerebral blood flow in patients. In those patients with underlying cerebrovascular disease, such reductions in cardiac output may produce brain damage in marginally perfused areas.

In addition to rhythm disturbances that produce bradycardias and tachycardias, another important abnormal heart rhythm is the development of complete heart block with Stokes-Adams episodes or loss of consciousness. Although patients may tolerate complete heart block and extremely slow heart rates without circulatory or neurological symptoms, the disorder is often complicated by transient changes in pacemaker activity when the abnormal focus of impulse formation changes location in the heart. Usually, a period of asystole or ventricular tachycardia fibrillation ensues, and either of these extreme disturbances in heart beat can produce syncope. The extreme reduction in cardiac output, cerebral blood flow, and syncope can produce neurological damage unless therapeutic interventions are prompt.

In a healthy person, cerebral blood flow is usually not significantly reduced until the heart rate exceeds 180 to 200 beats per min. However, the most serious rapid heart rhythms are ventricular tachycardia and ventricular fibrillation which are often associated with loss of consciousness and potential brain damage. Although these rhythm disturbances may occur in the absence of heart disease, there is usually evidence of coronary artery disease with ischemia in either of the ventricles. These rhythm disturbances often complicate the early phase of acute myocardial infarction. The cardiac output and cerebral blood flow are critically reduced and loss of consciousness and brain damage may quickly follow unless restoration to an effective slower heart rate is promptly produced.

Rarely, patients with external carotid artery disease may exhibit syncope owing to sensitivity of the carotid sinus which is located at the bifurcation of the internal and external carotid artery. Normally, massage of the carotid sinus produces transient slowing of the heart rate owing to the mechanism of baroreceptor stimulation and reflex bradycardia. This mechanism may become more sensitive in patients with carotid artery disease or in those patients that have been maintained on digitalis for various cardiac disorders. This clinical entity can produce syncope and if sufficient cerebral vascular disease is present, areas of brain damage may result.

CARDIAC RESUSCITATION

In recent years, the development and availability of emergency rescue squads for patients sustaining sudden cardiovascular collapse or loss of consciousness has increased the number of successful resuscitations (Table 14.4). Also, the availability of resuscitation teams in hospitals has provided prompt reaction to such events within the hospital. However, those situations in which cardiac function and cerebral blood flow are not restored within a critical period of time, the resuscitation may only be

Table 14.3
Cardiac Arrhythmias

1. Sinus node disease
2. Complete heart block
3. Ventricular tachycardia
4. Ventricular fibrillation
5. Carotid sinus sensitivity

Table 14.4
Cardiac Resuscitation

1. Etiology
   A. Cardiac arrhythmia
   B. Acute myocardial infarction
2. Cardiac massage
3. Cerebral hypoxia

successful in restoring cardiac performance with resulting hypoxic damage to the nervous system. The cerebral hypoxia can be localized or diffuse depending on the duration of the impaired cardiac performance, the effectiveness of the resuscitation, and the extent of underlying cerebral vascular disease. When intracranial or extracranial cerebral vascular disease is present, the transient interruptions in cardiac output and cerebral blood flow can produce localized or diffuse cerebral hypoxic damage even though cardiac function may be restored.

TREATMENT

Cerebral emboli that develop from underlying rheumatic heart disease or coronary artery disease generally are treated by systemic anticoagulation (Table 14.5). Experimental and clinical evidence suggest that certain cerebral infarctions may occur without hemorrhage while others may be associated with diffuse hemorrhage. This consideration becomes important in the decision as to the institution of anticoagulation and the selection of rapid or slow induction of anticoagulation. Intravenous heparin provides prompt therapeutic anticoagulation whereas the oral coumadin derivatives provide slower alterations in the clotting system which require 24 to 72 hours. For many years, anticoagulation in patients with bacterial endocarditis was considered a potential complication. Although the complications of bacterial endocarditis prior to the antibiotic era were due to infectious problems, the incidence of cerebral emboli in bacterial endocarditis persists as a major complication. Even though effective antimicrobial agents are available, the cerebral emboli may be sterile. Nevertheless, clinicians have remained somewhat reluctant to anticoagulate patients with bacterial endocarditis.

Patients with coronary artery disease may develop cerebral emboli as the result of an acute myocardial infarction and a mural thrombus. Anticoagulation remains the therapy of choice. Although the ventricular aneurysm and mural thrombus can be surgically removed, anticoagulants are still retained in the management of these problems. The

TABLE 14.5
Treatment of Cardiac Factors in Stroke Syndrome

1. Emboli
   - A. Source
   - B. Anticoagulation
   - C. Surgery
2. Vascular occlusion
   - A. Surgery
3. Cardiac arrhythmias
   - A. Medical management
   - B. Surgical procedures

ventricular aneurysm may be associated with serious cardiac arrhythmias, and isolated reports have described successful elimination of the arrhythmias after removal of the aneurysm. Intracardiac tumors and infected heart valves can be removed by open heart surgical techniques, and these sources of cerebral emboli can be managed surgically. The rapid progress and continued technical improvements in cardiac surgical techniques have reduced the incidence of cerebral emboli during open heart surgery and extracorporeal circulation.

The management of extracranial atherosclerosis in the production of the stroke syndrome continues to be an important area for recognition and surgical intervention. Patients presenting with the stroke syndrome should have careful examination of the carotid arteries for the detection of murmurs. Carotid arteriography has demonstrated a high incidence of extracranial lesions which are operative in the production of the stroke syndrome. Surgical interventions with removal or bypass of the stenosis is an important therapeutic consideration in these patients.

The medical control of hypertension remains a major problem in cardiovascular disease since the stroke syndrome is one of the most common complications of this chronic vascular disease. A number of effective agents are available for the control and management of hypertension. Caution must be exerted in the management of hypertension in older patients. Excessive reduction in arterial pressure or orthostatic hypertension can cause syncope and possible strokes.

The control of rhythm disturbances that alter cerebral blood flow may require both medical and surgical management. Atrial or ventricular ectopic activity and tachycardias can be medically treated with agents such as quinidine, pronestyl, and lidocaine. Lidocaine remains the intravenous agent of choice for the management of acute rhythm disturbances. Bradycardias and complete heart block may respond immediately to an infusion of intravenous isoproterenol. However, continued management requires insertion of a temporary pacemaker and preparation for replacement with a permanent device. The permanent cardiac pacemakers can be introduced through the jugular veins, or in selected situations a thoracotomy may be necessary. Cardiac pacemakers have proved to be highly effective for several years with a significant reduction in technical complications.

Recent experimental and clinical studies have suggested that the infusion of certain metabolic substrates may be useful during the temporary interruption of blood flow that can occur either in the heart or the brain (Table 14.6). In acute myocardial infarction, although the blood supply may be impaired to the area of damaged muscle, there is evidence that marginal zones of the ischemic tissue are still perfused

TABLE 14.6
Metabolic Support of Ischemic Tissue

1. Experimental evidence
2. Substrate sources
   A. Succinate
   B. Glucose — insulin — potassium
3. Monitoring requirements

during the early phase. Similarly, collateral flow in the brain may develop around the margins of injured tissue owing to deprived or severely reduced cerebral blood flow. Previous experimental studies have shown that the simultaneous aortic and vena cava occlusion in animals produces a 50% decrease in cerebral ATP in less than 4 minutes after the occlusion (1). Efforts directed at the preservation of the biological energy source ATP both in the heart and in the brain have employed hypothermia, perfusion techniques, and the infusion of substrates that may augment metabolism and ATP generation. In the brain, the glutamate succinate pathway may serve as a secondary support system in the maintenance of brain energy levels (4). Succinate has been shown to protect against hyperbaric toxicity of hyperbaric oxygenation and also preserve ATP levels prior to the development of seizure activity (5). Cardiovascular studies on experimental and clinical myocardial infarction have shown that infusions of solutions containing glucose-insulin-potassium can provide electrical and mechanical stability in hearts that were rendered ischemic. Although the brain primarily uses glucose as a source of biological energy, the heart can utilize lipids and other ketone bodies besides the glucose. The increase in anaerobic metabolism with availibility of glucose and insulin can support marginal ischemic issues of the heart during periods of temporary interruption of blood supply (3). Experimental studies have demonstrated that the glucose-insulin-potassium infusion can support the levels of ATP even in the necrotic and ischemic myocardium (2). Preliminary clinical studies suggest that an infusion of glucose-insulin-potassium may not only benefit the myocardium in patients sustaining acute myocardial infarction but also support the attendant cerebral hypoxia that can occur in patients resuscitated by rescue squads. The glucose-insulin-potassium solution has been infused as long as 3 weeks in a patient who had sustained cerebral damage following cardiac resuscitation. The infusion of substrates to support metabolic and biochemical pathways in marginally ischemic areas is an exciting area for future exploration.

SUMMARY

The cardiogenic factors which may contribute to the stroke syndrome have been discussed (Table 14.7). Pathophysiological mechanisms in-

TABLE 14.7
Cardiogenic Factors in Stroke Syndrome

1. Emboli
2. Atherosclerosis
3. Cardiac arrhythmias
4. Cardiac resuscitation
5. Treatment

clude emboli from rheumatic coronary and congenital heart diseases. Atherosclerotic disease and hypertension can involve both intracranial and extracranial arteries. Disturbances in cardiac rhythm can significantly reduce cerebral blood flow. The development of cerebral hypoxia with resuscitation is described. Treatment of these disorders is reviewed, and the potential role of metabolic support of the ischemic tissue both with cerebral and myocardial damage has been presented.

REFERENCES

1. Kramer, R. S., Sanders, A. P., Lesage, A. M., Woodhall, B., and Sealy, W. C. The effect of profound hypothermia on preservation of cerebral ATP content during circulatory arrest. J. Thorac. Cardiovasc. Surg., *56:* 699–709, 1968.
2. Opie, L. H., Bruyneel, K., and Owen, P. Effects of glucose, insulin and potassium infusion on tissue metabolic changes within first hour of myocardial infarction in the baboon. Circulation, *52:* 49–57, 1975.
3. Rogers, W. J., Stanley, A. W., Jr., Breinig, J. B., Prather, J. W., McDaniel, H. G., Moraski, R. E., Mantle, J. A., Russell, R. O., Jr., and Rackley, C. E. Reduction of hospital mortality of acute myocardial infarction with glucose-insulin-potassium infusion. Am. Heart J. In press.
4. Sanders, A. P., Currie, W. D., and Woodhall, B. Protection of brain metabolism with glutathione, glutamate, aminobutyrate and succinate. Proc. Soc. Exp. Biol. Med., *130:* 1021–1027, 1969.
5. Woodhall, B., Kramer, R. S., Currie, W. D., and Sanders, A. P. Brain energetics and neurosurgery. A review of recent studies done at Duke University. J. Neurosurg., *34:* 3–14, 1971.

CHAPTER

15

Epidemiology and Prevention of Stroke

WILLIAM S. FIELDS, M.D.

Data regarding the epidemiological characteristics of cerebrovascular disease are extremely difficult to obtain and more difficult to validate. Studies which present incidence rates by age, sex, and race differ widely with respect to the methods used to ascertain the information, the definition of the clinical disease, and the size of the population base under consideration (7). In many reports there has been no attempt made to distinguish between different etiological categories such as subarachnoid hemorrhage, intracerebral hemorrhage, and cerebral infarction. Ideally one should be able to consider, in addition, the severity of disease among the cases recorded, but unfortunately one is unable to achieve this goal by examining available data. The various manifestations of stroke are known largely from series of clinical cases, and data obtained from these sources cannot be appropriately extrapolated to a general population (8).

Even fewer data are available with respect to prevalence of stroke. The prevalence of any disease is the joint function of incidence, rate of recovery, and duration of survival. Information regarding prevalence would be invaluable in the planning of any health care delivery system for stroke patients and, therefore, knowledge of the extent of residual disability becomes a very critical consideration. Although very little definitive information is currently available, a recent survey suggests that of every 100 persons who survive the acute illness, 10 will be able to return to work virtually without impairment, 40 will have mild residual disability, 40 will be so disabled that they require special services, and 10 will need institutional care (11).

Mortality figures for a variety of specific populations can be found in published reports but there is little or no precise information with respect to the relative distribution of fatal stroke among the generally accepted clinical categories. Most epidemiological studies have been based on hospital cases or on postmortem examination and, therefore, it is likely that those individuals with less severe cerebrovascular disorders are seriously under reported. Unfortunately, these are the cases about which we need to know the most if we are to understand the role played by various risk factors, particularly those that influence the development of atherosclerosis and the mechanisms of coagulation.

Because of limitations of time, attention will be directed only to risk factors and prevention as they relate to ischemic cerebrovascular disease and not to hemorrhage.

Since stroke, particularly ischemic stroke, is considered generally to be a clinical consequence of atherosclerosis, investigators have been led to look for causative factors similar to those associated with ischemic cardiac disease. Regrettably, all that can be said with any degree of accuracy is that the risk of stroke increases sharply with increasing age, and that in most white populations, it occurs about 10 years later than myocardial infarction (6). It is almost impossible, however, recognizing the competing risks for the two diseases, namely myocardial and cerebral infarction, to be certain how many persons who died of the former might have suffered the latter had they survived for the additional 10 years. The harvesting effect of the first illness influences one's ability to obtain information about a concomitant serious vascular disorder which characteristically manifests itself clinically later in life.

Numerous factors have been considered as possibly being related to the occurrence of stroke. The evidence for some is minimal so that it is difficult to put a specific degree of priority on each in the present state of our knowledge. The problem in discussing risk factors and stroke prevention becomes even more difficult when one takes into consideration the fact that cerebral infarction due to intravascular occlusion has quite a different pathogenesis from that of intracranial hemorrhage of either the intracerebral or subarachnoid type. Furthermore, cerebral infarction may be due to either atherosclerotic occlusion *in situ* of an extracranial or intracranial artery, to an embolus originating from an ulcerated atheromatous plaque in an internal carotid artery, or an embolus from a cardiac source.

It is evident, however, that the most important concerns with regard to stroke prevention are the identification and treatment of individuals with: (1) hypertension, (2) transient cerebral ischemic attacks, and (3) cardiac disorders that are frequently associated with cerebrovascular complications (14). Consequently, in this presentation no attempt will be made to discuss all risk factors which might conceivably be involved but to devote attention to those which are most frequently implicated and most readily identifiable and treatable.

Hypertension appears to be the most important alterable factor that is associated with nonembolic cerebral infarction, but the information is far from complete at present. From the best available data, it appears that strokes are from 2 to 4 times as frequent in hypertensive as in comparable normotensive individuals (11). Actuarial data indicate that mortality from cerebrovascular disease increases as blood pressure elevates, starting with the lowest levels at which hypertension may be suspected. Diastolic pressures appear to be no more reliable than systolic pressures as indicators of risk for stroke, and no reliable information concerning individuals with systolic hypertension in the absence of diastolic elevation is available at the present time.

It is reasonable to ask whether control of existing hypertension lowers subsequent stroke incidence. Information regarding this question is known only from studies of individuals who have already had an identifiable cerebral infarction and then allocated in a random fashion to antihypertensive therapy or placebo (1, 5, 12). It is generally accepted that sufficient evidence has accumulated to indicate that hypertension is not only a significant cause of stroke but also the most readily treatable risk factor for this condition. It would appear justified, therefore, to undertake extensive drug trials in hypertensive populations with the view to preventing cerebral infarction and hemorrhage.

Induced hypotension of an excessive or prolonged degree from any cause, including shock, severe hemorrhage, surgery, dehydration, various medications, and diagnostic procedures may lead to diffuse cerebral ischemia. In the presence of atherosclerotic arterial disease, the reduction of blood flow may become critical in a region supplied by a vessel, the lumen of which has been severely compromised. Whenever procedures which may cause such hypotension are undertaken, careful monitoring of blood pressure is of critical importance.

Transient cerebral ischemic attacks and *amaurosis fugax* are recognized generally as precursors of ischemic stroke since the best available evidence suggests that approximately one-third of affected individuals are likely to have a cerebral infarct within 5 years of the onset of such episodes (13). This is more than 10 times the rate of expected stroke incidence for persons of the same age and sex in the general population. Conversely, approximately three of every four persons with cerebral infarction and four of every five with documented internal carotid artery occlusion will give a history of one or more transient ischemic attacks (9).

Some physicians hold to the belief that long term anticoagulant therapy with coumarin type drugs in patients with transient ischemic attacks prevent stroke in a high percentage of cases (10). However, many others consider that the possibility of serious hemorrhagic complications from the protracted use of such agents outweighs any potential advantage, or that the anticoagulant drugs are ineffective. Numerous other medical treatments including agents presumed to be cerebral vascular dilators (so-called vasoactive drugs) have been recommended for patients with transient ischemic attacks, but there is absolutely no substantiating data, although these agents are widely employed both in Europe and North America.

Transient ischemic attacks are associated in a high percentage of cases with angiographic evidence of severe stenosis of the extracranial portion of the appropriate internal carotid artery or with ulcerated plaque in a similar location. Arterial reconstructive surgery with removal of the offending lesion has been shown to be beneficial in preventing subsequent cerebral infarction in the territory supplied by that vessel (2). Usually a person with transient ischemic attacks who is a candidate for carotid endarterectomy will have either a well localized bruit over the carotid bifurcation in the midcervical region or decreased ipsilateral retinal artery pressure as measured by ophthalmodynamometry or some similar noninvasive procedure. Individuals with this combination of symptoms and signs should be studied carefully by arteriography and, if an appropriate lesion is demonstrated, a carotid endarterectomy would be considered to be an appropriate method of treatment. However, since symptomatic patients seldom have a solitary lesion it would seem reasonable to recommend medical therapy postoperatively.

Platelet-fibrin emboli in retinal arterioles either with or without associated cholesterol emboli may also arise from an ulcerated plaque. In all probability they occur more commonly than cholesterol emboli but are not observed as often. They are the type of emboli usually seen when the fundus of the eye is examined during the transient episodes of monocular blindness. Presumably if these emboli originate from a lesion proximal to the ophthalmic artery, it is likely that others from the same source may pass further downstream and obstruct cerebral vessels as well.

Observation of either cholesterol emboli or platelet-fibrin emboli in the retinal arteries associated with symptoms of monocular blindness or cerebral ischemia is considered presumptive evidence of a lesion correctable by surgery; therefore, arteriography should be done in all such patients.

Many authorities recommend no further studies or treatment for an asymptomatic patient with normal or even decreased ipsilateral retinal artery pressure who has a localized systolic bruit over the carotid bifurcation. However, others advise angiography and surgery in selected persons with asymptomatic carotid bruit, especially those in whom major surgical procedures are contemplated either in the thorax or abdomen. Recognizing, however, that there is surgical risk involved, carotid procedures should be carried out only in the facility where the operative team is experienced in arterial surgery and capable of managing any ensuing complications (4).

In the past several years, evidence has been accumulating that transient ischemic attacks may be eliminated or reduced in frequency by administration of nonsteroidal anti-inflammatory drugs which modify platelet function in intra-arterial coagulation (3). This is based upon the assumption that most transient ischemic attacks are due to downstream embolization of fibrinoplatelet emboli formed on irregular, roughened, or ulcerated atherosclerotic plaques. Prevention by suppressing platelet aggregation seems promising in transient ischemic attacks, but there is no certainty that the pathogenesis of such attacks is the same as that for cerebral infarction. One could conceivably eliminate the former without reducing the risk of the latter. Several studies are currently underway, one in Canada and the other in the United States, to study this problem. Thus far, no definitive report has been released.

Embolic infarction characteristically presents as a single, abrupt event which reaches its peak very quickly. Recent advances in the prevention and treatment of many cardiovascular diseases have changed the incidence of stroke associated with these disorders. For example, the use of prophylactic antibiotics has reduced the incidence of rheumatic heart disease and subacute bacterial endocarditis and consequently has reduced the incidence of cerebral embolism. Cerebral infarction following the insertion of a prosthetic heart valve is now one of the common neurological problems encountered by cardiovascular specialists. Most authorities agree, however, that the frequency of stroke from this cause can be reduced by employing judicious postoperative anticoagulant or platelet suppressive therapy.

The highest correlation between embolic cerebral infarction and prior cardiac rhythm disorder occurs with atrial fibrillation. Patients with either chronic or intermittent fibrillation should be considered as stroke prone. Anticoagulant therapy should be considered for all patients with long standing atrial fibrillation, especially when there is evidence of valvular heart disease.

When an acute myocardial infarction occurs, there are usually no detectable physical findings suggestive of endomural thrombi unless the patient already demonstrates evidence of an embolus to the brain or elsewhere. On the other hand, myocardial infarction is occasionally recognized only after the occurrence of a stroke and, therefore, it is advisable in all acute stroke patients to obtain an electrocardiogram as soon as possible after the onset of the neurological disorder.

Public education should be provided in terms of the known risk factors for cerebrovascular disease in order to facilitate early institution of medical or surgical care in the potential stroke victim. Furthermore, those persons who are considered stroke prone should be urged to have proper evaluation and treatment. It has been adequately demonstrated beyond any doubt that people vary in their patterns of response to dangerous situations. The person who does not seek attention when threatened with any illness may be weighing different competing risks. The average individual assumes that most preventive health measures are excessively expensive, and if there is a low risk of acquiring a certain disease, he may not wish to pay the cost involved in avoiding the potential disorder. He seldom considers, however, that its treatment may be far more expensive than the preventive care he could have obtained initially. Usually it is only after the patient has become ill that he and his family are susceptible to health education. At that time he may be willing to examine all aspects of the predisposing causes and learn how to avoid another incident or be more amenable to following suggestions which may lead to a satisfactory recovery.

In spite of the fact that there are limitations in our knowledge with regard to stroke prevention, the public should know this also and be made aware of the available diagnostic measures and treatment. A continuing campaign should be conducted which will focus on the responsibility of the individual for changing his own health habits, particularly in relation to the prevention of serious illness.

REFERENCES

1. Carter, A. B., and Barham, A. Hypotensive therapy in stroke survivors. Lancet. *1:* 485–497, 1970.
2. Fields, W. S. Selection of stroke patients for arterial reconstructive surgery. Am. J. Surg., *125:* 527–529 1973.
3. Fields, W. S., and Hass, W. K. (eds): Aspirin, Platelets and Stroke. 163 pp. Warren H. Green, Inc., St. Louis, 1971.
4. Fields, W. S., Maslenikov, V., Meyer, J. S., Hass, W. K., Remington, R. D. and MacDonald, M. Joint study of extracranial arterial occlusion: V. Progress report of prognosis following surgery or nonsurgical treatment for transient cerebral ischemic attacks and cervical carotid artery lesions. J.A.M.A. *211:* 1993–2003, 1970.
5. Hypertensive Stroke Cooperative Study group. Effect of antihypertensive treatment on stroke recurrence. J.A.M.A. *229:* 409–418, 1974.
6. Kannel, W. B., Dawber, T. R., Cohen, M. E. and McNamara, P. M. Vascular disease of the brain: epidemiologic aspects: The Framingham Study. Am. J. Public Health, *55:* 1355–1366, 1965.
7. Kuller, L., Cook, L. P. and Friedman, G. D. Survey of stroke epidemiology studies. Draft report by the Committee of Criteria and Methods, Council on Epidemiology, American Heart Association, 1971.
8. Kurtzke, J. F., Epidemiology of Cerebrovascular Disease, 197 pp. Springer-Verlag, Berlin, 1969.

9. *In* Cerebral Vascular Diseases; Transaction of the Fourth Conference, edited by C. H. Millikan, R. G. Siekert, and J. P. Whisnant, pp. 221–235, Grune & Stratton, New York, 1965.
10. Millikan, C. H. Reassessment of anticoagulant therapy in various types of occlusive cerebrovascular disease. Stroke, *2:* 201–208, 1971.
11. Stallones, R. A., Dyken, M. L., Fang, H. C. H., Heyman, A., Seltser, R., and Stamler, J. Report of the Joint Committee for Stroke Facilities I. Epidemiology for Stroke Facilities Planning. Stroke, *3:* 359–371, 1972.
12. Veterans Administration Cooperative Study Group on Antihypertensive Agents. Effects of treatment on morbidity in hypertension: results in patients with diastolic blood pressures averaging 115-129 mm. Hg. J.A.M.A., *202:* 1028–1034, 1967.
13. Whisnant, J. P., Anderson, E. M., Aronson, S. M., Harrison, C. E., Haynes, M. A., Kurtzke, J. F., Lindsay, W. H., Ostfeld, A. M., Rentz, L. E., and Sundt, T. M. Jr. Report of the Joint Committee for Stroke Facilities V. Clinical Prevention of Stroke. Stroke, *3:* 803–825, 1972.
14. Whisnant, J. P. Matsumoto, N., and Kurland, L. T. Transient cerebral ischemic attacks in a community: Rochester, Minn., 1955–1969. Circulation, *44*(Suppl. 2)*:* 94, 1971.

CHAPTER

16

Strokes in Children

JOHN SHILLITO, JR., M.D.

In children, a sudden neurological deficit, or "stroke" may be caused by hemorrhage, vascular insufficiency, or by neither. The variety of causes is greater than in adulthood. With the one exception of arteriosclerotic cardiovascular disease, a child is subject to all the adult problems, plus a great number peculiar to the young. For example, certain congenital anomalies are of such a nature that they must cause trouble early in life: metabolic defects such as hemophilia and homocystinuria; anatomic anomalies such as those of the heart and great vessels. Bleeding from aneurysms and arteriovenous malformations (AVMs) may occur even in infancy. Furthermore, some diseases which are common to childhood may affect the blood vessels or the blood clotting mechanism, as does leukemia.

To illustrate some of the many problems, nine cases from the Boston Children's Hospital will be presented, not under any diagnostic heading, but as they presented themselves. Each child had suffered a sudden neurological deficit which suggested a cerebrovascular accident. Some attacks were transient, others progressive. We will let you be the diagnostician, as each story unfolds.

In trying to sort out the diagnostic clues, a neurosurgeon may find himself facing one of the problems of his veterinarian colleague—the patient is not always a good historian and in fact may not speak at all!

CASE HISTORIES

Case 1. *Sudden hemiplegia and coma.* This 10-year-old boy had been playing at school, walked up two flights of stairs, sat down at his desk, and began to cry because he could not move his right arm or leg. He vomited and became unconscious. After hospitalization, he gradually awakened, but the hemiplegia persisted. A hemihypalgesia was also noted as he became more lucid. Although right-handed, he was not aphasic. Skull films were normal. A lumbar puncture showed grossly bloody fluid. A left carotid arteriogram (Fig. 16.1) showed only slight displacement of midline vessels to the right. There were no occlusions and no recognizable sources of bleeding. He remained stable. The next day a pneumoencephlogram was done, which showed downward displacement of the posterior portion of the left lateral ventricle (Fig. 16.2) and suggested a parietal mass (Fig. 16.3). Since this occurred in 1956, some of today's diagnostic tests were unavailable. Some centers in Boston were just

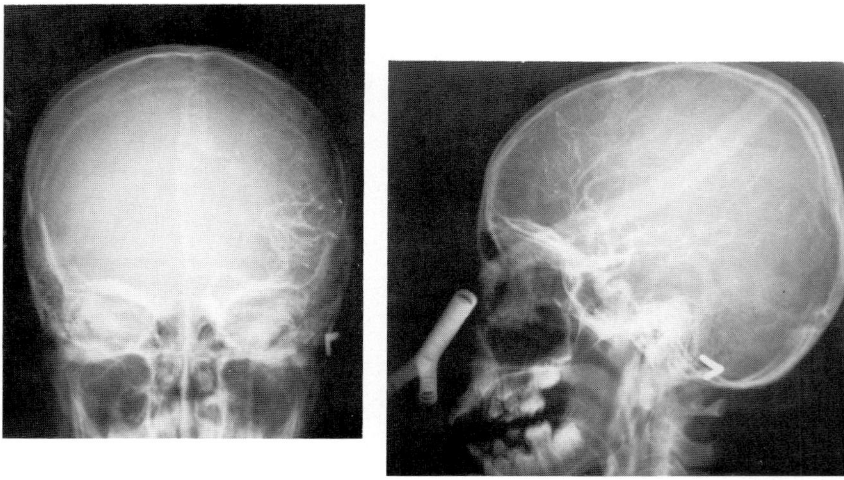

FIG. 16.1. Case 1. Left carotid arteriogram, showing subtle evidence of a parietal mass, but no abnormal vasculature.

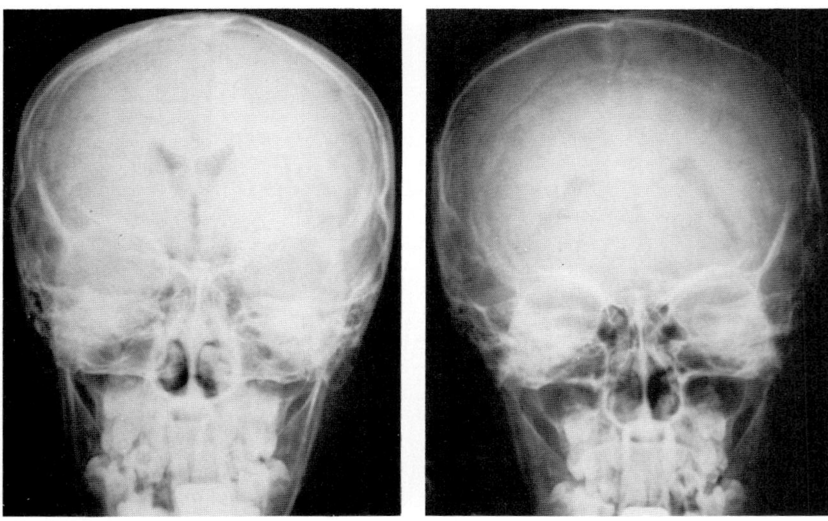

FIG. 16.2. Case 1. Pneumoencephalography confirms presence of left parietal mass.

beginning to scan with radioactive arsenic. The Electronic Musical Instrument Company was not then making computers.

Because the studies indicated a mass lesion, the boy was explored. On the surface of the left parietal area was a small vascular lesion 1.5 cm. in diameter which appeared to contain clot. There was some staining of the arachnoid nearby but no surface clot nor widespread subarachnoid hemorrhage. Careful dissection around this mass revealed that it was supplied by three small arteries and about the same number of veins which drained toward the midline. These were not thrombosed and were seen to contain arterial blood. After tying, clipping, and dividing the feeding vessels, the lesion literally fell out into the operator's hand (Fig. 16.4). Beneath it within the parietal lobe was a clot estimated at 50 ml. This was removed through two small cortical incisions. The boy recovered the use of his right side but still had a severe seizure problem when last seen 11 years later.

Diagnosis: Thrombosed AVM with intracortical clot.

Here a mass and lack of diagnosis prompted exploration. At operation there appeared to be still a trickle of blood through the malformation, although it did not show on the arteriogram. More often lesions of this size are angiographically demonstrable. Not only may they hemorrhage but they may come to attention in a multitude of ways: headache, dilated scalp veins, asymptomatic bruits (which the pediatrician then wishes he had never heard!), slowly progressive neurological deficit, seizures, or hydrocephalus. They can mimic brain tumors and even multiple sclerosis (1).

Once discovered, what to do with them? Our understanding of the natural history of these malformations is at best inaccurate for we do not

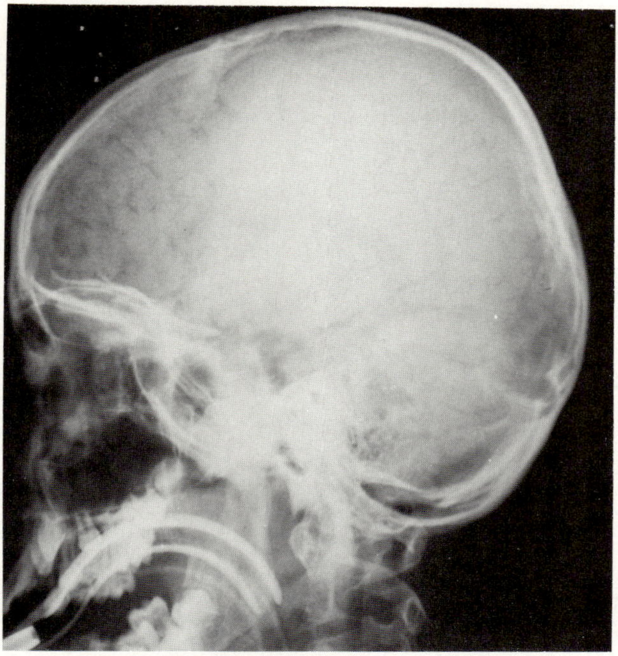

FIG. 16.3. Case 1. Pneumoencephalography showing distortion of body of lateral ventricle.

know how many undiscovered lesions exist. Variation in their size, pattern, and location is infinite. We find it hard to predict for patient or parents which malformation will ever bleed not to mention which will bleed again. The size of the malformation does not correlate with its propensity to hemorrhage. Massive lesions which involve almost an entire hemicranium may not produce symptoms of any kind until adulthood. Microscopic arteriovenous malformations found in surgically evacuated intracortical clots are not even apparent on preoperative arteriograms.

In general, if you can obliterate the shunt without hurting the patient, do so. The likelihood of doing some harm and the nature and extent of that deficit which the patient might have to exchange for eradication can only be decided on an individual basis. Certainly prophylactic ablation is desirable if the price to be paid is nonexistent or small, for a child has a long life ahead and the possibility of getting into trouble is greater than when such a malformation is discovered in middle age.

Successful treatment of these lesions necessitates interruption of the shunt or shunts. Ideally, this should be done at the point or points of entry of arterial feeders into the venous system. Ligation of the arterial feeders far proximal to the site of the shunt must ultimately fail unless there happens to be no collateral channel between the site of ligation and

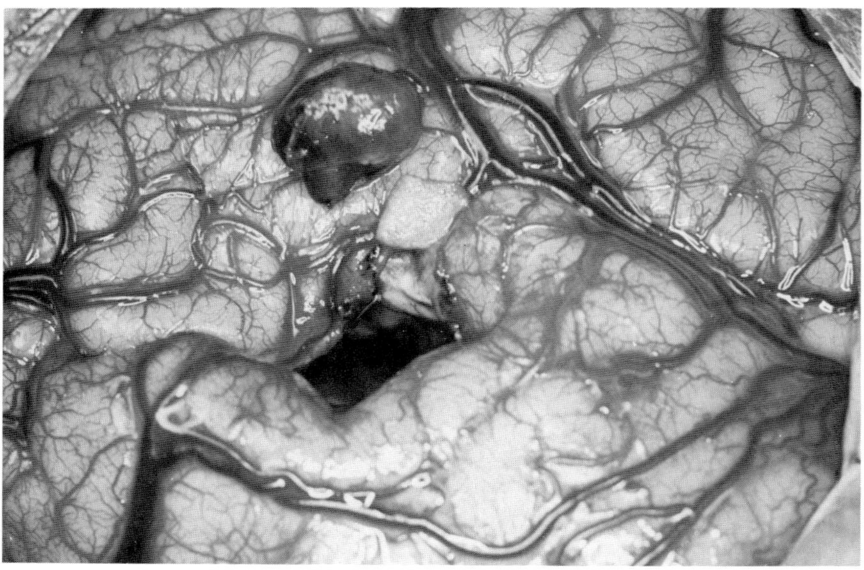

FIG. 16.4. Case 1. Operative photograph of small superficial AVM and cavity in parietal lobe from which clot was evacuated.

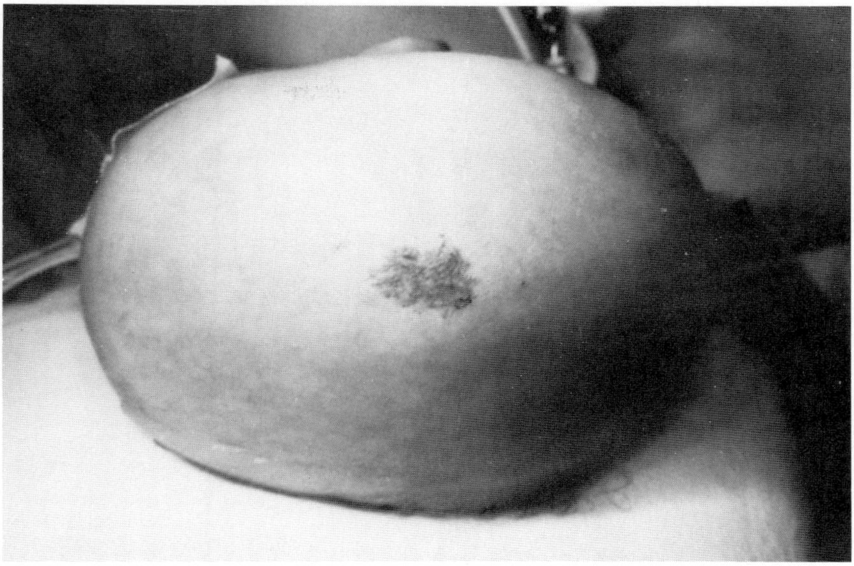

FIG. 16.5. Angioma of scalp of 5½-week-old girl with large AVM of right parietal lobe.

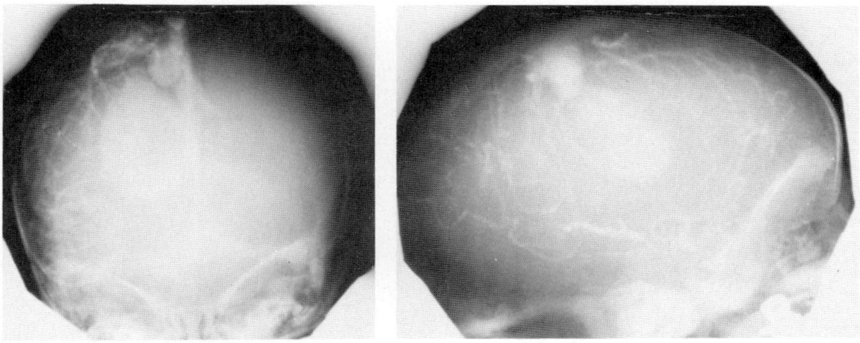

FIG. 16.6. Right carotid angiogram of patient shown in Figure 16.5; AVM appears tri-lobed. Deep large lobe fills and drains from above.

the lesion. This is rarely the case. Ideally, a tie or clip must be placed exactly at the lesion, as, for example, in controlling primary malformations of the vein of Galen (3). The same principle applies to embolization techniques: occlude the shunt without occluding an important artery and without making the occlusion too proximal. Surgery, embolization, or a combination of both, aided by the operating microscope and all the instrumentation that it has brought, are our best tools at the moment.

Some lesions are awesome but manageable. A 5½-week-old girl

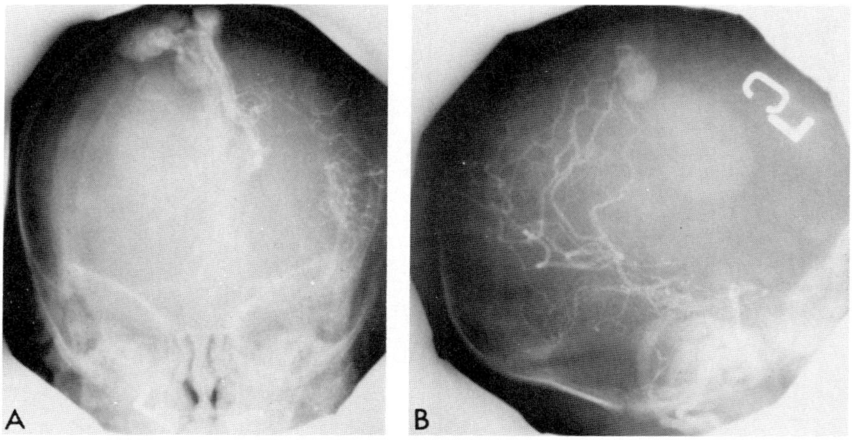

Fig. 16.7. (A) Left carotid and (B) vertebral angiograms of same patient as in Figures 16.5 and 16.6.

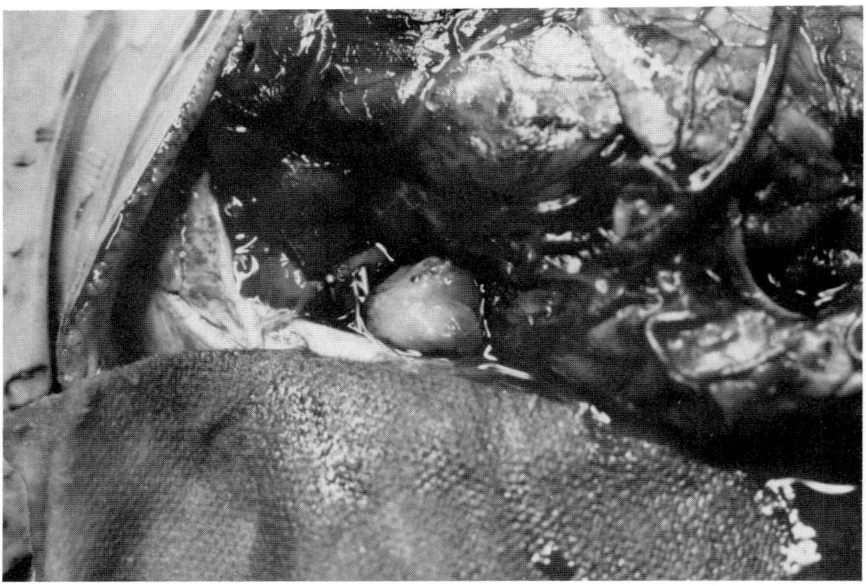

Fig. 16.8. Operative photograph showing superficial sac of AVM shown in Figures 16.6 and 16.7.

developed seizures. There was an angioma on the right parietal scalp (Fig. 16.5). Her right carotid arteriogram (Fig. 16.6) showed a trilobed sac. Two small superficial sacs were recipients of several arterial feeders from the carotid and also the vertebral arteries (Fig. 16.7). The larger sac was apparently a blind pseudoaneurysm of one of the others. At craniotomy it was apparent that there had been extensive hemorrhage into the right hemisphere, presumably venous in origin, for damage was quite remote from the lesion (Fig. 16.8). It was eradicated without excision by securing the feeders at the smaller sac (Fig. 16.9). She was later shunted for a communicating hydrocephalus.

Some massive lesions are compatible with long life. A 14-year-old girl

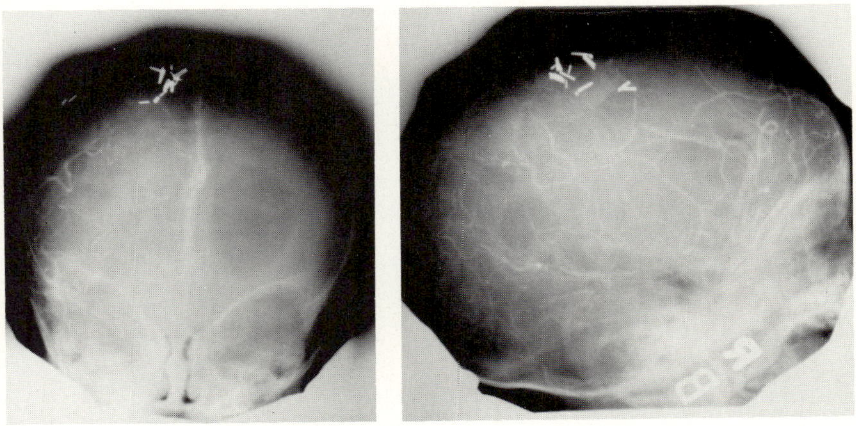

FIG. 16.9. Post-operative angiogram showing obliteration of the AVM. Note hydrocephalus.

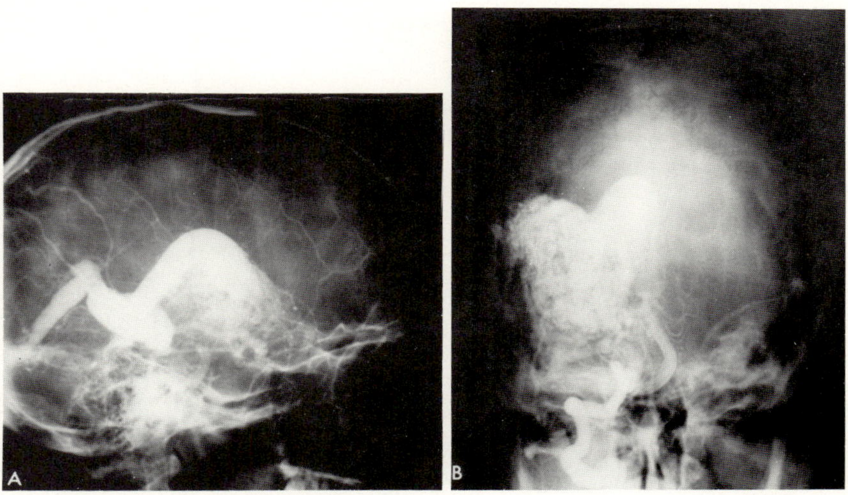

FIG. 16.10. (A and B). Angiograms showing massive right hemisphere AVM in a 14-year-old girl. Venous drainage into the vein of Galen has enlarged it, but the shunt is diffuse and intracortical.

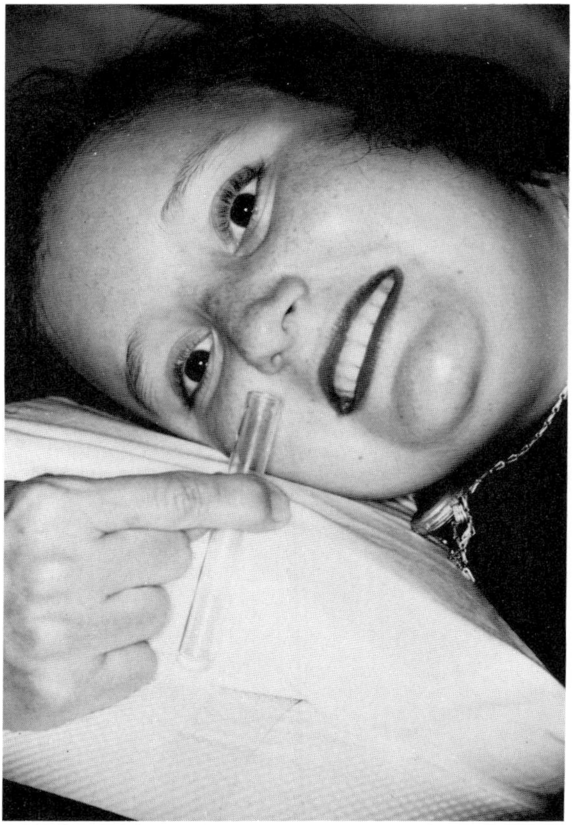

FIG. 16.11. CSF rhinorrhea in girl shown in Figure 16.10; hydrocephalus secondary to vein of Galen enlargement produced spontaneous, intermittent leak.

presented with headache and was found to have an enlarged sella turcica. It was said that she had "cerebral palsy" because of a very slowly progressive hemiparesis. A loud bruit was heard over the right posterior cranium. Arteriograms (Fig. 16.10) showed that a massive malformation occupying much of the right hemisphere secondarily involved the vein of Galen. Rhinorrhea (Fig. 16.11) prompted a shunting procedure. She is little changed 12 years after discovery of this inoperable lesion which has never bled. Her bruit has actually lessened. Although blood is shunted into the vein of Galen which is greatly enlarged, this is not an example of the operable primary malformation involving that vein.

Another girl (CD #83-52-03) suffered a subarachnoid hemorrhage at age 21. She was found to have an occipital AVM (Fig. 16.12). It was resected using loupes and bipolar forceps without leaving any residual neurological deficit.

One AVM will always be remembered. A 16-year-old boy suffered an intracranial hemorrhage which led to arteriographic studies (Figs. 16.13 and 16.14) made shortly after his first hemorrhage. Plans had been made at another center for an elective stereotactic ablation of the lesion. Prior to that appointment, however, the boy had a lesser hemorrhage from which he recovered readily. The parents were understandably quite concerned and sought help elsewhere. It was elected first to perform a pneumoencephalogram and with air still in the ventricles to repeat the arteriographic studies to show the relationship of the lesion to the ventricle to aid in its localization. To our great surprise and joy, the

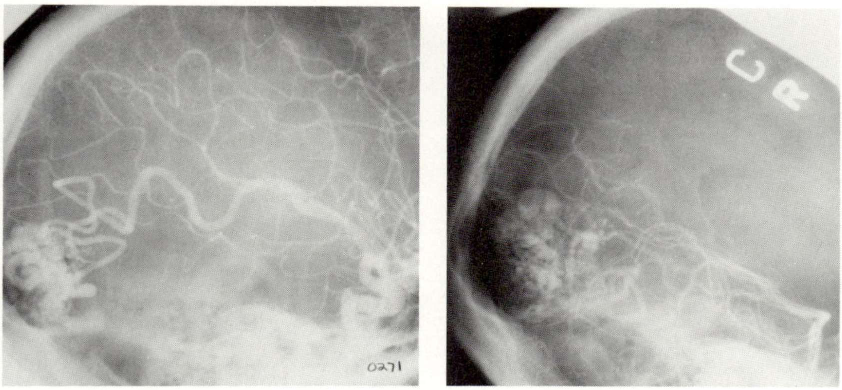

FIG. 16.12. Occipital AVM in a 21-year-old girl (C.D. #83-52-03), resected without neurological deficit. Blood supply was from carotid and vertebral circulation.

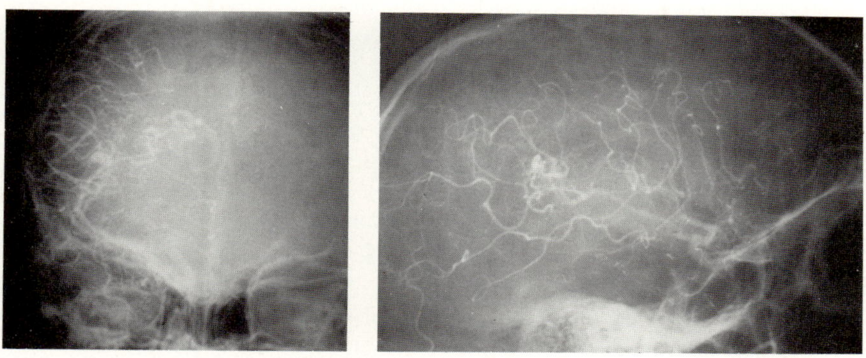

FIG. 16.13. Small deep AVM in dominant hemisphere of a 16-year-old boy. Hemorrhage prompted this first study. Arterial phase.

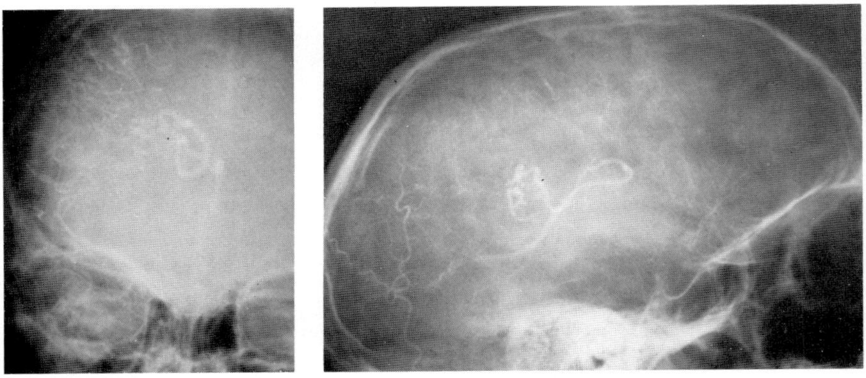

FIG. 16.14. Same patient as in Figure 16.13, venous phase.

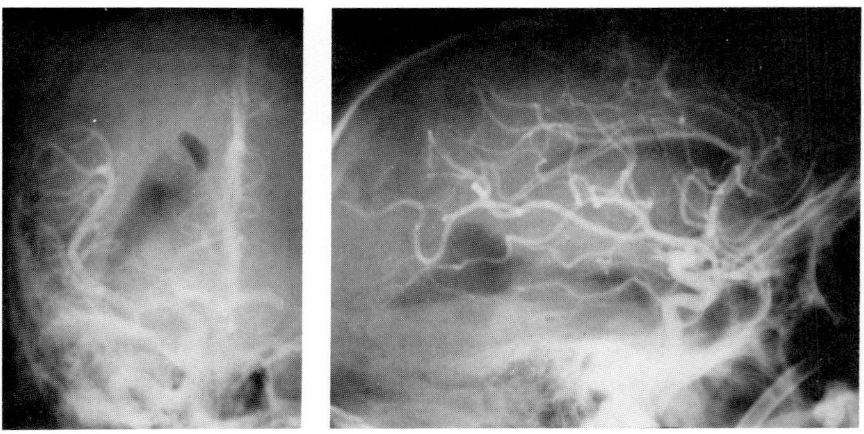

FIG. 16.15. Combination pneumoencephalogram and arteriogram in same patient as in Figures 16.13 and 16.14, after second hemorrhage had destroyed the malformation. Arterial phase.

malformation had disappeared (Figs. 16.15 and 16.16)! Neither we nor the parents could believe this good fortune so the arteriograms were repeated 6 months later. Still no sign of the malformation! The second bleeding episode apparently destroyed it completely.

In the cooperative study (17) of 52 children presenting with subarachnoid hemorrhage, 29% were found to have AVMs.

In the Children's Hospital Medical Center experience there have been 65 patients (Table 16.1). In his text *Neurosurgery of Infancy and Childhood* (19), Dr. Matson reported 34 confirmed AVMs between 1952 and 1966. These were exclusive of primary malformations of the vein of Galen, which were dealt with separately, as were post-traumatic malformations, and the cryptic malformations which he considered hamartomas.

To this group has been added another consisting of 31 patients treated in the period 1967 to the present, October 1975, making a total series of 65 patients. The mortality rate associated with ligation or excision of the lesion has fallen from 24% to zero. The mortality rate in the group not dealt with surgically except by shunt has fallen from 53 to 7.5%. What this really means is hard to know without studying each patient's history and each patient's lesion.

Case 2. *Shoveling snow; collapsed.* This 11 2/12-year-old boy was shoveling snow when he collapsed with a headache and soon became stuporous. Arteriograms showed a deep

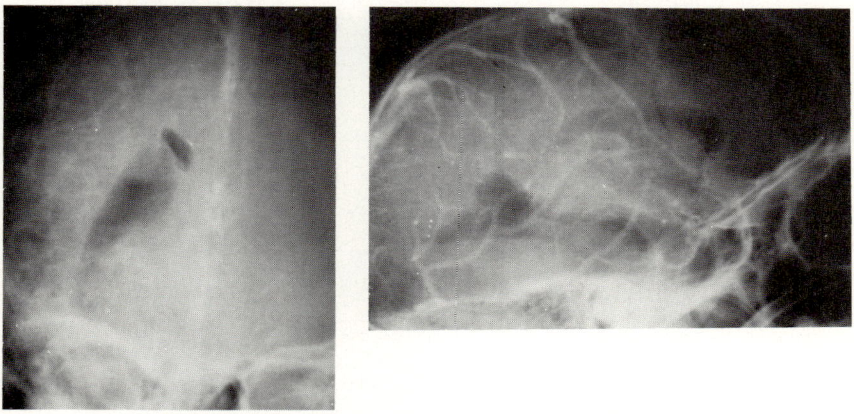

FIG. 16.16. Same patient as in Figures 16.13–16.15, venous phase. No sign of malformation.

TABLE 16.1.

Summary of Intracranial Arteriovenous Malformations Diagnosed at the Children's Hospital Medical Center, Boston, 1952–1975. Cryptic Microscopic and Primary Vein of Galen Malformations are not Included.

	OPERATED			UNOPERATED	
PATIENTS	LIGATION	CLOT ONLY	FEEDERS	SHUNT	NONE
34	12	4	1	3	14
1952-1966	MORTALITY 24 %			MORTALITY 53 %	
31	15	0	1	1	14
1967-1975	MORTALITY 0			MORTALITY 7.5 %	
65	33 TOTAL OPS, MORTALITY 12 %			32 PATIENTS, MORTALITY 34 %	

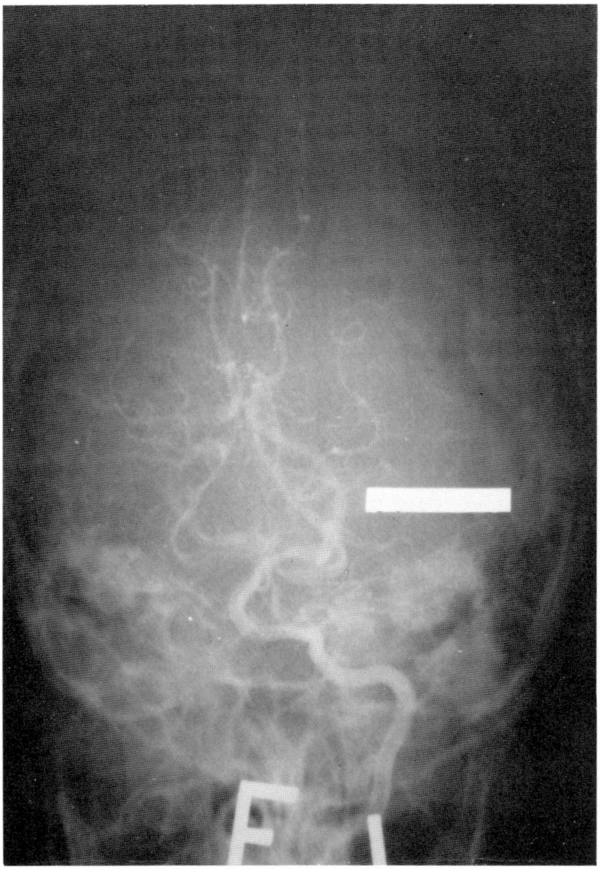

FIG. 16.17. Case 2. Arteriograms show a deep posterior parietal mass but no abnormal vasculature. Anteroposterior view.

posterior mass (Fig. 16.17) but no abnormal vasculature (Fig. 16.18). Clot was removed from the area within 24 hours of his first symptoms. He never awakened and died at the end of the week.

At autopsy, a microscopic AVM (Fig. 16.19) was found 1 cm. deeper than a piece of Gelfoam which had been placed on the wall of the cavity containing the clot.

Diagnosis: Cryptic vascular hamartoma of the parietal lobe.

All such lesions in our series have presented with hemorrhage, usually massive and sometimes fatal. The lesion has not been demonstrable angiographically. Usually the presence of a large amount of clot demands evacuation at which time the malformation may be found in the specimen. Repeated smaller bleeding episodes have been documented from such lesions and have been very puzzling. A 19-year-old girl had three episodes over a period of as many years which were thought by their subtle and rapidly clearing nature to be indicative probably of multiple sclerosis (1). On the occasion of the third episode, however, unexpected xanthochromia of her spinal fluid prompted a pneumoencephalogram which showed a mass in her left thalamus (Fig. 16.20). Transparietal, transventricular exploration showed that this mass was only blood (Fig. 16.21). It was elected not to biopsy the wall of the cavity in this important area so what is left of the presumed malformation remains cryptic. Nine years later she is well, almost normal neurologically, is married, and has one child. Such malformations may be infratentorial also. One 13-year-old girl had numerous small bleeding episodes over a 2-year period, and many studies revealed no source. She ultimately died from a more massive hemorrhage. At autopsy a tiny subependymal malformation was found in the floor of the fourth ventricle (Fig. 16.22).

Case 3. *Minor dashboard bump; headache and hemiparesis.* A 2 1/12-year-old girl bent over to pick up an object which had fallen to the floor of her parents' Volkswagen. On the way up she bumped her head on the dashboard with no immediate sequela.

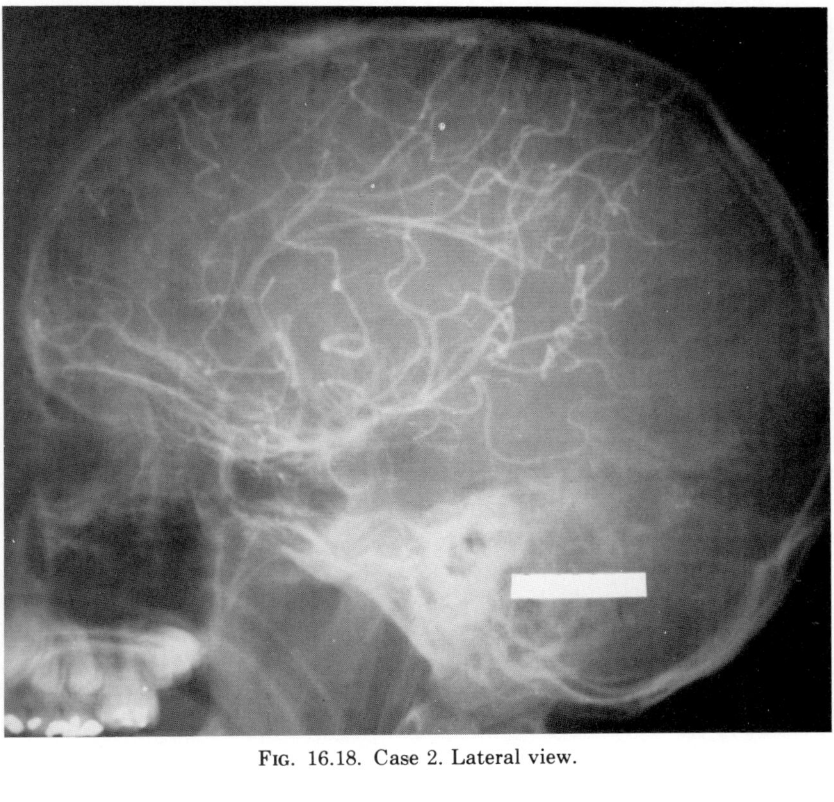

FIG. 16.18. Case 2. Lateral view.

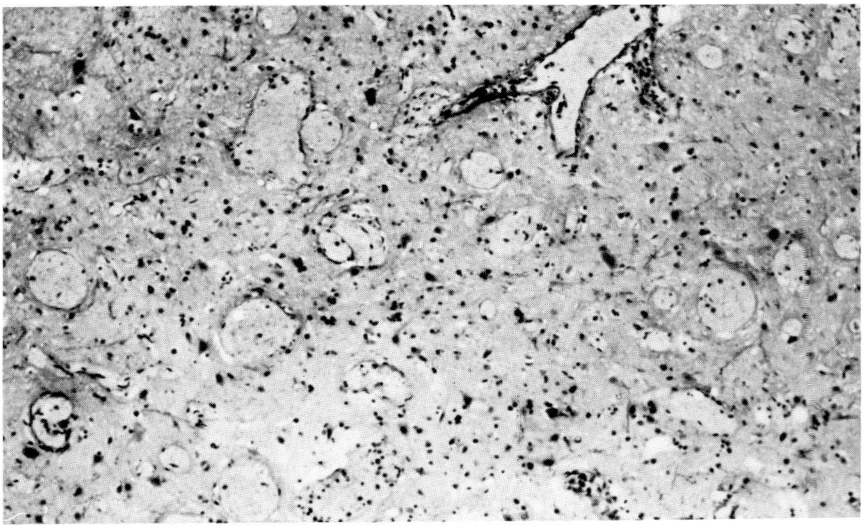

FIG. 16.19. Case 2. Microscopic arteriovenous malformation found at autopsy.

That night, 6 hours later, she awakened with severe headache, vomited, and developed a left hemiparesis. She had a history of generalized febrile convulsions. There was a "port wine" stain on the parietal scalp. She was still being treated with ampicillin because of a respiratory infection and otitis of 1 week's duration. A cousin had died in childhood because of a ruptured intracranial aneurysm.

A computerized axial tomography (CAT) scan showed right temporal lobe clot and an arteriogram showed an aneurysm of the middle cerebral artery deep to the clot (Fig. 16.23). She had a respiratory arrest which was fortunately reversible but which prompted emergency evacuation of the clot at which time the aneurysm was clipped. She survived. Four months later her hemiparesis was still improving.

Diagnosis: Congenital berry aneurysm of the middle cerebral artery.

In the cooperative study (17), of 52 children under 15 years presenting with subarachnoid hemorrhage, 27% were found to have aneurysms. The youngest child reported in whom an aneurysm has been successfully dealt with was 4 weeks old (13). The Children's Hospital Medical Center surgical experience with aneurysms over a 21-year period is shown in Table 16.2. The youngest patient was 16 months old; his middle cerebral aneurysm was clipped, but he did not survive. The youngest to survive rupture and surgery was 23 months old; the aneurysm was on the posterior inferior cerebellar artery.

The distribution of aneurysms, their gross appearance, and the relation to parent vessels is similar to those found in adults. Even an arteriosclerotic "sentinal plaque" was found in a 6½-year-old boy's carotid artery at the base of the bifurcation aneurysm.

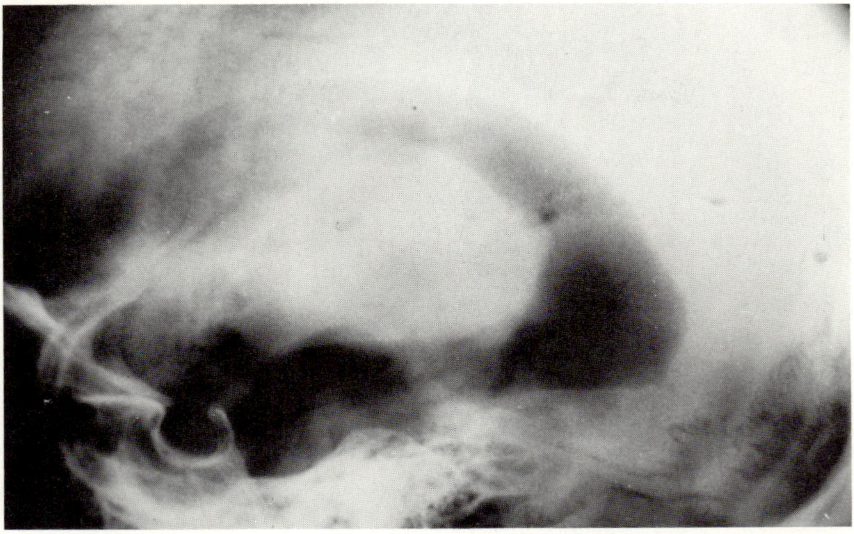

FIG. 16.20. Pneumoencephalogram of a 19-year-old girl thought to have multiple sclerosis. Mass lesion occupies left thalamus.

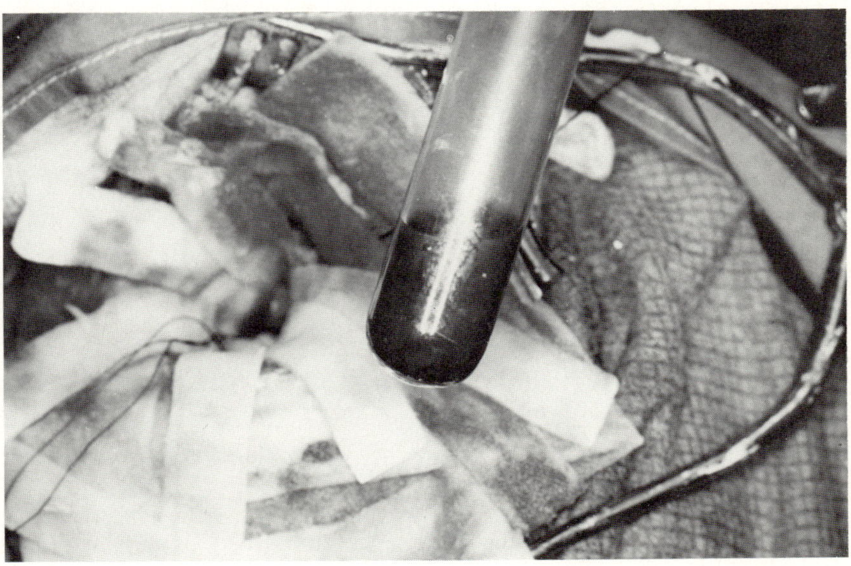

FIG. 16.21. Operative photograph of girl shown in Figure 16.20. Thalamus contained old, unclotted blood.

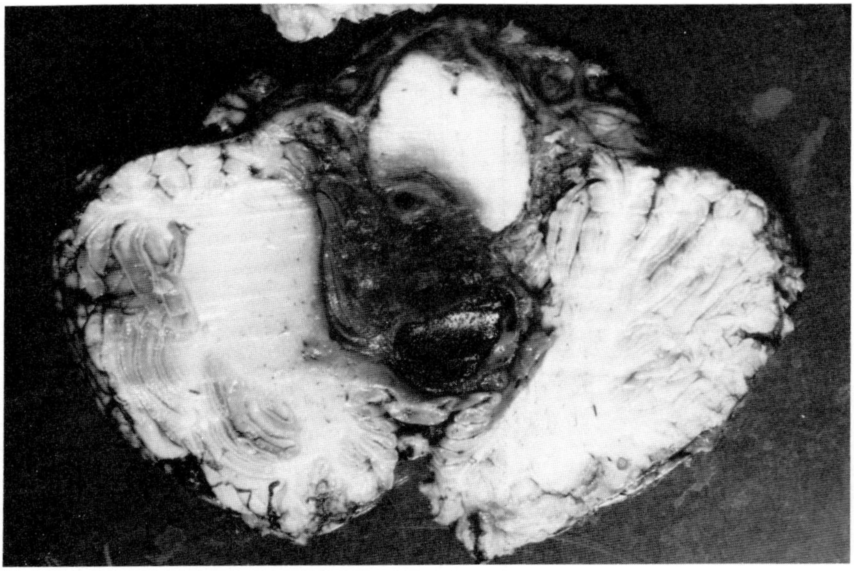

FIG. 16.22. Autopsy specimen of 13-year-old girl who died of hemorrhage from cryptic AVM in floor of 4th ventricle after many lesser hemorrhages.

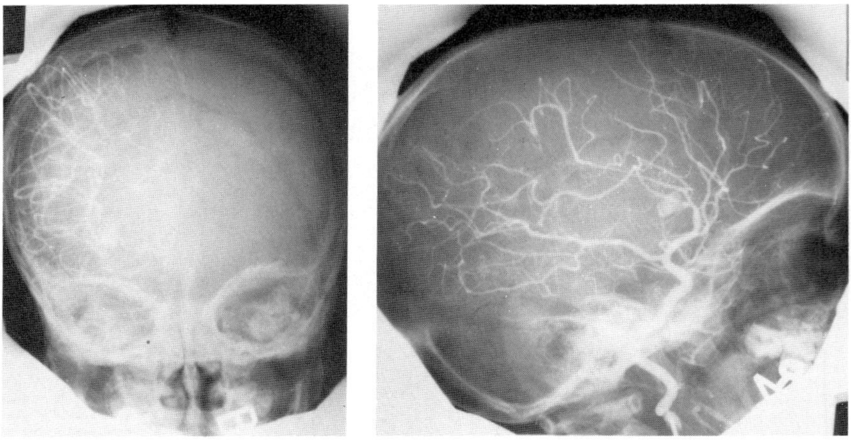

FIG. 16.23. Case 3. Right carotid arteriogram of 2½-year-old girl who hemorrhaged from middle cerebral aneurysm.

Spasm is just as prevalent in children as in adults. A 5½-year-old boy who bled from his apical basilar aneurysm (Fig. 16.24), showed marked widespread spasm which produced devastating neurological deficits (Fig. 16.25). He had a second aneurysm on his left posterior cerebral artery.

After waiting several weeks for the spasm to subside, the aneurysms were coated. He died several years later of complications of shunted hydrocephalus.

In children, other undiscovered congenital anomalies may be present, such as coarctation of the aorta and polycystic kidneys, and a search

TABLE 16.2.
Summary of Congenital Intracranial Aneurysms Diagnosed at the Children's Hospital Medical Center, Boston, 1954–1975

INTERNAL CAROTID	-----	5
ANT. COMM., ANT. CEREBRAL	-----	8
MIDDLE CEREBRAL	-----	4
VERTEBROBASILAR	-----	3
TOTAL		20

AGES 1 4/12 - 17 7/12 YRS.

19 OPERATED UPON

16 SURVIVORS

16 % OPERATIVE MORTALITY

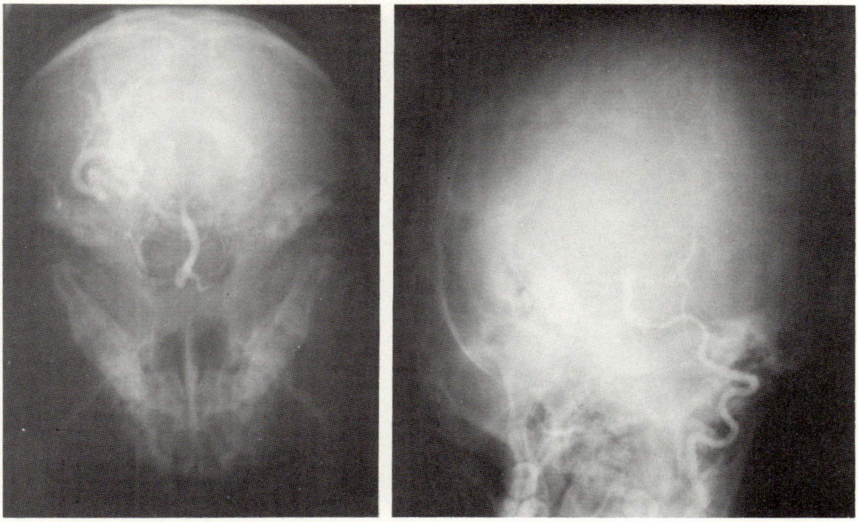

FIG. 16.24. Two aneurysms on the posterior circulation of a 5½-year-old boy. Apical basilar aneurysm had bled; second on left posterior cerebral had not. Oblique and basal views.

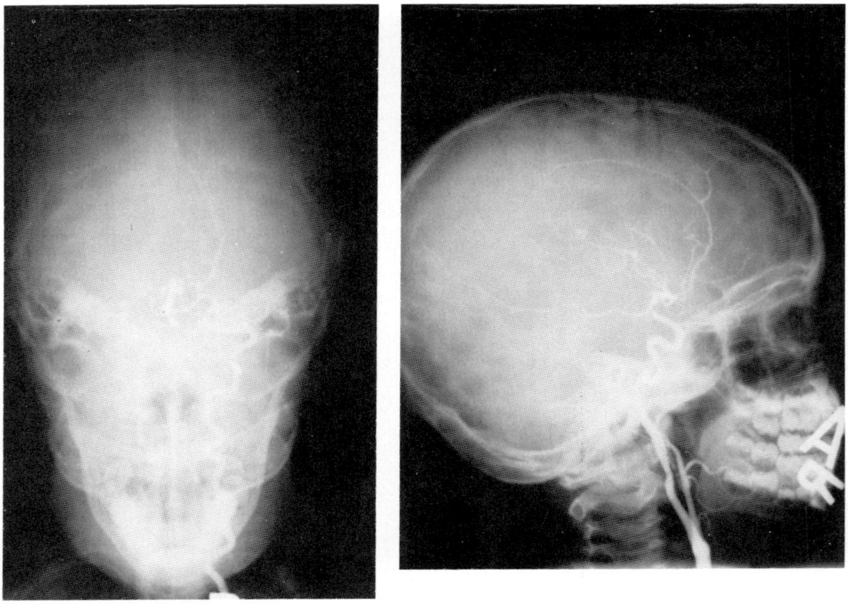

FIG. 16.25. Same boy as in Figure 16.24, showing marked spasm. Anteroposterior vertebral and lateral right carotid injections.

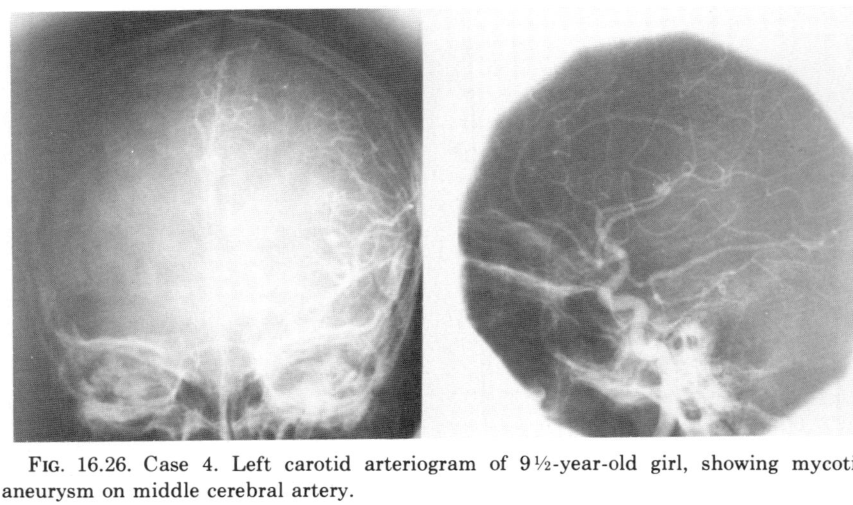

FIG. 16.26. Case 4. Left carotid arteriogram of 9½-year-old girl, showing mycotic aneurysm on middle cerebral artery.

should be made for these conditions whenever a child presents with an intracranial aneurysm.

In newborn infants, massive intracranial hemorrhage may occur from the choroid plexus or, in premature infants, from the ganglionic eminence, an area on the ventricular surface of the caudate nucleus. Both regions have been shown by Gilles (9) to be high in fibrinolytic activity which may propagate hemorrhage once it has occurred. The great susceptibility of premature and newborn infants to hemorrhage of this type is not fully understood. High venous pressure and venous stasis resulting from immaturity of the pulmonary vascular bed or from hyaline membrane disease may play a role. The neurosurgeon must be alert to rule out subdural hematoma caused by head molding at delivery and also retrocerebellar hemorrhage from tears of the venous sinuses (10). If the infant survives the bleeding episode, hydrocephalus or chronic subdural effusions may require action.

Children may suffer from spontaneous intracranial hemorrhage because of congenital abnormalities of the clotting mechanism, such as in hemophilia (15, 20, 23) or disease processes such as leukemia (21). Idiopathic thrombocytopenic purpura has been reported in children (18). Sickle cell disease can lead to intracranial hemorrhage as well as occlusion of intracranial vessels (2, 6).

Case 4. *Meningitis, endocarditis, osteomyelitis, and sudden headache.* A 9½-year-old girl developed staphylococcus meningitis. During therapy she was found to have acute bacterial endocarditis and osteomyelitis of one metacarpal bone. This area was drained surgically. One month after the onset of her initial symptoms, she had a spontaneous intracerebral hemorrhage. Arteriography (Fig. 16.26) that day revealed an aneurysm of the left middle cerebral artery with proximal spasm. She was treated with epsilon-aminocaproic acid (Amicar, Lederle, Pearl River, N. Y.), 1.5 gm. intravenously every 2 hours , a dose of 0.7 mg. per kilogram per day.

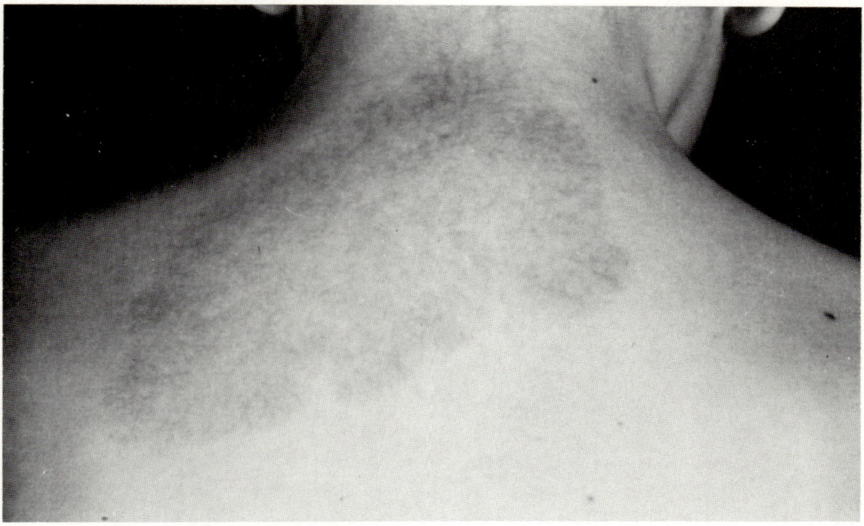

FIG. 16.27. Case 5. Cutaneous hemangioma at base of neck.

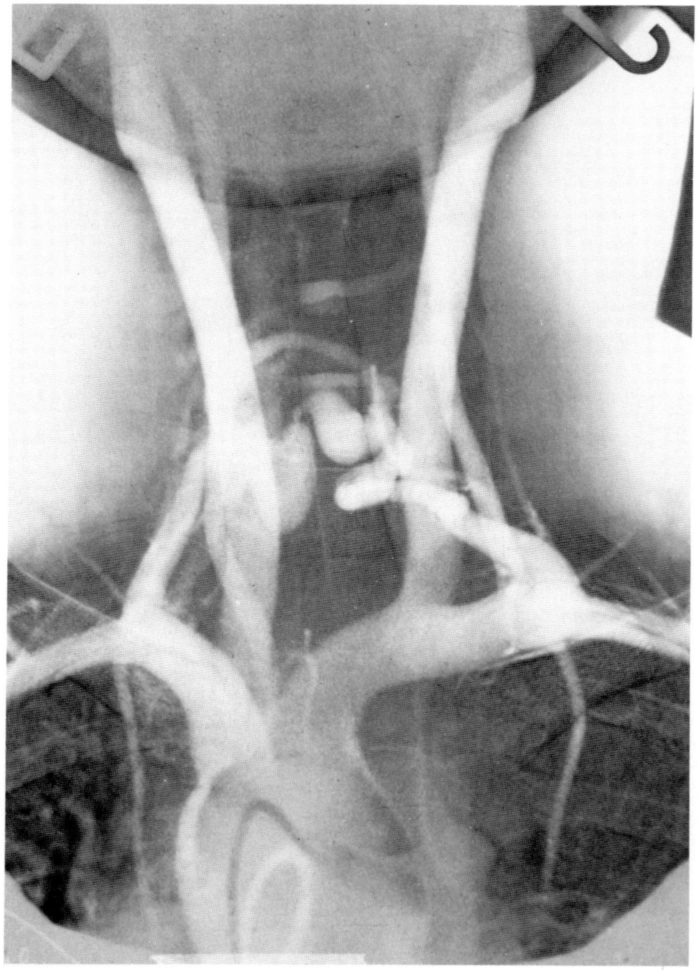

FIG. 16.28. Case 5. Arch aortagram. Intraspinal AVM is fed by a cervical artery on each side.

She improved neurologically and her CSF and blood cultures became negative. A second arteriogram suggested enlargement of the aneurysm and therefore craniotomy was performed 4 weeks after the hemorrhage. The pia arachnoid in the Sylvian fissure was significantly thickened and densely adherent to the middle cerebral vessels. An aneurysm 5 mm. in diameter was found, dissected free, and coated with plastic by the technique of Selverstone (24, 25). The girl has done well and 2 years later is normal except for a seizure tendency and some learning disability.

Diagnosis: Mycotic aneurysm, middle cerebral artery.

Case 5. *Riding bike, severe headache, tingling arms, weak legs.* This 8 10/12-year-old boy was riding his bike when he developed a severe headache which promptly spread to his neck and back. He noticed a heaviness of his arms and could no longer easily ride. He walked the bike home. The headache persisted until he arrived in the emergency ward where he was found to have nuchal rigidity but was neurologically normal except for an equivocal response in the left great toe. Lumbar puncture yielded grossly pink fluid, a pressure of 210 mm., 39,000 red cells per cubic millimeter and a protein of 109.5 mg. per 100 ml. There were multiple pink flat hemangiomata of his trunk and extremities, the largest of which was at the base of his neck posteriorly (Fig. 16.27). He gave a history of having been hit on the head by a friend 2 days prior to admission.

By the next day his headache was gone. Skull films, EEG, technetium scan, and flow studies were all normal. On the following day, cerebral angiography was performed and was completely normal. Because of the cervical hemangioma, an arch study was done and the neck filmed (Fig. 16.28). An intraspinal AVM was demonstrated. It was fed by two enlarged cervical arteries (Fig. 16.29) arising from the region of the thyrocervical trunk on each side just distal to the origins of the vertebral arteries. A loud bruit was then noted over the C-7 area!

An elective procedure was carried out 2 weeks later. It was very much a joint effort between the patient's neurologist, the neuroradiologist, and the neurosurgeon. With the boy sedated but awake, the procedure began in the x-ray department. Through the right axillary artery a #6 French catheter with a balloon near its tip was passed into the right feeding artery. Through the left femoral artery, a similar catheter was passed into the left feeding vessel. A third catheter was passed through the right femoral artery to the aortic arch.

While the boy's neurological state was carefully and frequently tested, first one and then the other balloon was inflated with Renografin. The boy did not show any change, except that his bruit disappeared. Test injections into the arch showed no filling of the AVM (Fig. 16.30). The boy was observed for a total of 1 hour with the balloons inflated without showing any neurological change.

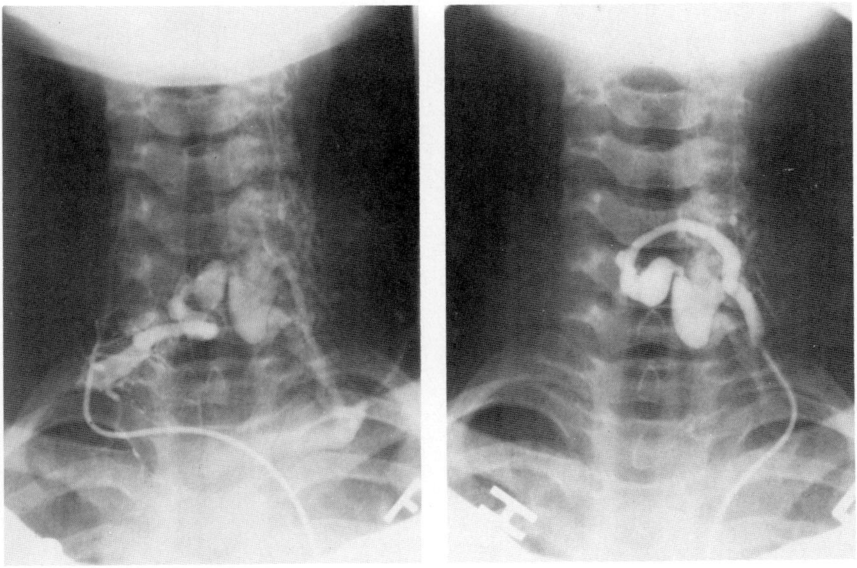

FIG. 16.29. Case 5. Detail of left and right feeding vessels.

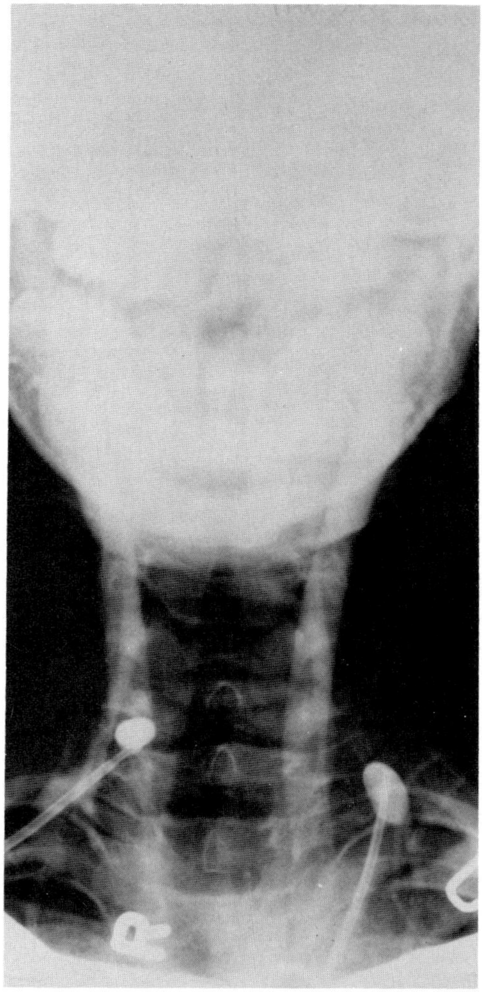

FIG. 16.30. Case 5. Arch aortagram after occluding both feeding vessels with balloon catheters. AVM no longer fills.

Next, in the operating room, catheters still in position and balloons inflated, the boy was anesthetized and each feeding vessel isolated and ligated. The balloon catheters were felt to be invaluable in the localization of the feeding vessels. The bruit has not recurred and the boy has remained well and fully active.

Follow up angiography was performed about 5 months following surgery. Injection of dye near the origin of the right thyrocervical trunk showed no evidence of the malformation. To our dismay, a similar injection on the left side showed the feeding vessel intact and the malformation still filling from it! Whether the balloon catheter changed its position during the trip to the operating room or whether the surgeon imagined he felt the catheter in the vessel he ligated will always be a mystery. At this time, our plans are to embolize the shunt through the remaining feeding vessel.

Diagnosis: Intraspinal AVM.

Case 6. *Episodic vomiting, recent papilledema, acute hemiparesis.* An 11 9/12-year-old

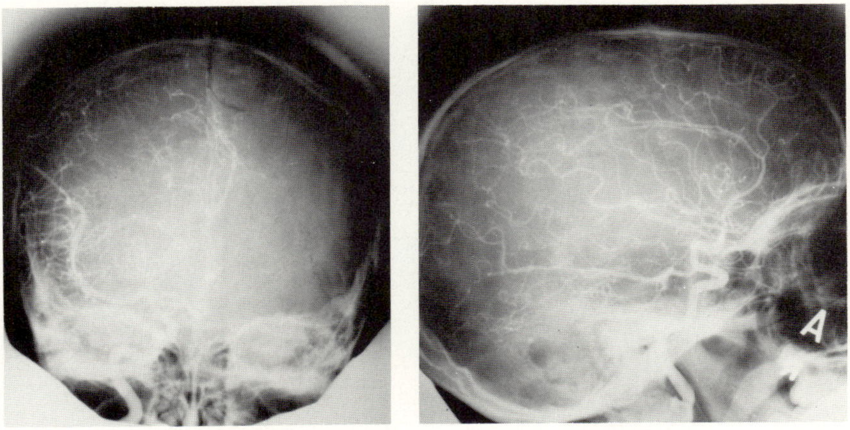

FIG. 16.31. Case 6. Right carotid arteriogram showing mass effect but no abnormal vasculature.

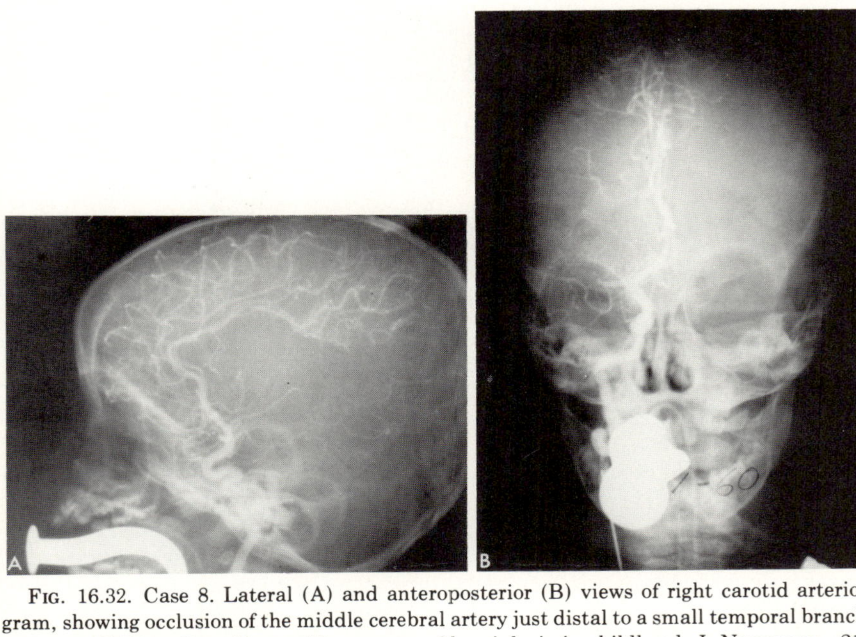

FIG. 16.32. Case 8. Lateral (A) and anteroposterior (B) views of right carotid arteriogram, showing occlusion of the middle cerebral artery just distal to a small temporal branch (From J. Shillito: Carotid arteritis; a cause of hemiplegia in childhood. J. Neurosurg., *21:* 540–551, 1964.)

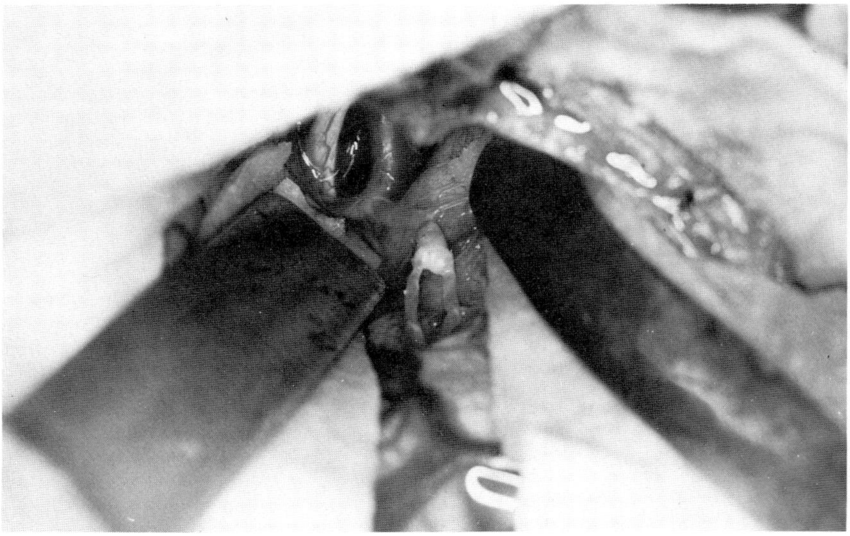

FIG. 16.33. Case 8. Operative photograph showing occluded middle cerebral artery. Right subfrontal approach (From J. Shillito: Carotid arteritis; a cause of hemiplegia in childhood. J. Neurosurg., *21:* 540–551, 1964.)

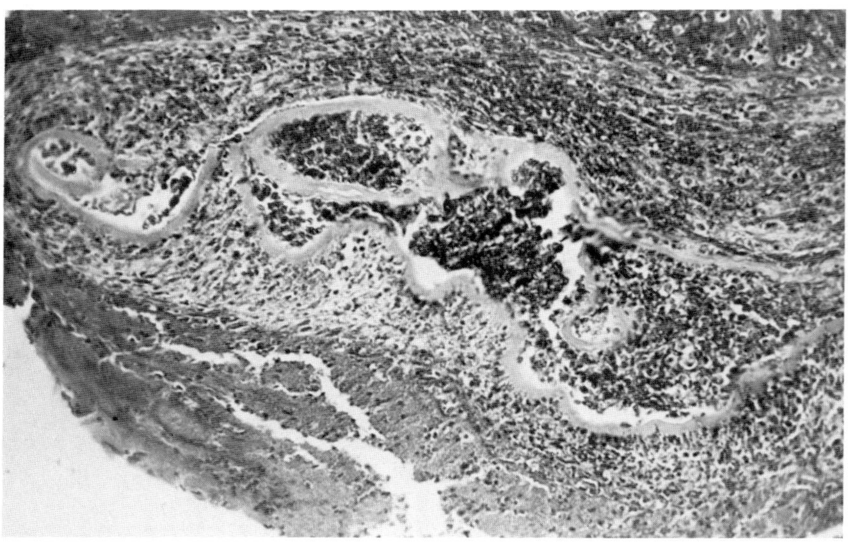

FIG. 16.34. Case 8. Microscopic view of specimen removed. Thrombus is surrounded by what appears to be displaced internal elastic membrane and a surrounding zone of arteritis (From J. Shillito: Carotid arteritis; a cause of hemiplegia in childhood. J. Neurosurg., *21:* 540–551, 1964.)

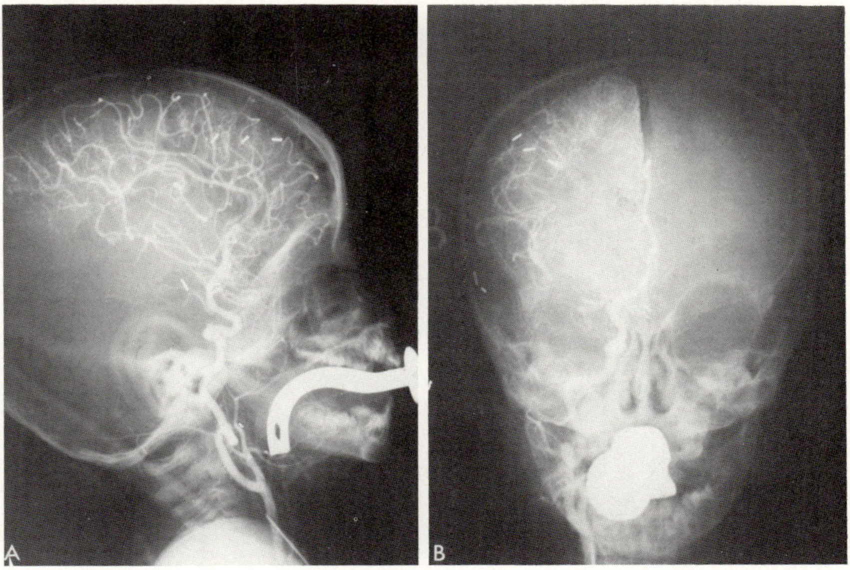

FIG. 16.35. (A and B). Case 8. Postoperative arteriograms show persistence of the block at site of arteriotomy, but good collateral filling of middle cerebral artery (From J. Shillito: Carotid arteritis; a cause of hemiplegia in childhood. J. Neurosurg., *21:* 540–551, 1964.)

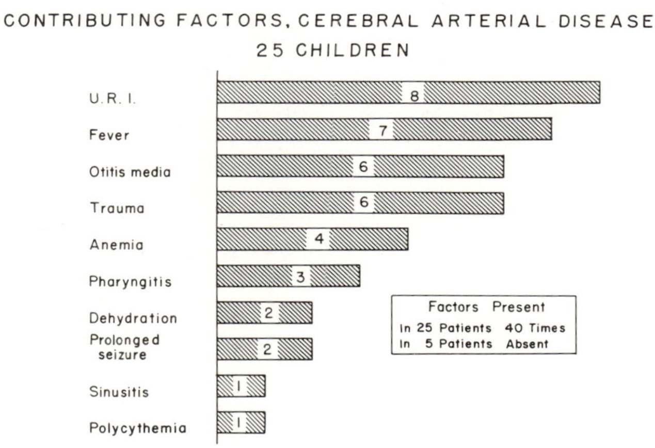

FIG. 16.36. Possible contributing factors in cerebral arterial disease of 25 children (From J. Shillito: Carotid arteritis; a cause of hemiplegia in childhood. J. Neurosurg.,*21:* 540–551, 1964.)

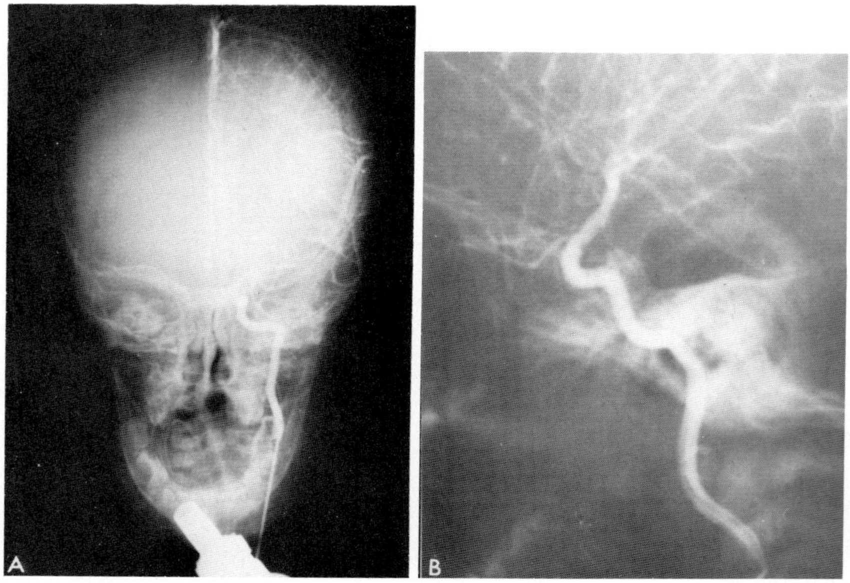

FIG. 16.37. (A and B). Left carotid arteriogram of a 1 2/12-year-old girl who had a right hemiparesis. Flow is retarded at carotid intracranially, where vessel appears irregular and somewhat narrowed (From J. Shillito: Carotid arteritis; a cause of hemiplegia in childhood. J. Neurosurg., *21:* 540–551, 1964.)

boy developed a right hemiparesis within the 1½ hours necessary to get from his pediatrician to the neurosurgeon. The referral was made because of a change in the appearance of his optic discs compared to examination 1 week earlier and because of some difficulty which he was experiencing with vision. He had had several episodes of vomiting during the previous 2 months. On the first occasion, gastroenteritis was prevalent and he was thought to have this. Ten days prior to admission the second transient episode prompted a gastrointestinal series which was normal. His third episode prompted the current visit to the pediatrician.

When first seen by the neurosurgeon he had 4 diopters of papilledema, no hemorrhages, and enlarged blind spots. New in the past 1½ hours were the neurological findings: a left hemiparesis, left paresthesias with extinction on sensory examination, and an upgoing left toe. He could not stand and moved his left arm only by lifting it with his right. Dexamethasone (Decadron, Merck, Sharp & Dohme, West Point, Pa.) and mannitol were started immediately and a technetium scan and arteriogram performed. These showed an avascular mass deep in the right parietal area (Fig. 16.31). Because of worsening of his condition a few days after admission, an emergency craniotomy was performed which revealed a large glioblastoma, partly cystic and partly within the right lateral ventricle. Strangely enough, there was no sign of recent hemorrhage nor was that ventricle enlarged as though acutely obstructed. Subtotal resection of the tumor was followed by radiation therapy. The boy died 9 months later.

Diagnosis: Malignant tumor of the right cerebral hemisphere.

Brain tumors have mimicked strokes by bleeding or by acutely obstructing a lateral ventricle. This tumor appeared to have done

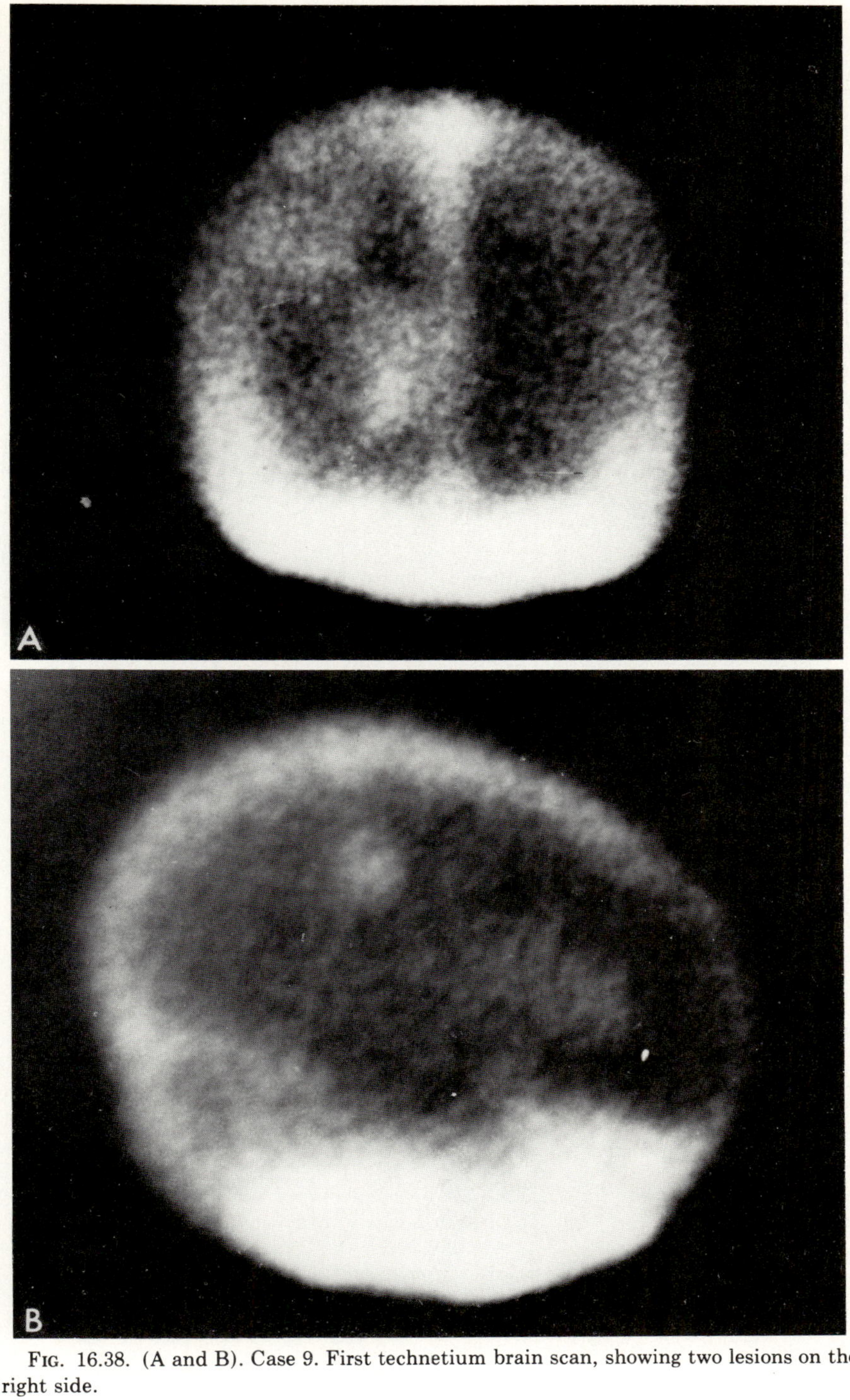

FIG. 16.38. (A and B). Case 9. First technetium brain scan, showing two lesions on the right side.

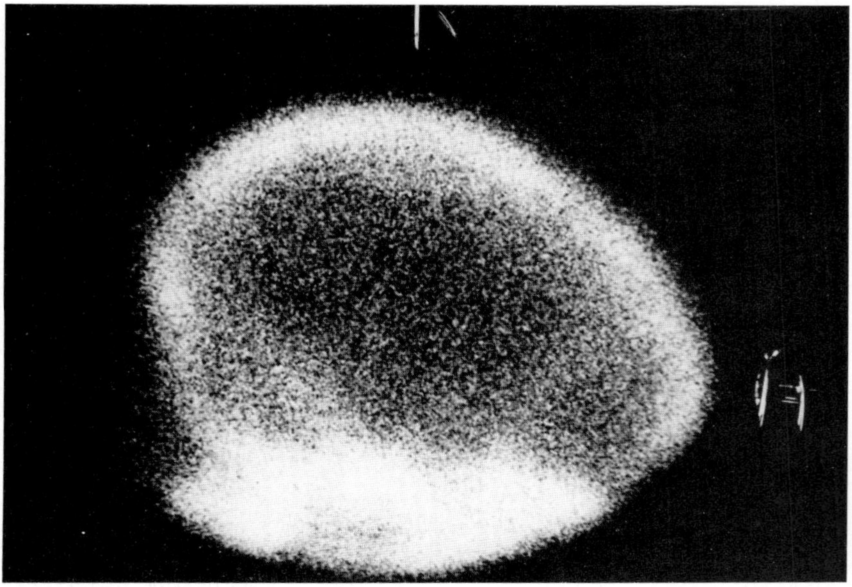

FIG. 16.39. Case 9. Second Tc scan 3 days later—previous lesions are not seen!

neither. Usually the tumors which bleed are intraventricular, such as the choroid plexus papilloma, malignant, or both. Recently, acute cerebellar hemorrhage in a child was found to have originated from a malignant tumor. These possibilities must be kept in mind when planning studies for the elucidation of what may appear superficially to have been a cerebrovascular accident.

Case 7. *Catching football; fell hemiplegic.* An 11 2/12-year-old boy was running to catch a football thrown by his father when he suddenly fell to the ground. He had not tripped and had no headache but said his left leg had simply buckled and given way. He tried to stand but his leg would not support him. He could not make a fist with his left hand. There had been no alteration in consciousness and no seizure activity had been witnessed.

Three hours later in the hospital he could just wiggle his left big toe and could get his left arm up over his head briefly. Throughout the night his hemiparesis continued to improve. He admitted to putting his head down on his desk at school the day before because he just didn't feel quite right and to having had a few ill defined headaches during the past few months.

The next day he was further improved. A technetium static scan and flow study both were normal. A cerebral angiogram was completely within normal limits, including the vessels in the neck! The boy was discharged and within 10 days he was back to normal.

Two months later he experienced dizziness, tingling of his *right* arm and leg, and weakness of the *right* side. The left side, which had been previously involved, remained completely normal. He could walk but limped. By the time he arrived in the hospital, he was already improving. His lumbar puncture showed 57 red cells, 35 mg. per 100 ml.

protein, 1.2 mg. per 100 ml. gamma globulin. There was no evidence of cardiac vegetations or intraventricular myxoma by echocardiogram. Technetium scan and flow studies again were normal. A CAT scan was normal. The episode cleared slowly with a little residual even 2 months later. He has presented once since that time with headache but no new neurological deficit.

Diagnosis: Hemiplegic migraine.

This has been reported in children under 3 years of age (32).

Case 8. *Awoke with weak arm.* A 1-year-old boy awoke on the day prior to admission with a weak left arm. During the previous 2 weeks he had had a minor fall without head injury and a nonproductive cough. On admission he had a left hemiparesis, slight reddening of the right ear drum, and a hemoglobin of 7.4 gm. per 100 ml.

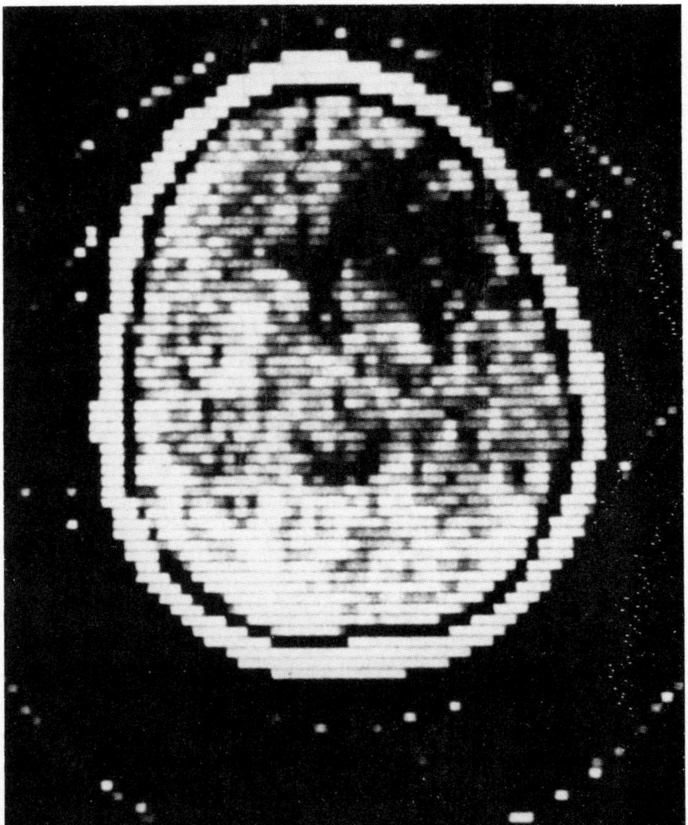

FIG. 16.40. Case 9. First CAT scan, at about the time of negative Tc scan, shows a heterogeneous mass of low mv in the right frontal lobe, displacing the ventricular system to the left and partially amputating the right frontal horn.

After transfusion, arteriography was performed on the 2nd hospital day. The right middle cerebral artery was occluded just distal to a small temporal branch (Fig. 16.32). At craniotomy immediately thereafter, a firm white obstruction was found straddling a major bifurcation of the middle cerebral artery (Fig. 16.33). It was removed with some difficulty; the arterial wall was thickened and the mass was adherent to it. After closing the arteriotomy, blood filled the distal branches which then pulsated. Microscopically (Fig. 16.34), it appeared that part of the wall of the vessel had been removed in the specimen, for one area showed thrombus in a narrowed lumen where an unusual density of round cells and some neutrophils surrounded a stripped internal elastic membrane. This was considered either reaction to a clot present for several days or a primary process which caused the thrombosis. It is quite similar to reported cases of cerebral-dissecting aneurysms. Arteriography, 3 weeks postoperatively (Fig. 16.35A), demonstrated excellent filling of all branches of the middle cerebral artery, but closer inspection of the films, particularly the anteroposterior view (Fig. 16.35B), showed that the obstruction had recurred at the operative site and demonstrated a remarkable collateral circulation *via* the small temporal branch of the middle cerebral artery and *via* the anterior cerebral circulation. The child has recovered with minimal dysfunction of the left hand.

Diagnosis: *Arteritis, etiology unknown.*

In 1964, 25 patients from the Children's Hospital Medical Center files were reported who had had sudden ischemic strokes followed by arteriographic study (26). Twenty showed total arterial occlusion, 4 partial occlusion, and the study in one case suggested recannulization. In all but 5 of these patients there was some factor or combination of factors that might have contributed to inflammation of the carotid artery near the base of the skull (Fig. 16.36). These included upper respiratory infection, fever, otitis media, trauma, pharyngitis, and sinusitis. Arteritis was suggested by the radiographic appearance of one carotid artery incompletely occluded intracranially just at the carotid syphon (Fig. 16.37), by surgical specimens, and by one autopsy specimen. Surgery in no case permanently relieved the obstruction but current microsurgical techniques were not then employed. Those few cases which have come to attention since that report have been diagnosed several days after the onset of symptoms and exploration has not been carried out.

There are other causes of vascular occlusion in childhood. Taveras (29) reported 10 cases of multiple progressive intracranial arterial occlusions, 5 of which were in children under 16 years of age, one as young as 7 months.

The strange "moyamoya" disease (28) with its blush of tiny vessels near the base of the brain resembling a puff of cigarette smoke may be, in fact, rich anastomotic pathways developing early in life in response to carotid stenosis or occlusion. Polyarteritis (8), sickle cell disease (27), systemic lupus erythematosus (12) all can produce symptoms of stroke. In teenagers, one must also consider vascular problems associated with drug abuse (16) and contraceptive medications (4).

Occlusion of cerebral veins and venous sinuses can occur in children for many reasons (5, 14,): infection, anemia, and, particularly, congenital heart disease (31). An important warning: in children with cyanotic congenital heart disease, any sudden focal neurological deficit whether static or progressive must be considered as possibly due to a cerebral abscess (7) and studies planned to establish or rule out this diagnosis promptly and with safety (30).

We have found arteriography in the pediatric age group to be safe. Only in the presence of homocystinuria is the risk of cerebral angiography considered forbidding. There have been cases reported in which neurological worsening was apparently caused by cerebral angiography in children with multiple intracranial arterial occlusions and homocystinuria. We take the precaution of a urinary nitroprusside test before performing angiography on any child who is thought to have had

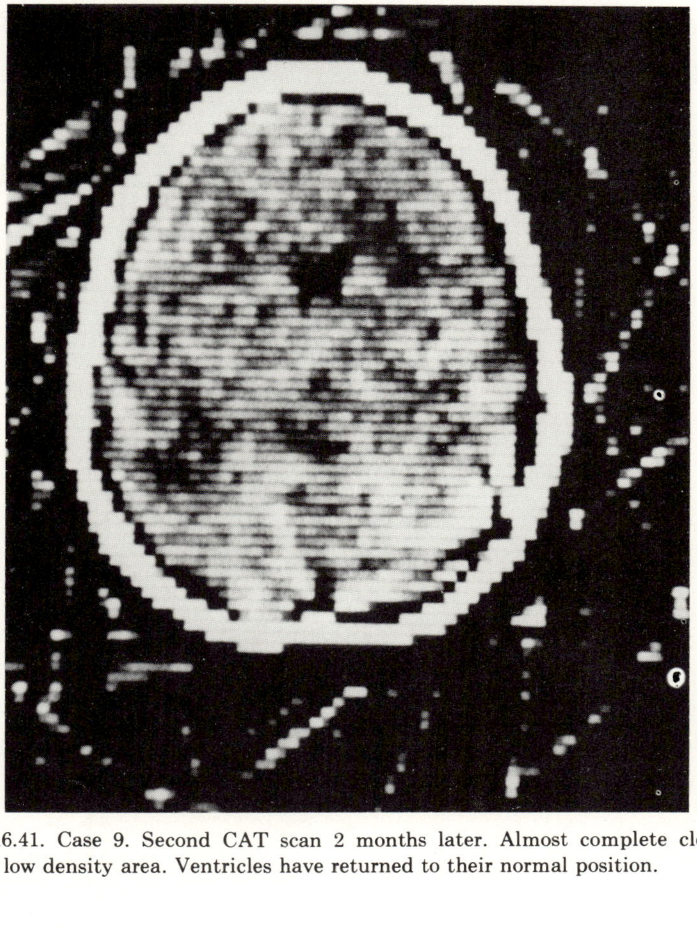

FIG. 16.41. Case 9. Second CAT scan 2 months later. Almost complete clearing of previous low density area. Ventricles have returned to their normal position.

an ischemic cerebrovascular accident. Angiography would not be performed in any child with the clinical features of homocystinuria (22).

Case 9. *Recurrent occipital headaches, facial weakness.* A 5 5/12-year-old girl had complained of occipital headaches several times during the preceding 5 months. Once, a month earlier, she rose from her nap drooling from the left corner of her mouth, seemed to be disoriented, vomited, and went back to bed again. After awakening 2 hours later, she appeared normal except for a fever which went as high as 102°F. and lasted for about 2 days. Two weeks prior to admission, she had again a severe occipital headache and a left facial weakness. She underwent several tests at that time, including an EEG and skull films, all of which were normal. Her symptoms subsided.

On the day of admission she again appeared with a left facial weakness, some awkwardness of left-sided coordination and was felt by some observers to have early papilledema. All tests including arteriograms were normal except a technetium brain scan which showed two areas of increased concentration of isotope in the right cerebral hemisphere (Fig. 16.38). The girl was placed on dexamethasone (Decadron), and a search was begun for a possible primary site of metastatic tumors. The search was not productive. A second technetium scan 3 days later was completely normal (Fig. 16.39)! A CAT scan, however, suggested a lesion deep in the right hemisphere (Fig. 16.40). The lesion was described as a heterogeneous mass of low mu in the right frontal lobe which displaced the ventricular system to the left and partially amputated the right frontal horn. It was felt to be consistent with a glioma. To define this in relation to the ventricular system, a pneumoencephalogram was performed. This showed only diffuse expansion of the deep portion of the right hemisphere. The spinal fluid protein was 20 mg. per 100 ml. and gamma globulin was normal. The girl was improving on dexamethasone (Decadron) and, because of this and the improving technetium scan, it was decided simply to observe her further. Two months later the CAT scan was much improved (Fig. 16.41), and the patient was normally active!

Four months after the first hospitalization, she had recurrence of her left occipital headache lasting 1 to 2 hours, this time with a *right* facial weakness and slurred speech. The function of her entire right side appeared to be somewhat abnormal and she was felt to have early papilledema. She was readmitted for study. A lumbar puncture was 220 mm. of water with a total protein of 25 mg. per 100 ml. and the gamma globulin again was normal.

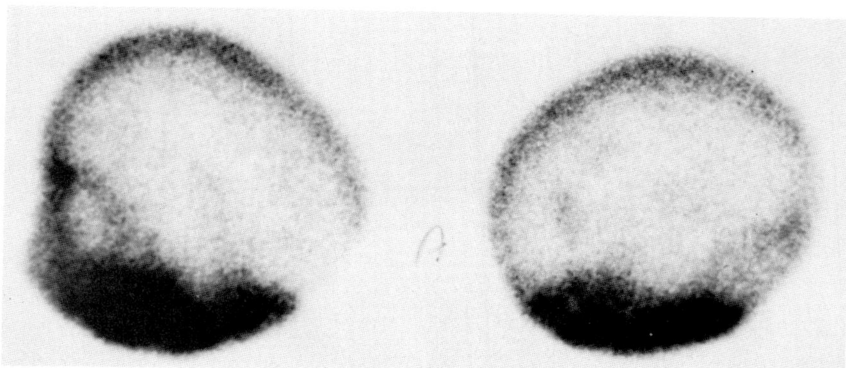

Fig. 16.42. Case 9. Third Tc scan at time of right-sided signs. Four lesions are suggested on the left side.

Technetium scan at this time showed *four* lesions in the left hemisphere (Fig. 16.42). She was again placed on dexamethasone (Decadron) and her neurological status and scans returned to normal. Two months later she complained of poor vision. There was no other neurological deficit. A central scotoma was found in her left eye and a lesser one in the right. A diagnosis of optic neuritis was made and her entire course now appears compatible with. . . .

Diagnosis: *Multiple sclerosis*.

SUMMARY

Nine cases have been presented in detail to illustrate some of the varied causes of sudden neurological deficit in childhood: arteriovenous malformation, cryptic hamartoma, berry aneurysm, mycotic aneurysm, intraspinal arteriovenous malformation, brain tumor, migraine, arteritis, and multiple sclerosis. The Boston Children's Hospital experience with aneurysms and intracranial arteriovenous malformation has been summarized.

It is noteworthy that a cutaneous hemangioma overlay one cranial and one intraspinal arteriovenous malformation.

One small but deep cerebral arteriovenous malformation apparently destroyed itself after its second hemorrhage.

Not only have multiple sclerosis and a brain tumor mimicked a vascular lesion, but a series of vascular accidents was misdiagnosed first as multiple sclerosis then as a thalamic tumor.

The many possible causes of childhood strokes has been thoroughly cataloged in the Report of the Joint Committee for Stroke Facilities in 1973 (11). Children may be more susceptible to strokes because of congenital abnormalities such as congenital heart disease, hemophilia, and sickle cell anemia, or by diseases which more commonly occur in this age group, such as leukemia.

The likelihood of brain abscess in cyanotic congenital heart disease is stressed. Arteriographic studies in our series have been safe; however, there have been reports of probable worsening of symptoms in children with multiple cerebral occlusive lesions in the presence of homocystinuria.

ACKNOWLEDGMENTS

The author would like to express thanks to the following: Dr. Roy Strand, neuroradiologist, provided all the recent studies and collaborated in the treatment of the intraspinal arteriovenous malformation; Dr. Michael Bresnan, neurologist, was in charge of that boy's care, collaborated in the care of Case 2 and has kindly allowed me to report this patient, Case 9; Dr. Keasley Welch was the surgeon in Case 4 and CD #83-52-03; Dr. Salador Treves, of Nuclear Medicine, Children's Hospital Medical Center, provided the Tc scans; Dr. Paul New, radiologist, Massachusetts General Hospital, interpreted the CAT scans in Case 9.

REFERENCES

1. Abroms, I. F., Yessayan, L., Shillito, J., and Barlow, C. F. Spontaneous intracerebral haemorrhage in patients suspected of multiple sclerosis. J. Neurol., Neurosurg. Psychiatry, *34:* 157–162, 1971.
2. Adeloye, A., Ogbeide, M. I., and Odeku, E. L. Massive intracranial hemorrhage in sickle cell anemia. Neurology, *20:* 1165–1170, 1970.
3. Amacher, A. L., and Shillito, J. Jr. The syndromes and surgical treatment of aneurysms of the great vein of Galen. J. Neurosurg., *39:* 89–98, 1973.
4. Atkinson, E. A., Fairburn, B., and Heathfield, K. W. G. Intracranial venous thrombosis as complication of oral contraception. Lancet, *1:* 914–918, 1970.
5. Byers, R. K., and Hass, G. M. Thrombosis of the dural venous sinuses in infancy and in childhood. Am. J. Dis. Child., *45:* 1161–1183, 1933.
6. Cheatham, M. L., and Brackett, C. E. Problems in management of subarachnoid hemorrhage in sickle cell anemia. J. Neurosurg., *23:* 488–493, 1965.
7. Fischbein, C. A., Rosenthal, A., Fischer, E. G., Nadas, A. S., and Welch, K. Risk factors for brain abscess in patients with congenital heart disease. Am. J. Cardiol., *34:* 97–102, 1974.
8. Ford, R. G., and Siekert, R. G. Central nervous system manifestations of periarteritis nodosa. Neurology, *15:* 114–122, 1965.
9. Gilles, F. H., Price, R. A., Kevy, S. V., and Berenberg, W. Fibrinolytic activity in the ganglionic eminence of the premature human brain. Biol. Neonate, *18:* 426–432, 1971.
10. Gilles, F. H., and Shillito, J. Jr. Infantile hydrocephalus: retrocerebellar subdural hematoma. J. Pediatr., *76:* 529–537, 1970.
11. Gold, A. P., Challenor, Y. B., Gilles, F. H., Hilal, S. P., Leviton, A., Rollins, E. I., Solomon, G. E., and Stein, B. M. Report of Joint Committee for Stroke Facilities. IX. Strokes in children. Part 1. Stroke, *4:* 835–894, 1973. Part 2. Stroke, *4:* 1009–1052, 1973.
12. Gold, A. P., and Yahr, M. D. Childhood lupus erythematosus: A clinical and pathological study of the neurological manifestations. Trans. Am. Neurol. Assoc., *85:* 96–102, 1960.
13. Jones, R. K., and Shearburn, E. W. Intracranial aneurysm in a four-week-old infant, diagnosis by angiography and successful operation. J. Neurosurg., *18:* 122–124, 1961.
14. Kalbag, R. M., and Woolf, A. L. Cerebral Venous Thrombosis, with Special Reference to Primary Aseptic Thrombosis, 280 pp. Oxford University Press, London, 1967.
15. Kerr, C. B. Intracranial haemorrhage in haemophilia. J. Neurol. Neurosurg. Psychiatry, *27:* 166–173, 1964.
16. Lignelli, G. J., and Buchheit, W. A. Angiitis in drug abusers. N. Engl. J. Med., *284:* 112–113, 1971.
17. Locksley, H. B. Report on the cooperative study of intracranial aneurysms and subarachnoid hemorrhage. V., Part 1. Natural history of subarachnoid hemorrhage, intracranial aneurysms and arteriovenous malformations. J. Neurosurg., *25:* 219–239, 1966.
18. Lusher, J. M., and Zuelzer, W. W. Idiopathic thrombocytopenic purpura in childhood. J. Pediatr., *68:* 971–979, 1966.
19. Matson, D. D. Arteriovenous Malformation. *In* Neurosurgery of Infancy and Childhood, Ed. 2, Chapter 48, Charles C Thomas Springfield, Ill., 1969.
20. Olsen, E. R. Intracranial surgery in hemophiliacs, report of a case and review of the literature. Arch. Neurol., *21:* 401–412, 1969.

21. Pierce, M. I. Neurologic complications in acute leukemia in children. Pediatr. Clin. North Am., *9:* 425–442, 1962.
22. Schimke, R. H., McKusick, V. A., Huang, T., and Pollack, A. D. Homocystinuria. Studies of 20 families with 38 affected members. J.A.M.A. *193:* 711–719, 1965.
23. Seeler, R. A., and Imana, R. B. Intracranial hemorrhage in patients with hemophilia. J. Neurosurg., *39:* 181–185, 1973.
24. Selverstone, B. Aneurysms at middle cerebral "trifurcation": treatment with adherent plastics. J. Neurosurg., *19:* 884–886, 1962.
25. Selverstone, B., and Ronis, N. Coating and reinforcement of intracranial aneurysms with synthetic resins. Bull. Tufts N. Engl. Med. Center, *4:* 8–12, 1958.
26. Shillito, J. Carotid arteritis; a cause of hemiplegia in childhood. J. Neurosurg., *21:* 540–551, 1964.
27. Stockman, J. A., Nigro, M. A., Michkin, M. M., and Oski, F. A. Occlusion of large cerebral vessels in sickle cell anemia. N. Engl. J. Med., *287:* 846–849, 1972.
28. Suzuki, J., and Takaku, A. Cerebrovascular "moyamoya" disease; disease showing abnormal net-like vessels in base of brain. Arch. Neurol., *20:* 288–299, 1969.
29. Taveras, J. M. Multiple progressive intracranial arterial occlusions: a syndrome of children and young adults. Am. J. Roentgenol. Radium Ther. Nucl. Med., *106:* 235–268, 1969.
30. Treves, S. Pediatric aspects of nuclear medicine. Postgrad. Med., *57:* 125–132, 1975.
31. Tyler, H. R., and Clark, D. B. Cerebrovascular accidents in patients with congenital heart disease. Arch. Neurol. Psychiatry, *77:* 483–489, 1957.
32. Verret, S., and Steele, J. C. Alternating hemiplegia in childhood; A report of eight patients with complicated migraine beginning in infancy. Pediatrics, *47:* 675–680, 1971.

CHAPTER

17

Hypertensive Brain Hemorrhage*

ROBERT G. OJEMANN, M.D. and J. P. MOHR, M.D.

INCIDENCE AND RELATED FACTORS

Parenchymatous brain hemorrhage attributed to hypertension continues to be a discouragingly frequent cause of stroke. This problem accounts for 2 to 4% of all deaths (50, 58), and estimates of its frequency among cerebrovascular causes of death range from 16 to 26% (18, 26). In patients with a diagnosis of hypertensive hemorrhage, fatal outcome approximates 50% in large hematomas and 21% in smaller superficial hematomas (33, 46).

As a cause of stroke, irrespective of the issue of mortality, hypertensive hemorrhage accounts for approximately 14 to 16% of the cases, exceeding the reported frequency of subarachnoid hemorrhage by factors ranging from 1.3 to 2.0 (20, 26, 35, 48). Support for hypertensive etiology of the hemorrhage includes a high incidence of left ventricular hypertrophy in the autopsied cases (49) and an elevated admission blood pressure compared to other forms of stroke (Fig. 17.1). There may be other etiological factors of the hemorrhage in addition to hypertension (31) (see "Differential Diagnosis"). Findings which have been inferred to coincide with hypertension and its complications in the individual cases include a slight familial tendency (10), greater prevalence among American Blacks (18), and a shift from age 70 for other strokes to 10+ years younger for hypertensive hemorrhages (19, 20). Sex differences appear insignificant (26). Therapy for hypertension is thought to have reduced the incidence of related hemorrhage (57) and might prove wholly preventative, if vigorously pursued.

PATHOLOGY

The exact source of the hemorrhage remains a controversial subject. It has long been known that these hemorrhages arise principally in the arterial territories of the penetrating arteries from the circle of Willis (the lenticulostriate and thalamoperforant arteries) and from similar

* Supported in part by grants 5 PO1 NS 10828-02, HL 14888, and HS 00188 from the U. S. Public Health Service and by a grant from the United Chairitable Trust.

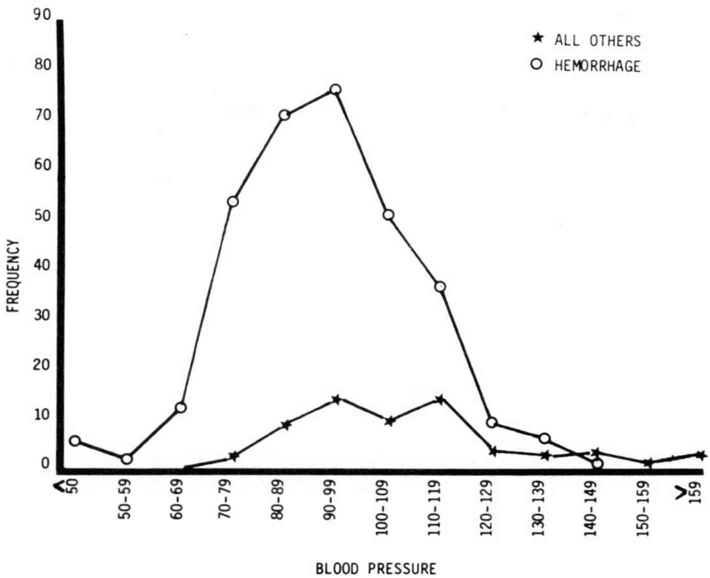

FIG. 17.1. Comparison of diastolic blood pressure in cases of stroke due to hypertensive hemorrhage *versus* all other types of stroke.

branches (the paramedian) of the basilar artery. In a few cases, angiographic dye has even been filmed escaping from these arteries and puddling in the hematoma confirming the arterial branch origin of the hematomas, but not settling the mechanism of the rupture (25).

The normal cerebral arterial walls have proven remarkably resistant to rupture even under pressures up to 1520 mm. Hg in studies using autopsy material (27). Many theses have been put forward to account for pathological weakness of the walls to permit rupture under the lesser pressures met clinically in hypertension. The two main theories involve leakage from microaneurysms or from an area of the vessel wall altered by the segmental fibrinoid necrosis seen in hypertension. Rupture of microaneurysms was considered the likely mechanism for almost a century (4, 6–8, 11, 50, 53), although many later authors also entertained the likelihood that some hemorrhages arose directly from nonaneurysmal walls weakened by fibrinoid necrosis (2, 8, 10, 30, 50, 59). Other authors have doubted a role of the miliary aneurysms in the rupture (5, 14). Direct microscopic examination of the site of arterial rupture in cases of hemorrhage was long considered a useless endeavor because the rupture site was envisioned to have destroyed itself in the process of hematoma formation. However, Fisher, by using serially sectional material, has reported one of the few studies demonstrating the rupture sites in both pontine and putaminal cases. Numerous examples of rupture sites were found but in none was a microaneurysm seen although unruptured miliary microaneurysms were found in a few vessels, " . . . all at a distance from the large hemorrhage" (16). He suggested that the changes in the arterial wall produced by hypertension and referred to as lipohyalinosis, hyalinosis, hyaline arterionecrosis, hyaline fatty change, fibrinoid necrosis, fibrinoid arteritis, angionecrosis, plasmatic vascular destruction, and atherosclerosis of small arteries might cause ischemia in some instances and be associated with arterial rupture and hemorrhage in others.

The final triggering mechanism for the rupture itself is not known, although speculations have been put forward that a sudden increase in blood pressure coincident with exertion, emotional stress, and the like may serve to exceed the vessel wall pressure limits (59). This notion is supported by the finding that the setting for the hemorrhages is usually during periods of activity, and infrequently during sleep, but little additional data bear on this issue.

The hemorrhage appears to produce both destruction and displacement of tissue. This latter effect is often more evident than is the disruption. It provides the basis for hope that the ultimate outcome may be much less than the acute deficit.

The hemorrhage is inferred to be of short duration in most cases, irrespective of its size when the bleeding ceases. The mass then awaits the slow mechanism of macrophage resorption for its removal, accounting for the static and nonfluctuant clinical course usually followed. Rehemorrhage appears rare at the site of the original hemorrhage. Using chromium-labeled red cells, injected on hospital admission for hypertensive hemorrhage, Herbstein and Schaumburg found that cases of fatal hematomas contained virtually no evidence of labeling in the original hemorrhage, although the Duret hemorrhages that reflected the postadmission fatal cerebral herniations were easily labeled by this method (21). Once the hemorrhage has ceased, edema appears the main mechanism of subsequent worsening, if any. No correlation has been found between the hematoma size and the blood pressure (10).

In the nonfatal cases, considerable reduction in the hematoma size is accomplished by reparative mechanisms over several months. The process is understandably somewhat slow because macrophage activity must go on along the rim of the mass and slowly whittle down the hematoma rather like the sculptor does with a block of marble. Within a year, in most cases, the hemorrhage site has been considerably reduced in size and forms a cavity whose orange-stained walls are filled with hemosiderin-laden macrophages around which the surrounding tissue appears more or less normal.

Hypertensive hemorrhage most commonly arises in the basal ganglia with an average incidence of 69%, varying from 59 to 82%. Other sites of hemorrhage include the pons 10%, ranging from 6 to 17%, the cerebellum 8%, ranging from 4 to 13%, with the remainder in other sites including subcortical regions (1, 6, 19, 23, 31, 40, 42, 48).

Utilizing modern diagnostic methods, the Massachusetts General Hospital (M.G.H.) cases have been collected prospectively since 1972 as part of the Harvard Cooperative Stroke Registry (H.C.S.R.). The M.G.H. cases show the distribution of hypertensive hemorrhage to be: putamen—53%, thalamus—13%, pons—5%, cerebellum—10%, and other sites—19% (20). The greatest controversy relates to the further specification of hemorrhages within the basal ganglia regions. Little argument has arisen over hemorrhage medial to the internal capsule as most occur in the thalamus, while few, if any, occur in the head of the caudate. Laterally, including the internal capsule, hemorrhages have been considered to arise in the external capsule, putamen, and claustrum (9), these regions including the internal capsule (40), external capsule predominantly (33), internal capsule (58), and putamen (13, 14). Experience at the M.G.H. supports Fisher's original views of putaminal and thalamic sites and is also supported by computorized tomographic (CT) scan data (Fig. 17.2). Virtually none of the hemorrhages occur in the surface gray matter itself.

HEMORRHAGE SYNDROMES

Putamen

Most cases appear to arise in the posterior half of the putamen. The direction of spread varies considerably for reasons poorly understood, but is not merely a function of the ultimate size of the hematoma (12). The hemorrhage may expand in a ball-like fashion with its center remaining at the site of origin, extend front to back within the cerebral white matter, spread upward through the corona radiata into the centrum semiovale and stretch thin the overlying surface gray matter, arc through the isthmus of the temporal lobe to produce a large mass in the posterior temporal lobe white matter, or rupture into the ventricular system. It seems possible that the outcome and therapy for each circumstance may ultimately differ considerably; at present there is insufficient experience with the individual variations to settle this issue.

The prognosis varies directly with size and is predictable by the motor deficit. In a recent study by Hier, Davis, and Mohr, all cases with clear CSF and slight motor deficit had an excellent result (22). Those showing at least some form of voluntary motor function in the affected side lived and experienced a fairly satisfactory outcome. Those flaccid on admission showed little improvement in motor function, while those comatose from huge hemorrhages all died.

The clinical picture in the typical case is well known (17). The patient characteristically is up and active when he suddenly becomes aware something is wrong, shortly after which a hemiparesis begins emerging smoothly and steadily, accompanied by a hemisensory syndrome and hemianopia, dysphasia if the dominant hemisphere is affected, unawareness of the deficit if the nondominant hemisphere is involved. Conjugate horizontal gaze deviation occurs to the side of the hemorrhage, away from the side of the hemimotor deficit. The syndrome may cease further development at any stage or continue to death in a few hours.

The details and variations noted in 27 consecutive cases studied at the M.G.H. and entered in the H.C.S.R. allow for further clarification of the syndrome. A smooth onset characterized 62% of these cases, while 30% developed so rapidly the observers felt the deficit was maximal at onset. None experienced fluctuation of the deficit, a point that supports the maxim that any immediate improvement rules out a hypertensive hemorrhage. Headache affected only 14% at onset, and only 28% at any time, leaving fully 72% free of headache even in the presence of substantial focal deficit. Similarly, only 12% suffered a stiff neck. Vomiting, an infrequent sign in other causes of stroke, affected 39% of patients, all within 12 hours of onset. On examination, none showed papilledema or subhyaloid preretinal hemorrhages, a diagnostic point which, when present, favors ruptured aneurysm or arteriovenous malformation. Some form of motor deficit affected all cases, varying from mild to complete paralysis. Sensory disorder was not fully assessed in some cases, but almost 35% of cases tested showed little, if any, disorder in sensation to pinprick. Eye movement disorders followed the expected pattern of conjugate horizontal gaze deviation in 52%, but 37% showed no impairment in eye movements, at a time when motor function varied from mild paresis to hemiplegia. The 11% showing other disorders of eye movements were all at a stage of midbrain compression, coma, and hemiplegia. The dysphasia encountered has generally been of the total (complete) variety (38); only one case has shown by evidence of a syndrome of so-called conduction aphasia (3). This finding suggests the hemorrhages are either too large for specific dysphasic syndromes or that the disruption of the deep insula white matter does not produce conduction aphasia. This last point would be contrary to the traditional predictions of the pathological mechanism of conduction aphasia, mechanisms based entirely on cases of cerebral surface embolism and not further tested by cases of subcortical hemorrhage such as are encountered in putaminal hemorrhage. Fever, a rise in sedimentation rate, and a rise in the peripheral white blood cell count as high as 21,000 cells per cu. mm. has been observed frequently. Abnormalities in the electrocardiogram suggestive of subendocardial ischemia occur infrequently.

Cases 1, 2, and 3 reflect typical examples of the small, medium, and large sized hemorrhages, respectively.

Thalamus

Like putaminal hemorrhage, its classic features are well known (13, 17). The syndrome reflects spread of hemorrhage against and into the adjacent internal capsule producing a motor deficit which adds to the initial sensory syndrome. As the hemorrhage can enlarge laterally, conjugate horizontal gaze deviation can occur that mimics the putaminal hemorrhage, but thalamic hemorrhage classically produces a midbrain syndrome of vertical gaze palsy reflecting spread of the hemorrhage inferiorly into the upper brain stem. This thalamic-midbrain mass has produced a variety of other ocular motility and pupillary disorders as well, including retraction nystagmus, skew deviation of the eyes, absence of convergence, ipsilateral ptosis and miosis, inequality of the pupils, and absence of the light reaction (17). The thalamus is surrounded on several sides by cerebrospinal fluid and early, sometimes massive, blood staining of the spinal fluid regularly occurs.

The 12 prospectively studied cases contributed by the M.G.H. to the H.C.S.R. substantiate these points. Headache was present in only a few cases but in one patient was present for at least 30 minutes before the focal deficit emerged (see Case 4-A). Two experienced stiff neck. Only one showed subhyaloid preretinal hemorrhages, and none showed papilledema. Vomiting affected six of the 12, all within a few hours of onset. The motor deficit mimicked those of putaminal hemorrhage, while a sensory deficit affected all testable cases, often of striking severity and widely distributed over the limbs, face, head, and trunk on the affected side. A variety of ocular motility disorders occurred; two showed paralysis of upward gaze, one experienced additional oculomotor palsy, while another had the third nerve palsy alone, two showed conjugate horizontal gaze deviation, one showed skew, two had no eye movements and were in deep coma, while three had no impairment in eye movements. The dysphasia encountered in the dominant hemisphere cases appears better described as a fluctuant delirium-like state with disproportionate unwanted literal paraphasias (37).

The effects on temperature, peripheral white blood count, and other parameters are similar to that of putaminal hemorrhage. The spinal fluid has been bloody or xanthrochromic in all but the tiniest thalamic hemorrhages.

Case 4 describes an unusual thalamic hemorrhage.

Cerebellum

Hemorrhage in the cerebellum causes a syndrome whose frequently life-threatening evolution is subject to the most striking surgical reversals, both in the saving of life and in the longer term low morbidity outcome. Classically, the onset is described as sudden, with nausea, vomiting, and instability to stand and walk (15). The suddenness of the cerebellar disruption appears to preclude a worsening of the initial cerebellar deficit over the short course of the expanding hematoma, and the evidence of continuing hemorrhage comes in the form of brain stem compression, signs which appear suddenly and are often followed immediately by death. It is this lack of a smoothly evolving syndrome which makes management of the cerebellar hemorrhage so difficult.

In a recent study of 56 cases of cerebellar hemorrhage (45), no distinctive clinical features could be delineated in the acute state in noncomatose patients to predict those who would survive with minimal or mild disability from those who were to die in the acute stage from the hemorrhage. Surgical intervention has a low morbidity, is rarely followed by rehemorrhage, and usually is associated with a satisfactory outcome in cases operated on before coma occurs. These findings and the lack of modern, controlled data to evaluate the efficacy of surgical therapy prompted the suggestion that all cases diagnosed within the first 48 hours be operated.

The clinical picture, at one time considered uncertain (32), has been defined (15, 45). The onset is almost invariably sudden, with nausea and vomiting in 95%, inability to stand and walk in 94% questioned on this point, headache in 74%, dizziness in 55% of cases. By contrast, loss of consciousness at onset is rare, 14%. The clinical examination showed appendicular or gait ataxia in 78%, peripheral facial palsy in 61%, and ipsilateral gaze palsy in 54% of cases. Two or all three of these signs were present in 73% of cases tested. Other signs proved less useful in the diagnosis.

Cases 5 and 6 represent typical and complex examples of the syndrome, respectively.

Pons

This represents the most dramatic and least treatable of the hypertensive hemorrhages, as well as one of the more uncommon syndromes. A comparatively small sized hemorrhage occurs, precipitating prompt and deep coma within minutes of onset. Coma, total paralysis with striking decerebrate rigidity, and small—almost pin-point—pupils occur, the latter reactive to light when examined carefully with a hand lens and a bright light stimulus. More detailed examination frequently reveals a variety of ocular motility disturbances that include uni- or bilateral internuclear ophthalmoplegia, occasionally combined with uni- or bilateral sixth nerve palsy, hyperventilation, and facial or other cranial nerve palsies. The uncommon smaller hemorrhage may reveal the patient paralyzed but communicative *via* ocular movements (locked-in state). Survival of a few cases has extended for months, but most die in the acute phase. Surgical approach to the hemorrhage has been proved possible (39), but the influence on mortality is unknown.

Parietal—Occipital

Roughly 20% of hematomas occur in sites other than those described above. The parietal—occipital region is the most common. The "slit" hemorrhage is a condition rarely recognized in life prior to the advent of the CT scan. This uncommon hemorrhage develops at the junction of the gray and white matter producing a globular mass that separates the two. Late survival is common, and at autopsy, the remnant of the hemorrhage appears as a shallow orange-stained cavity, given the name "slit" hemorrhage. In the dominant hemisphere, the hemorrhage produces a dense central (Wernicke's) aphasia. To date, no features have been delineated clinically that separate the dysphasia of "slit" hemorrhage from that of other causes, but experience with the syndrome is limited. Case 7 is one of the few examples diagnosed in life.

DIAGNOSTIC STUDIES

Computerized Tomographic Scan

The advent of this test (24, 41, 45) has completely changed methods of evaluating patients with brain hemorrhage. The scan gives a precise localization of the hemorrhage; outlines its size and configuration; displays the degree of hydrocephalus, ventricular shift, or compression; shows the presence of blood in the ventricular system; gives an indication of the degree of edema in the adjacent brain tissue; and gives a precise indication of the residual hematoma following medical and surgical therapy (Figs. 17.2–17.7).

This study is the procedure of choice immediately on admission in all patients suspected of having brain hemorrhage. Even in urgent situations with increasing intracranial pressure, two or three tomographic cuts can be obtained within 10 to 15 minutes.

When available, CT scanning should take precedence over other tests and may permit avoidance of lumbar puncture, arteriography, and radionuclide brain scanning.

Coagulation Studies

Every patient with a spontaneous intracranial hemorrhage should have a platelet count, prothrombin time, and partial thromboplastin

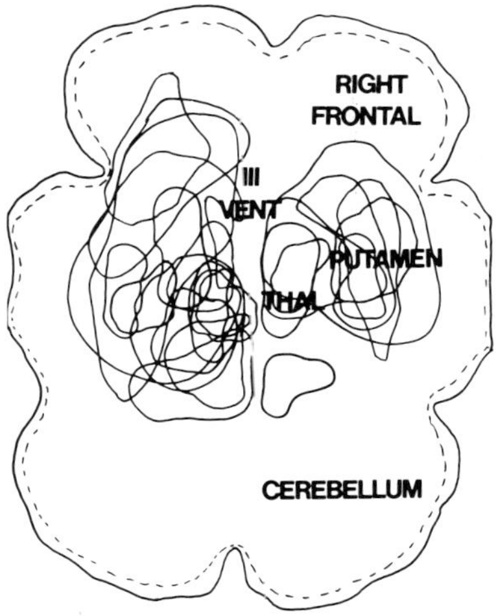

FIG. 17.2. Configuration of hypertensive hemorrhages involving the putamen, thalamus, and adjacent structures in 24 consecutive cases as shown by CT scan in a section through the basal ganglia.

time to assess coexisting disorders of coagulation mechanisms, which, however, are rarely found to be abnormal.

Lumbar Puncture

In order to confirm the clinical diagnosis, a lumbar puncture may be necessary. However, in the early phases of a hemorrhage or in small hemorrhages at any phase of the illness, the CSF may be clear and colorless. When clear, the protein is also usually normal. When bloody, the fluid shows varying degrees of xanthrochromia and protein values from normal to as high as 1200 mg. per 100 ml. Symptoms of herniation have followed lumbar puncture in cases of large putaminal hemorrhage (Case 3), may occur in thalamic or cerebellar hemorrhage, and have not been an issue in pontine or "slit" hemorrhage.

Arteriography

When the CT scan is available, arteriography is principally utilized to exclude a vascular anomaly or neoplasm as the cause of the hemorrhage. It should be performed in all patients with a hemorrhage outside the basal ganglia or cerebellum even when hypertension is present. In cases of hypertensive hemorrhage, the principal finding reflects the mass effect of the hematoma (56). Extravasation of contrast media may be noted rarely early in the course of the illness (25). In putaminal hemorrhage, the course of the lateral lenticulostriate arteries on angiography has been used as a prognostic sign (36).

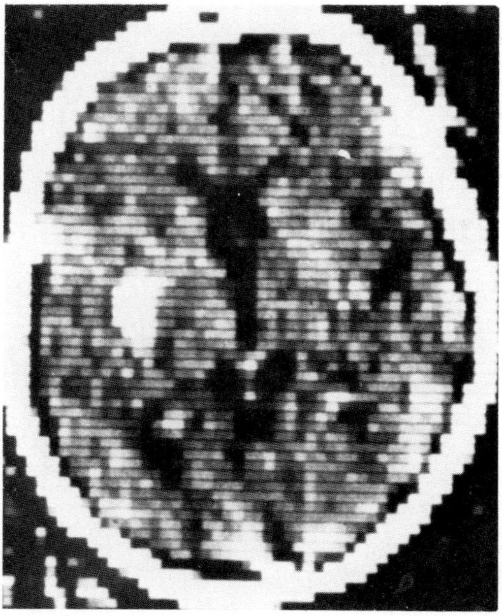

FIG. 17.3. Case 1. CT scan shows small left putaminal hemorrhage. There is no ventricular compression or displacement.

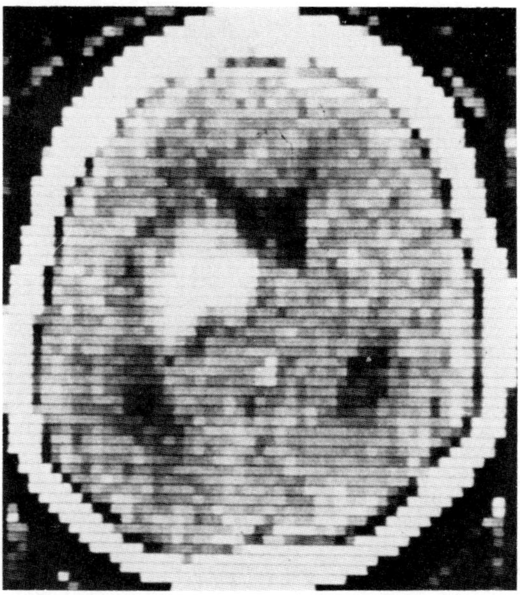

FIG. 17.4. Case 2. CT scan shows moderate left putaminal hemorrhage. Compression of left frontal horn of lateral ventricle is noted.

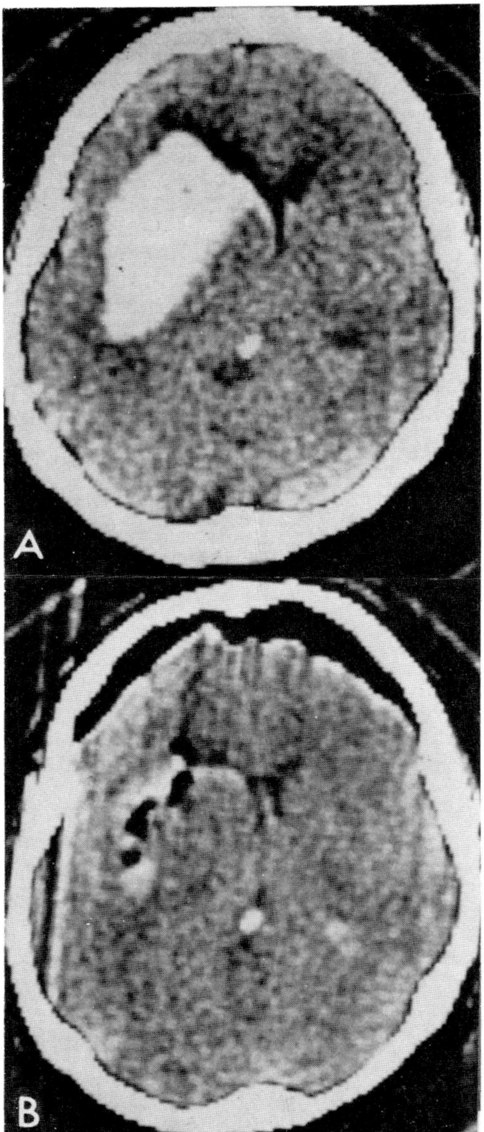

FIG. 17.5. (A) Case 3. CT scan shows large left putaminal hemorrhage which has extended laterally and posteriorly. There is ventricular compression and displacement. (B) Case 3. Postoperative CT scan 2 hours after removal of the large hematoma seen in (A). Note expansion of the compressed basal ganglia tissue. The small high density area along the edge of the hematoma cavity represents a few fragments of clot left on the adjacent cerebral tissue. The dark area anterior to both frontal lobes is subdural air.

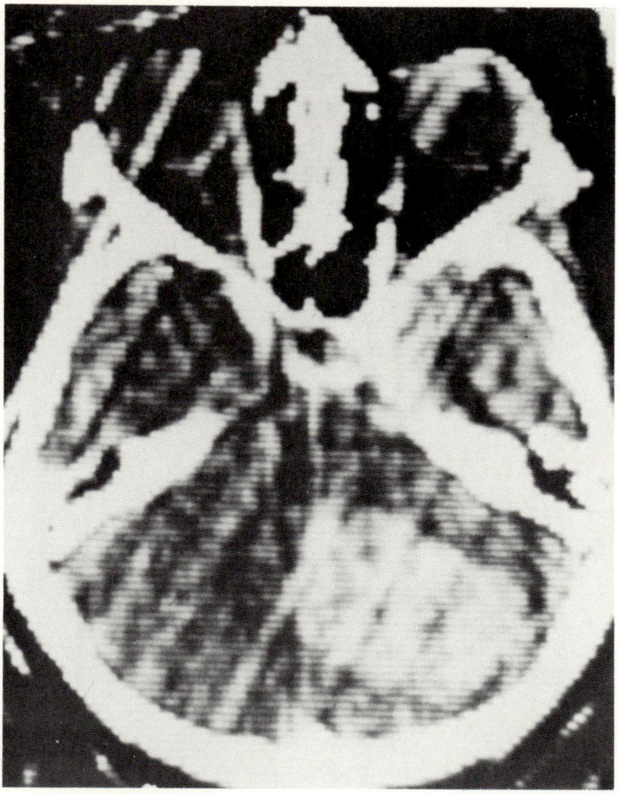

FIG. 17.6. CT scan of large right cerebellar hemorrhage extending from midline out into the cerebellar hemisphere.

Radionuclide Brain Scan

Prior to the advent of the CT scan, this procedure was found to localize about 75% of hematomas large enough to produce a neurological deficit, even in the acute stages (44). With the development of the CT scan, it has fallen into disuse.

Air Study

In the past, pneumoencephalography or ventriculography were utilized to evaluate posterior fossa or intraventricular hematomas. Arteriography has proved a safer means of obtaining the same information, and the CT scan has eclipsed this study in evaluating brain hemorrhages.

DIFFERENTIAL DIAGNOSIS

A detailed clinicopathological study of 118 adults with massive nontraumatic brain hemorrhage indicated that a specific cause (aneu-

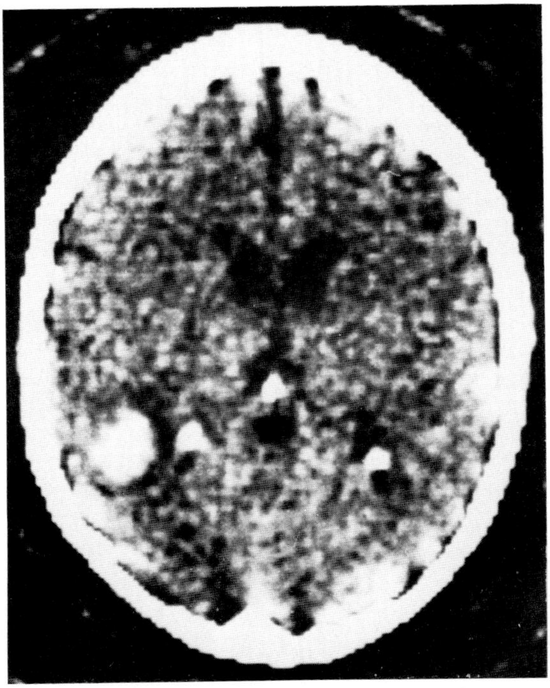

FIG. 17.7. Case 7. CT scan shows a small left temporal parietal subcortical hemorrhage.

rysm, angioma, arteritis, neoplasms, blood dyscrasia) was present in one-half. In 21 of 58 hypertensive patients, a specific cause of the hemorrhage in addition to hypertension was found. In one-third of the entire group, the hemorrhage was demonstrated to be due to only hypertension (31). It is, therefore, important to consider other etiological factors even when hypertension is present.

Aneurysms and Arteriovenous Malformations

Rupture of these lesions can be distinguished from hypertensive hemorrhage on several clinical points: Hypertension is not usually present; rupture precipitates headache and frequently syncope at onset (50% of cases of aneurysm, less so of malformations); initial neurological deficit tends to improve; the cerebrospinal fluid shows heavy staining from hemorrhage; early smooth evolution of the syndrome over time rarely occurs; and rerupture is common. Electrocardiographic abnormalities often occur in subarachnoid hemorrhage (54), but only rarely in hypertensive hemorrhage.

Hemorrhagic Infarction

This occasionally mimics brain hemorrhage but is rarely misdiagnosed when a careful history is taken that indicates the abrupt onset with maximal deficit at onset that characterizes embolus. Experience with the CT scan indicates hemorrhagic infarction may be evident within hours, in several cases before anticoagulant therapy was begun. The cerebral surface is usually prominently involved. The density characteristic of hemorrhage can be observed to follow the surface gyral pattern, and it fades patchily into adjacent tissues. The uniformity at some sites raises the question of frank hemorrhage but is thought to reflect the inability of the scan to distinguish dense hemorrhagic infarction from frank hemorrhage. At times, hemorrhagic infarction affecting the lenticulostriate territories takes the appearance of frank hemorrhage, but in such cases, symptoms reflecting embolic etiology and signs indicating cerebral surface involvement, such as Wernicke's aphasia, permit the proper interpretation of the data. With CT scanning becoming a routine in acute stroke, a better idea of the incidence of hemorrhagic infarction is now being acquired.

Bland Infarction

This is rarely mistaken for hemorrhage in the cerebrum, but prior to the availability of the CT scan, it posed a problem in the management of acute cerebellar infarcts whose occasional dramatic mass effect often closely mimicked cerebellar hemorrhage. Despite the easier differentiation using the CT scan, ischemic cerebellar infarction occasionally requires surgical decompression to relieve the pressure syndrome produced by edema in the infarct (28).

Anticoagulant Disorders

These occur in iatrogenic and endogenous forms. In anticoagulant therapy, there is a constant risk of hemorrhage, but the actual incidence is low, on the order of 1% (31, 34, 51, 52, 55). In the H.C.S.R. (20), 12 cases from the M.G.H. have been recorded in the past 2 years. Anticoagulant therapy accounted for six, four of whom were hypertensive. In four of the six, treatment was in the therapeutic range, while two in excess of the therapeutic range showed hemorrhage into the skin as well as into the brain. Five of the six experienced hemorrhage in the sites typical for hypertension, the sixth in the occipital pole. The therapy is presumed to have assisted in precipitating a typical hypertensive hemorrhage, but only in those with skin hemorrhages or hemorrhages in unusual sites is the causal relationship clear. The symptoms, signs, and course seem essentially the same as ordinary hypertensive hemorrhage in those observed personally. Prompt correction of the anticoagulant effect is done.

Endogenous disorders include the coagulopathies, purpuras, and leukemias (31), the latter group being the most common. Sites affected vary but those typical for hypertension are usually involved, and simultaneous multiple sites are common, a phenomenon almost unknown in hypertension.

Brain Tumors

Rarely is hemorrhage the first sign of a tumor. Glioblastoma multiforme, oligodendrogliomas, and pituitary adenomas are the tumors most prone to hemorrhage, while metastases produce few hemorrhages. The clinical features are virtually indistinguishable from those of hypertensive hemorrhage. Occurrence of the hemorrhage in a site uncommon for hypertensive hemorrhage is the most frequent sign that raises suspicion of tumor. Angiography should be done in such circumstances. If the wall of the hemorrhage cavity appears abnormal at operation, a biopsy should be taken.

TREATMENT

Medical Therapy

Following confirmation of the hemorrhage, efforts are undertaken to stop the hemorrhage, reduce the mass effect, prevent complications (seizures, in particular), and reduce the elevated pressure that set the stage for the hemorrhage. As most hemorrhages appear to have ceased before the patient has arrived at the hospital, assessment of efforts to stop the hemorrhage have proved difficult. Direct methods include compression of the ipsilateral carotid artery and acute lowering of the blood pressure. Methods to encourage coagulation include the correction of abnormalities in coagulation factors and use of aminocaproic acid (Amicar, Lederle, Pearl River, N. Y.). None have been tested sufficiently to ascertain their value, and all would depend, in the end, on documentation that the hemorrhage is, in fact, continuing. Efforts to reduce the mass effect focus principally on the use of edema-modifying factors, particularly corticosteroids, usually given in huge doses. The benefit from this therapy has not been demonstrated (47). Seizures are uncommon, but prophylactic therapy with diphenylhydantoin (Dilantin, Parke, Davis and Co., Detroit, Mich.) is routine. Lowering of the blood pressure appears prudent, although no clear relationship exists between the absolute height of the blood pressure and hemorrhage size (10). Rehemorrhage from the same site is almost unknown, and prompt subsequent hemorrhage from another site is rare. Therapy with methyldopa (Aldomet, Merck, Sharp and Dohme, West Point, Pa.) is often deferred because of drowsiness produced in the early stages in favor of hydralazine (Apresoline, Ciba, Summit, N. J.) which does not usually produce this effect.

Unless the patient declines in function or level of consciousness early, the medical therapy is continued and surgery deferred. In a few cases, decline in function is evident from the time of arrival at the hospital, and under such circumstances, it has been our practice to assume such patients will continue to worsen unless some method is found to cause the hemorrhage to cease. To date, none of the methods outlined above have clearly modified the progress in these cases and surgery has been the main alternative. In cases of cerebellar hemorrhage, special considerations apply, as discussed above, and all such cases are operated if encountered within the first 48 hours of the hemorrhage.

Surgical Therapy

General guidelines for surgical therapy have been summarized in a previous report (43). Hematomas in the putamen, subcortical white matter, and cerebellum are amenable to surgical therapy while those in the thalamus and pons are rarely operated.

If the patient is drowsy or showing signs of increasing neurological deficit or decreasing state of consciousness, surgical removal of the hematoma is considered. Several reports have attempted to determine the indications and timing of operation. The best guide to prognosis has been the state of consciousness (2, 33). Benefit of delayed operation has been reported by some (2, 46, 47) and of immediate operation by others (29). Whether morbidity can be lessened by removal of a hematoma in a patient with a stable moderate or severe neurological deficit several days after onset has not been established.

If there are signs of severe increased intracranial pressure and brain stem compression, emergency surgery is considered depending on the findings on the CT scan and the physical examination. Mannitol (Abbott, North Chicago, Ill.) (100 gm. in 500 ml.) is given intravenously over 15 or 20 minutes while the CT scan is being done. Surgery is not undertaken if there is massive hemorrhage with loss of pupillary reaction and brain stem function.

Operative Technique

Prior to induction of anesthesia, a radial artery catheter is placed for continuous monitoring of intra-arterial blood pressure and intermittent blood gas determinations. Care is taken to avoid aggravating the hypertension during induction of anesthesia. Blood pressure is maintained in a normal range either with anesthetic drugs such as halothane or intravenous sodium nitroprusside or trimethaphan camsylate (Arfonad, Roche Lab., Nutley, N. J.). Arterial blood gas determinations are done and the pCO_2 is kept in the low 30 range. While the skin incision is being made and the bone flap elevated, 100 gm. of Mannitol (Abbott, North Chicago, Ill.) is given.

The hematoma is exposed through a cortical incision and must be removed under direct vision using magnifying lens and headlight or the operating microscope. Needle aspiration is ineffective and is associated with poor results. The bulk of the mass of blood is removed, but a few fragments of clot may be left on the edematous walls of the hematoma cavity in order to avoid further injury to the surrounding brain tissue. As the hematoma is carefully removed, an area of arterial hemorrhage may be noted and is probably the source of the hematoma. This is controlled with bipolar coagulation or a clip. If the hematoma is in an unusual location or the history is atypical, the walls of the cavity are carefully inspected for any localized pathology such as tumor or small arteriovenous anomaly. No drain is used.

Prior to closing the dura, the blood pressure is temporarily elevated for 5 to 10 minutes to a hypertensive level (180 mm. Hg) to be sure that hemostasis is complete. On more than one occasion, a small area of hemorrhage has developed when using this technique.

Postoperative Care

At the conclusion of the operative procedure, care must be taken to prevent rapid return of blood pressure to an elevated level as the anesthesia agents wear off. The intra-arterial blood pressure is monitored continuously in the Recovery Room and, if necessary, intravenous antihypertensive agents, sodium nitroprusside or trimethaphan camsylate (Arfonad) are utilized until intramuscular or oral agents have become effective. Steroids and anticonvulsants are continued.

If there is any question of recurrent hemorrhage, the CT scan is repeated.

Case 1. *Putaminal Hemorrhage. History.* A 61-year-old hypertensive woman, under inpatient therapy for depression but not for hypertension, awoke aware of right arm weakness and clumsiness as she attempted to turn off a ringing alarm clock. Her right leg would not support her weight when she rose from the bed. Her speech was heavily dysarthric. No headache occurred. The deficit worsened steadily over several hours, prompting transfer to the M.G.H.

Examination. Four hours after onset, the blood pressure was 160/90. Language function was normal, but her speech was almost incomprehensibly dysarthric. She showed diminished blink to threat from the right side, impaired conjugate voluntary gaze to the right, dense right central facial weakness, difficulty swallowing, weakness of the left sternomastoid muscle, flaccid proximal and distal right arm and leg, an extensor plantar response on the right side, and slightly blunted sensation to pin prick on the right side.

Course. Lumbar puncture was clear and colorless, with 5 RBCs in the sample, and a protein of 36 mg. per 100 ml. CT scan showed a small left putaminal hemorrhage (Fig. 17.3). Corticosteroid therapy was begun.

By that evening, evidence of the visual field defects and her extraocular movement disturbance had vanished, the limbs could be freely lifted from the bed, and the dysarthria had improved enough to certify intact repetition from dictation, even from complex polysyllables.

Steady improvement occurred over the succeeding days, first with disappearance of the sensory abnormality, then with improvement in the motor strength, proximally more than distally, and she walked by the 3rd day. Legible writing was possible with the right hand by the 5th day. In 8 days, virtually no deficit was evident, steroids were tapered, and the patient was discharged.

Case 2. *Putaminal Hemorrhage. History.* A 27-year-old right-handed homemaker, hypertensive for 5 years, but on no therapy, stumbled and appeared to stub her right foot while climbing the stairs in the company of her husband. She was helped in walking for a few moments and then developed complete right-sided hemiparalysis that evolved smoothly over a several minute period. The evolution was so rapid as to be considered almost sudden. She was transferred to the M.G.H. for further evaluation within hours of the development of hemiplegia.

Examination. The blood pressure was 230/130 with a pulse of 100 and regular cardiac rhythm. The general physical examination was normal. She was alert but unable to follow simple spoken commands and made no efforts at spontaneous speech. A right homonymous hemianopia was evident to confrontation testing with threat stimuli. The optic fundi were normal. The pupils were symmetrical with normal reactions to light. A flaccid dense right hemiplegia involved the face, arm, and leg, including proximal as well as distal appendicular movements. Sensory response on the right side of the body was limited to decorticate movements of the right arm following painful stimuli.

Course. Lumbar puncture revealed grossly bloody spinal fluid with 3,600 RBCs, the fluid xanthrochromic to 3/10, and total protein 330 mg. per 100 ml. Bilateral selective internal carotid arteriogram performed *via* the transfemoral route demonstrated a left hemisphere mass effect with a 3-mm. shift to the right of the left internal cerebral vein. CT scan (Fig. 17.4) revealed a deeply placed, moderate sized hemorrhage situated near the posterior putamen, apparently involving the posterior capsule and possibly the lateral portion of the left thalamus.

Antihypertensive therapy was instituted. The neurological deficit worsened for approximately a 1-day period, principally by appearance of slight stupor. From the time of admission throughout the entire hospital course, full extraocular movements were evident, and no evidence of conjugate deviation occurred at any time. Corticosteroids were added to the treatment program.

By the 3rd hospital day, she was awake and fully alert, speaking softly with a dysphonic and dysarthric voice, showing persisting severe facial paresis, but many aspects of language function were remarkably intact, including the repeating from dictation of short sounds and words, action from dictated to visual choices using the left hand with the stimulus materials, including short three-letter words and pictures, and pointing to body part names on dictated command, including a few praxic responses with the left hand. The motor deficit in the right upper and lower extremities was unchanged.

By the 5th day, the right homonymous hemianopia to threat stimulus had disappeared. Language function was further improved slightly, but no change was noted in the motor examination. By the end of 2 weeks, she articulated much more smoothly, but no essential change had occurred in the motor deficit otherwise. Steroid therapy was gradually reduced.

At 1 month, the patient had spontaneous speech, essentially normal in its language content, contaminated only by occasional hesitancies. She read aloud easily from complex printed material, named and spelled the names of objects at sight, performed a number of dictated praxic commands, and repeated complex polysyllables smoothly and easily. No evidence of homonymous hemianopia was present. Sensory deficit had improved slightly, and she was capable of moving the right leg to some extent proximally.

By 6 weeks, she was capable of sitting erect, resisting moderately well with the right thigh and elevating the arm above horizontal at the shoulder. At 6 months, the patient was ambulating by means of a short leg brace, the right arm held in a stiff flexion at the elbow, and a moderate central facial weakness still present. No evidence of sensory disturbance, visual field abnormalities, extraocular motility disturbances or language function disturbance was present.

Comment. The case is of unusual interest because of the documentation of the evolution of language deficit independent of the outcome of motor deficit in a case of major putaminal hemorrhage. At no time did evidence of conduction aphasia appear.

Case 3. *Putaminal Hemorrhage. History*. A 46-year-old hypertensive man drove off from the automobile agency in his new car and was found shortly thereafter with complete hemiplegia and total aphasia.

Examination. One hour after onset, the blood pressure was 130/80. The neck was supple, and he vomited twice while being examined. He was awake, frequently moving the head, body, left arm and left leg, but not the right side. With the left arm, he was observed to rub the forehead, scratch the face, pull up his shorts, rub his belly, grip the examiner's hand when placed in his left, and flex and extend the leg. The eyes tended to stay closed, but when open, moved conjugately and freely to each side and down, but not up. Attempts to augment eye movements by means of oculocephalic tests did not succeed in achieving upward gaze, although horizontal and downward gaze were easily augmented. He was remarkably unresponsive to any form of noxious stimulus delivered to the left side, including the face, ear, neck, trunk, shoulder, finger, groin, thigh, ankle, and toe, not even showing extensor movements on the right side of the body, although such movements occurred promptly to similar, even lighter, noxious stimulation delivered over similar sites on the right side. Pupillary reactions were normal, and the optic fundi were normal.

Course. As part of the initial evaluation to establish the diagnosis, lumbar puncture was done and revealed an opening pressure of 460 mm. of water, and 4 ml. of uniformly bloody fluid were taken off, followed 15 seconds thereafter by enlargement of the left pupil, during which time no other changes occurred in the examination. Resuscitative measures, including intubation and intravenous Mannitol therapy were instituted. Within 5 minutes, the pupil was back to normal size. CT scan revealed a large left cerebral hemorrhage, principally situated in the putamen, but involving the caudate as well (Fig. 17.5A).

His clinical appearance remained essentially unchanged on corticosteroid and epsilon-amino-caproic acid therapy for the next 72 hours. Then, over a period of approximately 10 minutes, the left pupil became larger than the right and unreactive to direct or consensual light response, at which time the left side of the body became less spontaneously active. Prompt infusion of Mannitol was followed by reversal of this state within a period of 4 to 5 minutes. Repeat CT scan revealed displacement of the midline from left to right side by several millimeters, but no detectable change in size of the large hemorrhage.

Operation was done through a high frontal approach, hoping to evacuate the hemorrhage and spare direct additional injury to the remaining potentially functional fibers in the left Sylvian region that might mediate eventual recovery of language function. The postoperative CT scan (Fig. 17.5B) done within 2 hours of operation revealed restoration of structures toward their normal midline positions and removal of the hematoma.

Postoperative course was essentially uneventful, but very little significant change occurred in the patient's clinical state for the next 2 weeks. Gradually, motor function began to emerge, then echoic repetitive spoken naming responses, followed by gradual improvement in auditory and visual comprehension, but little spontaneous speech apart from a few simplistic stereotypic words. In the long term follow up, the patient became able to stand with the support of a leg brace, the right arm remained essentially useless in the distal functions of the hand and elbow, although he was able to elevate the arm against gravity. The right side of the face remained weak, the tongue deviated slightly to the right. Visual field and extraocular movements, pupillary reactions, and funduscopic examinations were normal.

The patient is now at home under the care of his wife.

Comment. This case illustrates the hazard of lumbar puncture and the need to do a CT scan as the initial diagnostic study. There is considerable difference of opinion regarding timing of surgery in such a patient. The postoperative CT scan shows the immediate effect of removing the large hematoma.

Case 4. *Thalamic Hemorrhage. History.* A 56-year-old hypertensive untreated lawyer complained bitterly of bilateral generalized headache for approximately 30 minutes while ambulating and active in his office, then paused to hold his head, sat down in his chair, vomited, and became paralyzed and comatose over a period of 2 minutes.

Examination. One hour after onset, the blood pressure was 190/110 mm. Hg. The patient was completely comatose. A small subhyaloid hemorrhage was noted at the edge of the right optic disc. The pupils were not reactive to light. The right eye was deviated 5 mm. to the right in the horizontal plane, while the left varied from the same position back to the midline. No upward gaze occurred, even in response to oculocephalic testing. The limbs were immobile, with extensor posturing bilaterally, but response to noxious stimulus was slightly greater on the right arm and right leg compared with the left side. The plantar responses were bilaterally extensor.

Course. The unusual presentation was considered more likely from ruptured aneurysm or malformation than from primary hemorrhage, and an arteriogram was the first study undertaken. Findings of a mass effect in the left thalamus region with moderate hydrocephalus, but no aneurysm, prompted a CT scan that revealed the left thalamic hematoma situated high in the thalamus.

Ventricular drainage was carried out in the hopes that correction of the hydrocephalus would improve the clinical state. Despite adequate ventricular decompression, neither improvement nor worsening resulted.

No major changes in the clinical condition occurred in the 14-day course before death. Autopsy findings corroborated the site and size of the hematoma, located high in the left thalamus.

Comment. The case was considered unusual because of the comparatively long duration of headache before the evolution of focal signs.

Case 5. *Cerebellar Hemorrhage. History.* A 72-year-old man under medical therapy for hypertension was attending an evening party in the home of friends when he suddenly became dizzy, vomited, and was unable to walk unassisted. En route to the M.G.H., he developed diplopia on horizontal lateral gaze, became somewhat drowsy, and vomiting and dizziness continued over a period of approximately an hour.

Examination. The blood pressure was 180/100 mm. Hg. He was drowsy, but arousable to a clear mental state without dysphasia or memory loss. The pupillary reactions and the appearance of the optic fundi were normal. Eye movements were fully conjugate, but right lateral conjugate gaze was not fully accomplished, lacking 2 or 3 mm. of gaze deviation on voluntary efforts. A distinct, but mild right peripheral facial weakness was evident, accompanied by slight reduction in pin-prick over the right side of the face. Strength, bulk, tone, and deep tendon reflexes were normal, but he showed gross disturbance in fine coordination and rapid alternating movements affecting the right upper and lower extremities compared with the left. The plantar responses were bilaterally extensor.

During the 1st hour after arrival, the patient became somewhat more stuporous, the right lateral conjugate gaze became increasingly difficult to produce voluntarily, and the right leg became weak. A lumbar puncture was performed, revealing fluid containing 5,000 RBCs with 2+ xanthrochromia.

Under a diagnostic impression of right cerebellar hematoma, the patient was taken directly to surgery where a 25-ml. hematoma was removed from the right cerebellar hemisphere. Postoperatively, the patient was alert with a clear spinal fluid, but the face and limb paresis persisted for several weeks.

Comment. This case would now have a CT scan performed immediately and the risk of lumbar puncture would be avoided. Prompt surgical intervention prevented a fatal or disabling outcome.

Case 6. *Cerebellar Hemorrhage. History.* A 58-year-old hypertensive man suddenly developed dizziness, followed within moments thereafter by vomiting, nausea, unsteadiness, and bilateral occipital headache while working as a groom at a local race track.

Examination. Four hours after onset, blood pressure was 225/110 mm. Hg. He was alert and fully conversational. The cranial nerves on initial examination were intact except for spontaneous vertical nystagmus with the eyes in the primary position. There was severe appendicular ataxia of the left extremities as well as an ataxic gait requiring assistance from the examiners for support in attempted walking.

A lumbar puncture revealed an opening pressure of 170 mm. of water and grossly bloody fluid. A left cerebellar hemorrhage was suspected and preparations made for craniectomy. Two and one-half hours after admission, he became drowsy but remained easily arousable by voice. A right internuclear ophthalmoplegia appeared, and over the next 20 minutes he became intermittently comatose, with ocular bobbing, irregular respirations, and apneic periods between the irregular respirations. He was taken directly to the operating room where suboccipital craniectomy revealed a large left cerebellar hematoma that had extended into the brain stem and 4th ventricle. Postoperatively, his brain stem function remained severely impaired, coma persisted, and he died on the 6th postoperative day.

Comment. This case compares favorably with Case 5 up to the point of sudden worsening and serves to illustrate the lack of warning prior to disastrous worsening that characterizes these cases and re-emphasizes the recommendation for prompt surgical intervention.

Now, a CT scan would be done promptly on admission and would have an appearance similar to that seen in Fig. 17.6.

Case 7. *Subcortical Hemorrhage. History.* A 64-year-old right-handed homemaker with a 5-year history of hypertension, but no therapy, conversed in a paraphasic fashion over the telephone with her husband in the late afternoon, prompting the husband to return home from work immediately to find his wife speaking paraphasically, but walking about freely, admitting to no headache. Her husband drove her immediately to the M.G.H. During the 30-minute trip the patient was unusually silent and stared to the left side of space.

Examination. Blood pressure was 240/140 on admission. She was awake and fully alert, oriented her face and eyes toward the examiner and participated in a few tasks involving mimicry of gesture, but she made no reliable response to dictated command or to printed commands placed in front of her face. She read the commands aloud in a ludicrous fashion, the word spoon read as "s-p-a-a-s-n, spas." She could not be made to write. The dense right homonymous hemianopia was evident to confrontation testing with threat stimuli. The extraocular movements were full. Motor examination was normal bilaterally, but the right plantar response was extensor.

Course. Lumbar puncture revealed slightly xanthrochromic fluid with no red cells, and a total protein of 66 mg. per 100 ml. She was suspected to be a middle cerebral artery lower division embolic infarct and underwent selective left internal carotid arteriogram *via* the transfemoral route. A mild mass effect was evident in the lower parietotemporal region on the left side. This mass effect prompted a CT scan (Fig. 17.7) which demonstrated a left parietotemporal hemorrhage near the junction of the cerebral surface gray matter and the underlying white matter.

By the next day, the patient spelled a variety of dictated words but continued to speak aloud in literal paraphasic errors, "That's what's bothering me. I'll say the wrong work, work, w-o-r-k, see?" Within 3 days, she had shown further remarkable improvement and gave an umprompted, unperseverative direct narrative of the events of the day of admission, beginning with plans to go to a meeting, the development of her left temporal headache throughout the day, development of dysphasic speaking errors, but she ended the history during the time when she was riding to the hospital. She readily recalled events from distant memory, named the presidents, their circumstances of death, salient information concerning their family lives, showed two fingers in response to the dictated command to show on her fingers the numerical position in the alphabet for the first letter in the name of this city (Boston), spelled the name of the city forward and backward, pointed to various cities on the map, described thematic pictures, repeated complex polysyllables, and named manipulable objects at sight, by touch, and from dictated description. Persisting errors occurred for several days in conversation, such as, "With this headache between, behime, behine my eye, head, eye."

Repeat CT scans over several days, then weeks, demonstrated steady diminution in the size of the mass.

In the weeks that followed, her only neurologic abnormality was the easy disruption of performance when tests were conducted quickly, yet she showed excellent performance on virtually all language tests carried out in a slow and deliberate fashion. She was discharged home, eventually free of deficit, and within 3 months had no evidence of language disturbance.

REFERENCES

1. Adams, R. D., and Vander Eeken, H. M. Vascular diseases of the brain. Ann. Rev. Med., *4:* 213–252, 1953.
2. Beneš, V., Koukoík, F., and Obrovská, D. Two types of spontaneous intracerebral hemorrhage due to hypertension. J. Neurosurg., *37:* 509–513, 1972.
3. Benson, D. F., Sheremata, W. A., Bouchard, R., Segarra, J. M., Price, D., and Geschwind, N. Conduction aphasia: a clinicopathological study. Arch. Neurol., *28:* 339–346, 1973.
4. Bramwell, B. Clinical and pathological memoranda. Edinburgh Med. J., *32:* 4, 97, 243, 911, 1886–1887.
5. Cappell, D. F. Muir's Textbook of Pathology, Ed. 7, Edward Arnold, London, 1958.
6. Charcot, J. M., and Bouchard, C. Nouvelles recherches sur la pathogénie de l'hémorrhagie cérébrale. Arch. Physiol., *1:* 110–127, 643–665, 725–734, 1868.
7. Cole, F. M. Spontaneous intracerebral hemorrhage; a review. West Indian Med. J., *18:* 129–137, 1969.
8. Cole, F. M., and Yates, P. O. Pseudo-aneurysms in relationship to massive cerebral hemorrhage. J. Neurol. Neurosurg. Psychiatry, *30:* 61–66, 1967.
9. Courville, C. B. Pathology of the Central Nervous System, Ed. 3, 473 pp. Pacific Press, Mountain View, Calif., 1950.

10. Dinsdale, H. B. Spontaneous hemorrhage in the posterior fossa. Arch. Neurol., *10:* 200–217, 1964.
11. Ellis, A. G. The pathogenesis of spontaneous cerebral hemorrage. Proc. Path. Soc. (Phila.), 12 (N.S.), *3:* 197–235, 1909.
12. Fasano, F. A., and Broggi, G. Aspect clinique et chirurgical de l'hemorragie cerebrale. à propos de 9 cas d'hematomes intracérébraux spontanés. Neurochirurgie (Paris), *2:* 357–387, 1956.
13. Fisher, C. M. The pathologic and clinical aspects of thalamic hemorrhage. Trans. Am. Neurol. Assoc., *84:* 56–59, 1959.
14. Fisher, C. M. Clinical syndromes in cerebral hemorrhage. *In* Pathogenesis and Treatment of Cerebrovascular Disease, edited by W. S. Fields, pp. 318–338. Charles C Thomas, Springfield, Ill., 1961.
15. Fisher, C. M., Picard, E. H., Polak, A., Dalal, P., and Ojemann, R. G. Acute hypertensive cerebellar hemorrhage: diagnosis and surgical treatment. J. Nerv. Ment. Dis., *140:* 38–57, 1965.
16. Fisher, C. M. Pathological observations in hypertensive cerebral hemorrhage. J. Neuropathol. Exp. Neurol., *30:* 536–550, 1971.
17. Fisher, C. M., Mohr, J. P., and Adams, R. D. Cerebrovascular diseases. *In* Harrison's Principles of Internal Medicine, edited by M. M. Wintrobe, G. W. Thorn, R. D. Adams, E. Braunwald, K. J. Isselbacher, and R. G. Petersdorf, Ed. 7, pp. 1743–1780. McGraw-Hill, New York, 1974.
18. Florey, C. du V., Senter, M. G., and Acheson, R. M. A study of the validity of the diagnosis of stroke in mortality data. I. Certificate analysis. Yale J. Biol. Med., *40:* 148–163, 1967.
19. Freytag, E. Fatal hypertensive intracerebral haematomas: a survey of the pathological anatomy of 393 cases. J. Neurol. Neurosurg. Psychiatry, *31:* 616–620, 1968.
20. Goldstein, R. J., Bleich, H. L., Caplan, L. R., Melski, J. W., Mohr, J. P., Pessin, M., and Duncan, G. W. Computer stroke registry and diagnosis program. Neurology, *25:* 356, 1975.
21. Herbstein, D. S., and Schaumburg, H. H. Hypertensive intracerebral hematoma. An investigation of the initial hemorrhage and rebleeding using chromium Cr51-labeled erythrocytes. Arch. Neurol., *30:* 412–414, 1974.
22. Hier, D. B., David, K. R., Richardson, E. P., and Mohr, J. P. Hypertensive putaminal hemorrhage. (Submitted for publication.)
23. Johansson, S. H., and Melin, H. S. Spontaneous cerebral haemorrhage and encephalomalacia. Acta Psychiatr. Neurol. Scand., *35:* 457–479, 1960.
24. Kistler, J. P., Hochberg, F. H., Brooks, B. R., Richardson, E. P., Jr., New, P. F. J., and Schnur, J. Computerized axial tomography: clinicopathological correlation. Neurology, *25:* 201–209, 1975.
25. Kowada, M., Yamaguchi, K., Matsucka, S., and Ito, Z. Extravasation of angiographic contrast material in hypertensive intracerebral hemorrhage. J. Neurosurg., *36:* 471–473, 1972.
26. Kurtzke, J. F. Epidemiology of Cerebrovascular Disease, 197 pp. Springer, Berlin, 1969.
27. Lampert, H., and Müller, W. Bei welchem Druck kommt es zu einer Ruptur der Gehirnfasse? Frankfurt Z. Pathol., *33:* 471–477, 1926.
28. Lehrich, J. R., Winkler, G. F., and Ojemann, R. G. Cerebellar infarction with brain stem compression: diagnosis and surgical treatment. Arch. Neurol., *22:* 490–498, 1970.
29. Luessenhop, A. J., Shevlin, W. A., Ferrero, A. A., McCullough, D. C., and Barone, B.

M. Surgical management of primary intracerebral hemorrhage. J. Neurosurg., *27:* 419–427, 1967.
30. Matsuoka, S. Histopathological studies on the blood vessels in apoplexia cerebri. *In* Proceedings of the First International Congress of Neuropathology, Vol. 3, pp. 222–231, Rosenberg and Sellier, Turin, 1952.
31. McCormick, W. F., and Rosenfield, D. B. Massive brain hemorrhage: a review of 144 cases and an examination of their causes. Stroke, *4:* 946–954, 1973.
32. McKissock, W., Richardson, A., and Walsh, L. Spontaneous cerebellar hemorrhage: a study of 34 consecutive cases treated surgically. Brain, *83:* 1–9, 1960.
33. McKissock, W., Richardson, A., and Taylor, J. Primary intracerebral hemorrhage: a controlled trial of surgical and conservative treatment in 180 unselected cases. Lancet, *2:* 221–226, 1961.
34. MacMillan, R. L., and Brown, K. W. G. Haemorrhage in anticoagulant therapy. Can. Med. Assoc. J., *69:* 279–283, 1953.
35. Merritt, H. H. A Textbook of Neurology, Ed. 4, 175 pp. Lea & Febiger, Philadelphia, 1967.
36. Mizukami, M., Araki, G., and Mihara, H. Angiographic sign of good prognosis for hemiplegia in hypertensive intracerebral hemorrhage. Neurology, 120–126, 1974.
37. Mohr, J. P., Watters, W., and Duncan, G. W. Thalamic hemorrhage and aphasia. Brain Language, *2:* 3–17, 1975.
38. Mohr, J. P., and Sidman, M. Aphasia: behavioral aspects. *In* American Handbook of Psychiatry, edited by M. Reiser, Vol. 4, Basic Books, New York, (in press).
39. Murphy, M. G. Successful evacuation of acute pontine hematoma. J. Neurosurg., *37:* 224–225, 1972.
40. Mutlu, N., Berry, R. G., and Alpers, B. J. Massive cerebral hemorrhage: clinical and pathological correlations. Arch. Neurol., *8:* 644–661, 1963.
41. New, P. F. J., Scott, W. R., Schnur, J. A., Davis, K. R., and Taveras, J. M. Computerized axial tomography with the EMI scanner. Radiology, *110:* 109–123, 1974.
42. Odom, G. L., Bloor, B. M., and Woodhall, B. Intracerebral hematomas; a survey of 106 verified cases. South. Med. J., *45:* 936–942, 1952.
43. Ojemann, R. G. Intracerebral and intracerebellar hemorrhage. *In:* Neurological Surgery, edited by J. R. Youmans, Vol. 2, pp. 844–851. W. B. Saunders Co., Philadelphia, 1973.
44. Ojemann, R. G., Aronow, S., and Sweet, W. H. Scanning with positron-emitting radioisotopes: aneurysm, arteriovenous malformation and intracerebral hemorrhage. J. Neurosurg., *22:* 489–498, 1965.
45. Ott, K. H., Kase, C. S., Ojemann, R. G., and Mohr, J. P. Cerebellar hemorrhage: diagnosis and treatment. A review of 56 cases. Arch. Neurol., *31:* 160–167, 1974.
46. Paillas, J. E., and Alliez, B. Surgical treatment of spontaneous intracerebral hemorrhage. Immediate and long-term results in 250 cases. J. Neurosurg., *39:* 145–151, 1973.
47. Richardson, A. Surgical therapy of spontaneous intracerebral hemorrhage. *In* Progress in Neurological Surgery, edited by H. Krayenbuhl, P. Maspes, and W. H. Sweet, Vol. 3, pp. 397–418, Karger, Basel, 1969.
48. Russell, D. S. The pathology of spontaneous intracranial haemorrhage. Proc. R. Soc. Med., *47:* 689–693, 1954.
49. Stehbens, W. E. Aneurysms and anatomical variation of cerebral arteries. Arch. Pathol., *75:* 45–64, 1963.
50. Stehbens, W. E. Pathology of the Cerebral Blood Vessels. 661 pp. C. V. Mosby, St.

Louis, 1972.

51. Stephens, C. A. L., Jr., Anticoagulant therapy in private practice. Circulation, *9:* 682–686, 1954.
52. Tulloch, J., and Wright, I. S. Long-term anticoagulant therapy: further experiences. Circulation, *9:* 823–834, 1954.
53. Turner, F. C. Arteries of the brain from cases of cerebral haemorrhage. Trans. Path. Soc. London, *33:* 96–102, 1882.
54. Weidler, D. J. Myocardial damage and cardiac arrhythmias after intracranial hemorrhage: a critical review. Stroke, *5:* 759–764, 1974.
55. Wells, C. E., and Urrea, D. Cerebrovascular accidents in patients receiving anticoagulant drugs. Arch. Neurol., *3:* 553–558, 1960.
56. Yamaguchi, K., Uemura, K., and Takahashi, H. An angiographic study of sequential changes in hypertensive intracerebral hemorrhage. Br. J. Radiol., *46:* 125–130, 1973.
57. Yates, P. O. A change in the pattern of cerebrovascular disease. Lancet, *1:* 65–69, 1964.
58. Zimmerman, H. M. Cerebral apoplexy: mechanism and differential diagnosis. N.Y. State J. Med., *49:* 2153–2157, 1949.
59. Zülch, K. J. Pathological aspects of cerebral accidents in arterial hypertension. Acta Neurol. Belg., *71:* 196–220, 1971.

CHAPTER

18

The Radionuclide Cerebral Angiogram in Stroke Diagnosis

JOHN F. ROCKETT, M.D.

The results of nuclear angiography in confirming the early diagnosis of stroke are reported in this presentation.

METHODS AND MATERIALS

The charts of all patients admitted to the Baptist Memorial Hospital in Memphis, Tennessee, between August, 1974 and February, 1975 with acute cerebrovascular accidents were reviewed. Seventy-eight patients who had radionuclide cerebral studies and adequate clinical and laboratory data for the diagnosis of acute stroke form the basis of this communication. All patients had nuclear studies within 10 days of the onset of symptoms. The age range was from 38 years to 87 years. Those with transient ischemic attacks and residua from earlier cerebrovascular accidents were excluded from this report. Division into internal carotid and vertebrobasilar groups was made on the basis of clinical and contrast angiographic evidence.

All patients were studied with the Anger scintillation camera following the intravenous injection of 15 to 20 millicuries of ^{99m}Tc-pertechnetate in a 1- to 2-ml. bolus. The patient's chart was reviewed prior to administering the radiopharmaceutical to determine the appropriate position for the radionuclide cerebral angiogram.

If occipital lobe pathology or a vertebrobasilar arterial abnormality was suspected, the patient was studied in the posterior projection. Otherwise, the subject was positioned to obtain an anterior view of the head and neck.

When the isotope was demonstrated in the carotid arteries, eight rapid serial scintiphotographs were recorded on hand-pulled Polaroid film at 2-second intervals.

Initially, symmetrical streams of radioactivity are seen in the neck in the normal radionuclide cerebral angiogram (Fig. 18.1). This activity primarily represents the first arterial transit of the radiopharmaceutical through the right and left carotid arteries.

Arterial, capillary, and venous phases are seen as the isotope passes

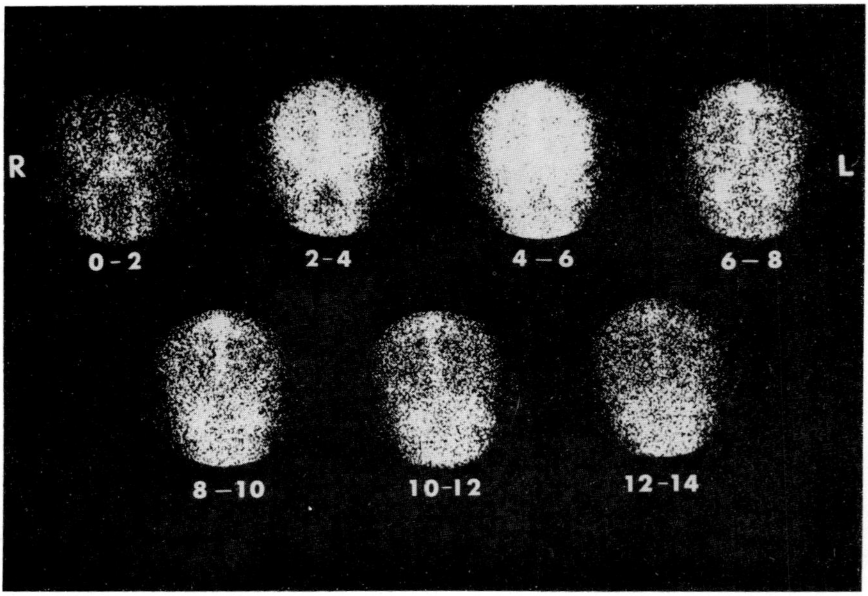

FIG. 18.1. Normal anterior radionuclide cerebral angiogram. Numbers denote time range in seconds.

through the intracerebral circulation. The right and left middle cerebral arterial areas and overlapping anterior cerebral arterial areas are demonstrated. Symmetrical and homogeneous perfusion is present during the arterial and capillary phases in the hemispheres. Asymmetrical activity when seen during the venous portion of the dynamic study is usually due to a dominant transverse sinus.

The static brain scan is then obtained from 1 to 3 hours after the radionuclide cerebral angiogram has been performed depending upon clinical information and findings on the nuclear cerebral angiogram.

RESULTS

The typical abnormality on the nuclear cerebral angiogram in a patient with an acute stroke was a reduction of tracer activity in an arterial distribution compared to the opposite side. The reduced perfusion usually persisted throughout the study (Fig. 18.2). In this 56-year-old male, occlusion of the M-1 segment of the left middle cerebral artery was demonstrated. Decreased activity in the left middle cerebral arterial distribution was present throughout the dynamic study. Contrast arteriography verified the findings shown by rapid sequential scintiphotography (Fig. 18.3).

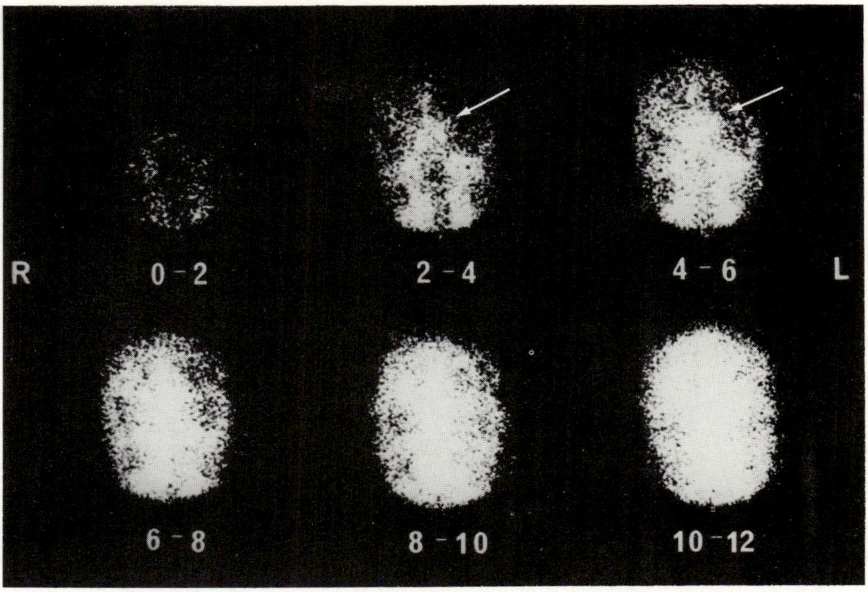

FIG. 18.2. Middle cerebral artery obstruction. Anterior radionuclide cerebral angiogram demonstrating left middle cerebral artery occlusion. Arrows point to the lesion site. Numbers denote time range in seconds.

In some individuals with cerebral vascular occlusive disease, late in the dynamic study, the involved hemisphere showed greater activity than the normal hemisphere. This apparently was due to delayed filling of the abnormal area of the brain by collateral vessels.

Another abnormal perfusion pattern seen in patients with acute stroke was vascular displacement due to an intracerebral hemorrhage. An example of the scintiphotographic changes in a hemorrhagic stroke victim is shown in Figure 18.4. The individual was a 61-year-old hypertensive female who had suffered a sudden onset of severe left frontal headache, nausea, and vomiting. She had become aphasic and while attempting to walk, fell, striking her head on the floor. She had been maintained on oral sodium warfarin for a year following a pulmonary embolus. Upon her admission to the hospital, the attending neurosurgeon asked for immediate radionuclide studies of the brain.

Absence of deep left frontal activity persisted throughout the anterior radionuclide cerebral angiogram. The left middle cerebral vessels appeared displaced laterally, and the anterior cerebral arteries were felt to be slightly shifted to the right. Peripheral depression of the convexity branches of the left middle cerebral artery was also suspected. Postflow images were interpreted as normal.

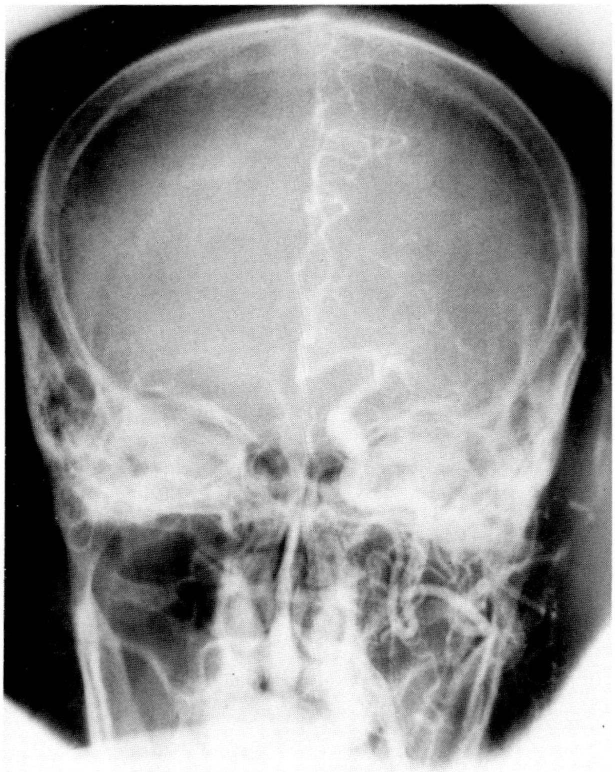

Fig. 18.3. Left direct common carotid angiogram. Anterioposterior view, showing occlusion of the left middle cerebral artery.

The nuclear cerebral angiogram appeared to detect a hypovascular mass deep in the left frontal region, most likely an intracerebral hemorrhage. It was thought a small left subdural or extradural hematoma might also be present.

The neurosurgeon was immediately notified of these impressions, but before carotid arteriography could be performed, 2-hour postinjection static brain images were made.

No definite abnormalities were detected by the conventional brain scintiphotos.

A left direct carotid arteriogram (Fig. 18.5) showed the hypovascular left frontal mass. The acute left-sided subdural hematoma which had caused the depression of the peripheral vessels on the radionuclide cerebral angiogram was also visualized.

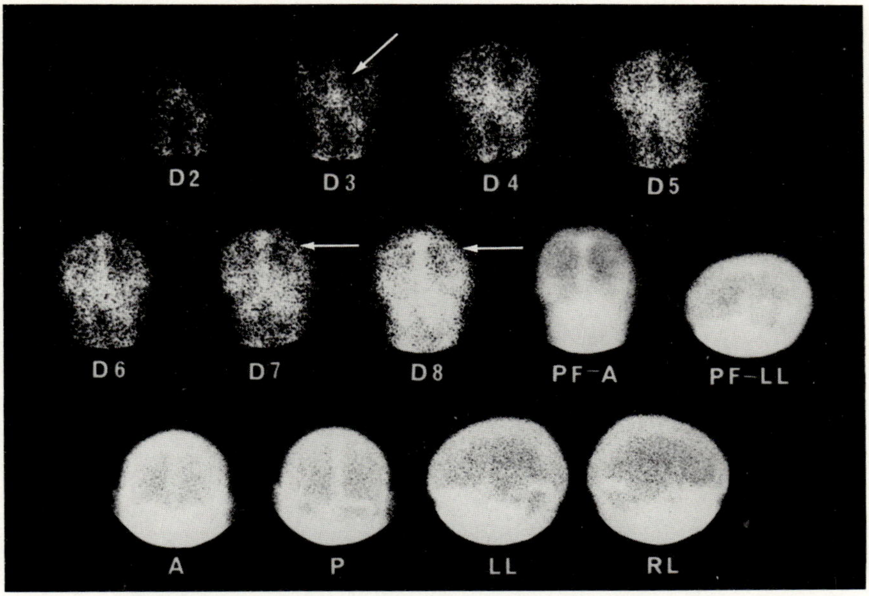

FIG. 18.4. Intracerebral hemorrhage and acute subdural hematoma. D2-D8, scintiphotos from anterior radionuclide cerebral angiogram, taken at 2-second intervals, show avascular left frontal lesion and peripheral compression of convexity branches of the left middle cerebral artery. Arrows point to the abnormalities. PF-A, post "flow"—anterior view; and PF-LL, post "flow"—left lateral view, appeared normal. A, anterior; P, posterior; LL, left lateral; and RL, right lateral 1 hour post-injection static brain scans fail to demonstrate any abnormal areas.

The same day, a 20-ml. deep left frontal intracerebral hemorrhage and a 15-ml. acute subdural hematoma were surgically evacuated.

A definite abnormality in perfusion during the arterial phase of the neck vessels and/or arterial-capillary phases of the cranial vessels was present in 47 of the 78 patients (60%) with acute strokes. The deficit had to persist on at least two successive scintiphotos to be considered significant.

In 29 individuals with acute strokes, the radionuclide cerebral angiograms were abnormal, and the conventional brain images were negative (Table 18.1). Abnormalities were present on both radionuclide studies in 12 patients. The static brain scan detected two infarcts in patients with normal radionuclide cerebral angiograms. One was a small middle cerebral stroke, the other an anterior cerebral branch infarct. Six additional stroke victims in whom no brain scan was requested had vascular deficits detected by the dynamic study.

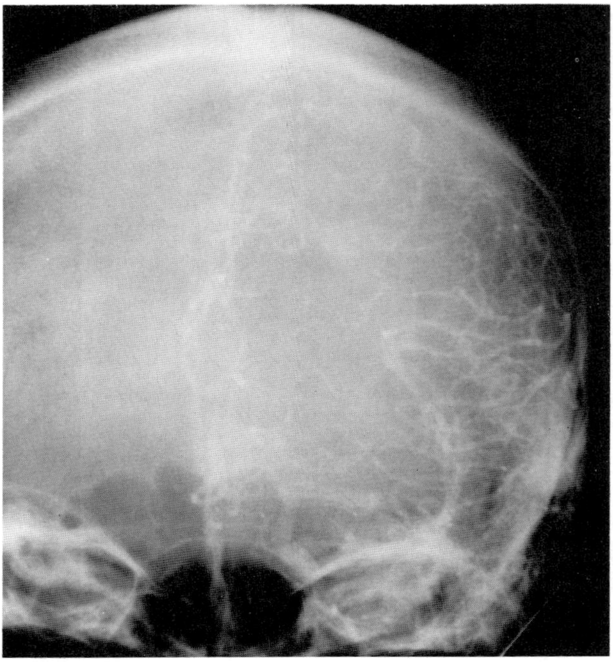

FIG. 18.5. Left direct common carotid angiogram showing left frontal intracerebral hemorrhage and left acute subdural hematoma.

TABLE 18.1
Radionuclide Cerebral Angiogram (NCA)–Brain Scan Correlation

Results	No.
NCA + scan	29
NCA + scan+	12
NCA − scan+	2
NCA + no scan	6
NCA − no scan	2

Static brain scans were not performed in two patients with false negative isotopic perfusion studies.

The nuclear cerebral angiograms were not technically satisfactory in 6 of the 78 patients in this series. These studies were assumed to be normal.

Radionuclide angiography was interpreted as abnormal in 45 of 68 patients with acute strokes involving the internal carotid artery or its branches (Table 18.2).

Only two dynamic studies in patients with vertebrobasilar system disease were abnormal. One patient had unilateral vertebral artery disease. The other individual had a posterior cerebral artery occlusion. The static brain images failed to detect any additional strokes in those with negative radionuclide angiography. Eight patients with vertebrobasilar system strokes failed to show a perfusion defect on cerebral angioscintiphotography.

Static brain images were abnormal in 14 of 70 (20%) patients with acute strokes. Patients had nuclear studies an average of 2.8 days after the onset of symptoms. All abnormal brain scans were in regions of the brain supplied by the internal carotid artery. One patient with a posteror cerebral infarct had positive dynamic and static studies. Her right posterior cerebral artery originated from the carotid system, rather than the basilar artery.

The detection rate of acute strokes in this series is shown in Table 18.3. The radionuclide cerebral angiogram was abnormal in 66% of acute carotid system strokes. Blood flow abnormalities were seen in 20% of patients with strokes in the vertebrobasilar distribution. The two abnormal brain scans in patients with normal nuclide angiography raised the detection rate in acute carotid system strokes by nuclide studies to 69%. No additional vertebrobasilar cerebrovascular accidents were detected on static brain scans.

Of the 31 stroke patients who had arteriographically proven cerebral vascular disease, 23 had abnormal radionuclide cerebral angiograms (74%). Contrast arteriography detected vascular lesions in the neck in six patients that had normal anterior radionuclide cerebral angiograms. The carotid obstruction was less than 70% of the arterial lumen. Verte-

TABLE 18.2
Stroke Distribution

	Carotid System	Vertebrobasilar System
Radionuclide cerebral angiogram abnormal	45	2
Radionuclide cerebral angiogram normal	23	8
Total	68	10

TABLE 18.3
Acute Stroke Per Cent Detected

	Carotid System	Vertebrobasilar System
Radionuclide cerebral angiogram abnormal	66%	20%
Radionuclide cerebral angiogram and/or brain scan abnormal	69%	20%

brobasilar disease or bilateral carotid lesions were present in these six false negative isotopic patients.

An anterior projection nuclear angiogram failed to detect a posterior cerebral artery occlusion.

The radionuclide perfusion study was not technically satisfactory for interpretation in one patient with an abnormal radiocontrast arteriogram. This tracer examination was counted as a false negative study.

Three patients with acute strokes in the middle cerebral distribution had abnormal radionuclide cerebral angiograms and normal contrast angiograms. The tracer study detected a vascular lesion while the radiographic examination did not.

Division of the patients into hemorrhagic and ischemic strokes could not always be made from the clinical information available. In five of seven patients with proved intracerebral hemorrhages, vascular displacement was present on the radionuclide cerebral angiogram.

DISCUSSION

The radionuclide cerebral angiogram provides an assessment of the cerebral circulation that is unattainable by other noninvasive radiologi-

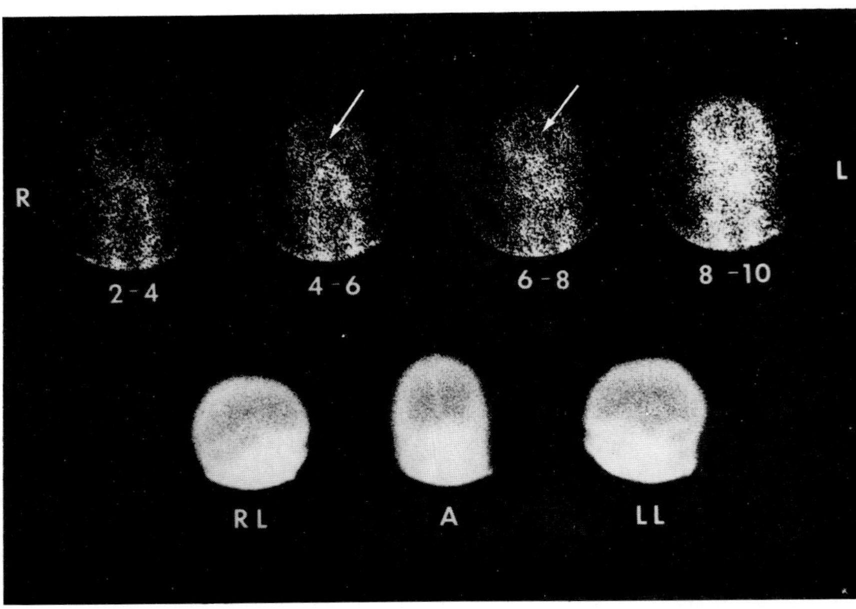

FIG. 18.6. Bilateral anterior cerebral occlusions. Anterior radionuclide cerebral angiogram portraying reduction of radioactive transit through the anterior cerebral arteries. (*Arrows*) denote the reduced activity. On the 8- to 10-second scintiphoto the region has filled, probably by collateral vessels. Static scintiphotos at 1 hour were negative. RL, right lateral; A, anterior; and LL, left lateral projections.

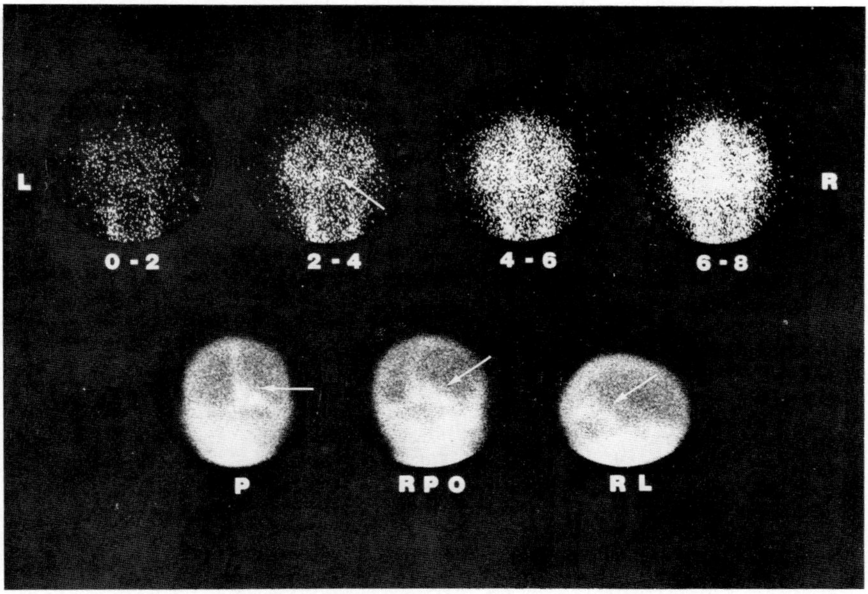

FIG. 18.7. Posterior cerebral infarct. Posterior radionuclide cerebral angiogram demonstrating reduction in activity in the right occipital area. Numbers denote time range in seconds. Static scintiphotos 2 hours after injection showing abnormal concentration of radiopertechnetate in the left posterior cerebral distribution. P, posterior; RPO, right posterior oblique; RL, right lateral views. Arrows point to pathology.

cal techniques, including computed tomography (6). It can detect abnormalities, particularly occlusive vascular lesions, that are not shown on the static brain images. For example, in this study, 35 of 47 patients with isotopic perfusion defects either had normal static images or did not have brain scans performed. Use of the radionuclide cerebral angiogram approximately doubles the isotopic detection rate of cerebrovascular disease (2, 4). This is partly because most static brain images are negative for the first 7 to 10 days after a cerebrovascular accident.

The isotopic perfusion study is most effective in detecting middle cerebral and carotid artery occlusive disease. Significant obstruction of the carotid artery, usually 70% or greater, will result in decreased blood flow (1). This degree of carotid occlusion will usually be detected by the radionuclide cerebral angiogram (10). In the present study, the nuclear cerebral angiogram detected all unilateral carotid stenoses when greater than 70% of the vessel's lumen was occluded.

Some difficulty in detecting bilateral carotid ischemic lesions has also been experienced by other investigators (2, 3, 5). Low cardiac output, slow intravenous injection of the radiopharmaceutical, and interfering external carotid flow may cause one to miss bilateral carotid cerebrovas-

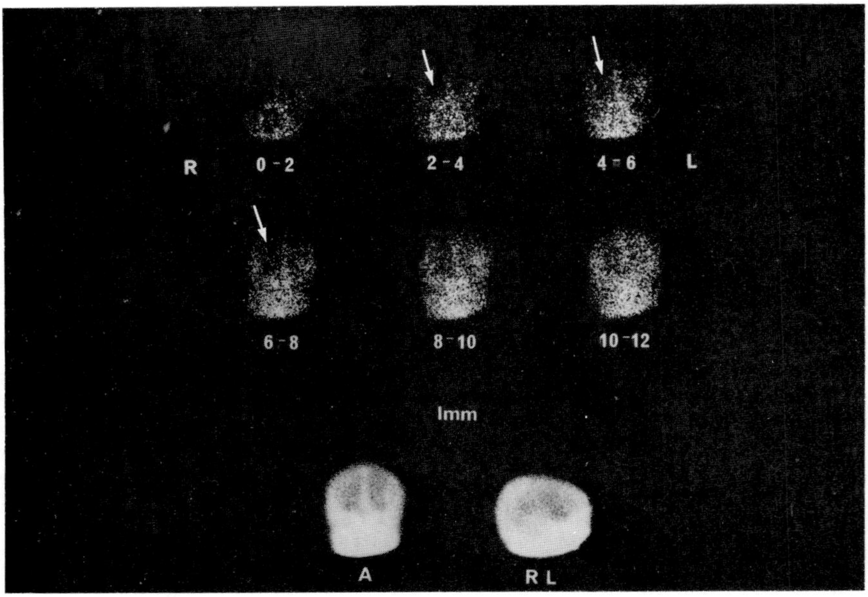

FIG. 18.8. Right intracerebral hemorrhage. Anterior radionuclide cerebral angiogram showing decreased transit of the radiopertechnetate through the right hemisphere and lateral displacement of the middle cerebral vessels due to the centrosylvian mass. Arrows point to the pathology. Numbers denote time range in seconds. Imm, immediate postradionuclide cerebral angiogram; A, anterior; and RL, right lateral scintiphotos are negative.

cular disease. Increased intracranial pressure also may cause slow but symmetrical passage of the radiopharmaceutical through the neck arteries.

Unilateral anterior cerebral artery ischemic lesions are difficult to visualize with the dynamic radioisotopic technique. The rarer bilateral anterior cerebral occlusions are readily recognized by nuclear angiography, however (8) (Fig. 18.6). Absence of early perfusion in the anterior cerebral artery distribution was evident in this stroke victim.

We did not find the radionuclide cerebral angiogram to be an effective means of detecting most vertebrobasilar vascular occlusions. Cowan and associates had a similar experience (2). Posterior cerebral strokes should usually be detected if the patient is studied in the posterior projection. This patient's posterior cerebral infarct was detected on both dynamic and static radionuclide studies (Fig. 18.7). The posterior radionuclide cerebral angiogram showed decreased activity in the right occipital region. Two-hour static brain images demonstrated the infarction in the calcarine region of the right cerebral hemisphere. As stated earlier, this posterior cerebral vessel originated from the carotid system.

The radionuclide cerebral angiogram can also detect vascular pathology not seen with contrast arteriography. The radioisotopic study visualizes the vasculature below the resolution of the contrast angiogram, or the microcirculation (9). Three acute middle cerebral stroke victims had definite vascular abnormalities demonstrated by the dynamic isotopic procedure while contrast angiography was interpreted as normal.

Detection of intracerebral hemorrhages by the nuclear cerebral angiogram alone has been reported (7). We have been successful in demonstrating frontal and temporal lobe hematomas on anterior cerebral angioscintigrams. An emergency radionuclide cerebral angiogram was requested on this comatose 16-year-old female (Fig. 18.8). It showed decreased activity in the right hemisphere throughout the anterior perfusion study. The right middle cerebral complex appeared displaced

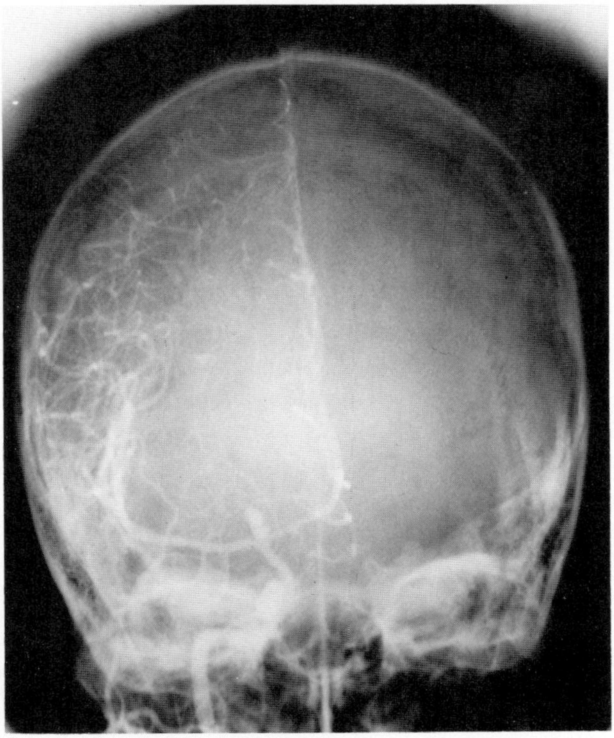

FIG. 18.9. Right direct common carotid angiogram. Anterioposterior view. Avascular centrosylvian mass and a lobulated aneurysm at the bifurcation of the right internal carotid artery.

laterally. The superior sagittal sinus was never demonstrated; therefore, it was believed the cerebral circulation was slowed, probably due to increased intracranial pressure. Immediate postinjection views were normal.

It was our impression that there was a large right frontal mass present, most likely an intracerebral hematoma. A low grade glioma or abscess could cause similar findings on the dynamic study.

A right direct common carotid arteriogram was performed immediately. An avascular right frontal lesion and a large lobulated aneurysm at the bifurcation of the internal carotid artery were shown (Fig. 18.9).

A right frontal craniotomy was then performed. The internal carotid aneurysm was clipped and the huge intracerebral hematoma evacuated.

The over-all stroke detection rate of 60% in the present series from the Baptist Memorial Hospital would have been improved considerably if the six patients with technically inadequate studies has not been included. All six unsatisfactory examinations occurred in patients with carotid system disease. If these isotopic studies had been excluded, the radionuclide cerebral angiogram detection rate in carotid system strokes would have increased to 71%.

Other investigators in not altogether comparable studies have reported from 45% to 83% cerebrovascular disease detection with nuclear angiography (2–5, 9).

SUMMARY

The radionuclide cerebral angiogram using intravenous radiopertechnetate has been found to be of value in confirming the early diagnosis of stroke. The isotopic perfusion study is of value in detecting ischemic carotid and middle cerebral lesions. It can also provide a rapid means of demonstrating intracerebral hemorrhages. Nuclear angiography is not recommended for detection of vertebrobasilar artery disease unless a posterior cerebral artery occlusion is suspected.

REFERENCES

1. Brice, J. G., Dowsett. D. J., and Lowe, R. D., Haemodynamic effects of carotid artery stenosis. Br. Med. J., *2:* 1363–1366, 1964.
2. Cowan, R. J., Maynard, C. D., Meschan. I., Janeway, R., and Shigeno, K. Value of the routine use of the cerebral dynamic radioisotope study. Radiology, *107:* 111–116, 1973.
3. Fischer, R. J., and Miale, A., Jr. Evaluation of cerebral vascular disease with radionuclide angiography. Stroke, *3:* 1–9, 1972.
4. Fish, M. B., Barnes, B., and Polycove, M. Cranial scintiphotographic blood flow defects in arteriographically proven cerebral vascular disease. J. Nucl. Med., *14:* 558–564. 1973.
5. Moses, D. C., James, A. E., Jr., Strauss, H. W., and Wagner. H. N., Jr. Regional

cerebral blood flow estimation in the diagnosis of cerebrovascular disease. J. Nucl. Med., *13:* 135–141, 1972.

6. Pendergrass, H. P., McKusick, K. A., New, P. F. J., and Potsaid, M. S. Relative efficacy of radionuclide imaging and computed tomography of the brain. Radiology, *116:* 363–366, 1975.
7. Rockett, J. F., Kaplan, E. S., Hudson, J. S., and Moinuddin, M. Intracerebral hemorrhage demonstrated by nuclear cerebral angiogram: case report. J. Nucl. Med., *16:* 459–461, 1975.
8. Rockett, J. F., Kaplan, E. S., Ray, M., Buchignani, J. S., and Gardner, H. C. Scintiphotographic demonstration of bilateral infarction in the distribution of the anterior cerebral arteries. Radiology, *112:* 135–137, 1974.
9. Rosenthall, L., Chan, J., Sidhu, R., and Stratford, J. Combined radiocontrast and radionuclide cerebral angiography. Radiology, *92:* 1223–1228, 1969.
10. Wise, G., Brockenbrough, E. C., and Marty, R. The detection of carotid artery obstruction: a correlation with arteriography. Stroke, *2:* 105–113, 1971.

CHAPTER

19

Techniques of Cerebral Revascularization

S. J. PEERLESS, M.D., F.R.C.S. (C)

INTRODUCTION

The current epidemic of atherosclerotic and thromboembolic vascular disease has resulted in an increasing number of individuals dead or severely disabled from cerebral ischemia. Despite the widespread and successful application of reconstructive vascular surgery to the arch of the aorta and extracranial segments of the carotid and vertebral arteries, there remains a large number of individuals whose disease is primarily, if not entirely, localized to the intracranial vasculature. It has been estimated that in somewhat more than 50 per cent of ischemic lesions of the brain, the vascular disease is limited to intracranial or to inaccessible sites of the extracranial vessels or both. Pharmacological manipulation of the cerebral blood vessels has proven to be of limited value in halting or reversing the atherosclerotic disease or improving collateral flow. Until recently, with the development of microvascular surgical methods, cerebral revascularization and intracranial vascular reconstruction has been an unfulfilled but tantalizing goal.

In the past, intracranial reconstructive vascular surgery has been performed in isolated cases without the surgical microscope by Welsh (11), Shillito (10), Driesen (3), Chou (1), and Woringer (12) in the early part of the last decade. In 1960, Jacobson and Suarez demonstrated the value of the surgical microscope in ensuring consistent patency in vascular anastomosis and endarterectomies of arteries and veins as small as 1 mm. in diameter (5). Their pioneer work stimulated the development of new instruments and ultrafine suture materials for microsurgery. In the early 1960's, these new techniques were refined and adapted for neurosurgery and a small number of reconstructive procedures on intracranial arteries were attempted by Jacobson and Donaghy (6), Lougheed (7), and Yasargil (13, 14).

Henschen, in 1944, attached a pedicle of temporalis muscle to the surface of the brain in an attempt to fashion a unique source of collateral circulation from the extracranial vasculature (4). Using this model and the newly developed techniques of microvascular surgery, Donaghy and

Yasargil in 1967 perfected a direct anastomosis between the extracranial and intracranial vessels using the superficial temporal artery and a cortical branch of the middle cerebral artery (STA-MC) (13, 14). In 1970 and 1972, Yasargil and Donaghy reported the first human cases with this procedure, and since that time many procedures have been done in centers around the world with an acceptably high rate of patency of the anastomosis and although unproven, encouraging clinical results (2, 14).

In 1971, Lougheed described a technique of a long bypass from the extracranial to intracranial carotid circulation using an interposed vein graft (8). Although technically feasible, the procedure has not gained wide acceptance primarily because of the great difficulty in carrying out the intracranial anastomosis on diseased vessels in the confined space at the base of the brain. The technique also suffers from the prospect of having to interrupt cerebral blood flow to gain sufficient length of the intracranial carotid artery to carry out the anastomosis. Although capable of delivering large volumes of blood to the hemisphere and indeed to the whole brain, prolonged patency is less certain due to intimal hypertrophy of the vein in response to arterial pressure and early occlusion.

The technique of anastomosing branches of the superficial temporal or occipital artery to cortical branches of the middle cerebral, vertebral, or basilar circulation has proven to be a safe procedure. Dissection into or under the surface of the brain is not necessary and interruption of flow through a branch of a cortical vessel even for prolonged periods is well tolerated. Furthermore, in that the procedure need not be lengthy nor require complex anesthetic techniques. one may minimize the hazards to a group of patients who by nature of their disease must be considered a high surgical risk. The technique suffers fundamentally from being able to supply relatively small volumes of blood to the hemisphere.

Central to the success of the STA-MC anastomosis is the development of the necessary techniques of microvascular surgery. These skills, gained in the laboratory, require a thorough familiarity with the operating microscope, microinstruments and microsuturing techniques. Once mastered, these skills are easily transferred to the operating room ensuring a high incidence of patency of the anastomosis.

Anesthesia

All patients have been operated upon under general endotracheal anesthesia using light doses of Halothane and controlled respiration to maintain pCO_2 values of 35 mm. of mercury and blood pressure in excess of 85 mm. of mercury mean. Blood loss is usually minimal and none of our cases have required transfusion. Preoperatively, care is taken to ensure a normal circulating blood volume and every effort is made to prevent episodes of hypotension during the procedure. Anticoagulants are not used pre- or postoperatively, but all patients have been started on sulfinpyrazone (Anturan, Geigy, Dorval, Quebec, Canada) and acetylsalicylic acid at least 48 hours before the operation and have been maintained on these platelet suppressive agents for at least 3 months.

The Procedure

With the patient supine and head turned to place the temporal region in a horizontal plane, the site of the superficial temporal artery is marked on the skin after clipping of hair and suitable preparation of the scalp with iodine and alcohol. The superficial temporal artery divides approximately 3 cm. above the zygomatic process into an anterior and temporal branch. We have found the anterior branch most suitable for anastomosis in that it usually has a large diameter over a greater length permitting a greater freedom of anastomosis site. Furthermore, the skin and scalp which it normally supplies has a rich collateral blood supply from frontal and periorbital arteries thereby decreasing the chance of ischemic damage to the wound edges.

In our early cases, we followed the example of Yasargil in fashioning a conventional frontotemporal or temporal skin and bone flap, sparing the dissection of the superficial temporal artery until such time as the dura had been exposed. The superficial temporal artery was then dissected from the under surface of the scalp flap. Experience with this technique, however, proved that it added considerable time to the operation and ran some risk of leaving a portion of the skin flap avascular. In our hands, it has been more satisfactory to make a gentle curvilinear incision over the course of the anterior branch of the superficial temporal artery and immediately commence dissection of the artery and its periarterial structures including vena comitantes (Figs. 19.1 and 19.2). This dissection may be aided with magnifying loops or with the operating microscope and is done with a scalpel to avoid picking up or crushing the artery with forceps. The small side branches of the superficial temporal artery are coagulated with the bipolar cautery at least 1 to 2 mm. away from the main stem vessel, again to avoid damage to the main vessel. The larger branches are doubly ligated with 6-0 silk and divided. Dissection is continued until the vessel is entirely freed from its subcutaneous position throughout the length of the incision but is left in continuity both proximally and distally to permit continuous blood flow in the superficial temporal artery. The vessel is then displaced to one side of the skin incision and suitable flaps are fashioned undermining the scalp in the subgaleal layer (Fig. 19.3). Most often, the superficial temporal artery

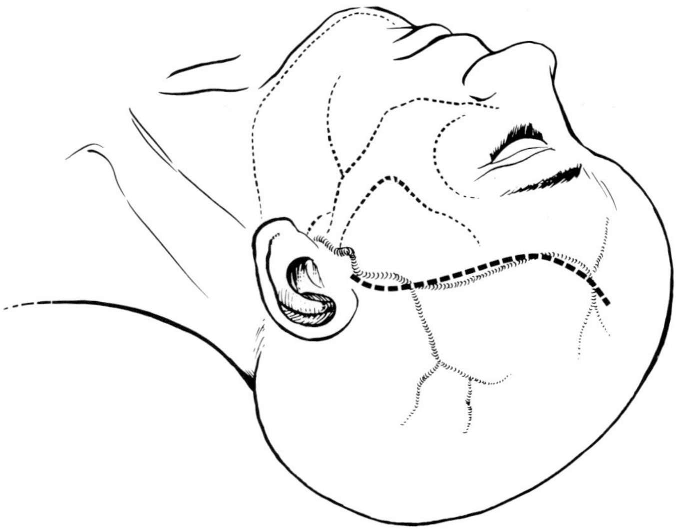

FIG. 19.1. Position of patient and scalp incision to expose the anterior branch of the superficial temporal artery.

will range between 1.0 and 2.0 mm. in diameter. Vessels with diameters greater than 1.5 mm. are relatively easy to suture and have a long term patency rate in excess of 90%. Vessels with diameters less than 1.25 mm. are more difficult to handle, deliver much smaller volumes of blood to the hemisphere, and have a patency rate of about 70%. If the superficial temporal artery is of narrow caliber or branches early resulting in too small a vessel for successful anastomosis, a length of short saphenous vein or cephalic vein of the forearm may be interposed between the external carotid or the main stem superficial temporal artery and the cortical vessel. Short segments of vein graft are more likely to result in long term patency.

The temporalis fascia and underlying temporalis muscle are divided in a cruciate fashion, leaving a narrow cuff of attachment of fascia and muscle on the superior temporal line to facilitate closure. The temporalis muscle is subperiosteally reflected from its attachment in the temporal fossa and then using a 3.5-cm. diameter trephine centered on the Sylvian fissure, a disc of bone is removed and stored in a bacitracin solution (Figs. 19.4 and 19.5). The position of the trephine opening depends upon the length of superficial temporal artery available, the clinical circumstances, and prior knowledge of the accessibility of the cortical branches of the middle cerebral artery.

In a study of 100 human brains at autopsy, the major cortical branches

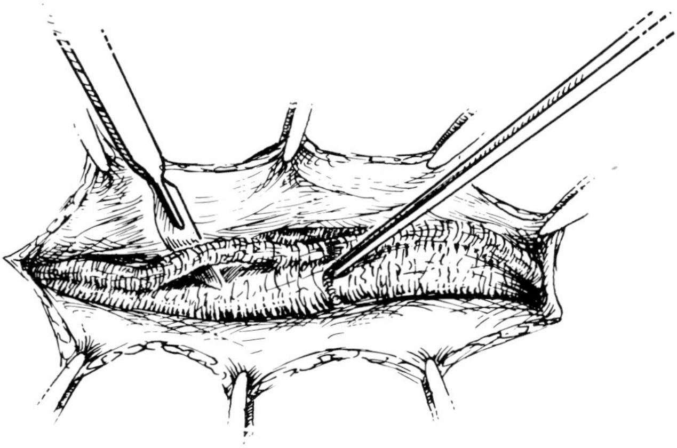

FIG. 19.2. Sharp dissection of superficial temporal artery.

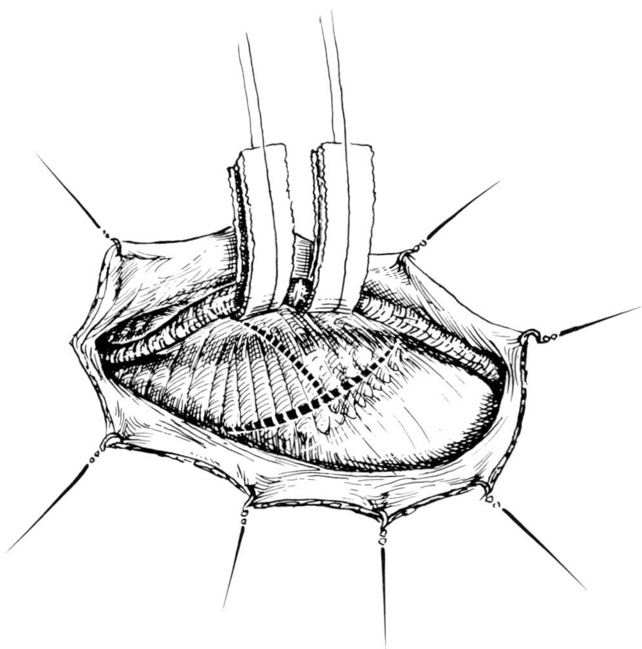

FIG. 19.3. Superficial temporal artery dissected free from the subcutaneous tissue but left in continuity. Dotted line marks incision in temporalis fascia and muscle.

of the middle cerebral artery were exposed by three overlapping trephinations along the Sylvian fissure (Fig. 19.6). In all specimens the angular artery was visible and was the largest of the cortical branches with a mean diameter of 1.3 mm. The second and third largest arteries,

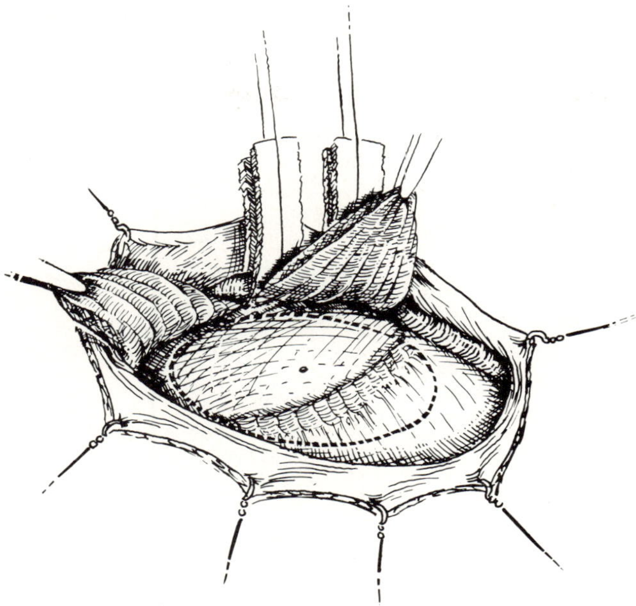

FIG. 19.4. Trephine craniotomy and exposure of Sylvian fissure.

with a mean diameter of 1.2 and 1.1 mm., were the temporal and central sulcus branches respectively and were visible in more than 95 per cent of the specimens. At the anterior end of the fissure, one or more orbitofrontal branches were constantly present and easy to locate but tend to be small with a mean diameter of 0.8 to 1.0 mm. In the specimens studied, the location of the posterior and accessory parietal arteries and the temporal artery was variable and often hidden in sulci. Similarly, the caliber and location of the operculofrontal arteries was not constant (9).

We have attempted, whenever possible, to carry out the anastomosis at a site closest to the area of transient cerebral dysfunction as indicated by clinical or radiological evidence of hypoperfusion. Recognizing that relatively small volumes of blood will be delivered by this technique, it would seem desirable to ensure the perfusion of a limited area of cortex rather than hope to improve flow to the whole middle cerebral territory.

After selecting a suitable cortical artery, the operating microscope is brought into position and using ultrafine forceps and microscissors, the arachnoid and pia surrounding the cortical vessel are meticulously removed. A small square of glove rubber is then fashioned to cover the craniotomy opening and in its center a 2-cm. linear incision is made through which the recipient cortical artery is delivered (Fig. 19.7). This

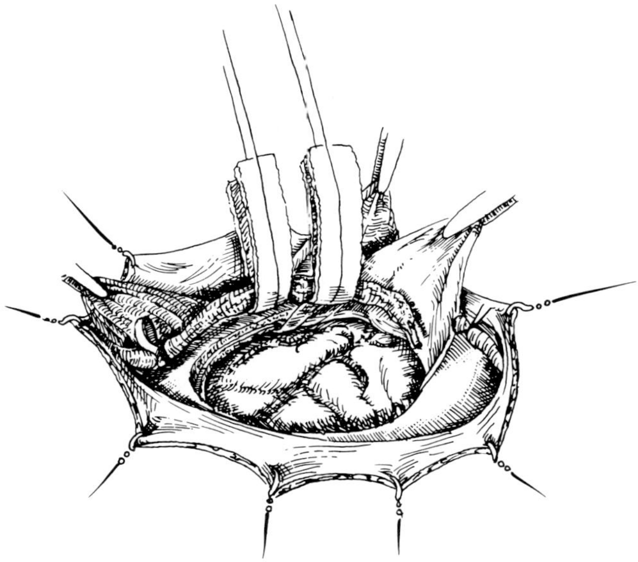

FIG. 19.5. Trephine craniotomy and exposure of Sylvian fissure. Note position of temporary clip on the superficial temporal artery.

rubber dam isolates the vessel while protecting the surrounding surface of the brain.

The superficial temporal artery is clamped across its base by a Kerr-Lougheed clip (Kerr Adjustable Tension Clip, 184 Clark Avenue, Thornhill, Ontario, Canada) designed to close with a tension of 2 gm. The distal end of this vessel is divided at the extremity of the flap and at a point distal to a main branch. Through this side branch, a fine polyethylene catheter (PE 50 polyethylene tubing Intramedic, Clay Adams, Division of Becton, Dickinson & Co., Parsippany, New Jersey 7054) is inserted a short distance into the vessel and secured by a ligature. The polyethylene catheter is attached to a 50-ml. syringe containing heparin and saline (10,000 units in 50 ml.). This arrangement permits flushing of the artery of contained blood and continuous gentle irrigation of the vessel and the anastomosis site during the period that it is occluded.

Under 12 to 20 magnification, the distal 2 cm. of the superficial temporal artery is carefully prepared by removing all the surrounding adventitial tissue down to the outermost layers of the media. This very important step is necessary to discard the highly thrombogenic adventitial tissue which would otherwise be caught up in the suture material and carried into the lumen, and thereby greatly increasing the chance of early thrombosis and obliteration of the anastomosis. Great care is taken during the preparation of the end of the superficial temporal artery not to squeeze or damage the media or intima with forceps. The vessel should be secured and manipulated by handling the periadvential tissue at some distance from the site of anastomosis.

Attention should then be directed back to the cortical artery which may be clamped with two small Kleinert-Kutz microclamps (Weck Surgical Company, Division of E.R. Squibb & Sons Ltd., 39 Klondike Drive, Weston, Ontario) separated by about 1 cm. With the cortical vessel occluded, a small 1.2-mm. elipse is removed from the wall of the cortical vessel using curved microscissors. Although a linear arteriotomy may be used to open the cortical vessel, it has proven to be more satisfactory to remove a tiny elipse which aids visualization of the lips of the arteriotomy and facilitates suturing during the anastomosis. We usually do not divide any of the small side branches of the cortical vessel and with the clamps in place, there is a small amount of bleeding. This has proved useful in that it allows one to easily visualize the lumen of the cortical vessel. The small amount of bleeding is not a problem when continually irrigated with heparin saline. Furthermore, by sparing the numerous small branches, the potential run off at the site of anastomosis is improved.

The end of the superficial temporal artery is trimmed obliquely. Using

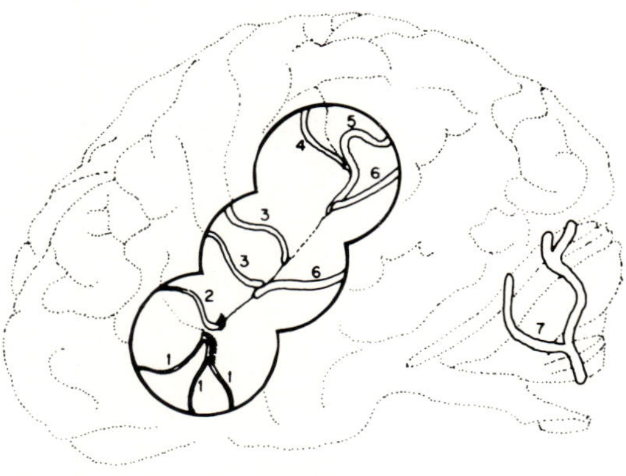

1 ORBITOFRONTAL A
2 OPERCULOFRONTAL A
3 CENTRAL SULCUS A
4 POSTERIOR & ACCES. PARIETAL A
5 ANGULAR A
6 TEMPORAL A
7 PICA

FIG. 19.6. Diagram of the surface anatomy of the major cortical branches of the middle cerebral artery and the posterior inferior cerebellar artery.

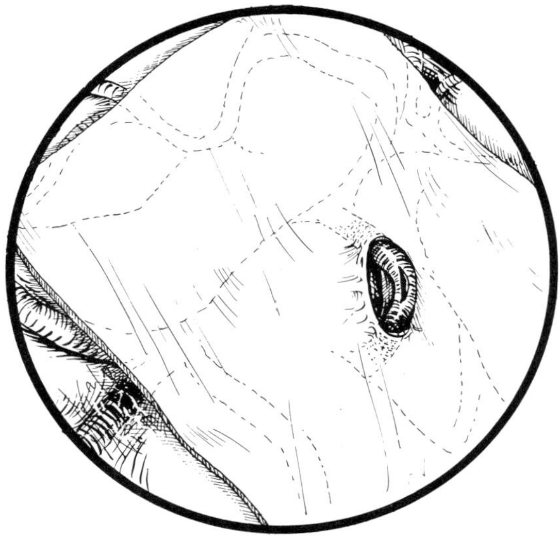

FIG. 19.7. Cortical branch of the middle cerebral artery exposed through a slit in a rubber dam. Elipitical longitudinal arteriotomy is visible.

10-0 monofilament nylon, anchoring sutures are placed through the superficial temporal artery and tied to the ends of the arteriotomy aligning the vessels to favor anterograde or retrograde flow as seems appropriate to the clinical circumstances. The anastomosis is then completed with 9 to 14 interrupted 10-0 nylon sutures approximating first the back and then the front wall. The needle is always passed first through the superficial temporal artery; the edges of both vessels must be gently supported as the suture is drawn through. The microsuture is facilitated by leaving the superficial temporal artery somewhat long so it can be turned from one side to the other allowing easy access to both the front and back walls of the anastomosis. With a little experience, the clamp time on the cortical artery averages between 20 to 40 minutes. With the last suture tied, a few small pledglets of Gelfoam are gently packed around the anastomosis and the clamps on the cortical artery released. After a few minutes, the clamp on the proximal superficial temporal artery is released to establish flow. After packing the area of anastomosis with cottonoid patties, the superficial temporal artery is carefully inspected and oozing from small branches on the graft vessel is stopped with bipolar coagulation (Fig. 19.8).

When complete hemostasis has been affected, the graft site is re-examined and the cottonoid, Gelfoam pledgets, and rubber dam removed. The dura is closed with interrupted 4-0 silk, leaving a small gap for the entering superficial temporal artery, and the bone disc is replaced again after cutting a notch on one side to allow the superficial temporal artery to enter the skull (Fig. 19.9). We have usually fixed the bone plug in this position with two or three stainless steel wires. The temporalis fascia and muscle are repaired followed by the skin and scalp in the usual fashion.

With slight variation of the technique, the occipital artery may be joined to a branch of the middle cerebral artery, or the occipital artery may be joined with relative ease to the large primary branches of the posterior inferior cerebellar artery on the lateral surface of the cerebellar hemisphere. On occasion, both major branches of the superficial temporal artery may be anastomosed to separate cortical vessels. However, we have considered it more desirable to establish a high volume of flow through a single artery rather than a smaller volume through two branches of the artery. Surgical anastomosis between the superficial temporal and middle cerebral arteries is most likely to succeed where the diameters of the vessels joined are greater than 1.5 mm. and there is a significant pressure differential between the external carotid and intracranial circulation. Long term patency of more than 90% can be expected in these instances with progressive enlargement of the bypass with time. Moreover, we have experienced no operative mortality and no significant morbidity in our series of 50 cases.

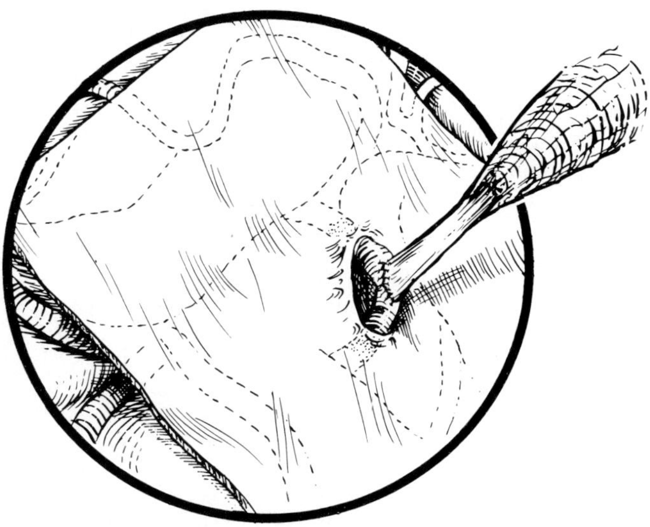

FIG. 19.8. Completed STA-MC anastomosis. Note the adventitia has been entirely removed from the distal end of the superficial temporal artery.

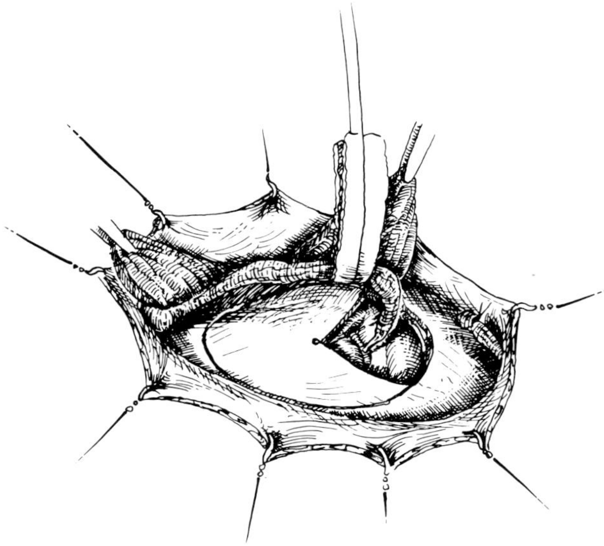

FIG. 19.9. Completed anastomosis. Trephine flap repositioned.

Although clear indications and the value of cerebral revascularization procedures are yet to be established, it is clear that the surgical techniques are now available to provide additional collateral blood flow to the brain. Whether these procedures will improve the natural history of individuals suffering from cerebral obliterative vascular disease remains to be seen, but the present results appear promising.

REFERENCES

1. Chou, S. N. Embolectomy of middle cerebral artery. Report of a case. J. Neurosurg., *20:* 161–163, 1963.
2. Donaghy, R. M. P. Neurologic surgery. Surg. Gynecol. Obstet., *134:* 269–271, 1972.
3. Driesen, E. Erfolgreiche Naht der linken A. cerebri media nach Verletzung bei Tumorresektion. Acta Neurochir., *10:* 462–465, 1962.
4. Henschen, C. Operative Revascularization des zirkulatorisch geschadigten Gehirns durch auflage gestielter Muskellappen (Encephalo-Myo-Synangiose). Langenbecks Arch. Chir., *264:* 392–401, 1950.
5. Jacobson, J. H., II, and Suarez, E. L. Microsurgery in the anastomosis of small vessels. Surg. Forum, *11:* 243–245, 1960.
6. Jacobson, J. H., II, Wallamn, L. J., Schumacher, G. A., Flanagan, M., Suarez, E. L., and Donaghy, R. M. P. Microsurgery as an aid to middle cerebral endarterectomy. J. Neurosurg., *19:* 108–115, 1962.
7. Lougheed, W. M., Gunton, R. W., and Barnett, H. J. M. Embolectomy of internal carotid, middle and anterior cerebral arteries. Report of a case. J. Neurosurg., *22:* 607–609, 1965.
8. Lougheed, W. M., Marshall, B. M., Hunter, M., Michel, E. R., and Sandwith-Smyth,

H. Common carotid to intracranial internal carotid bypass venous graft. Technical note. J. Neurosurg., *34:* 114–118, 1971.

9. Peerless, S. J., and Clayman, J. Surface anatomy of the cortical branches of the middle cerebral artery. In press.
10. Shillito, J., Jr. Indications for surgery in cerebrovascular accidents. Postgrad. Med., *30:* 537–544, 1961.
11. Welch, K. Excision of occlusive lesions of the middle cerebral artery. J. Neurosurg., *13:* 73–80, 1956.
12. Woringer, E. and Kunlin, J. Anastomose entre la carotide primitive et la carotide intra-cranienne ou la sylvienne par greffon selon la technique de la suture suspendue. Neurochirurgie, *9:* 181–188, 1963.
13. Yasargil, M. G. Experimental small vessel surgery in the dog including patching and grafting of cerebral vessels and the formation of functional extra-intracranial shunts. *In* Micro-Vascular Surgery, edited by R. M. P. Donaghy and M. G. Yasargil, pp. 87–126, Mosby, St. Louis, 1967.
14. Yasargil, M. G., Krayenbuhl, H. A., and Jacobson, J. H., II. Microneurosurgical arterial reconstruction. Surgery, *67:* 221–233, 1970.

CHAPTER

20

Blood Flow and Cerebral Revascularization*

PETER SCHMIEDEK, M.D., OTMAR GRATZL, M.D., HARALD STEINHOFF, M.D., VLADIMIR OLTNEANU-NERBE, M.D., AND FRANK MARGUTH, M.D.

Microvascular extraintracranial arterial bypass surgery has established itself as a new approach in the treatment of ischemic cerebrovascular disease. The principle of this procedure is to increase collateral circulation to the ischemic brain (13). Patency rates of approximately 90% have established the technical feasibility of this procedure (1–3, 8). The problem, however, is in selecting those (patients with cerebrovascular disease) that may benefit from surgery and in evaluating the postoperative results. For this purpose, we have employed regional cerebral blood flow (rCBF) measurements over the last 6 years (10–12), the results of which we are presenting.

METHODS

Regional cerebral blood flow was measured using the intra-arterial xenon-133 injection method (4, 6) (Fig. 20.1). The procedure was carried out in the following way: under local anesthesia the common carotid artery was punctured and a small catheter inserted into the internal carotid artery. Correct placement of the catheter was verified by injection of 5 ml. of saline resulting in a pale area corresponding to the supraorbital branch of the internal carotid artery. Then 3 mCi of xenon-133 dissolved in 5 ml. of saline were rapidly injected and the uptake and subsequent clearance of the isotope recorded over the hemisphere. The gamma activity clearance rates were monitored with 16 small collimated sodium iodide scintillation detectors. These data were then stored on magnetic tape and thereafter semilogarithmically displayed on a chart recorder. CBF was calculated by the initial slope index (ISI) method (7). This analytical method requires only a 2-minute period of data collection. A value of 50 ml/100 gm./min., plus or minus 10%, was considered as normal flow. In most patients the CO_2 response was measured by repeating rCBF studies during inhalation of an 8% CO_2-air mixture or hyperventilation. In selected cases autoregula-

* Supported in part by DFG-Sonderforschungsbereich 51: Medizinische Molekularbiologie und Biochemie.

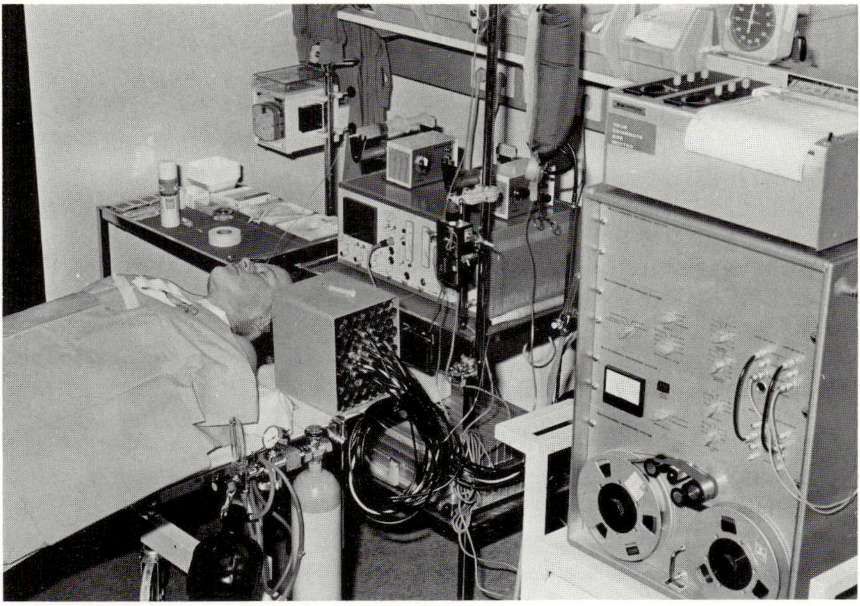

FIG. 20.1. General view of the CBF laboratory. The left hemisphere of the patient is being studied by 16 detectors arranged in a 'honeycomb'-holder. To the right is seen the multichannel analyzer with a chart recorder on top. In the background there is a monitoring unit for visual display of the EKG and measurement of arterial blood pressure.

tion of CBF was tested by elevating the systemic blood pressure with intravenous injection of angiotensin. All rCBF measurements included monitoring of the blood pressure and arterial pCO_2. At the end of the study which usually lasted 60 to 80 minutes, the position of three detectors in relation to the lateral aspect of the hemisphere was marked with small pieces of lead for exact localization of the counting fields on a lateral skull x-ray. When indicated, the patient then underwent serial cerebral angiography using the same catheter. Minor variations of the above described method were used in the following situations. In patients with unilateral internal carotid artery occlusion, rCBF was usually measured over both hemispheres provided a well functioning interhemispheric collateral flow was present *via* the circle of Willis. For postoperative rCBF studies, the external carotid artery was alternatively injected, allowing the isotope to reach the brain by way of the extraintracranial anastomosis.

MATERIAL

This series comprises 173 patients; 129 male and 44 female. The age ranged from 18 to 73 years, averaging 52 years. All patients were admitted with symptoms of cerebrovascular disease and were considered as potential candidates for extraintracranial bypass surgery. The indication for the procedure was then made on the basis of general physical, laboratory, and neurological examinations as well as cerebral angiography and rCBF studies. Our more recent patients also underwent radioisotope arteriography with intravenous ^{99m}Tc-sodium pertechnetate and axial computerized tomography (CT). Out of the 173 patients studied, 88 underwent bypass surgery. In 3 patients a bilateral bypass operation was performed. In the nonoperated group of 85 patients, there are 91 CBF studies, whereas 162 studies are available from the surgical group. In 65 patients rCBF measurements were carried out preoperatively, in 44 patients postoperatively, and in 15 patients two postoperative measurements were obtained (Table 20.1).

PREOPERATIVE rCBF MEASUREMENTS

The following classification has emerged from the analysis of preoperative rCBF measurements in 146 patients (Table 20.2 and Fig. 20.2). Seventeen patients had a severe general reduction of CBF with a mean hemispheric flow of less than 60% of normal. Moderate general reduction of flow was present in 13 patients and is defined as a CBF of 60 to 80% of normal. In the largest group, including 44 patients, a flow pattern was found for which we have introduced the term relative focal ischemia. Characteristically, in these patients, in addition to a moderately reduced mean hemispheric blood flow, a focal area of ischemia was also present. In the next group of 24 patients, only focal ischemia was present. In these two groups, the focal impairment of CBF was exacerbated by repeating

TABLE 20.1
rCBF Studies in 88 Patients with Extra-intracranial Bypass

Preoperative	65
Postoperative	44
Pre- and postoperative	38
Follow-up	15

TABLE 20.2
Results of Preoperative rCBF Studies in 65 Patients

Severe general reduction	4
Moderate general reduction	4
Relative focal reduction	35
Focal reduction	22
Acute disorders	0
Normal	0

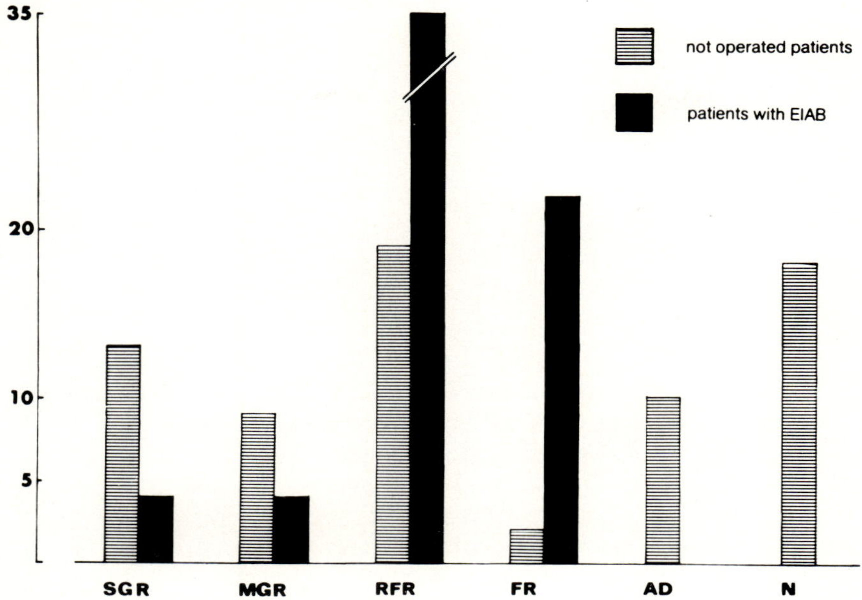

FIG. 20.2 The results of 146 initial rCBF studies were divided into 6 groups: severe general reduction of CBF (SGR), moderate general reduction of CBF (MGR), relative focal reduction of CBF (RFR), focal reduction of CBF (FR), acute disorders of CBF (AD), normal CBF (N). In the majority of the operated cases (black columns-EIAB), CBF findings were either consistent with a relative focal reduction or a focal reduction of CBF alone.

the study during CO_2 inhalation. The next group includes 10 patients with acute disorders of the CBF, such as loss of autoregulation, relative hyperemia, or paradoxical flow reactions in response to changes of the arterial pCO_2, reflecting a functional derangement of the cerebral vasoregulation and thereby indicating acute damage to the nervous tissue. This type of CBF can be seen in patients studied only a few days following onset of acute cerebral ischemia (5). Finally, in 18 patients, normal CBF was found, despite the fact that symptoms of cerebrovascular ischemia were present.

We have attempted to use this classification of rCBF results in establishing the indication for microneurosurgery. The predictive value of rCBF measurements was established through the analysis of the clinical results and the pre- and postoperative flow studies in our initial 30 cases. From this analysis, two groups of patients have emerged which we no longer consider for operation. These are the patients having either normal or a severe general reduction of CBF. That the operation is contraindicated in patients with a severely reduced CBF is based on our experience that there is a high occlusion rate in these cases. Furthermore, these patients commonly present with diffuse neurological deficit of long standing related to arteriosclerotic brain disease. Hence, their low CBF reflects primarily a lowered metabolic demand of the entire hemisphere as opposed to inadequate collateral blood supply. Patients with a moderate reduction of CBF are not optimal candidates for a bypass procedure and additional criteria, based on angiographic findings, clinical symptoms, and the age of the patient, are used to determine selection for surgical candidates. In patients belonging to the group with acute CBF disturbances, we recommend repeat CBF measurement at a later date. In our own early material, we operated on three patients only hours following an acute cerebrovascular accident. As all three patients died during the early postoperative period from intractable brain swelling, as ascertained at autopsy, we no longer operate on patients during the acute phase of a cerebral infarct. The most satisfying results were obtained in the two CBF groups with either relative ischemia or focal ischemia alone (Fig. 20.3). As the effect of the surgical anastomosis is regional, it follows then that only a regional impairment of CBF such as focal or relative focal cerebral ischemia can be adequately corrected. In order to illustrate the usefulness of CBF measurements for selecting surgical candidates, two representative case reports are presented.

Case 1. This 29-year-old woman was admitted to the Department of Neurosurgery 9 months following an acute cerebrovascular accident resulting in a right hemiplegia and aphasia. Cerebral angiography performed at that time disclosed occlusion of the left middle cerebral artery. During the following months there was gradual improvement of her neurological symptoms. On her present admission, the neurological examination revealed a hemiparesis of the right side and minor speech disturbances. Following our present program for evaluating potential candidates for a microneurosurgical bypass procedure, the patient first underwent radionucleotide arteriography. A normal perfusion of the brain was reported from this study. Measurement of regional cerebral blood flow and cerebral angiography were then performed using the same catheter. The CBF study revealed very slightly reduced flow values over an area corresponding to the territory of the middle cerebral artery, but still within normal range (Fig. 20.4A). The angiogram was within normal limits (Fig. 20.4B). Computerized x-ray scanning of the brain showed a large infarction on the left side with extensive involvement of the region normally supplied by the middle cerebral artery (Fig. 20.4C). As the patient had a normal rCBF study, it was decided not to operate.

Case 2. Two years prior to admission, this 38-year-old woman had an acute right-sided hemiparesis with expressive aphasia due to an occlusion of the middle cerebral artery on the left as proven by angiography. Her subsequent recovery was incomplete, but she was able to work in an office until an intermittent deterioration of the hemiparesis had occurred. On admission, she presented with neurological deficits of the right side consistent with a completed stroke of a moderate degree. The perfusion brain scan was normal. The left carotid angiogram showed a complete occlusion of the middle cerebral artery (Fig. 20.5A). There was also extensive collateral flow to the distal middle cerebral area *via* leptomeningeal anastomoses. The blood flow study revealed only insignificantly reduced flow values over the central region with an otherwise normal CBF (Fig. 20.5B). Computerized tomography disclosed a small area of low density localized within the deep

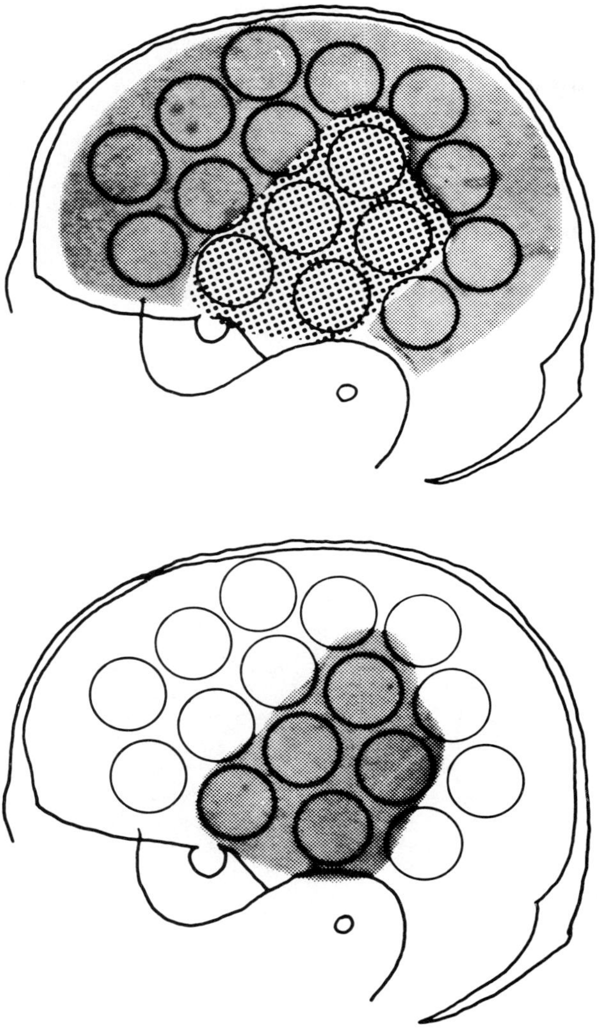

FIG. 20.3. Schematic presentation of preoperative rCBF pattern most likely to benefit from microvascular bypass surgery, above: relative focal ischemia; below: focal ischemia.

structures of the left hemisphere (Fig. 20.5C). Despite the rCBF results which indicated that the patient was not a candidate, she nevertheless underwent extraintracranial bypass surgery. This decision was based on the patient's age and on family pressure. Postoperative external carotid angiography failed to show any signs of a functioning bypass. When the patient was discharged from the hospital, her neurological status was unchanged.

These examples were chosen to emphasize the difficulty in the clinical selection of surgical candidates. In spite of the fact that the angiogram

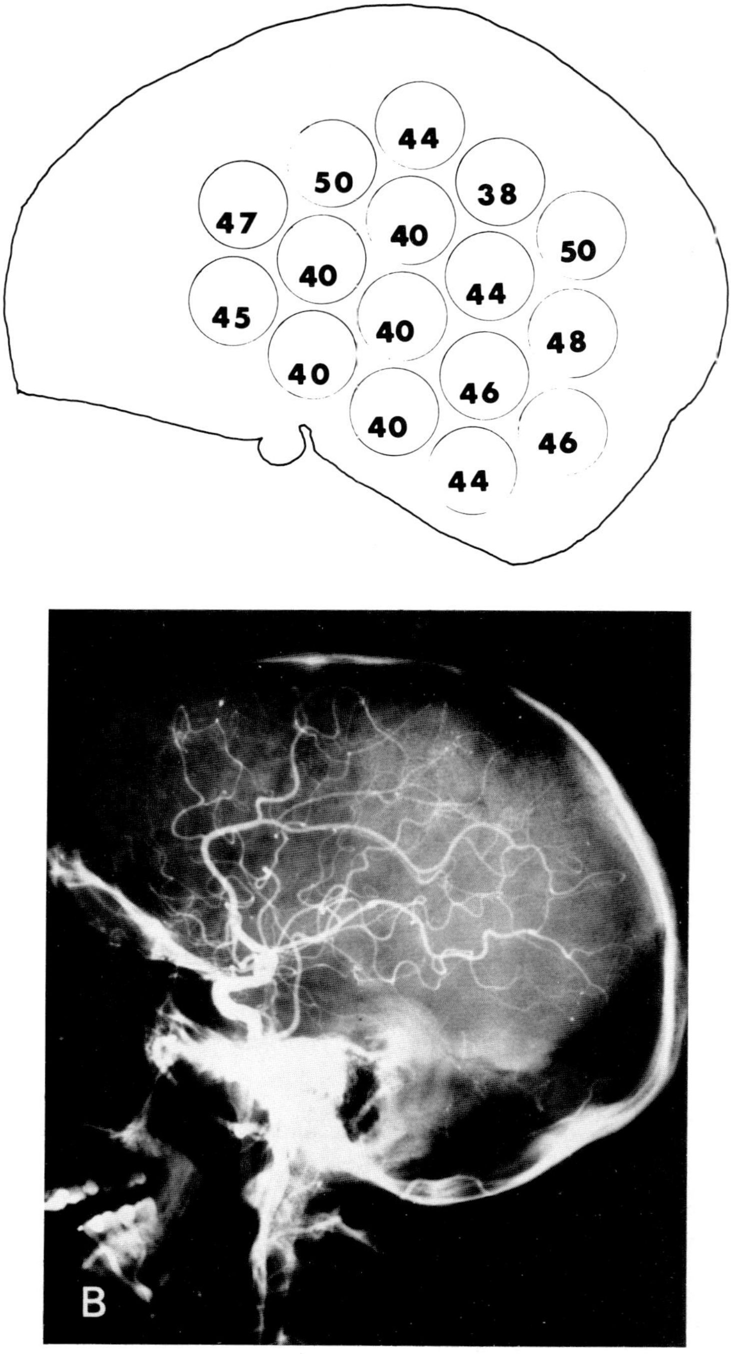

FIG. 20.4 (A–B) Case 1. See text.

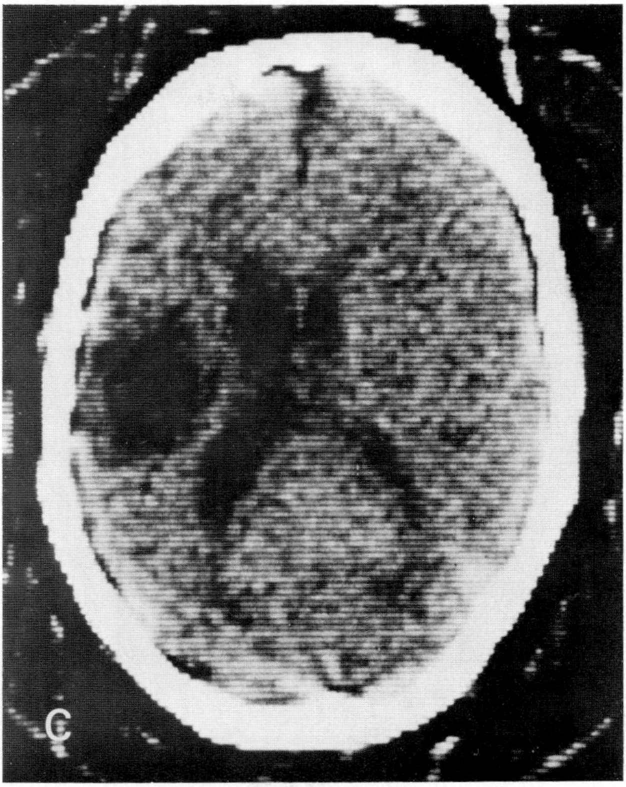

FIG. 20.4 (C) Case 1. See text.

and the CT varied markedly in these two cases, the rCBF results were almost identical. Although the discrepancy of the CT scan and the CBF measurements appear contradictory, the explanation is quite simple. The CT scan illustrates the change in density that occurs with infarction, whereas the CBF measurements only reflect cortical blood flow of perfused tissue. Thus the CBF measurements reveal areas of reduced perfusion but give no data on areas of absent perfusion as in the first case with a severe infarction. This again illustrates the usefulness of the CBF technique as it differentiates with the aid of the CT scan, an infarct which is complete and will not benefit from surgery from an infarct associated with an area of decreased perfusion which may, in fact, benefit from surgery. In the second case the CT scan revealed a small infarct in the deep structures of the brain, again with normal CBF measurements. Despite the angiographic findings of a complete occlusion of the middle cerebral artery, the CBF study indicated that the patient had sufficient collateral blood supply making an anastomosis superfluous. This was evidenced by the failure of the anastomosis, probably due to an insufficient pressure gradient between the two vessels. This resulted in insufficient flow at the site of the anastomosis leading to subsequent occlusion.

It should be emphasized, however, that the rCBF study is not performed unless there is sufficient evidence from other diagnostic procedures being suggestive for surgery (Fig. 20.6). We have performed a total of 365 CBF studies. Two of our early cases had transient neurological deficits following the examination. Although the procedure appears safe and is warranted in evaluating a potential surgical candidate, it is not feasible as a screening test because of the potential risk to the patient associated with the need for a carotid puncture.

We tried to correlate CBF findings with clinical data but we found no consistency. We also correlated rCBF data with angiography with the same disappointing results. Although it is too early to speculate on the value of computerized tomography in the selection of appropriate

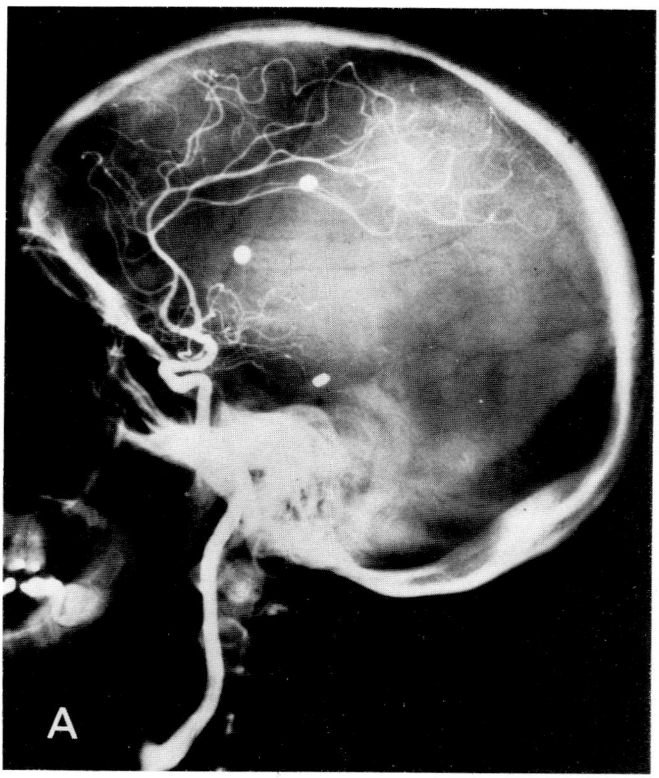

FIG. 20.5 (A) Case 2. See text.

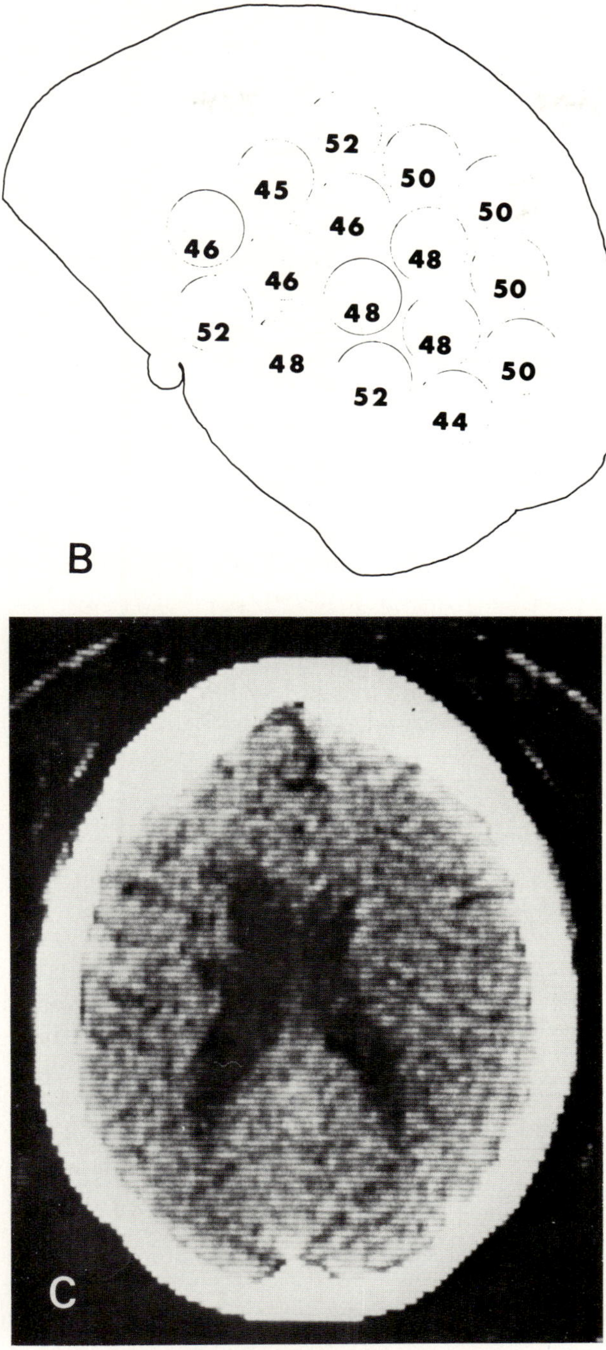

FIG. 20.5 (B–C) Case 2. See text.

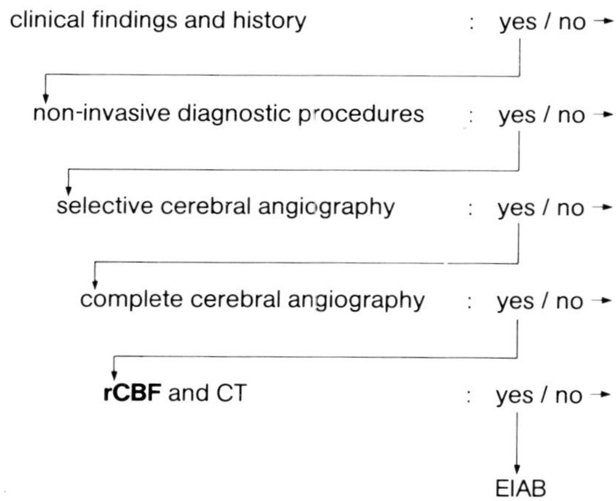

FIG. 20.6. Schematic presentation of the sequence-diagnostic procedures are employed in order to establish the indication for extra-intracranial bypass surgery (EIAB).

candidates for a microvascular procedure, it has greatly aided in explaining a patient's clinical presentation despite normal rCBF findings.

Measurement of rCBF in the preoperative situation, however, is not only useful for the selection of patients but it is, moreover, helpful in planning the surgical procedure (Fig. 20.7A and 20.7B). It is possible with this method to detect and localize the low perfusion area within the cerebral cortex thus providing a more anatomical placement of the extracranial vessel (9).

POSTOPERATIVE rCBF MEASUREMENTS

Our postoperative rCBF measurements show that in patients selected by the above outlined criteria a microvascular anastomosis will result in a measurable increase of rCBF. (Table 20.3). At present, 44 out of a total of 88 operated cases have undergone postoperative rCBF measurements. In 22 patients the external carotid artery was used for flow studies. In two of these cases, the bypass did not function postoperatively. Following injection of xenon-133 into the external carotid artery in these patients, no radioactivity could be detected over parts of the scalp normally supplied by the superficial temporal artery. Over the temporal region, however, values in the range of 15 to 20 ml./100gm./min. were obtained, suggesting clearance from extracerebral tissue. Both patients had a severe generally decreased CBF on their preoperative rCBF studies. Both of them were done early in our study, neither patient would be a surgical candidate with our present criteria. In the other 20 patients, the function of the anastomosis was clearly established (Fig. 20.8A, 20.8B, and 20.8C). The CO_2 inhalation test was routinely used in all postoperative

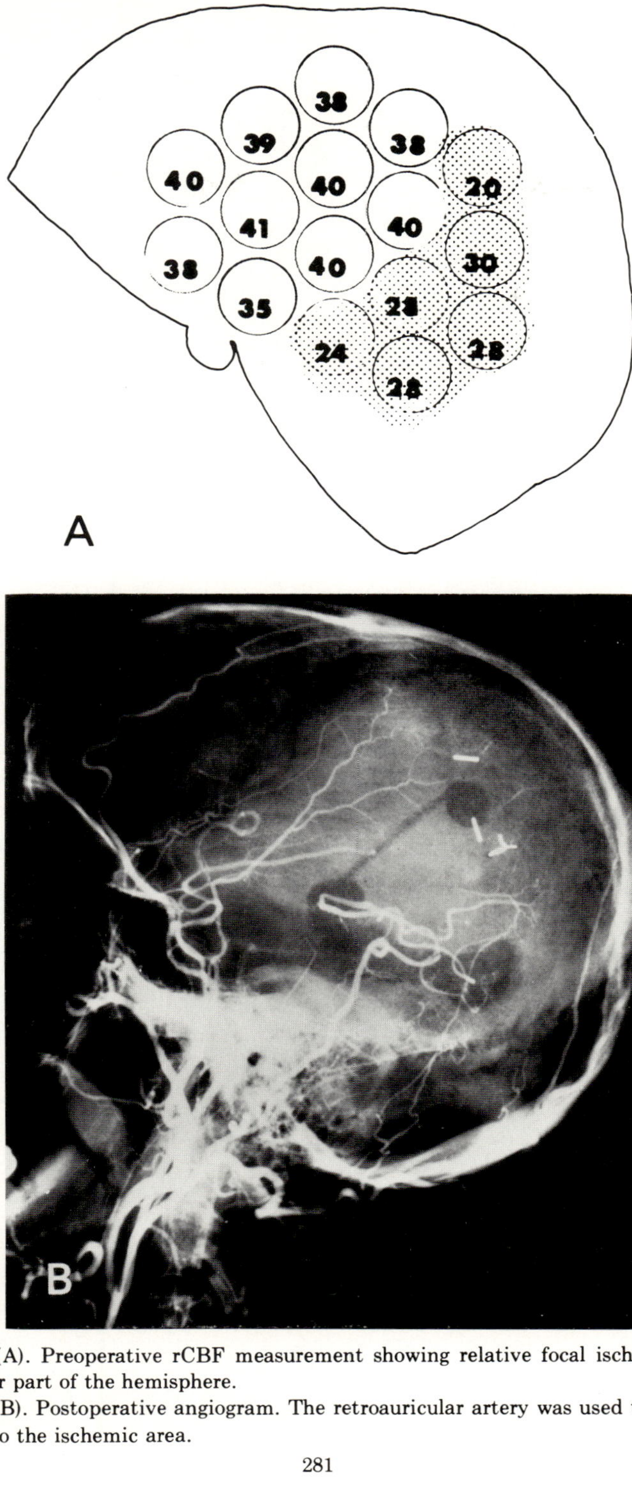

FIG. 20.7(A). Preoperative rCBF measurement showing relative focal ischemia within the posterior part of the hemisphere.

FIG. 20.7(B). Postoperative angiogram. The retroauricular artery was used to direct the blood flow to the ischemic area.

TABLE 20.3
Results of Postoperative rCBF Studies in 44 Patients

No function of bypass	2
(Secondary occlusion	3)
Function of bypass established	20
Improvement of rCBF	22
Within small area	8
Within extended area	14

studies as an additional measure for evaluation of bypass function. During hypercarbia, blood flow in the extracerebral compartment remained constant or revealed only a very slight increase whereas in the intracerebral compartment, there was a significant increase in flow. This established the cerebrospecific flow response to an elevated arterial pCO_2.

In 22 patients the internal carotid artery was used for injection of the isotope. In all cases cerebral hemodynamics were restored. In 8 patients postoperative, rCBF study disclosed a relatively small area—including not more than 3 counting fields—with an improved blood supply as compared with the preoperative rCBF measurement. In 14 patients the microvascular bypass increased blood flow over an extended area, that is, over more than three adjacent detector fields. Only flow changes exceeding 15% were considered a significant improvement of CBF. Further evidence of a postoperative improvement of the previous ischemic cerebral circulation was derived from a comparatively higher increase of rCBF values during CO_2 inhalation.

We have now stopped doing rCBF measurements as a routine in the early postoperative period as selective external carotid angiography has revealed good correlation with postoperative rCBF results (Fig. 20.9). The practical reason for not performing postoperative rCBF studies in all patients is that we are too busy now with preoperative rCBF studies, doing at least two patients every week. Furthermore, we are more interested in continuing late postoperative CBF follow-up studies in order to assess the lasting effect of the anastomosis. So far the rCBF measurements have been repeated in 15 patients on a late follow-up basis. The time interval between the two postoperative studies has varied from 2 to 28 months with an average of 11 months. A secondary occlusion of the bypass was found in 3 patients in whom the early postoperative study had shown a function of the bypass. Preoperatively, two of these patients had a severely reduced blood flow of the entire hemisphere under study, while the third case had only very slight focal

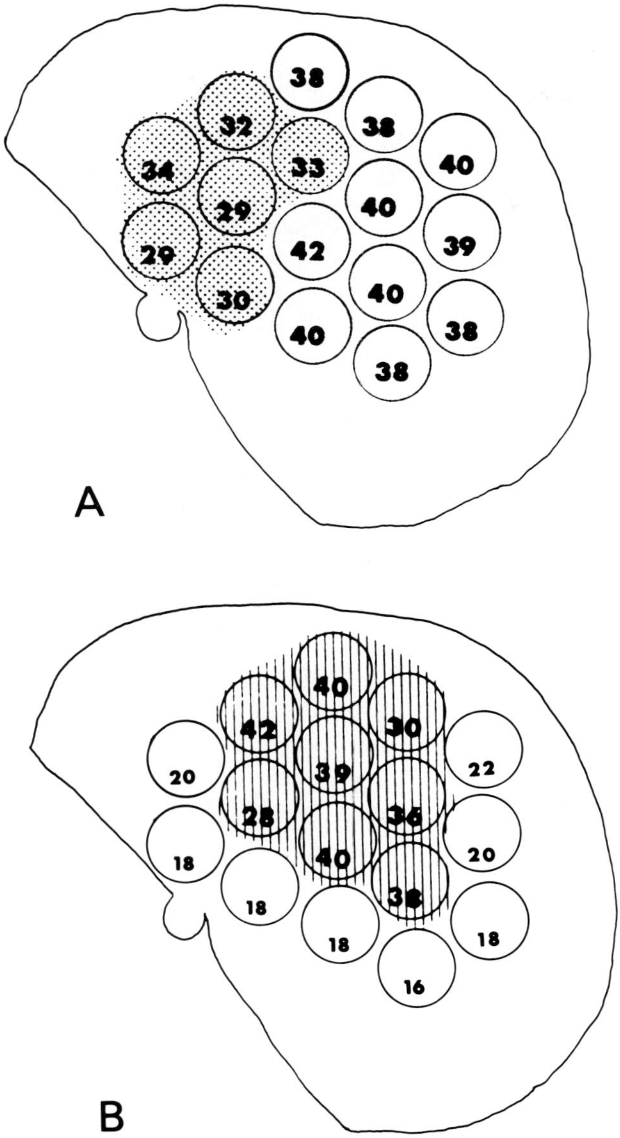

FIG. 20.8(A). Preoperative rCBF study in a patient with relative focal ischemia over the left central region of the brain.

FIG. 20.8(B). External carotid rCBF study performed 8 days postoperatively. High flow values are seen over the central area indicating a good function of the bypass. The lower values within the surrounding counting fields represent clearance from extracranial tissue.

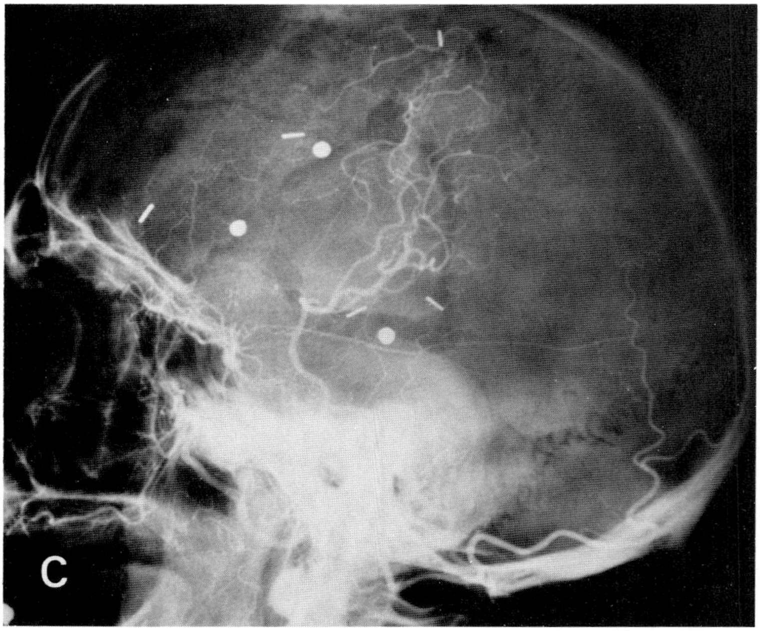

FIG. 20.8(C). External carotid angiography demonstrating an excellent functional result of the anastomosis.

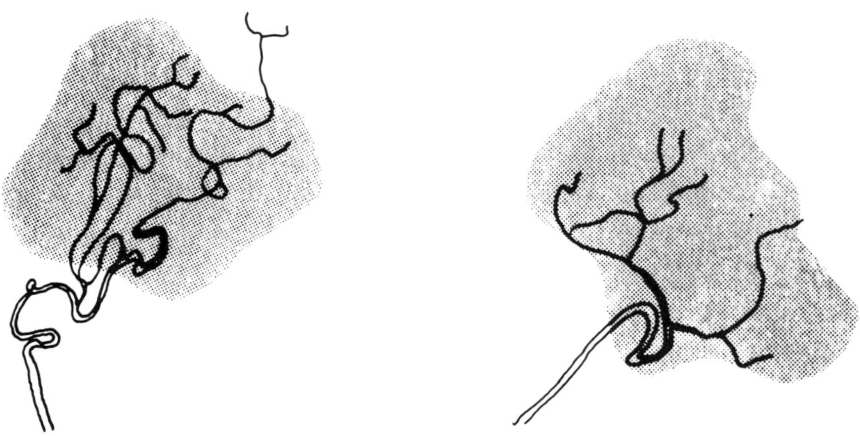

FIG. 20.9 Composite presentation showing the correlation of postoperative rCBF measurement with the angiographic appearance of the new bypass on a lateral view. On the right, there are 4 counting areas (dotted) with an increased CBF; on the left, CBF improved within 5 counting areas.

disturbances of his rCBF. Again, none of these patients would be a surgical candidate with our present criteria. In six patients, the two postoperative measurements revealed virtually identical results. In the remaining six patients, further improvement of CBF could be demonstrated. In these patients there was also a significant increase in size of the anastomosis as demonstrated by angiography.

From these follow-up studies we have learned that it takes considerable time before the collateral effect of the bypass can be established with certainty. Therefore, the final assessment of the operative result should await at least a 3-month period following the operation. The possibility of a secondary occlusion of the anastomosis should be taken into consideration, a result that can be missed when reference is made only to an early postoperative study, as well as the finding of a subsequent increase of rCBF as demonstrated in six of our patients.

In summary, the rCBF measurements offer another tool in evaluating potential surgical candidates. It by no means replaces any of the other studies now commonly employed, but with guarded optimism, I believe it provides scientific criteria for patient selection by which improvement of postoperative results can be achieved.

REFERENCES

1. Austin, G., Laffin, D., and Hayward, W. Microcerebral anastomosis for the prevention of strokes. *In* Microneurosurgery, edited by H. Handa, pp. 47–67. Igaku Shoin Ltd. Tokyo, 1975.
2. Chater, N. Neurosurgical microvascular bypass for stroke—current status. Presented at the Fifth Annual Neurosurgical Postgraduate Course, University California Medical Center, San Francisco, May, 1975.
3. Gratzl, O., Schmiedek, P., Spetzler, R., Steinhoff, H., and Marguth, F. Clinical experience with extra-intracranial arterial anastomoses in 65 cases. J. Neurosurg., *44:* 313–324, 1976.
4. Høedt-Rasmussen, K. Regional cerebral blood flow. The intra-arterial injection method. Acta Neurol. Scand. (Suppl.), *43:* 1–81, 1967.
5. Ingvar, D. H., Regional cerebral blood flow in cerebrovascular disorders. Prog. Brain Res., *30:* 57–61, 1968.
6. Lassen, N. A., Høedt-Rasmussen, K., and Sorensen, S. C. Regional cerebral blood flow in man determined by krypton. Neurology (Minneap.), 13: 719–727, 1963.
7. Olesen, J., Paulson, O. B., and Lassen, N. A. Regional cerebral blood flow in man determined by the initial slope of the clearance of intra-arterially injected 133-Xe. Stroke, *2:* 519–540, 1971.
8. Reichman, O. H., Anderson, R. E., Roberts, T. S., and Heilbrum, M. P. The treatment of intracranial occlusive cerebrovascular disease by STA-cortical MCA anastomosis. *In* Microneurosurgery, edited by H. Handa, pp. 31–46. Igaku Shoin Ltd. Tokyo, 1975.
9. Spetzler, R., and Chater, N. Occipital artery-middle cerebral artery anastomosis for cerebral artery occlusive disease. Surg. Neurol., *2:* 235–238, 1974.
10. Schmiedek, P., Steinhoff, H., Gratzl, O. Steude, U., and Enzenbach, R., rCBF

measurement in patients treated for cerebral ischemia by extra-intracranial vascular anastomosis. Eur. Neurol. *6:* 364–368, 1971/72.

11. Schmiedek, P., Gratzl, O., Steinhoff, H., Steude, U., Baethmann, A., and Enzenbach, R. Microvascular surgery of the brain and regional cerebral blood flow. *In* Cerebral Circulation and Metabolism, edted by T. W. Langfitt, L. C. McHenry, Jr., M. Reivich, and H. Wollman, pp 285–288, Springer, New York—Berlin, 1975.
12. Schmiedek, P., Gratzl, O., Spetzler, R., Steinhoff H., Enzenbach, R., Brendel, W., and Marguth, F., Selection of patients for extra-intracranial arterial bypass surgery based on regional cerebral blood flow measurements. J. Neurosurg., *44:* 303–312, 1976.
13. Yasargil, M. G., Krayenbühl, H. A., and Jacobsen, J. H., Microneurosurgical arterial reconstruction. Surgery, *67:* 221–233, 1970.

CHAPTER

21

Patient Selection and Results of Extra to Intracranial Anastomosis in Selected Cases of Cerebrovascular Disease

NORMAN CHATER, M.D.

INTRODUCTION

More than 2 decades have passed since C. Miller Fisher suggested that surgeons investigate the possibility of extra to intracranial anastomosis in problems of occlusive cerebrovascular disease (27). The concept of surgical collateral augmentation was proposed again by Wolff at the Princeton Conference on Cerebrovascular Disease in 1961.

Yasargil and Donaghy performed the initial experimental studies in 1967, establishing the feasibility of an arterial bypass from scalp to brain vessels in dogs (71). This surgical approach was then applied clinically to two patients for the first time by Yasargil and Donaghy 8 years ago; it involved the microsurgical anastomosis of the superficial temporal artery, a branch of the external carotid artery, to a cortical branch of the middle cerebral artery on the surface of the brain (19, 70, 72).

In the past several years a number of papers have described the indications for and preliminary results of such a neurosurgical microvascular bypass operation designed to augment the collateral blood supply to ischemic areas of the brain in patients suffering from symptomatic occlusive cerebrovascular disease. In the patients selected, the symptoms were felt to be due to episodic hemodynamic insufficiency rather than recurrent embolization (10–12, 14, 15, 26, 31, 32, 38, 49, 50, 54, 55, 73).

Since the early reports were published concerning the neurosurgical procedure described above, it is estimated that seven to eight hundred such operations have been performed for cerebrovascular occlusive disease (26, 56). Although the initial results are promising, a longer follow-up study is required to observe the ultimate effect of this type of surgery on the future clinical course of these patients. The postoperative patency rates in the vessels must be evaluated arteriographically in a large series of bypass patients. Operative morbidity and mortality rates require further evaluation also (14).

The fundamental issue to be discussed here is whether surgical extracranial to intracranial collateral blood flow augmentation can be justified on the basis of currently available clinical data and theoretical principles. When the medical profession evaluates any mode of therapy, especially when it is a new surgical procedure, several evaluative criteria should be fulfilled in order to justify its continued clinical application.

CRITERIA FOR A RATIONAL SURGICAL PROCEDURE

Criteria for a rational surgical procedure extend from basic theoretical principles on one hand to successful evaluation of those principles during clinical application on the other. These criteria are:

1. A need exists for therapeutic innovation in response to an unsolved medical problem.
2. Prediction of results of the new operation is based on sound theoretical principles.
3. The surgical technique is reliable; reproducible results have been obtained at several independent centers by others.
4. The operative morbidity and mortality rates are acceptably low.
5. The surgical results are observed during an adequate postoperative follow-up period, *i.e.*, long term anastomotic patency with improvement in preoperative symptoms.
6. The natural history of the untreated disease is altered in a positive fashion by (a) improving the quality of life defined herein as decreasing transient ischemic attacks (TIA) or recovery of neurological deficit, and (b) by decreasing the complications of the disease process, that is, permanent ischemic damage to the brain.
7. The surgical treatment results in prolongation of anticipated patient longevity.

Stroke as a Clinical Problem and the Need for Improved Therapy

INCIDENCE

The incidence of stroke in the United States is slightly less than 2 per 1000 population but rises sharply with advancing age (36, 37, 45). In Middlesex County, Connecticut, for example, the adjusted incidence was 1.7 per 1000 (22). Approximately 400,000 new strokes occur per year in the United States of which 80% are due to cerebral vascular occlusive disease (66). In contrast, only 5 to 10% are due to subarachnoid hemorrhage, a major area of interest to the neurosurgeon. It is estimated that two million people in America are presently disabled and unemployable as a result of stroke (30). The majority of individuals in that two million are under 65 years of age and are in the so-called "preretirement" or productive years (25). Consequently, it is well recognized that stroke is a leading cause of death and disability in the U.S.A. Stroke is third in frequency after heart disease and cancer as a medical cause of suffering in this country (60). Stroke, therefore, is the most prevalent neurological health problem occurring in the world today (28).

Reported Natural History of Cerebral Vascular Transient Ischemic Episodes or Fate of Untreated Cases

Patients who have developed TIA have a 13 to 60% chance of developing a completed stroke within 4 years (1, 6, 24, 36, 44, 62, 74). A comprehensive study recently published from Rochester, Minnesota, reports an annual incidence of TIA of 0.31 in 1000 with a 40% chance of a completed stroke in 48 months. Fifty per cent of these strokes were completed within the initial 12 months after occurrence of the first warning attack (67). The overriding aim of stroke therapy, therefore, is to prevent such disasters and, if possible, to improve the over-all quality of life following the onset of symptomatic cerebrovascular disease.

Arteriographic Findings

ANATOMICAL BASIS OF TRANSIENT STROKES

In a series of 100 consecutive patients presenting with TIA (or TIA with a mild completed stroke) 33% of those studied by arteriography demonstrated significant obstructive lesions classified as "inaccessible or inoperable" by traditional vascular surgery techniques (43). Other arteriographic studies have reported 33% of obstructive lesions to be intracranial (8).

In a recent analysis of 123 consecutive patients presenting with only transient ischemic symptoms at one university vascular clinic, arteriograms revealed that 19% (N = 23) had a completely occluded internal carotid artery as the cause of their hemodynamic cerebrovascular insufficiency. Such lesions are, in general, considered inoperable (7). In a short follow-up period three of these 23 patients suffered a completed stroke (40).

Results of the National Cooperative Cerebrovascular Disease Study

Haas and associates catalogued cerebrovascular arteriographic lesions as surgically accessible, inaccessible, or inoperable according to traditional criteria which limit surgical treatment to stenotic or ulcerating extracranial lesions involving the cervical vessels (34).

INACCESSIBLE

Arteriographic investigations from the National Cooperative Study revealed that 6% of the patients studied had purely inaccessible intracranial lesions and an additional 33% demonstrated inaccessible lesions combined with accessible extracranial vascular obstruction, the so-called "tandem lesion." Insofar as cerebrovascular atherosclerotic disease is a multifocal entity, this is an expected finding (34).

INOPERABLE

An additional 16% of patients studied for cerebrovascular symptoms were shown to have chronic internal carotid occlusion (39), which at the present time is not subjected to surgical exploration by vascular surgeons because of the low success rate in reopening the occluded vessel (23, 61, 68). However, vascular surgeons are also loathe to operate on an acute internal carotid occlusion because of the reported high incidence of complications due to ensuing hemorrhagic infarction (69). Computer analyses of follow-up data relevant to the natural history of patients suffering from internal carotid occlusion from the National Cooperative Study revealed that this is not a benign condition and that the outlook is poor (39). A similar result suggesting a poor prognosis in patients with internal carotid occlusions has been reported also by Gurdjian and his colleagues (33).

In summary, 20% of cerebrovascular disease patients studied by arteriography demonstrated lesions which are "inoperable or inaccessible" according to present surgical criteria. This figure amounts to approximately 14,000 individuals per year presenting with transient ischemic attacks without permanent neurological deficit.

Theoretical Basis of Proposed Surgical Procedure

Based on Baker's extensive research on the distribution of atherosclerotic cerebral vascular occlusive lesions (amount of atherosclerosis deposited = blood pressure × radius of vessel), microvascular surgery has the potential to bypass the major obstructive pathology and surgically supply an additional collateral blood supply to ischemic areas (51). Since symptoms of cerebrovascular insufficiency in some cases may be the result of insufficient collateral supply distal to the site of vascular obstruction rather than the result of recurrent embolization, a surgical collateral augmentation procedure should theoretically correct this problem (16–18, 35, 41). Whether such a surgical operation can partially or completely improve mild neurological defects remains to be tested. Some pathological studies have suggested that minor neurological deficits, at least theoretically, could be improved with the restoration of normal perfusion pressures to the areas of marginal blood flow (52, 59). At the present time, however, no reliable clinical method exists to determine in advance which neurons are poorly functioning because of partial anoxia or which neurons are, in fact, dead.

INDICATIONS FOR INTRA-EXTRACRANIAL ARTERIAL BYPASS

Clinical Presentation

TRANSIENT ISCHEMIC ATTACKS

The diagnosis of a TIA is based solely on an adequate history obtained from the patient or the relatives. TIA are characterized by transient episodes of neurological dysfunction due to a temporarily inadequate blood supply to a region of the brain. The duration of an episode may vary from a few minutes to several hours, although 15 to 30 minutes is the usual duration of the TIA. During the attack neurological abnormalities are found upon examination; between attacks the patient appears normal. The attacks vary in frequency and number. In a given patient the episodes tend to be similar, though varying in severity. The attacks come on quickly and are maximal in degree within a few seconds. Abatement of the attack is rapid. As noted previously, the prognosis in patients with TIA's is guarded as the patients are likely to sustain a significant cerebral infarction (65, 67). Reversible ischemic neurological deficit (RIND) is simply an attack as described above that lasts over 24 hours.

PROGRESSIVE STROKE

This is a separate category that is commonly encountered in stroke evaluation. The accumulation of the neurological deficit may be smooth or stepwise. The degree of hemiparesis is a useful principal indicator of progression. Occasionally, one deficit, such as homonymous hemianopsia, may be complete while another deficit, such as hemiparesis, is still increasing in severity. Examination reveals evidence of focal cerebral damage. The diagnosis of progressive stroke is based on the finding of signs pointing to a focal cerebral lesion which has developed and is continuing to develop over a period of a few hours and which is not the result of some other cause, such as hemorrhage or tumor. Computerized axial tomography (CAT) scan is particularly helpful in confirming the absence of a mass lesion. In our series of strokes in evolution, all patients had internal carotid occlusions as the cause of the progressive neurological deterioration of their clinical course. This deterioration was arrested by the surgical bypass in all cases.

COMPLETED STROKE

This stage is characterized by a focal neurological deficit that is stable and persistent over a period of hours or days. The word "complete" means that the clinical effects of the ischemic process are completed; however, some improvement may occasionally be seen within hours after onset. Many patients with marked recovery of their initial neurological deficit continue to exhibit a fluctuating daily course. They may complain of "good days and bad days" with varying amounts of dysphasia; hand or arm clumsiness, varying difficulty in writing day to day; and varying amounts of sensory loss. These patients, if significant obstructive lesions can be demonstrated arteriographically, can be improved in many instances by improving the collateral supply and cerebral perfusion with a surgical bypass.

GENERALIZED LOW PERFUSION SYNDROMES

Patients who suffer from a generalized ischemic cerebrovascular syndrome due to multiple large vessel occlusive disease constitute a smaller group. These individuals may complain of symptoms such as intermittent dizziness, incoordination, staggering, blurred vision, syncope, mental deterioration, and transient motor or speech or sensory deficits (48, 68). These symptoms are often of such severity that daily activities may be markedly affected. Microvascular bypass surgery in such cases may diminish the symptomatology dramatically.

ADDITIONAL DIAGNOSTIC STUDIES

Ocular Pneumoplethysmography in Cases of Carotid Artery Occlusion

One potential type of candidate for a superficial temporal artery-middle cerebral artery (STA-MCA) bypass suffers from an internal carotid occlusion with ipsilateral TIA felt to be due to hemispheric hypoperfusion.

The determination of the collateral hemispheric blood pressure (CHBP) is an accurate, objective method of assessing the adequacy of collateral blood flow to a given cerebral hemisphere. This technique, more commonly known as the internal carotid back pressure or stump pressure, is regularly used by neurosurgeons and vascular surgeons to determine the tolerance of a cerebral hemisphere to temporary or permanent occlusion of the common or internal carotid artery prior to cervical carotid thromboendarterectomy (46). A noninvasive method of measuring the CHBP has been devised and evaluated by Gee, the ocular pneumoplethysmograph (OPG) (29, 53). This technique combines accepted methods of ophthalmodynamometry and ocular plethysmography. Measured with a scleral suction cup elevation of the intraocular pressure to a level which exceeds the systolic blood pressure of the ophthalmic artery results in recording of a cessation in blood flow in the retinal and choroidal branches of the ophthalmic artery. This procedure thus provides an indirect measure of retinal artery pressure which can be equated with internal carotid pressure derived solely from collateral sources when the carotid is ligated or thrombosed proximally (9).

Clinical Examples

Case 1. A 58-year-old man suffered a right hemispheric stroke 10 years prior to admission to our hospital. Arteriography at that time revealed a right internal carotid occlusion. The patient completely recovered from the stroke and remained asymptomatic until 1 year prior to admission. During the year prior to admission, the patient noted transient numbness of his left hand and these TIA had increased in frequency, severity, and duration with the onset of weakness and apraxia. He underwent an STA-MCA shunt and he has been asymptomatic since operation. Figure 21.1 shows the preoperative and postoperative arteriograms. Figure 21.2 shows the OPG's obtained preoperatively and 6 weeks postoperatively. Figure 21.3 shows the OPG's with and without compression of the right superficial temporal artery obtained 6 months after operation. The data of Table 21.1 clearly document the contribution of the shunt to the collateral hemispheric blood pressure and resultant cerebral blood flow.

Case 2. A female patient who underwent a shunt procedure presented with ischemic TIA of the cerebral hemisphere ipsilateral to her internal carotid occlusion consisting of dysphasia and difficulty writing. The CHBP was 60 mm. Hg at a systemic blood pressure of 175/85. After operation the CHBP was 102 mm. Hg, at a systemic blood pressure of 160/80. In this case the shunt resulted in the elevation of the CHBP of 42 mm. Hg (from 60 mm. Hg before operation to 102 mm. Hg after operation), in spite of the fact that the postoperative

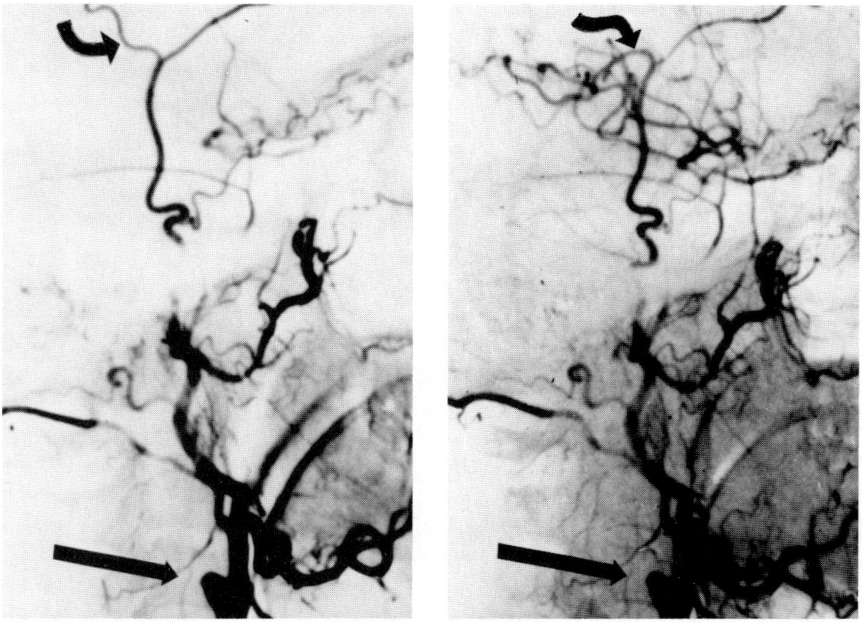

FIG. 21.1. Arteriogram on the left is a lateral projection of the preoperative study. The straight arrow indicates the stump of the occluded internal carotid artery. The curved arrow indicates the posterior branch of the superficial temporal artery. The arteriogram on the right is a lateral projection of the postoperative study. Note that the posterior branch of the superficial temporal artery (curved arrow) now curves downward and inward. Its anastomosis with a cortical branch of the middle cerebral artery has resulted in arteriographic filling of the latter vessel. (Courtesy of William Gee, M.D.)

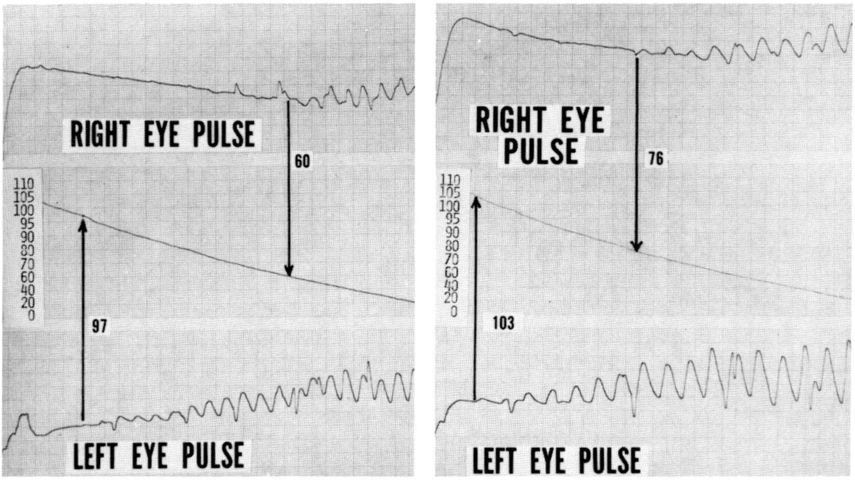

FIG. 21.2. The preoperative OPG tracing is on the left. Note that no pulse is noted in the right eye (upper tracing) until the applied intraocular pressure (middle tracing) has fallen to 60 mm Hg. The postoperative OPG is on the right. Note that the right eye pulse (upper tracing) is now noted at an applied intraocular pressure (middle tracing) of 76 mm Hg. (Courtesy of William Gee, M.D.)

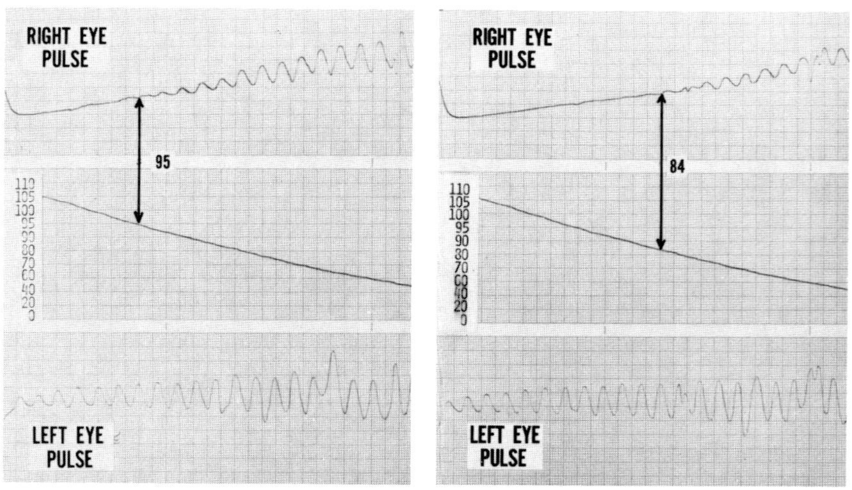

FIG. 21.3. OPG tracings obtained 6 months after operation. The tracing on the left was taken *without* compression of the right superficial temporal artery. The pulse in the right eye (upper tracing) commences at an applied intraocular pressure (middle tracing) of 95 mm. Hg. The tracing on the right was taken *with* right superficial temporal artery compression. The pulse in the right eye (upper tracing) does not start until the applied intraocular pressure (middle tracing) has fallen to 84 mm Hg. Also note that the pulse amplitude in the right eye is reduced with the arterial compression. (Courtesy of William Gee, M.D.)

TABLE 21.1
Ocular Pneumoplethysmography (OPG)—Case 1

OPG*	Systemic Blood Pressure (Cuff)	Collateral Hemispheric Blood Pressure†	
		Left eye ICA patent	Right eye ICA occluded
		mm. Hg	*mm. Hg*
Postoperative	158/85	97	60
Postoperative (6 weeks)	146/86	103	76
Postoperative (6 months)			
With shunt compression	180/90	110+	84
Without shunt compression	180/90	110+	95

* OPG studies performed courtesy of William Gee, M.D.
† ICA = internal carotid artery.

systemic blood pressure was lower than that noted preoperatively. The patient has been completely asymptomatic since operation. The bypass is patent and enlarging after 36 months.

Thus, two patients who had a CHBP of 60 mm. Hg or less underwent a STA-MCA shunt and both have been asymptomatic since operation. The OPG documented the postoperative elevation of the CHBP in both patients. In one of the patients presented, the contribution of the STA-MCA shunt to the collateral hemispheric blood pressure is clearly demonstrated by obtaining OPG records with or without compression of the superficial temporal artery. The OPG appears to be a valuable tool for the selection of patients for a STA-MCA shunt and for an objective, noninvasive documentation of one aspect of the operative result.

Regional Cerebral Blood Flow

This topic has been previously discussed in detail by my colleague, Peter Schmiedek, M.D. (see Chapter 20). Regional cerebral blood flow measurements, although technically difficult to obtain, promise to provide accurate and objective information for evaluating and selecting patients and for documenting the results of bypass surgery (4, 31, 32, 54, 55).

PRESENT ARTERIOGRAPHIC INDICATIONS FOR THIS COLLATERAL AUGMENTATION PROCEDURE

Lateralized Low Perfusion Syndromes

SYMPTOMS

The symptoms depend on the vessel involved (usually the middle cerebral artery) and the functional collateral supply available to a specific region of brain; symptoms may be transient or progressive.

Type of etiology:

1. Internal carotid occlusions with inadequate collaterals.

2. Inaccessible carotid stenosis with inadequate collaterals (petrous, cavernous, supraclinoid).

   a. Atherosclerotic.

   b. Extrinsic tumor (sphenoid wing meningioma).

   c. Aneurysm, wrapping, or clipping with postoperative narrowing of the parent vessel (21, 47).

3. Middle cerebral stenosis with inadequate collaterals.

   a. Atherosclerotic.

   b. Vasculitis (50).

   c. Extrinsic pressure secondary to tumor.

   d. Narrowing postaneurysm surgery (21, 47).

4. Middle cerebral occlusions with mild deficit and

   a. absent recanalization.

   b. inadequate collaterals.

5. Vertebral basilar lesions with inadequate collaterals (occipital artery employed) (64).

6. Giant aneurysms with inadequate collaterals (inoperable intracranially but unable to occlude internal carotid artery or trap the aneurysm without precipitating a neurological deficit (21, 47).

Generalized Low Perfusion Syndromes

Etiology:

1. Multiple vessel occlusions.

2. Multiple vessel inaccessible stenoses.

In cases of multiple vessel occlusion involving both internal carotid arteries and one or more vertebrals, bypass surgery may provide collateral augmentation to the anterior circulation thereby relieving symptoms of transient posterior fossa ischemia caused by shunting of blood flow to the cerebral hemispheres *via* the circle of Willis (35).

SUMMARY OF SURGICAL RESULTS

The surgical results are summarized in Tables 21.2–21.7.

CONTRAINDICATIONS

The contraindications are given in Table 21.8.

DISCUSSION

Morbidity

The primary risk of surgical morbidity stems from the necessity of clamping a portion of the recipient cortical artery for approximately 30 minutes in order to perform a satisfactory anastomosis in a bloodless

TABLE 21.2
Analysis of Bypass Status, January 1975 (N = 70)

No. of cases	70
Males	85%
Females	15%
Over 65	25% (retirement years)
Under 65	75% (working years)
Average age	In late 50's
Range	21–81 years
Minimal follow-up	6 months
Average follow-up	16 months

TABLE 21.3
Types—Clinical Presentation (N = 70)

	No. Cases	Per Cent
A) TIA or RIND	41	58
B) Completed stroke		
Mild	18	25
Moderate	3	5
Severe	5	7
C) Progressive stroke	3	5

TIA, dysfunction under 24 hours with complete recovery; RIND, dysfunction over 24 hours with complete recovery; mild, clumsiness of hand or leg, fluctuating at times, fluctuating dysphasia; moderate hemiparesis or monoparesis (fixed) dysphasia nonfluctuating; severe, hemiplegia, monoplegia, aphasia; and progressive, progressive loss of neurological function.

TABLE 21.4
*Arteriographic Findings (N = 70)**

	No. Cases	Per cent
1) BICO	11	16
2) a) ICO	25	35
b) CCS	13	19
3) a) MCS	6	8
b) MCO	6	8
4) MOS	9	13
Total	70	

* BICO, bilateral internal carotid occlusions; ICO, internal carotid occlusion; CCS, cavernous carotid stenosis; MCS, middle cerebral stenosis; MCO, middle cerebral occlusion; and MOS, multiple vessel occlusions and stenoses (intra- or extracranial).

field. Rarely minor neurological deficits do occur postoperatively; however, the vast majority tend to clear spontaneously if the cortical branch occlusion time is 30 minutes or less. An experienced surgical team is therefore a necessity.

TABLE 21.5
*Results of Surgical Therapy to Date, January 1975 (Criteria #6)**

	No. Cases	Asymptomatic or Improved‡
A) TIA or RIND	41	34/41 (83%)
B) Completed stroke		
Mild	18	10/18 (55%)
Moderate	3	1/3 (33%)
Severe	5	0/5 (0%)
C) Progressive	3	3/3 (100%)

* Previous tables presented data through January 1975. As of September 1975, 94 cases have been performed with no increase in morbidity and no further mortality.

‡ Improved—one TIA maximal postoperatively.

Mortality

The only death of a patient presented in this study occurring within the first week after surgery was from a stroke involving the opposite hemisphere from an embolic clot to the opposite carotid siphon. The case is included as an operative death. A second death occurred within the first month from gastrointestinal hemorrhage; this possibly now can be avoided by vigorous antacid regimes in all patients since they are usually placed on aspirin for several weeks postoperatively as an aid in avoiding platelet clumping at the fresh bypass anastomotic sites.

Patency

The anterior temporal lobe branches of the middle cerebral artery have been abandoned as recipient vessels. There were two cases of postoperative thrombosis of the bypass attributed to technical problems due to the small size (less than 1 mm.) (Table 21.8) of the available cortical artery in this location. The posterior temporal angular artery complex above the ear has been used exclusively in the past 90 cases and no major difficulties have been encountered in finding a suitable recipient vessel of sufficient size even though a small craniectomy was utilized (13) (Table 21.7).

Summary of Results

1. *TIA*. A significant percentage of patients suffering from transient ischemic attacks obtained symptomatic relief following the surgical bypass. Thus, the quality of their lives is improved (Tables 21.5 and 21.6).

The Mayo Clinic has followed extensively a series of 200 patients suffering from definite transient ischemic attacks. In the Mayo group the stroke occurrence rate after 16 months was 22% (67). In our operated

TABLE 21.6
Follow-up Studies

Type of Case	Number	Average Months Follow-up	Arteriographic Patency	No Symptoms or Improved Status	Later Stroke
Bilateral internal carotid occlusions	11	14	9/9	9/10 (90%)	1—progressive cerebral vasculitis, bilateral, 26 mos.
Multiple occlusions plus stenosis	9	16	6/7	6/9 (66%)	1—anastomosis closed 3 mos. 2—stroke on opposite side 5 mos., 5 days
Internal carotid occlusions	25	20	15/16	18/74 (75%)	
Cavernous carotid siphon stenosis	13	11	9/10	9/10 (90%)	
Middle cerebral stenosis	6	22	5/5	5/6 (83%)	1—stroke vertebral basilar, 5 mos., small vessel disease
Middle cerebral occlusion	6	16	3/3	3/6 (50%)	
Totals	70	16 mos. (average)	47/50 (94%)	49/65 (74%)	5/70 (7%)

TABLE 21.7
Patency (N = 70) (Criteria #3)

1) Doppler auscultation (42)	70/70
	65/70 = 93% apparently open
2) Postoperative arteriograms	50/70
	70% of total cases
3) Patent	47/70 = 94%

TABLE 21.8
Contraindications

1) Severe long standing neurological deficit
2) Marked hypertension with small vessel disease demonstrated by arteriography
3) Severe pulmonary disease
4) Severe cardiovascular disease
5) Inadequate diameter of donor temporal artery (smaller than 1 mm.) (58)*

* Potential alternative choices:
(1) Occipital artery (57)
(2) Free autografts
 a) Opposite temporal artery
 b) Radial artery
 c) Vein—saphenous (calf)
(3) Homograft
 Radial artery
 Umbilical artery (?)
 Saphenous vein (?)
(4) Synthetic grafts (?)

series to date (with a similar follow-up period) the stroke occurrence incidence was 7% including those patients who later suffered a stroke in the distribution of a vessel not supplied by the bypass. The incidence of stroke in the hemisphere supplied by the bypass is 3% at present and in one of these cases (N = 2) the bypass was occluded (Table 21.6). It may be that in the future, bilateral surgical arterial bypasses should be considered in patients with multiple vessel occlusive disease. However, to date bilateral procedures have not been advised prophylactically in asymptomatic patients after a unilateral bypass.

2. *Progressive and completed strokes.* The improvement rate in progressive and mild completed strokes was 62%. This statistic, of course, must be viewed cautiously as the natural history of spontaneous improvement in completed strokes is quite variable. Most of our cases of completed stroke were operated at least 3 months following the completed stroke (Table 21.5).

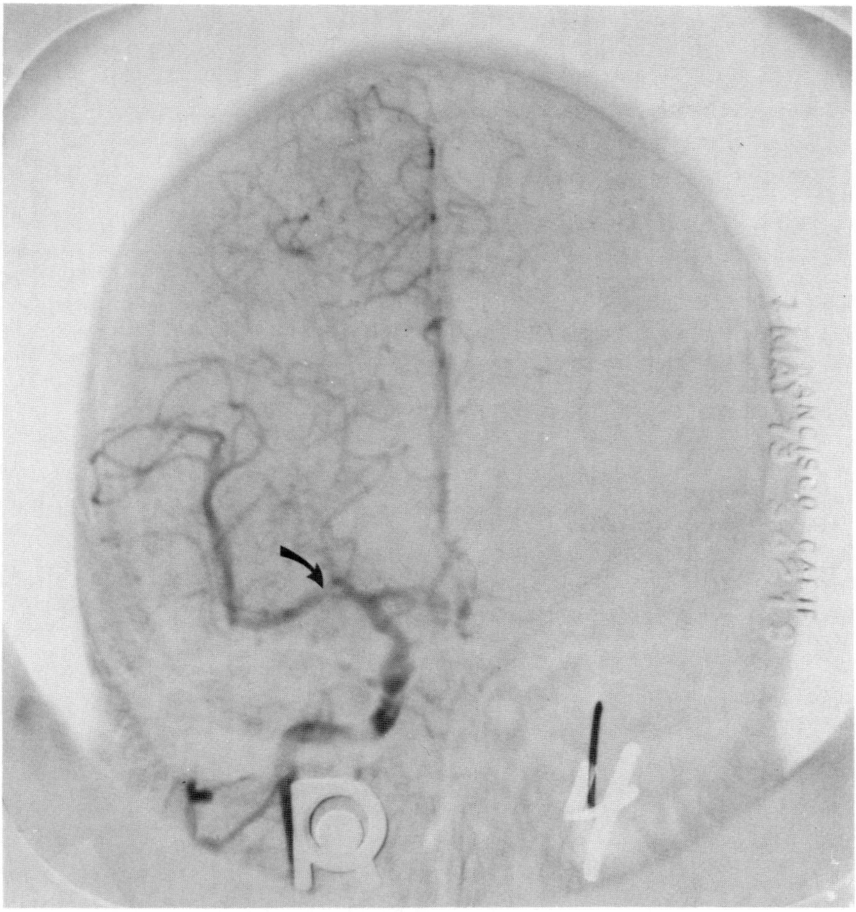

FIG. 21.4. Preoperative right internal carotid arteriogram reveals a marked right middle cerebral artery stenosis (black arrow).

3. No recurrent strokes have occurred to date in the group of patients (N = 21) with (1) completed stroke with mild neurological deficits or (2) progressive stroke. The reported incidence of recurrent stroke in such a group is estimated at 30 to 50%, most occurring within three years (36) (Table 21.5).

Despite the degree to which the data presented here satisfy our criteria for a rational surgical procedure, further objective evaluation of the effects of a new operation, such as this one, may be difficult to obtain. Several investigators have reported significant improvement in regional cerebral blood flow following such a bypass (4, 54, 55, 63) (allowing for the intrinsic errors implicit in the methods employed) (20). Additional supportive evidence has emerged in our series where follow-up arteriograms have revealed that a previous stenotic lesion in the intracranial vasculature had gone on to complete occlusion without the development of symptoms after a successful bypass.

Clinical Example. A 55-year-old black female school teacher developed two attacks of left-sided hemiparesis and numbness 3 months apart. Arteriograms performed on each occasion revealed a stenotic lesion of the right middle cerebral artery (Fig. 21.4). There was no source for emboli demonstrated on the arch study. She made a complete recovery from each episode and it was assumed that the attacks were due to inadequate collateral. A right superficial temporal to angular artery bypass was performed in February 1973. She remains asymptomatic 30 months later (September 1975). Routine arteriograms performed 10 days following surgery revealed a patent bypass. Arteriograms 1 year later demonstrated that the

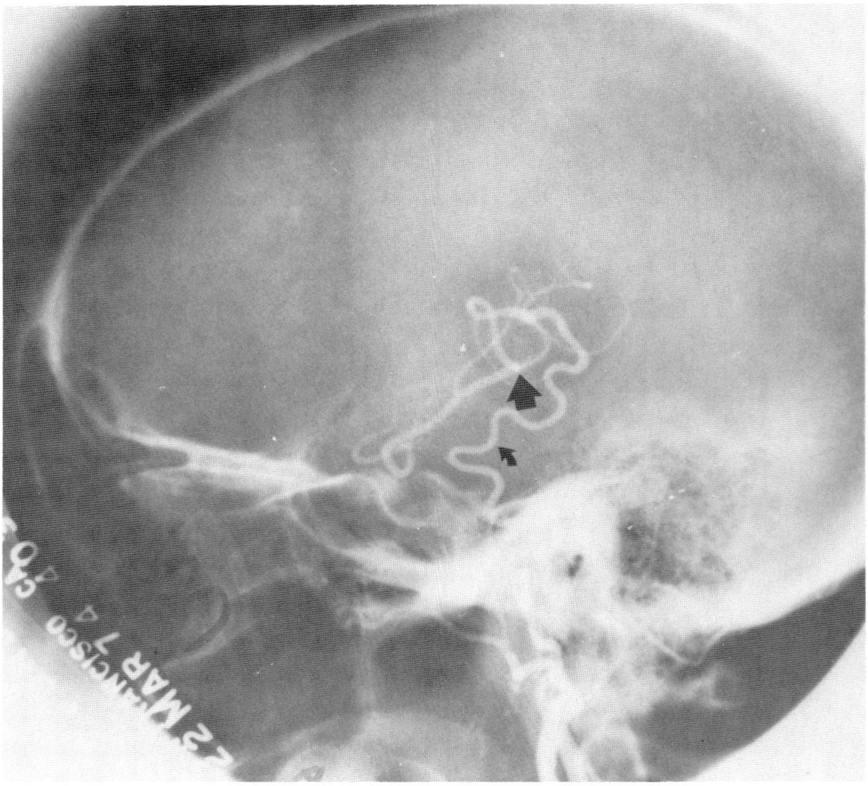

FIG. 21.5. One year postoperative arteriogram. The small arrow indicates the increased size in the superficial temporal artery. The large arrow marks the point of anastomosis.

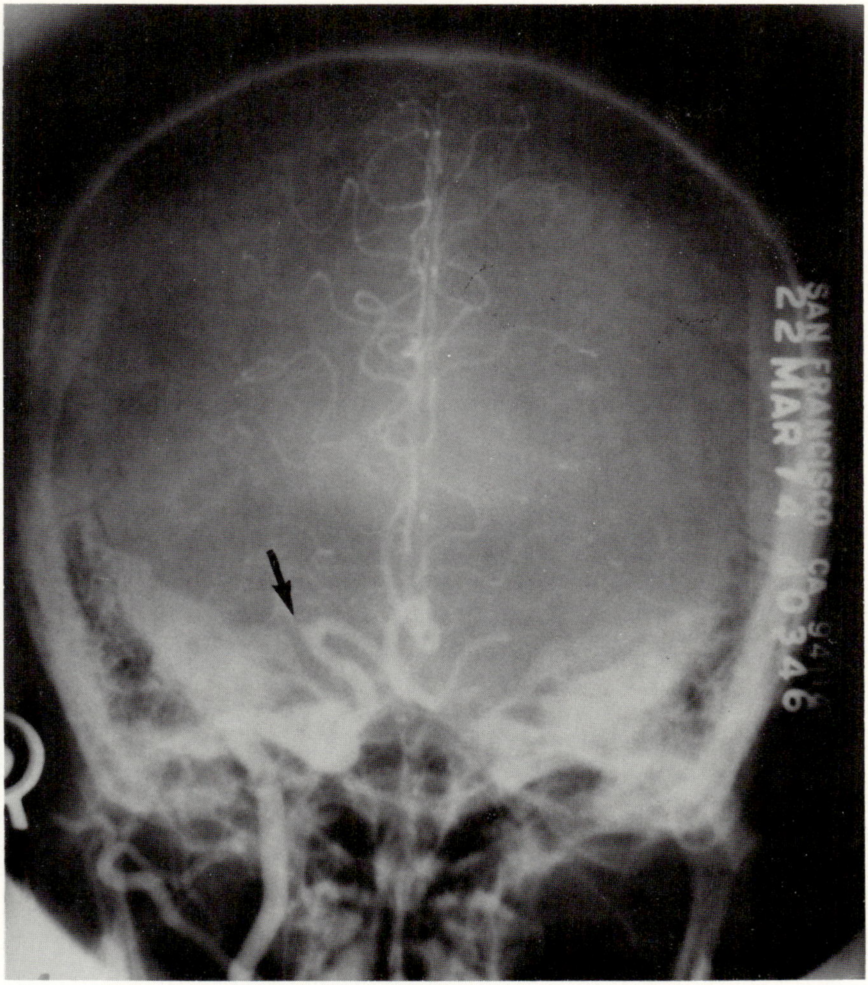

FIG. 21.6. Postoperative arteriogram 1 year followng surgery. Middle cerebral stenosis has progressed to complete occlusion.

middle cerebral stenosis had gone on to complete occlusion with the distal portion of the middle cerebral complex being sustained by an enlarging and patent bypass (Figs. 21.5–21.8). The operation in this clinical example may have prevented the serious stroke which would be expected to follow middle cerebral artery thrombosis.

Our over-all results in this group of 70 patients are quite similar to other series reported by Reichman, Gratzl, Yasargil, Austin and Peerless (2, 5, 11, 32, 50, 73). The ultimate test of whether this particular operative approach is clinically useful will be a comparison between

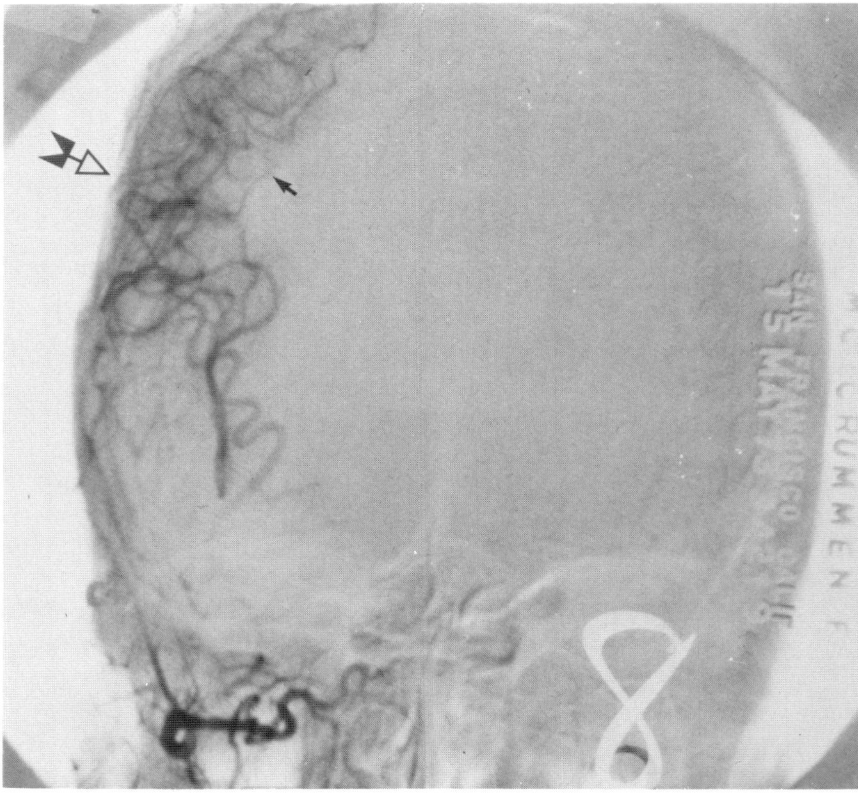

FIG. 21.7. Distal middle cerebral complex sustained by an enlarging and patent bypass 1 year postoperative. Anteroposterior view.

similar randomized groups of patients (operated *vs.* nonoperated) suffering from angiographically demonstrated inaccessible or inoperable cerebrovascular stenotic or occlusive lesions (3).

CONCLUSIONS

This paper describes the results of a neurosurgical microvascular bypass procedure in 70 patients with 6 to 48 months postoperative follow-up (Tables 21.2–21.4). The majority of cases in the group reported here were suffering from transient ischemic attacks or had suffered a "completed stroke" with marked recovery and subsequent mild residual neurological deficit. From our series of 70 patients the following observations have been made:

1. In cases of TIA with hemodynamic lesions previously considered inaccessible or inoperable results have been encouraging (Table 21.5).

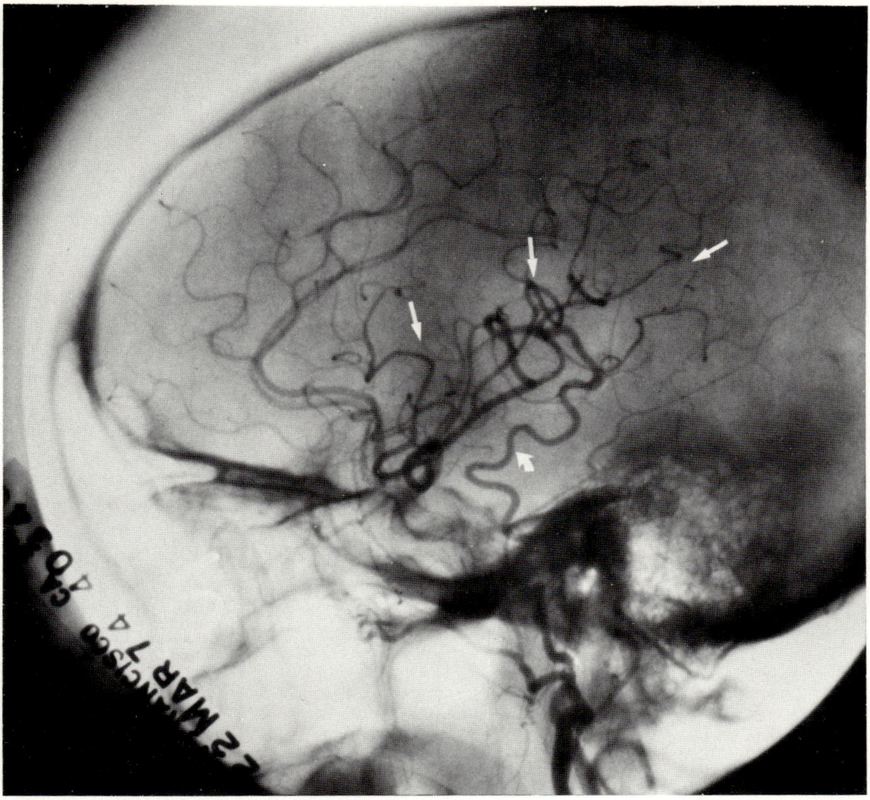

FIG. 21.8. Arteriogram 1-year postoperative showing patent and enlarging bypass filling middle cerebral.

2. Patients with mild fluctuating neurological deficits appear to improve in 50% of cases (Table 21.5).

3. It appears that a patient suffering from a severe completed stroke probably will not be aided by this procedure.

4. The permanent morbidity rate is acceptably low.

5. The operative mortality rate is 1.4%.

6. In analyzing the cases presenting with TIA, the total postoperative follow-up stroke rate of 7% in our series, including strokes occurring on the nonoperated side, falls below the predicted rate of stroke in the Mayo Clinic study. Our follow-up average is 16 months. The stroke occurrence rate to date in the hemisphere supplied by the bypass is 3% (N = 2) compared to the Mayo predicted rate for untreated patients at 16 months of 22%. In one of these patients the bypass was occluded.

7. The incidence of recurrent stroke in the hemisphere supplied by a patent bypass is low.; patency rates are high (Table 21.7).

Although these results are considered to be preliminary, neurosurgeons involved in this aspect of stroke therapy remain encouraged.

REFERENCES

1. Acheson, J., and Hutchison, E. C. The natural history of "focal cerebral vascular disease." Q. J. Med., *40:* 15–23, 1971.
2. Anderson, R. E., Reichman, O. H., and Davis, D. O. Radiological evaluation of temporal artery-middle cerebral artery anastomosis. Radiology, *113:* 73–79, 1974.
3. Annas, G. J. The Rights of Hospital Patients, 246 pp. Avon Books, New York, 1975.
4. Austin, G., Laffin, D., and Hayward, W. Physiological factors in the selection of patients for superficial temporal artery to middle cerebral artery anastomoses. Surgery, *75:* 861–868, 1974.
5. Austin, G., Laffin, D., Thompson, J., *et al.* Microsurgical anastomosis for brain ischemia. J. Neurosurg., in press.
6. Baker, R. N., Ramseyer, J. C., and Schwartz, W. S. Prognosis in patients with transient cerebral ischemic attacks. Neurology (Minneap.), *18:* 1157–1167, 1968.
7. Blaisdell, W. F., Clauss, R. H., Galbraith, J. G., Imparato, A. M., and Wylie, E. J. Joint study of extracranial arterial occlusion—IV. A review of surgical considerations. J.A.M.A., *209:* 1889–1895, 1969.
8. Blaisdell, W. F., Hall, A. D., Thomas, A. M., and Ross, S. J. Cerebrovascular occlusive disease—Experience with panarteriography in 300 consecutive cases. Calif. Med., *103:* 321–329, 1965.
9. Carney, A. L. Ocular plethysmography in the evaluation of cerebral vascular disease. Presented at Second International Conference on Neurosurgical Anastomoses for Cerebral Ischemia. Chicago, Illinois, June 1974.
10. Chater, N., Mani, J., and Tonnemacher, K. Superficial temporal arterial bypass for cerebrovascular occlusive disease. Calif. Med., *119:* 9–13, 1973.
11. Chater, N., and Peerless, S. J. The early effects of neurosurgical microvascular bypass operations on problems of cerebrovascular occlusive disease. Presented at American Academy of Neurology, San Francisco, Calif., April 1974.
12. Chater, N. L., Reichman, O., and Tew, J. Cerebral revascularization: Scientific Exhibit. American Association of Neurological Surgeons, Los Angeles, April 1973.
13. Chater, N. L., and Spetzler, R. Anatomical studies of the cerebral cortical vasculature of microvascular surgical significance. Presented at the International Symposium on Neurosurgery Through the Microscope. Mount Sinai School of Medicine, City University of New York, New York, June 1973.
14. Chater, N., Spetzler, R., Mani, J. The spectrum of cerebrovascular occlusive disease suitable for microvascular bypass surgery. Angiology, *26:* 235–251, 1975.
15. Chater, N. L., and Yasargil, M. G. Results of temporal artery bypass procedures in the treatment of cerebrovascular disease. Presented at Congress of Neurological Surgeons, Miami, Fl, October 1971.
16. Connolly, J. E., and Stemmer, E. A. Endarterectomy of the external carotid artery. Its importance in the surgical management of extracranial cerebrovascular occlusive disease. Arch. Surg., *106:* 799–802, 1973.
17. DeBakey, M. D., Crawford, E. S., Cooley, D. A., Morris, G. C., Garrett, E., and Fields, W. S. Cerebral arterial insufficiency: one to 11 year results following arterial reconstructive operation. Ann. Surg., *161:* 921–945, 1965.

18. Diethrich, E. B., Liddicoat, J. E., McCutchen, J. J., and DeBakey, M. E. Surgical significance of the external carotid artery in the treatment of cerebrovascular insufficiency. J. Cardiovasc. Surg., *9:* 213–223, 1968.
19. Donaghy, R. M. P., and Yasargil, M. G. Extra-intracranial blood flow diversion. Presented at the American Association of Neurological Surgeons, Chicago, Ill., April 1968.
20. Donley, R. F., Sundt, T. M., Anderson, R. E., and Sharbrough, F. W. Blood flow measurements and the "Look Through" artifact in focal cerebral ischemis. Stroke, *6:* 121–131, 1975.
21. Drake C. G. Giant intracranial aneurysms. Presented at Fifth Annual Neurosurgical Postgraduate Course, University California Medical Center, San Francisco, May 1975.
22. Eisenberg, H., Morrison J. T., Sullivan, P., and Foote, F. M. Cerebrovascular accidents: Incidence and survival rates in a defined population, Middlesex County, Connecticut. J.A.M.A. *189:* 883–888, 1964.
23. Fields W. S. Selection of stroke patients for arterial reconstructive surgery. Am. J. Surg., *125:* 527–529, 1973.
24. Fields, W. S., Maslenikov, V., Meyer, J. S., Haas, W. K., Remington, R. D., and McDonald, J. Joint study of extracranial occlusion. V. Progress report of prognosis following surgery or non-surgical treatment for transient cerebral ischemia attacks and cervical carotid artery lesions. J.A.M.A., *211:* 1993–2003, 1970.
25. Fields, W. S., North R. R., Haas, W. K., Galbraith, J. G., Ratinov, G., Burns, M. H., MacDonald, M. C., and Meyer, J. S. Joint study of extracranial arterial occlusion as a cause of stroke. I. Organization of study and survey of patient population. J.A.M.A., *203:* 955–960, 1968.
26. First International Symposium Microsurgical Anastomosis for Cerebral Ischemia, Loma Linda, California, June 1973. (Charles C Thomas, Springfield, Ill., in press.)
27. Fisher, M. Occlusion of the internal carotid artery. Arch. Neurol. Psych., *65:* 346–377, 1951.
28. Friedlander, W. J. About three old men: an inquiry into how cerebral arteriosclerosis has altered world politics. Stroke, *3:* 467–473, 1972.
29. Gee, W., Mehigan, J. T., and Wylie, E. J. Measurement of collateral cerebral hemispheric blood pressure by ocular pneumoplethysmography. Am. J. Surg., *130:* 121–127, 1975.
30. Gordon, E. E., and Kohn, K. H. Evaluation of rehabilitation methods in the hemiplegic patient. J. Chronic Dis., *19:* 3–16, 1966.
31. Gratzl, O., Schmiedek, P., Spetzler, R., Steinhoff, H., and Marguth, F. Clinical experience with extra-intracranial arterial anastomoses in 65 cases. J. Neurosurg., in press.
32. Gratzl, O., Steude, U., and Schmiedek, P. Indications for extra-intracranial anastomosis between the superficial temporal artery and a branch of the middle cerebral artery in man. *In* Present Limits of Neurosurgery. Proceedings of the Fourth European Congress of Neurosurgery, June 1971, pp. 375–379. Aviceum, Prague, 1972.
33. Hardy, W. G., Lindner, D. W., Thomas, L. M., and Gurdjian, E. S. Anticipated clinical course in carotid artery occlusion. Arch. Neurol. *6:* 138–150, 1962.
34. Haas, W. K., Fields, W. S., North, R. R., Kircheff, I. I., Chase, N. E., and Bauer, R. B. Joint study of extracranial occlusion; II. Arteriography, techniques, sites and complications. J.A.M.A., *203:* 961–968, 1968.
35. Humphries, A. W., Young, J. R., Beren E. G., LeFevre, F. A., and DeWolfe, V. G. Relief of vertebrobasilar symptoms by carotid endarterectomy. Surgery, *57:* 48–52, 1965.

36. Hutchison, E. C., and Acheson, E. J. Natural history of stroke-recurrence rate. *In* Strokes—Natural History, Pathology and Surgical Treatment, pp. 146–150. W. B. Saunders, Philadelphia, 1975 .
37. Kannel, W. B., Dawber, T. R., Cohen, M. E., *et al.* Vascular disease of the brain—epidemiologic aspects: The Framingham Study. Am. J. Public Health, *55:* 1355–1366, 1965.
38. Lazar, M. L., and Clark, K. Microsurgical cerebral revascularization: concepts and practice. Surg. Neurol., *1:* 355–359, 1973.
39. Lemak, H. Personal Communication. National Computer Analysis. Joint Study Computer Analysis and Follow-up. Houston, Texas, 1974.
40. Machleder, H. I., and Barker, W. F. External carotid artery shunting during carotid endarterectomy. Evidence of feasibility. Arch. Surg., *108:* 785–788 1974.
41. Machleder, H. I., and Barker, W. F. Stroke on the wrong side. Use of the Doppler ophthalmic test in cerebral vascular screening. Arch. Surg., *105:* 943–947, 1972.
42. Maroon, J. C., Pieroni, D. W., and Campbell, R. L. Ophthalmosonometry: An ultrasonic method for assessing carotid blood flow. J. Neurosurg., *30:* 238–246, 1969.
43. Marshall, J. Angiography in the investigation of ischaemic episodes in the territory of the internal carotid artery. Lancet, *1:* 719–721, 1971.
44. Marshall, J. The natural history of transient ischaemic cerebrovascular attacks. Q. J. Med., *33:* 309–324, 1964.
45. Melamed, E., Cahane, E., Carmon, A., and Lavy, S. Stroke in Jerusalem District. 1960 through 1967, An Epidemiological Study. Stroke, *4:* 465–471, 1973.
46. Moore, W. S., Yee, U. M., and Hall, A. D. Collateral cerebral blood pressure. An index of tolerance to temporary carotid occlusion. Arch. Surg., *106:* 520–523, 1973.
47. Morley, T. P., and Barr, H. W. K. Giant intracranial aneurysms: Diagnosis, course, and management. Clin. Neurosurg., *16:* 73–94, 1973.
48. Paulson, G. W., Kapp, J., and Cook, W. Dementia associated with bilateral carotid artery disease. Geriatrics, *21:* 159–166, Nov. 1966.
49. Reichman, O. H. Extracranial-intracranial arterial anastomosis. *In:* J. P. Whisnant and B. A. Sandok (eds.), Cerebrovascular Diseases (Ninth Conference), pp. 175–186. Grune & Stratton, New York, 1975.
50. Reichman, O. H. Extracranial-intracranial arterial anastomosis for occlusive cerebral ischemia. Presented at Annual Meeting of American College of Surgeons, San Francisco, Calif., October 1975.
51. Resch, J. A., Loewenson, R. B., and Baker, A. B. Physical factors in the pathogenesis of cerebral atherosclerosis. Stroke, *1:* 77–85, 1970.
52. Romanul, F. C. A., and Abramowicz, A. Changes in brain and pial vessels in arterial border zones: a study of 13 cases. Arch. Neurol., *11:* 40–65, 1964.
53. Sand, B. J. Barker, W. F., Freeman, L. W., and Hummell, S. Ophthalmic arterial blood pressures measured by ocular plethysmodynamography. Arch. Surg., *110:* 813–818, 1975.
54. Schmiedek, P., Gratzl, O., Spetzler, R., Steinhoff, H., Enzenbach, R., Brendel W., and Marguth, F. Criteria for the selection of patients for extra-intracranial arterial bypass surgery based on regional cerebral blood flow measurements. J. Neurosurg., in press.
55. Schmiedek, P., Steinhoff, H., *et al.* Refining the indication for microvascular brain surgery by measurement of regional cerebral blood flow. International Symposium on the Pathology of Cerebral Microcirculation, 1973.
56. Second International Symposium Microsurgical Anastomoses for Cerebral Ischemia. Chicago, Ill., June 1974.
57. Spetzler, R. and Chater N. Occipital artery-middle cerebral artery anastomosis for

cerebral artery occlusive disease. Surg. Neurol., *2:* 235–238, 1974.
58. Spetzler, R., and Chater, N. Superficial temporal artery-middle cerebral artery blood flow measurements. Presented at American Association of Neurological Surgeons, St. Louis, Mo., April 1975.
59. Symon, L., Crockard, H. A., Dorsch, N. W. C., Branston, N. M., and Juhasz, J. Local cerebral blood flow and vascular reactivity in a chronic stable stroke in baboons. Stroke, *6:* 482–492, 1975.
60. The President's Commission on Heart Disease, Cancer and Stroke. U. S. Government, Washington, D. C., 1964.
61. Thompson, J. E. Surgery for Cerebrovascular Insufficiency (Stroke); with Special Emphasis on Carotid Endarterectomy. 96 pp. Charles C Thomas, Springfield, Ill., 1968.
62. Toole, J. F., Janeway, R., Choi, K., Cordell, R., Davis, C., Johnston, F., and Miller, H. S. Transient ischemic attacks due to atherosclerosis. A prospective study in 160 patients. Arch. Neurol., *32:* 5–12, 1975.
63. Weinstein, P., Chater, N. L. Ocular plethysmography pre- and post-temporal artery bypass. Presented at Second International Conference on Neurosurgical Anastomoses for Cerebral Ischemia, Chicago, Ill., June 1974.
64. Weinstein, P., Chater, N. L., Ausman, J., and Lamond, R. Extra to intracranial bypass for occlusive vertebral basilar cerebrovascular disease. Presented at American Association of Neurological Surgeons, Miami, Fl., April 1975.
65. Whisnant, J. P. Controversies in the management of extracranial cerebrovascular disease. (Annual Postgraduate Course, "Present Concepts in Internal Medicine," Letterman General Hospital, San Francisco, Calif., October 1972.) Fort Sam Houston, Texas, Videotape, U. S. Army Academy of Health Sciences, Television Division, 1972.
66. Whisnant, J. P., Fitzgibbons, J. P., Kurland, L. T., and Sayre, G. P. Natural history of stroke in Rochester, Minnesota, 1945 through 1954. Stroke, *2:* 11–22, 1971.
67. Whisnant, J. P., Matsumoto, N., and Elveback, L. R. Transient cerebral ischemic attacks in a community, Rochester, Minnesota, 1955 through 1969. Mayo Clin. Proc., *48:* 194–198, 1973.
68. Wylie, E. J., and Ehrenfeld, W. K. Extracranial Occlusive Cerebrovascular Disease; Diagnosis and Management, 231 pp. W. B. Saunders Co., Philadelphia, 1970.
69. Wylie, E. J., Hein, M. F., and Adams, J. E. Intracranial hemorrhage following surgical revascularization for treatment of acute strokes. J. Neurosurg., *21:* 212–215, 1964.
70. Yasargil, M. G. Anastomosis between the superficial temporal artery and a branch of the middle cerebral artery. *In* Microsurgery Applied to Neurosurgery. pp. 105–155. Georg Thieme Verlag, Stuttgart (Academic Press, New York), 1969.
71. Yasargil, M. G. Experimental small vessel surgery in dog including patching and grafting of cerebral vessels and the formation of functional extra-intracranial shunts. *In* Microvascular Surgery, edited by R. M. P. Donaghy, and M. G. Yasargil, pp. 87–126. C. V. Mosby Co., St. Louis, 1967.
72. Yasargil, M. G., Krayenbuhl, H. A., and Jacobsen, J. H. Microneurosurgical arterial reconstruction. Surgery, *67:* 221–233, 1970.
73. Yasargil, M. G., Yonekawa, U., and Klarber, R. Intraoperative intra-arterial pressure measurement in cerebral ischemia in man. *In:* Cerebral Vascular Disease, edited by J. S. Meyer, H. Lechner, and J. Reivich. Seventh International Salzburg Conference, September 1974. Georg Thieme Verlag, Stuttgart, in press, 1975.
74. Ziegler, D. K., and Hassanein, R. S. Prognosis in patients with transient ischemic attacks. Stroke, *4:* 66–673, 1973.

CHAPTER

22

Factors Influencing Postoperative Vascular Patency*

DAVID G. PIEPGRAS, M.D.

In the field of vascular surgery, with its concerns about postoperative vascular patency, we as neurosurgeons have gained much from the past experiences of our colleagues in general surgery. Although Chiari (5) documented the clinical and pathological findings of cervical carotid artery disease in 1905, it is only slightly more than 20 years since the first successful carotid endarterectomy was performed for cerebrovascular insufficiency (7). Today, the procedure is often performed by vascular surgeons and neurosurgeons alike. More exclusively in the domain of the neurosurgeon, however, are the intracranial vascular procedures such as embolectomy and extracranial-to-intracranial arterial anastomoses that have largely been made possible through adaptation of the operating microscope and microsurgical techniques. It is to each of these types of arterial procedures that this discussion is directed.

PATHOGENESIS OF THROMBOSIS

Before considering specific factors that affect postoperative patency of a vessel, it is imperative that we establish basic understanding of the process of thrombosis and that we distinguish it from coagulation. Oversimplifying, coagulation is a sequence of physicochemical reactions (3), usually initiated by tissue injury and enhanced by stasis, in which plasma fibrinogen is converted to a fibrin network with haphazard entrapment of formed blood elements to result in a "red" clot. Thrombosis, on the other hand, is characterized by the focal adhesion and aggregation of platelets at the site of vascular injury to form a "white" thrombus. Particularly in arterial thrombi, platelets constitute a prominent portion of the depositing mass (18).

Comprehensive studies in recent years have given us a pathogenetic concept of the main sequences in thrombus formation, which proceeds as

* Supported in part by Research Grant NB-6663 from the National Institutes of Health, Public Health Service.

follows (21):

1. Vascular injury and endothelial damage result in exposure of subendothelial tissue to the bloodstream.

2. Platelets readily adhere to exposed collagen, basement membrane, and noncollagenous microfibrils.

3. Platelet contact with collagen induces a release reaction with discharge of many platelet constituents, including catecholamines, serotonin, platelet factors 3 and 4, and, most noteworthy, adenosine diphosphate (ADP).

4. The released ADP induces aggregation of new platelets to those already adherent. Parenthetically it should be mentioned that substances other than ADP can be released or be present in pathological states to induce platelet aggregation, these including epinephrine, serotonin, thrombin, fatty acids, endotoxins, and antigen-antibody complexes (9).

5. Simultaneous with these events, tissue thromboplastin liberated at the site of vascular injury and the developing platelet mass facilitate the evolution of thrombin, and this results in further consolidation of the platelet aggregates by the deposition of a fibrin network between platelets and around the periphery of the platelet aggregate. Failure of the coagulation component at this point (as might be induced with anticoagulants) would result in an unstable platelet mass, which could then readily be disaggregated and washed away in the flowing blood.

6. Further propagation of the thrombus or formation of a "red" clot is likely determined by the availability of more ADP and the rate of ADP degradation, the pattern of blood flow, and the activity of the coagulation mechanism.

7. Finally, fibrinolysis and thrombolysis occur.

FACTORS INFLUENCING THROMBOSIS

Changes in the coagulability of the blood, disturbance of blood flow, and abnormalities of the vessel wall (Virchow's triad) have long been recognized as factors predisposing to thrombosis. It is the last two factors that obviously assume great importance in vascular surgery, and we will now direct our attention to these.

RHEOLOGICAL FACTORS

Laminar blood flow will not facilitate the formation of platelet aggregates and will tend to break down those that form (19). Conversely, turbulent flow, with creation of eddies and vortices, has been shown to enhance the platelet release reaction and aggregation (11) and to facilitate the formation of thrombi (28). This is undoubtedly related in part to the liberation of ADP from, and induced by mechanical trauma to, both platelets and red cells. It is this mechanism that has been implicated in the formation of platelet thrombi on artificial heart valves and in arterial grafts and anastomoses (21).

With these facts in mind, vascular surgical procedures should be completed in such a way as to change as little as possible normal laminar flow. Abrupt constriction or dilatation of the vessel lumen should be avoided, bell-mouthed anastomoses are preferred to sharp edged orifices (29), and angles of bifurcation are best kept as acute as possible (10, 29). Also, it should be recalled that, as formulated in Poiseuille's law, conduit constrictions produce a reduction in flow which varies with the fourth power of the radius. Although blood vessels and the flowing blood therein do not constitute a system that follows this law exactly, the relationship nevertheless exists; and particularly with small diameter vessels, such as 1 to 2 mm, a relatively small compromise of the lumen may markedly reduce flow.

Recognizing that reduced flow and stasis are of paramount importance in facilitating thrombosis, we now routinely perform a saphenous vein patch graft angioplasty in the repair of small diameter internal carotid arteries after carotid endarterectomy to ensure good blood flow at this critical site. Although we have seen a small number of acute carotid occlusions after simple arterial suture in our patients, there have been none in those with a saphenous patch graft.

In addition, we feel strongly that hypotension, particularly in the immediate postoperative period, enhances the risk of thrombosis of an arterial reconstruction, and close attention should be given to adequate blood replacement and maintenance of good cardiac output.

VESSEL WALL

The importance of the vessel wall in the pathogenesis of thrombosis cannot be overemphasized. A normal vessel wall with intact endothelium will not initiate coagulation of blood or the adhesion of platelets (18, 27). Alteration of the vessel wall, however, is almost uniformly followed by adhesion of platelets and initiation of the thrombotic sequence. This has been widely studied in many different animal models, but common to all is intimal damage (8) with exposure of subendothelial elements, the importance of which has already been discussed. Furthermore, there is evidence to suggest that injury of the arterial wall may directly release ADP from the damaged tissue to enhance thrombus formation (15).

In clinical vascular surgery there is no doubt that the vessel wall is injured in the course of the procedure. It is the magnitude of this injury which varies and which may very well determine the difference between postoperative patency and thrombosis. In larger vessels, such as the extracranial carotid artery, rough handling and overzealous application of vascular clamps and tourniquets may induce severe disruption of the wall, particularly in an atherosclerotic segment.

In vessels of smaller diameter, seemingly minor injury, such as that produced by temporary occlusion, branch coagulation, or even careful suture with microtechniques, induces significant alteration in the vessel wall and in platelet-fibrin deposition. The recognition of these changes has been greatly facilitated by the scanning electron microscope (12, 16, 20).

Suture materials are of obvious importance in vascular surgery, particularly microvascular surgery, but good results are obtained with those presently available. Although the suture itself may be thrombogenic, our own observations in the laboratory indicate that its presence in the vessel lumen and its influence on thrombosis are of secondary importance to such factors as exposed subendothelial elements and compromised flow at the surgical site (22). It should be mentioned, however, that some attempts have been made to reduce the thrombogenicity of suture, Winfrey and Foster (35) having reported success with induction of a negative electric charge to a stainless steel suture line. This has theoretical merit because the cellular constituents of blood, including platelets, have a negative charge, and their adhesion has been shown to be retarded with induction of a negative charge to the vessel wall (26).

THERAPEUTIC AGENTS

As a final consideration of factors influencing postoperative vascular patency, I will review briefly several of the many agents (30) that have been popularized as antithrombotic agents because of their supposed effect either on the formed elements of the blood or on the coagulation system. Based on our understanding of the pathophysiology of thrombosis, it seems logical that agents that alter platelet function or fibrin stabilization of the platelet mass should be effective in preventing thrombus formation. Unfortunately, this has not proven to be wholly the case.

The dextrans, particularly dextran 70 (medium molecular weight) and dextran 40 (low molecular weight), have great appeal on theoretical grounds. Among their pharmacological and clinical effects are blood volume expansion; reduction of blood viscosity, not only through hemodilution but also through reduction of red cell rigidity and aggregation; reduction of platelet adhesiveness and aggregation; and, finally, coating of red cells, platelets, and endothelium which may give them similar electric charges and cause them to repel one another (1, 4). Although there have been many reports of beneficial effects of dextran against thrombosis in vascular surgery (4), it has not proven as effective in practice as one would expect on a theoretical basis (22, 30). Furthermore, the use of dextran carries with it some risks, not the least of which is bleeding diathesis (2, 6).

In the anticoagulant group of agents we should consider dicumarol and heparin. Dicumarol can be ignored as an arterial antithrombotic agent as it has no effect on platelet function and has been shown to be relatively ineffective in preventing arterial thrombosis (14, 17, 23, 36).

Heparin is a much more effective anticoagulant than is dicumarol, probably because of its multiple effects in the coagulation cascade. Of prime importance is its activation of plasma antithrombin and the inhibitors to Factor Xa, the latter action forming the basis for the effective "minidose" heparin therapy (32, 33). Further, heparin has been shown to affect platelet function (30), in part through its antithrombin effect (33), and to enhance fibrinolysis (31). As stated by Salzman (25) heparin is the ideal agent for preventing coagulation of stagnant blood distal to vascular clamps during arterial surgery or distal to a fresh embolus until the patient is in the operating room.

In endarterectomized cat carotid arteries, we found systemic heparin anticoagulation to be highly effective in reducing postoperative thrombosis—100% effective when anticoagulation was maintained for more than 4 hours (23). Translating this to the clinical situation, on occasion in patients in whom we have been fearful of postoperative arterial thrombosis, we have administered constant intravenous heparin solution drip over several days with apparent beneficial results (22). Obviously such treatment carries with it risks of hemorrhage, particularly in the craniotomy cases, and is not routinely indicated.

Lastly regarding heparin, I would advance my purely subjective opinion that, in vascular surgery, intermittent local irrigation of the operative site with a dilute heparin solution is efficacious in reducing thrombosis. Such therapy has logic based on the local inhibition of thrombin production. Further, there is some evidence to suggest that the heparin may be taken up locally in the endothelium (13) and could therefore exert an effect after vascular repair is completed and blood flow restored.

With the knowledge that platelet adhesion and aggregation constitute the basis for thrombus formation, there has been keen interest in the past 10 years, by researchers and clinicians alike, in the ability of "antiplatelet agents" to inhibit thrombosis. A multitude of these agents have been identified (30), most notably aspirin, sulfinpyrazone (Anturane), dipyridamole (Persantine), and also prostaglandin E_1. Many studies have been carried out, some showing benefit and others not; these have been reviewed elsewhere (9, 30). As yet there is no conclusive evidence that the antiplatelet agents presently available and suitable for clinical use are capable of significantly reducing thrombosis in the clinical situation.

Approaching the problem of vascular thrombosis with a different therapeutic rationale, fibrinolytic therapy, mainly using plasminogen activators such as urokinase or streptokinase, has been investigated. Again, results have been inconclusive (24). Reduced incidence of thrombosis after experimental endarterectomy with the use of plasmin, the fibrinolytic enzyme, was reported by Whitman *et al.* (34), but plasmin therapy is considered dangerous because of hemorrhagic complications (24).

SUMMARY

In summary, we have briefly examined the pathogenesis of arterial thrombosis, the importance of vessel wall injury and alteration of blood flow in this process, and finally the rationale for use of various agents in an attempt to promote postoperative vascular patency. At present, as in the past, the most important factor toward ensuring patency after arterial reconstruction is a technically perfect operation which allows vigorous inflow and runoff and rapid linear flow (25).

REFERENCES

1. Atik, M. The uses of dextran in surgery: A current evaluation. Surgery, *65:* 548–562, 1969.
2. Berliner, A. D., and Lackner, H. Hemorrhagic diathesis after prolonged infusion of low molecular weight dextran. Am. J. Med. Sci., *263:* 397–403, 1972.
3. Burton, A. C. Physiology and Biophysics of the Circulation: An Introductory Text, Ed. 2, 226 pp. Year Book Medical Publishers, Chicago, 1972.
4. Bygdeman, S. Prevention and therapy of thromboembolic complications with dextran. Prog. Surg., *7:* 114–139, 1969.
5. Chiari. Ueber das Verhalten des Teilungswinkels der Carotis communis bei der Endarteriitis chronica deformans. Verh. Dtsch. Ges. Pathol., *9:* 326–330, 1905.
6. Data, J. L., and Nies, A. S. Drugs five years later: Dextran 40. Ann. Intern. Med., *81:* 500–504, 1974.
7. DeBakey, M. E. Successful carotid endarterectomy for cerebrovascular insufficiency: nineteen-year follow-up. J.A.M.A., *233:* 1083–1085, 1975.
8. Didisheim, P. Animal models useful in the study of thrombosis and antithrombotic agents. Prog. Hemostasis Thromb., *1:* 165–197, 1972.
9. Didisheim, P., Kazmier, F. J., and Fuster, V. Platelet inhibition in the management of thrombosis. Thromb. Diath. Haemorrh., *32:* 21–34, 1974.
10. Ferguson, G. G., and Roach, M. R. Flow conditions at bifurcations as determined in

glass models, with reference to the focal distribution of vascular lesions. *In* Cardiovascular Fluid Dynamics, edited by D. H. Bergel, Vol. 2, pp. 141–156. Academic Press, New York, 1972.

11. Goldsmith, H. L. Blood flow and thrombosis. Thromb. Diath. Haemorrh., *32:* 35–48, 1974.
12. Gregorius, F. K., and Rand, R. W. Scanning electron microscopic observations of common carotid artery endothelium in the rat. II. Sutured arteries. Surg. Neurol., *4:* 258–264, 1975.
13. Hiebert, L. M., Jaques, L. B., and Millar, G. J. The study of heparin uptake on endothelium using the Häutchen preparation of rat endothelium (abstract). Proc. Can. Fed. Biol. Soc., *16:* 83, 1973.
14. Hladovec, J. The effect of some antithrombotics on the experimental arterial thrombosis (abstract). Fourth International Congress on Thrombosis and Haemostasis, p. 492. G. Gistel & Cie, Vienna, 1973.
15. Honour, A. J., and Mitchell, J. R. A. Platelet clumping in injured vessels. Br. J. Exp. Pathol., *45:* 75–87, 1964.
16. Kawamura, J., Gertz, S. D., Sunaga, T., Rennels, M. L., and Nelson, E. Scanning electron microscopic observations on the luminal surface of the rabbit common carotid artery subjected to ischemia by arterial occlusion. Stroke, *5:* 765–774, 1974.
17. Murphy, E. A., Mustard, J. F., Rowsell, H. C., and Downie, H. G. Quantitative studies on the effect of dicumarol on experimental thrombosis. J. Lab. Clin. Med. *61:* 935–943, 1963.
18. Mustard, J. F. Hemostasis and thrombosis. Semin. Hematol., *5:* 91–106, 1968.
19. Mustard, J. F., Jørgensen, L., Hovig, T., Glynn, M. F., and Rowsell, H. C. Role of platelets in thrombosis. *In* Pathogenesis and Treatment of Thromboembolic Diseases, Thromb. Diath. Haemorrh. (Suppl.), 21: 131–158, 1966.
20. Osgood, C. P. Comparative endothelial changes following microsurgical procedures. Presented at the Microneurosurgery Symposium, Cincinnati, May 29 to 31, 1975.
21. Owren, P. A. Developments in thrombosis research. Recent Adv. Thromb., pp. 1–16, 1973.
22. Piepgras, D. G., and Sundt, T. M., Jr. Unpublished data.
23. Piepgras, D. G., Sundt, T. M., Jr., and Didisheim, P. Effect of anticoagulants and inhibitors of platelet aggregation on thrombotic occlusion of endarterectomized cat carotid arteries. Stroke, *7:* 248–254, 1976.
24. Prentice, C. R. M., and McNicol, G. P. Fibrinolytic therapy. Recent Adv. Thromb., pp. 151–179, 1973.
25. Salzman, E. W. The limitations of heparin therapy after arterial reconstruction. Surgery, *57:* 131–137, 1965.
26. Sawyer, P. N., and Harshaw, D. H. Possible relationship of ionic structure of the blood-intimal interface to intravascular thrombosis. Surgery, *56:* 846–854, 1964.
27. Spaet, T. H., and Erichson, R. B. The vascular wall in the pathogenesis of thrombosis. *In* Pathogenesis and Treatment of Thromboembolic Diseases, Thromb. Diath. Haemorrh. (Suppl.), *21:* 67–86. 1966.
28. Stein, P. D., and Sabbah, H. N. Measured turbulence and its effect on thrombus formation. Circ. Res., *35:* 608–614, 1974.
29. Szilagyi, D. E., Whitcomb, J. G., Schenker, W., and Waibel, P. The laws of fluid flow and arterial grafting. Surgery, *47:* 55–73, 1960.
30. Vermylen, J., de Gaetano, G., and Verstraete, M. Platelets and thrombosis. Recent Adv. Thromb., pp. 113–150, 1973.
31. Von Kaulla, K. N., and McDonald, T. S. The effect of heparin on components of the human fibrinolytic system. Blood, *13:* 811–821, 1958.

32. Wessler, S., and Yin, E. T. Theory and practice of minidose heparin in surgical patients: a status report (editorial). Circulation, *47:* 671–676, 1973.
33. Wessler, S., and Yin, E. T. On the antithrombotic action of heparin. Thromb. Diath. Haemorrh., *32:* 71–78, 1974.
34. Whitman, N. L., Shohl, T., and Barker, W. F. Prevention of arterial thrombosis following experimental endarterectomy with plasmin (fibrinolysin). Ann. Surg., *153:* 533–536, 1961.
35. Winfrey, E. W., III, and Foster, J. H. Prevention of arterial thrombosis with a negatively charged wire suture. Surg. Forum, *13:* 229–231, 1962.
36. Zweifler, A. J. Thrombus growth under the influence of warfarin and after abrupt reversal of its effects. Angiology, *19:* 135–140, 1968.

CHAPTER

23

Complications of Cerebral Revascularization

O. Howard Reichman, M.D.

This report is based upon a 5-year experience (August 1970 to August 1975) with surgical anastomosis between the superficial temporal artery (STA) and a cortical branch of the middle cerebral artery (MCA) in 70 patients. An effort has been made to include all instances wherein less than ideal long term results have been achieved, for in the failures of the present lie the opportunities for future progress. (However, those patients with completed stroke and fixed neurological deficit, who were operated upon to prevent further worsening of neurological function and failed to improve after surgery, have not been considered since this situation is viewed as a separate problem.)

An evaluation of suboptimal results should be prefaced by a discussion of the prevalence of risk factors and other coexisting diseases in the population under consideration.

RISK FACTORS

As precursors of cerebral vascular disease, risk factors have been considered paramount (6), and their frequency as a major factor leading to subsequent morbidity and mortality was recognized early in this experience (10).

Hypertension

In this series significant hypertension was recognized in 30 patients. Seven were considered to have severe hypertension and another seven were considered to have moderately severe hypertension. Severe hypertension was recognized as a major factor leading to the death of three patients. Cases 4 and 10 have been reported (10–12). Case 34 is reported herein.

Cardiac Disease

Significant cardiac disease was recognized in 13 patients of this series. Eleven patients had previous myocardial infarction indicated by clinical manifestations and EKG findings. Two of these demonstrated left bundle branch block, one having had prior surgery for anastomosis between an internal mammary artery and the anterior descending branch of the left coronary artery. Three patients had experienced atrial fibrillation which was under control with quinidine sulfate. One patient had rheumatic heart disease and prior mitral valvuloplasty.

Diabetes

Fourteen patients of this series had diabetes. Its medical management was not a difficult problem in most cases, but it undoubtedly contributed to the development of cerebral arterial disease.

Hyperlipoproteinemia

Abnormal lipid metabolism was demonstrated in only seven patients of this series because this laboratory determination was not performed routinely. However, it was abnormal in the young patients with isolated intracranial occlusive arterial lesions.

COEXISTING DISEASES

Patients with occlusive vascular disease were found frequently to harbor other disease processes which vitally effected their long term outcome.

Systemic Diseases

Significant chronic pulmonary disease was recognized in three patients of this series. One patient had chronic idiopathic thrombocytopenia. One patient had chronic osteomyelitis in a lower extremity. Others had evidence of mild renal disease or minor abnormalities in hepatic function.

Cancer

Two patients were demonstrated subsequently to have cancer. One died 3 months postoperatively of pancreatic carcinoma, and the other died 5 months postoperatively of pulmonary carcinoma.

Atherosclerosis of Abdominal Aorta

Two of three patients with occlusion of the abdominal aorta had symptoms of the Leriche syndrome. Another patient had undergone resection of an abdominal aortic aneurysm.

Intracranial Aneurysm

During preoperative angiography, an asymptomatic intracranial aneurysm was demonstrated in two patients. One patient had transient ischemic attacks (TIA) with mild residual dysphasia and right hemiparesis associated with stenosis of the left middle cerebral artery and recent subarachnoid hemorrhage from an aneurysm of the left internal carotid artery at its posterior communicating branch. Two patients had a giant intracranial aneurysm as the primary reason for STA-cortical MCA anastomosis.

NONFATAL COMPLICATIONS

Permanent Worsening of Neurological Status

Three patients are currently worse in comparison with their preoperative clinical status:

Case 15. Patient had a giant aneurysm of the left middle cerebral artery. An STA-cortical MCA anastomosis was performed and the middle cerebral artery ligated distal to the aneurysm. As dissection was carried medially, the aneurysm ruptured. Hemostatic measures required clipping of the internal carotid artery resulting in no available source of irrigation for the lenticulostriate vessels. Postoperatively, the patient was dysphasic and hemiplegic. Arteriography 10 days after surgery demonstrated excellent perfusion of the middle cerebral territory by the STA bypass graft.

Case 31. Patient had extensive bilateral arterial occlusive disease which was interpreted by various observers as fibromuscular dysplasia, cerebrovascular "moyamoya" disease, or both. This patient had experienced transient ischemic attacks involving both cerebral hemispheres over a 3-year period, followed by a severe left cerebral insult manifest by aphasia and right hemiplegia. The patient made substantial improvement and STA-cortical MCA anastomosis was performed. The operation was tolerated well and the patient made further improvement over several months. Arteriography, performed 6 months after surgery, demonstrated excellent flow through the STA bypass graft with extensive perfusion of the left middle cerebral territory. Because of widespread arterial occlusive disease and previous ischemic events involving the right cerebral hemisphere, the possibility of surgery on the second (right) side was considered. However, the presence of an asymptomatic aneurysm of the basilar artery raised concern that subsequent surgery, if required by the aneurysm, would be complicated by the presence of bilateral STA bypass grafts. After extensive consultation, it was decided ultimately to proceed with elective surgery to obliterate the aneurysm (14 months after STA-cortical MCA anastomosis). The operation progressed smoothly, but, for unknown reasons, the patient did not tolerate the procedure and developed aphasia with hemiplegia on the left side.

Case 45. Patient developed aphasia and right hemiplegia after a 2-month history of transient ischemic events involving the left cerebral hemisphere. Considerable improvement followed during the next few months and an arteriogram demonstrated occlusion of the left internal carotid artery. Perfusion of the left middle cerebral territory resulted from a small posterior communicating artery which was irregularly stenosed by atherosclerotic disease. Right-to-left cross filling extended to the left anterior cerebral artery but not into the left middle cerebral artery, and there was no filling from the ophthalmic artery. Because it was supposed that disease of the posterior communicating artery placed the left cerebral hemisphere in jeopardy, STA-cortical MCA anastomosis was performed. The operation was tolerated well and the patient's condition was satisfactory following surgery. However, aphasia and right hemiplegia developed the next day. Arteriography demonstrated that the posterior communicating artery had closed and there was poor filling through the STA bypass graft.

Comment: This case suggests some similarities to Case 7 reported by Ojemann and co-workers wherein a right middle cerebral stenosis became symptomatic after endarterectomy for a left internal carotid artery stenosis (7).

Temporary Worsening of Neurological Status

Three patients were worse immediately after surgery than they had been preoperatively. One had experienced temporary worsening after previous arteriography and similarly, awakened from anesthesia with significantly increased right hemiparesis and dysphasia. This improved promptly and ultimately cleared beyond the preoperative status (minimal residual). The other two patients experienced only minimally increased weakness, which possibly was related to sacrifice of penetrating branches of the cortical artery selected for anastomosis (8). Both patients improved quickly and became essentially asymptomatic.

"RIND"

Only one patient (with long standing occlusion of the left internal carotid artery) experienced transient ischemic attacks after surgery. These were infrequent, but this individual did experience a moderately severe episode of reversible ischemic neurological deficit (RIND) 5 months after surgery even though arteriography demonstrated abundant flow through the STA bypass graft.

Pulmonary Embolus

Four patients developed a pulmonary embolus after surgery. Fortunately, none of these cases resulted in mortality. The circumstances of these patients are summarized in Table 23.1. This incidence is similar to that reported by Warlow and co-workers (13) in a series following stroke. The ever present threat of pulmonary embolus is emphasized by this experience and by recent studies of the frequent incidence of deep vein thrombosis following neurosurgical procedures (1, 4, 5). Perhaps with increased facility in performing STA-cortical MCA anastomosis and reduction of operating time, the incidence of pulmonary embolus will decrease. These patients were treated initially with heparin and subsequently maintained on warfarin. Case 38 developed a subdural hematoma which became symptomatic 7 weeks after surgery (Fig. 23.1).

Subdural Hematoma

Cases 38 and 44 developed chronic subdural hematomas after surgery (Fig. 23.1). Both had received anticoagulant therapy. Drainage of the hematoma was accomplished through burr holes in each case and a prompt recovery followed.

TABLE 23.1
Pulmonary Embolus

Case No.*	Age/ Sex	Clinical Features	Angiographic Features	Clinical Results	Duration of Surgery	Interval between Surgery and Pulmonary Embolus
29	45/M	Dysphasia and right hemiparesis–20 mos. (operated large farm)	ICA stenosis (supraclinoid) MCA stenosis MCA branch occlusion (lesions on left)	Unchanged	11 hrs. 50 min. (double branch anastomosis)	14 days
38	58/M	Dysphasia and right hemiparesis–5 years (operated janitorial service)	ICA occlusion (left)	Unchanged	7 hrs. 35 min.	4 days
53†	68/F	Bilateral visual loss (counted fingers inaccurately) Insertion of Crutchfield clamp–25 days after bypass surgery (in bed several weeks as clamp was closed)	Giant ICA aneurysm (right)	Right, slight improvement (counts fingers accurately) Left, marked improvement (reads newspaper)	9 hr. 35 min. (occipital artery graft)	58 days
63	74/F	Right hemiparesis–17 days (in bed–weak right leg)	MCA stenosis (left)	Slight improvement (not ambulating)	6 hrs. 25 min.	22 days

* Cases 1–26, aspirin used for analgesia, 27–70, acetaminophen (Tylenol, McNeal Laboratories, Inc., Fort Washington, Pa.) used for analgesia.

† Placed on sulfinpyrazone (Anturane, Geigy Pharmaceuticals, Ardsley, N.Y.) at the time of bypass surgery.

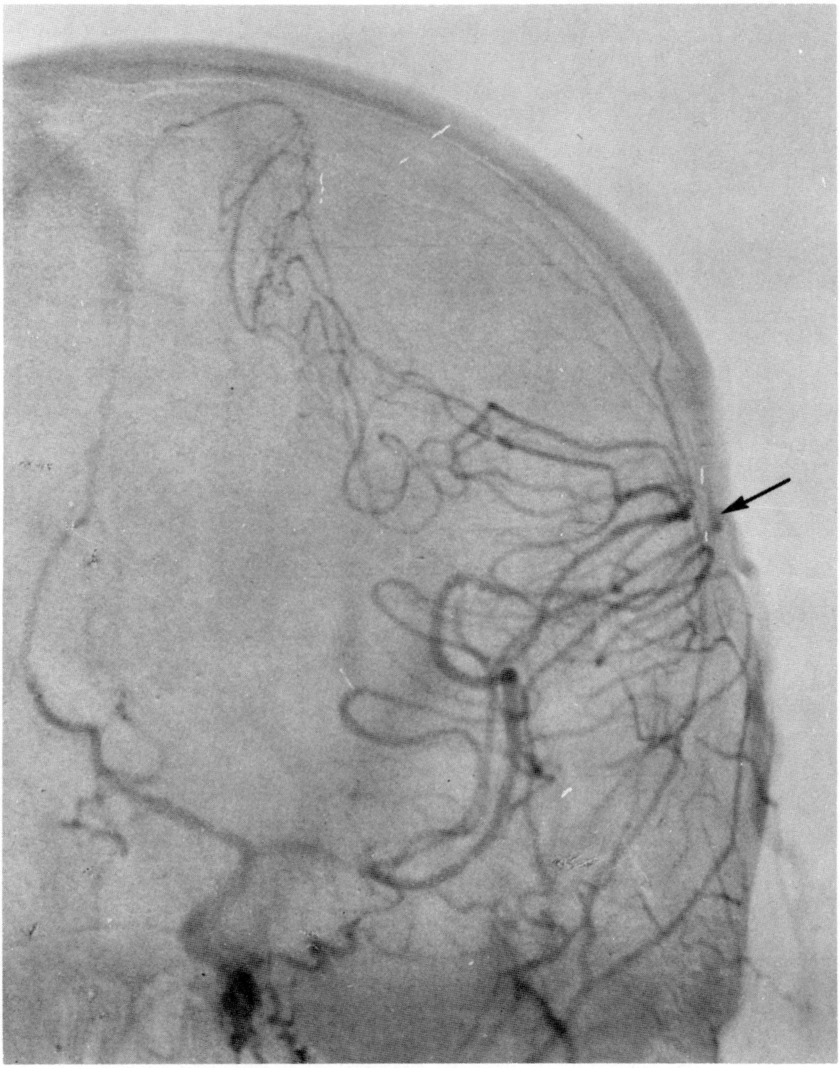

FIG. 23.1. Case 38. Frontal projection (subtraction version) of selective left external carotid arteriogram. Large avascular space over convexity of brain results from chronic subdural hematoma. Abundant left middle cerebral filling is derived from superficial temporal artery through anastomosis (arrow). Filling of internal carotid (intracranial) and anterior cerebral arteries is derived from ophthalmic and meningohypophyseal arteries. Patient had cervical occlusion of left internal carotid artery.

Seizures

Five patients experienced seizures preoperatively and again postoperatively. These cases are cited to indicate that in some individuals it is difficult, if not impossible, to distinguish between TIA and minor focal seizures. It is well known that both can result from cerebral ischemia and may coexist in the same patient. Treatment requires anticonvulsant medication in addition to the efforts designed to enhance cerebral perfusion.

Fever

One patient developed fever on the 5th postoperative day which continued for 4 days. This subsided spontaneously and no cause was identified, however, it resulted in a few additional days of hospitalization. There were no wound infections in this series.

Scalp Necrosis

Initially, when the major blood supply to the scalp was disconnected for use in developing new collateral circulation to the brain it was feared that scalp necrosis would be a frequent occurrence. Actually, this was

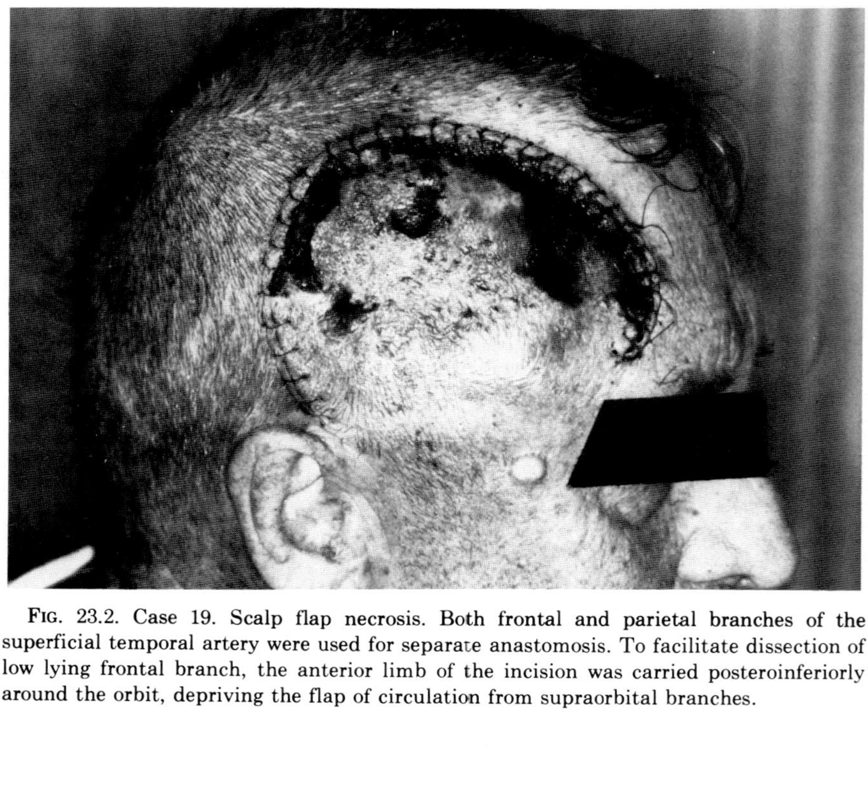

FIG. 23.2. Case 19. Scalp flap necrosis. Both frontal and parietal branches of the superficial temporal artery were used for separate anastomosis. To facilitate dissection of low lying frontal branch, the anterior limb of the incision was carried posteroinferiorly around the orbit, depriving the flap of circulation from supraorbital branches.

TABLE 23.2
Mortality

Case Number	Age/Sex	Hyper-tension	Heart Disease	Diabetes	Aortic Disease	Cause of Death	Interval Between Surgery and Death
4	60/M	+	+	+		Acute myocardial infarction	25 mos.
5	65/M				+	Brain stem ischemia	6 days
10	51/M	+			+	Acute bilateral subdural hematomas, spontaneous	17 days
27	60/F					Pulmonary carcinoma	5 mos.
30	43/M	+		+		Cerebral infarction, contralateral	2 mos.
34	57/M	+	+			Acute intracerebral hemorrhage (embolectomy of cortical artery)	1 day
37	57/M	+		+		Acute myocardial infarction	13 mos.
47	62/F	+		+		Pancreatic carcinoma	3 mos.
51	59/M		+			Acute myocardial infarction	5 mos.

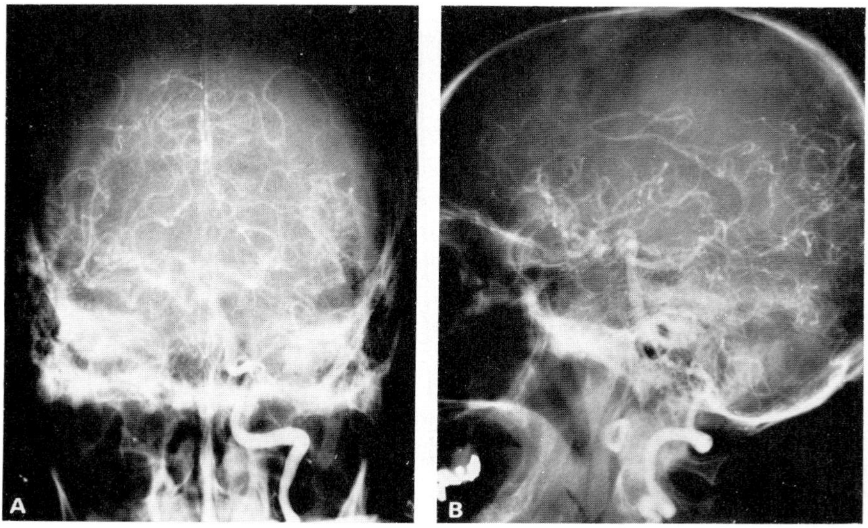

FIG. 23.3. Case 34. Selective left vertebral arteriogram. (A) Frontal projection. Bilateral middle cerebral perfusion arises from the vertebrobasilar system by posterior communicating arteries. (B) Lateral projection. Posterior communicating vessels are visualized and provide filling of middle cerebral arteries. Pericallosal filling extends anteriorly from posterior cerebral arteries.

observed in only five patients and was significant in only two. Both of these had anatomical variations in the arrangement of scalp vessels which led to the use of an unusual scalp flap. A double branch anastomosis was performed in one (Fig. 23.2). Only a single vessel was used in the other. All scalp problems healed spontaneously without the need for plastic surgery. It is thought that these problems can be avoided in the future.

Subgaleal Fluid Collection

One patient experienced subgaleal accumulation of CSF for a few weeks following surgery. This gradually subsided spontaneously.

Impaired Patency

Postoperative arteriography was performed in 42 patients (usually 5 to 8 months after surgery). All new collateral channels were patent, but poor filling was demonstrated in five patients. Two of these (Cases 8 and 12) ultimately closed (9, 11). Case 8 had adequate collateral circulation and did not require further surgery. Case 12 developed a recurrence of TIA which cleared after a second operation using the occipital artery as a

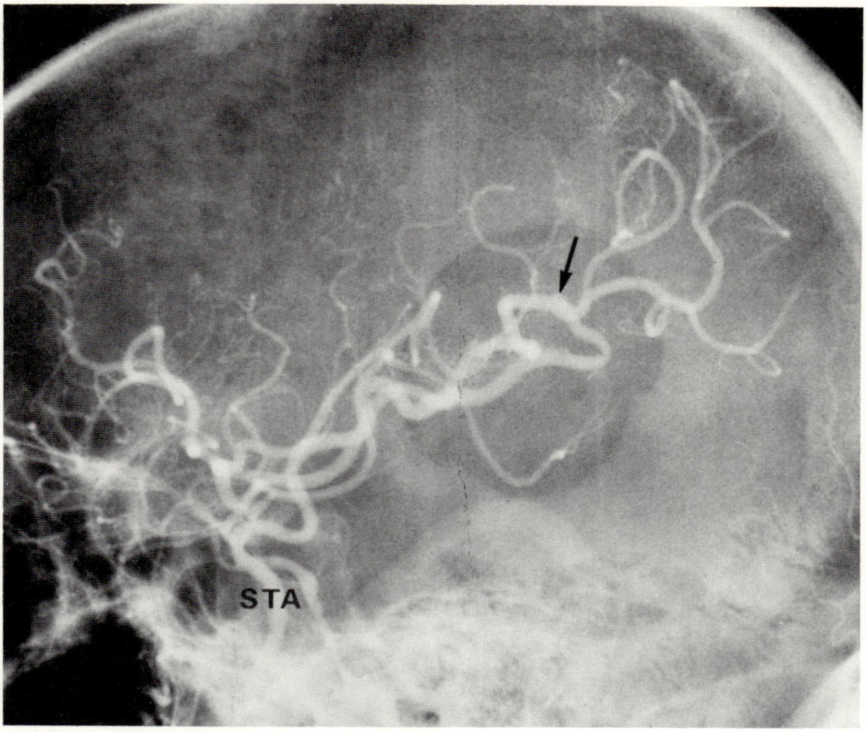

FIG. 23.4. Case 34. Lateral view of selective right external carotid arteriogram. Superficial temporal artery (STA) irrigates entire middle cerebral territory through anastomosis (arrow).

bypass graft. Excellent perfusion was subsequently demonstrated by arteriography (9).

MORTALITY

The nine deaths that have occurred in this series are summarized in Table 23.2.

Myocardial Infarction

Three patients were asymptomatic and had returned to work prior to developing an acute, fatal myocardial infarction. Case 4 expired 25 months after surgery, Case 37 at 13 months, and Case 51 at 5 months.

Cancer

A diagnosis of cancer was made postoperatively in two patients. Case 27 died of pulmonary carcinoma 5 months after surgery and Case 47 of pancreatic carcinoma at 3 months.

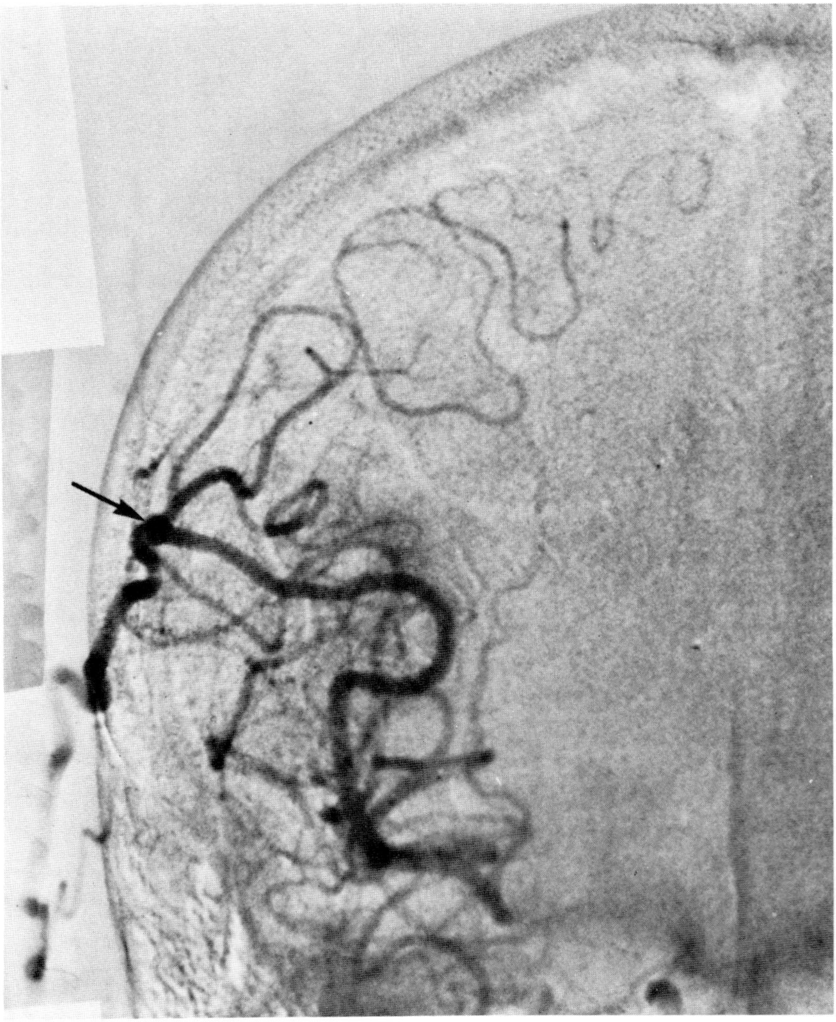

FIG. 23.5. Case 34. Frontal view (subtraction version) of selective right external carotid arteriogram. Superficial temporal artery enters cranial cavity to irrigate the middle cerebral territory through anastomosis (arrow).

Brain Ischemia

Two patients expired because of ischemia involving a region of the brain other than that served by the STA bypass graft.

Case 5 had experienced frequent transient ischemic attacks of the left cerebral hemisphere while anticoagulated with heparin. Surgery was

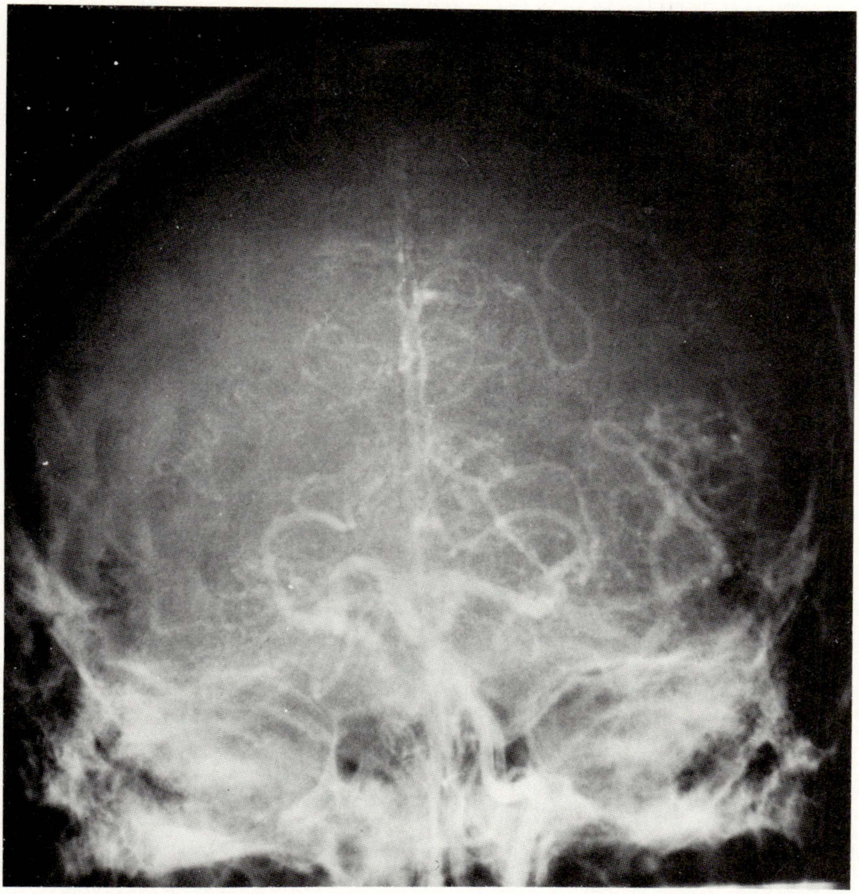

FIG. 23.6. Case 34. Frontal projection of selective left vertebral arteriogram. Significant perfusion of right middle cerebral territory is *not* present. Perfusion of the left middle cerebral territory is derived from the vertebrobasilar system.

tolerated without difficulty, but sudden death 6 days later was attributed to brain stem infarction (11).

Case 30 had dysphasia and right hemiparesis associated with left internal carotid artery occlusion. Surgery (STA-cortical MCA anastomosis) was performed on the left side and gradual improvement followed. A month later the patient became progressively lethargic and developed lack of awareness of the left side. Arteriography demonstrated poor perfusion through the STA bypass graft on the left, but normal findings on the right side. This patient had a progressive downhill course and

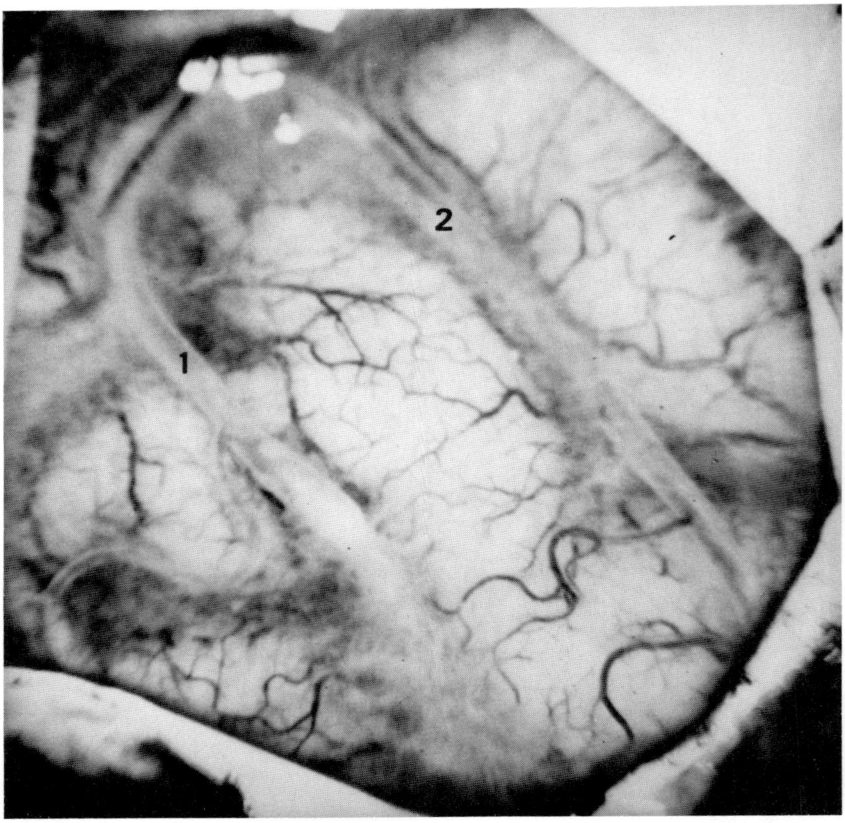

FIG. 23.7. Case 34. Operative exposure of cortical surface above left ear as viewed through operating microscope: (1) cortical artery containing embolus; (2) cortical artery selected as recipient for anastomosis.

expired a month later. Autopsy demonstrated several areas of infarction in both cerebral hemispheres, including a large, recent infarction within the right cerebral hemisphere that was considered responsible for the terminal events.

Intracranial Hemorrhage

Two patients died of intracranial hemorrhage.

Case 10 was asymptomatic following STA-cortical MCA anastomosis and had been discharged from the hospital. This patient had severe hypertension, but it was elected to treat this gradually. Seventeen days after surgery, the patient was awakened during the night with severe headache and vomited. The patient lapsed into deep coma, became decerebrate after a grand mal seizure, and expired a few hours later.

Autopsy demonstrated subdural hematoma over the superior surface of the tentorium and uniformly over both cerebral hemispheres. Thickness of the hematoma was not increased near the STA bypass graft which was not considered the source of bleeding (11).

Case 34 expired because of an acute intracerebral hemorrhage and is the only death in this series attributed to surgery. However, in addition to STA-cortical MCA anastomosis, an embolus was removed from a cortical vessel, and reflow into the ischemic brain, in the presence of severe hypertension, is considered the probable cause of hemorrhage. This case report follows.

Case 34. A 57-year-old man developed momentary weakness of his left leg during October 1973 and fell. Three days later he experienced transient numbness of his left 4th and 5th fingers. Eight days after the first episode, he developed clumsiness of his left hand

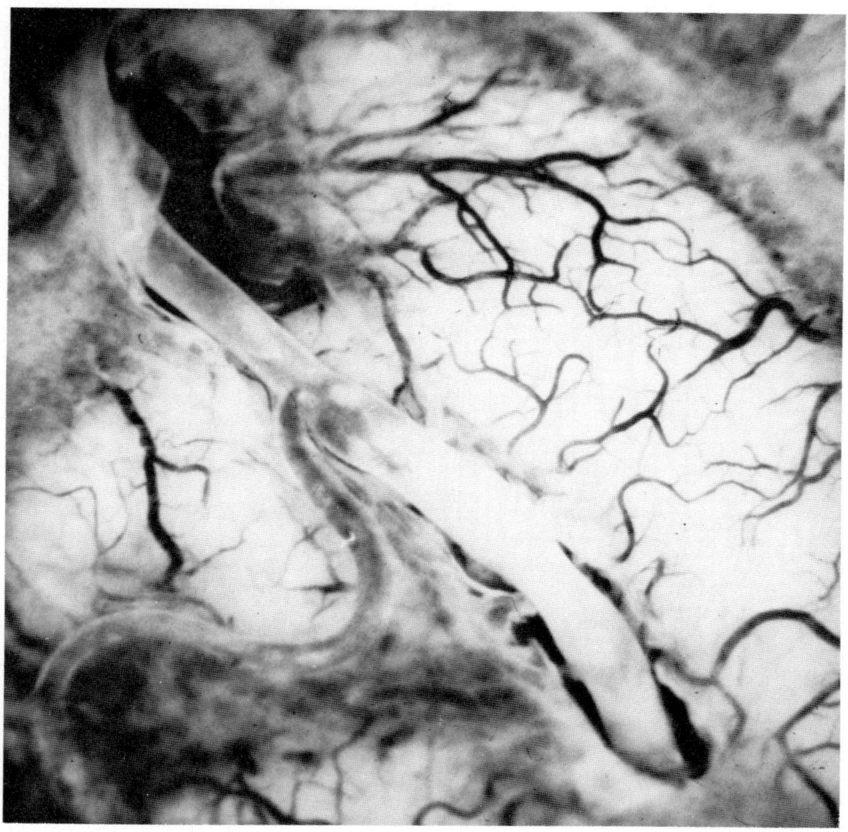

FIG. 23.8. Case 34. Higher power view of cortical artery containing embolus after dissection of arachnoidal investments.

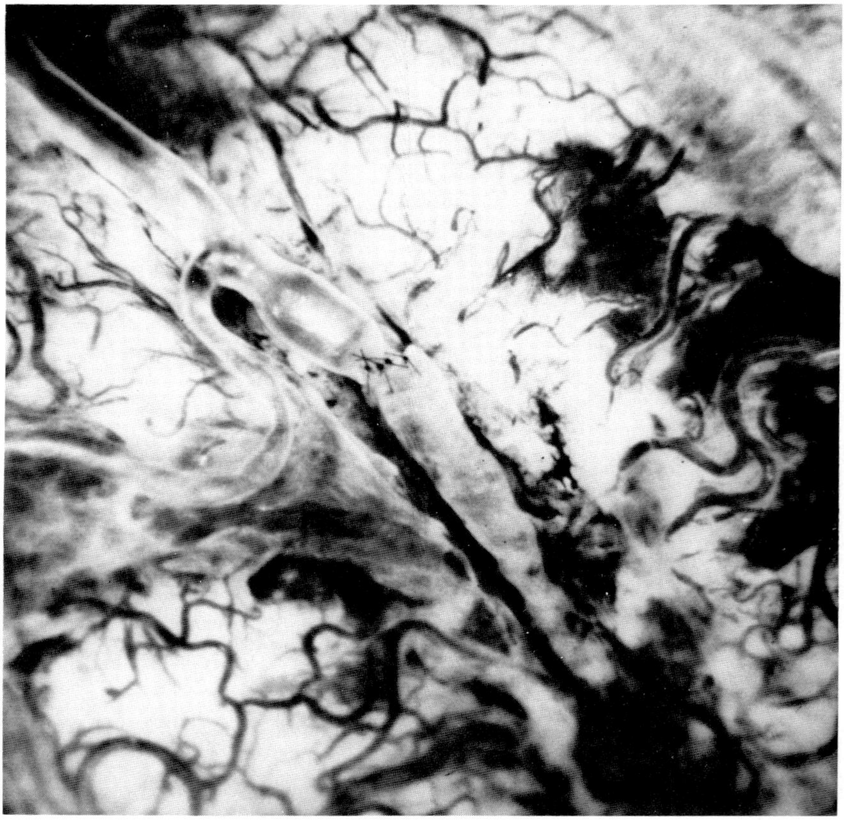

FIG. 23.9. Case 34. Flow re-established in cortical artery after removal of embolus.

and was unable to grasp a piece of paper between the thumb and index finger. This problem persisted and he noted numbness of his upper and lower lips on the left side. A week later he developed progressive numbness of his left leg and foot. During his evaluation he was shown to have chronic renal disease and hypertension. An arteriogram, performed January 4, 1974, demonstrated bilateral cervical internal carotid occlusion with some bilateral filling of internal carotid (supraclinoid) and middle cerebral arteries from the respective ophthalmic and posterior communicating arteries (Fig. 23.3).

On January 7, 1974 an STA-cortical MCA anastomosis was performed on the right side. The patient tolerated the procedure well but was hypertensive (190/110) for the next few days. The left hemiparesis gradually improved. Hypertension remained a difficult management problem because of symptoms of postural hypotension in response to treatment.

On March 12, 1974 he developed progressive numbness and weakness of his right hand and foot ("identical to prior difficulties on the opposite side"). On March 27, 1974 arteriography demonstrated that the STA bypass graft irrigated the entire right middle cerebral territory (Figs. 23.4 and 23.5). Significant contributions from the ophthalmic and posterior communicating arteries into the right middle cerebral territory were no longer visualized (Fig. 23.6). The left side appeared unchanged from the previous examination with middle cerebral perfusion derived primarily from the left posterior communicating artery (Fig. 23.6).

After considerable debate and in view of the good response to previous surgery, it was decided to proceed with a bypass graft on the second (left) side. This was performed March 28, 1974 and an excellent occipital artery was prepared for use as the graft artery. Upon exposing the cortical surface, an embolus was found occluding an angular branch of the left middle cerebral artery (Figs. 23.7 and 23.8). This filled a rather long segment of the cortical vessel and had the appearance of having been present for several days. An arteriotomy was performed, the embolus extracted, and flow re-established (Fig. 23.9). The proposed anastomosis was then accomplished between the occipital artery and another cortical branch of the middle cerebral artery. The patient tolerated the procedure well, but once again he had hypertension (250/140) postoperatively. The next morning his clinical condition was identical to that observed before surgery. However, by noon he had developed some slurring of speech and mild right hemiparesis. This gradually worsened during the day and he became comatose. He expired just before midnight. Autopsy demonstrated an enormous intracerebral hematoma beneath the surgical site (Fig. 23.10).

Comment. This case illustrates that embolization above chronic bilateral carotid artery occlusion is possible. A possible mechanism for an embolic cause of progressing stroke is retrograde propagation of thrombus with progressive occlusion of the orifices of penetrating

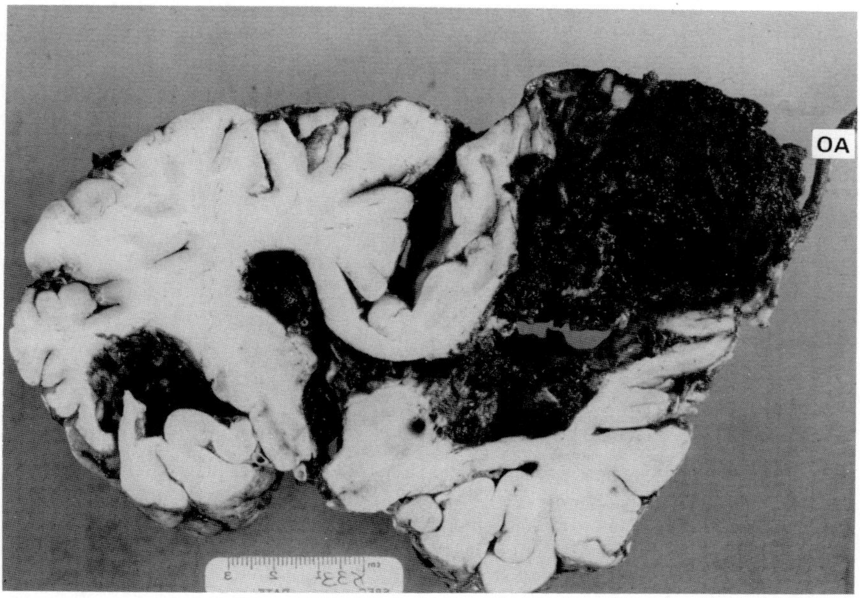

FIG. 23.10. Case 34. Cross section of brain at autopsy. Massive intracerebral hematoma lies beneath surgical site which includes occipital artery (OA) anastomosis.

branches (8). The re-establishment of flow directly into ischemic brain (particularly in the presence of hypertension) is a distinct risk as demonstrated by this case and a case of middle cerebral artery embolectomy (Case H. T.) reported by Yaşargil (14). This is the only operative mortality in this series and probably results from reflow into ischemic brain rather than STA-cortical MCA anastomosis.

CONCLUSIONS

Most patients in this series tolerated STA-cortical MCA anastomosis without difficulty and became asymptomatic. This operation is a reliable and reasonably safe method for establishing new pathways of collateral circulation to the brain. As with all neurosurgical procedures there are risks and potential complications (3). By itself, however, this operation does not pose unusual hazards and the minor problems that occurred during early development of this procedure can probably be eliminated or reduced in the future. The significance of risk factors cannot be overemphasized (6) and, if possible, they should be identified and adequately treated, particularly hypertension (2) and heart disease. The major problems experienced throughout this study have consistently occurred in the presence of complex situations resulting from generalized occlusive arterial disease, risk factors, or other coexisting disease processes. These will present a continuing challenge.

REFERENCES

1. Coppola, A. R. Deep vein thrombosis. J. Neurosurg. *43:* 510–511, 1975.
2. Freis, E. D. Effect of treatment of hypertension on the occurrence of stroke. *In* Cerebral Vascular Diseases. Ninth Princeton Conference, edited by J. P. Whisnant and B. A. Sandok, pp. 133–136. Grune & Stratton, New York, 1975.
3. Horwitz, N. H., and Rizzoli, H. V. Postoperative Complications in Neurosurgical Practice, 427 pp. Williams & Wilkins, Baltimore, 1967.
4. Joffe, S. N. Deep vein thrombosis, (Response to A. R. Coppola) J. Neurosurg., *43.* 511, 1975.
5. Joffe, S. N. Incidence of postoperative deep vein thrombosis in neurosurgical patients. J. Neurosurg., *42:* 201–203, 1975.
6. Kannel, W. B. Current status of the epidemiology of brain infarction associated with occlusive arterial disease. Stroke, *2:* 295–318, 1971.
7. Ojemann, R. G., Crowell, R. M., Roberson, G. H., and Fisher, C. M. Surgical treatment of extracranial carotid occlusive disease. Clin. Neurosurg., *22:* 214–263, 1975.
8. Penry, J. K., and Netsky, M. G. Experimental embolic occlusion of a single leptomeningeal artery. Arch. Neurol., *3:* 391–398, 1960.
9. Reichman, O. H. Extracranial-intracranial arterial anastomosis. *In* Cerebral Vascular Diseases. Ninth Princeton Conference, edited by J. P. Whisnant and B. A. Sandok, pp. 175–185, Grune & Stratton, New York, 1975.
10. Reichman, O. H., Anderson, R. E., Roberts, T. S., and Heilbrun, M. P. The treatment of intracranial occlusive cerebrovascular disease by STA-cortical MCA anastomosis. *In* Microneurosurgery, edited by H. Handa, pp. 31–46, Igaku Shoin, Ltd., Tokyo, 1975.

11. Reichman, O. H., Davis, D. O., Roberts, T. S., and Satovick, R. M. Anastomosis between STA and cortical branch of MCA for the treatment of occlusive cerebrovascular disease. *In* Reconstructive Surgery of Brain Arteries, edited by F. T. Mérei, pp. 201–218. Akadémiai Kiadó, Budapest, 1974.
12. Reichman, O. H., Satovick, R. M., Davis, D. O., and Roberts, T. S. Collateral circulation to the middle cerebral territory by anastomosis of superficial temporal and cortical arteries. *In* Present Limits of Neurosurgery, edited by I. Fusek and Z. Kunc, pp. 369–373. Avicenum, Czechoslovak Medical Press, Prague, 1972.
13. Warlow, C., Ogston, D., and Douglas, A. S. Venous thrombosis following strokes. Lancet, *1:* 1305–1306, 1972.
14. Yaşargil, M. G. Diagnosis and indications for operations in cerebrovascular occlusive disease. *In* Microsurgery Applied to Neurosurgery, edited by M. G. Yaşargil, pp. 95–119. Georg Thieme Verlag, Stuttgart, 1969.

CHAPTER

24

Complications of Carotid Endarterectomy

STEWART B. DUNSKER, M.D.

The first successful carotid endarterectomy was performed by DeBakey in 1953 (2). Since then the surgical techniques have improved and the morbidity and mortality have diminished. Yet indications for the procedure are still debated. If we accept the need for the operation, what are the complications that occur and what can be done to try to avoid them? Most discussions of complications try to compare the results of the operative and nonoperative methods in treatment of stroke, or they discuss them in general terms without revealing the incidence of most complications. Consequently, the frequency of most of these complications is unknown. In spite of that, we find that most complications involve one or more of the following:

1. General surgical principles, in exposing the vessel
2. Vascular problems: techniques of handling the artery
3. Dynamics of cerebrovascular perfusion
4. General physical condition of the patient.

Since 1968, the majority of carotid endarterectomies have been done with the aid of general anesthesia (10). This is not the place to debate the respective advantages of general and local anesthesia for carotid endarterectomies. However, I prefer to use general anesthesia because it does decrease the metabolic requirements of the brain and in most series, morbidity and mortality rates decreased when it was used (2).

PREPARATION OF THE PATIENT FOR SURGERY

Patients should be adequately hydrated. Many patients have suboptimal hydration preoperatively and in the early phase of anesthesia their blood pressure drops. In this group, with decreased cerebral and/or cardiac perfusion, a mild drop in blood pressure may be responsible for an acute stroke or myocardial infarction before the skin is scratched. In addition, these patients should not be sedated heavily with preoperative medication. The induced lethargy may produce a mild hypoxia and/or hypotension that leads to vascular occlusion.

COMPLICATIONS IN THE CERVICAL AREA

Infection

These patients often have some small hematomas from the use of anticoagulants in some phase of their operation or postoperative course. These hematomas may predispose to infection. Although cervical infections are usually eliminated rapidly by the body, in the face of vascular surgery, complications can be catastrophic. To help modify this problem, I recommend that absorbable suture be used in the deeper layers.

Hematoma

If a hematoma develops rapidly in the recovery room, pressure should be applied immediately. Re-exploration will probably be necessary. It is possible to have the trachea deviated so much by a hematoma that intubation is not possible. Therefore, it may be necessary to open the wound in the recovery room in order to maintain an adequate airway.

In my judgment, a drain will not prevent a massive hematoma from developing. If a small one forms, it is not necessary to drain it. Therefore, it is not my custom to drain the cervical wound.

Hypoglossal Paralysis

Paralysis usually develops from traction on the hypoglossal nerve and is usually reversible. Before performing the operation, it is of benefit to notice the origin of the occipital artery from the external carotid artery. To my knowledge, the hypoglossal nerve always courses around the occipital artery and is covered by the sternomastoid branch of the occipital artery. A high takeoff of the occipital artery does not guarantee that the hypoglossal nerve will cross the internal carotid that high, but a low origin will alert the surgeon to expect the nerve near the carotid bifurcation.

There are usually several small branches of the facial vein around the hypoglossal nerve. They are most easily eliminated by bipolar coagulation which will not injure the nerve.

Parotid Injury

The parotid gland may be injured during exposure of the superior portion of the internal carotid artery. This will cause a sharp pain when the patient eats sweet or sour foods. It is usually self-limited and of no major consequence.

Carotid Artery Disruption

Improper closure of the arteriotomy usually caused by not maintaining adequate tension on the continuous suture or by too much tension on the suture when the vessel is extremely thin will lead to a rupture of the suture line. This catastrophe will usually require immediate cervical compression and immediate evacuation of the hematoma.

Complications of Patch Grafts

False aneurysms are usually caused by infection of Dacron patch grafts or by improper closure. If Dacron patches are used, they should be sutured with Dacron sutures and not with silk (9).

Infection of a Dacron patch graft must usually be treated with large doses of antibiotics and replacement of the graft by a vein graft.

STROKE

The most frequent and dreaded complication of carotid artery surgery is an acute stroke which results in a new neurological deficit. Thompson (8) reported an incidence of 1.9% in 219 operations on patients with no preoperative neurological deficit. However, analysis of patients with greater risk, *e.g.*, with bilateral carotid stenosis has been more difficult to evaluate. One report even suggested that carotid endarterectomy should not be done in the face of bilateral carotid disease (1).

A general review of the literature produces conflicting information, often analyzed in different ways. Sundt and associates (7), however, published an excellent analysis of 331 carotid endarterectomies. These patients were separated into four categories (Table 24.1).

1. Neurologically stabile patients with no medical or angiographic risk, with unilateral or bilateral stenosis.
2. Neurologically stabile with no major medical risk, but with significant angiographic risks.
3. Neurologically stabile patients with major medical risks with or without significant angiographically defined risks.

TABLE 24.1
Morbidity and Mortality in Patients Undergoing Carotid Endarterectomy (7)

Group	No. of Procedures	Mortality (Myocardial Infarctions)	Morbidity		Total Morbidity and Mortality
			Myocardial Infarction	Stroke	
					%
1	129	0	0	1	1
2	56	0	0	1	2
3	76	2	3	(1)*	7
4	70	0	0	7	10

* This patient, with a cerebral infarct, also had a postoperative myocardial infarction (see text).

4. Neurologically unstabile patients with or without associated major medical or angiographically defined risks.

Medical risk factors were listed as angina pectoris, myocardial infarction of less than 6 months' duration, congestive heart failure, severe hypertension (blood pressure greater than 180/110 mm. Hg), chronic obstructive pulmonary disease, chronological age over 70 years, or severe obesity.

Neurological factors. A progressing neurological deficit of less than 24 hours' duration, frequent daily transient ischemic attacks, or neurological deficits secondary to multiple cerebral infarctions.

Angiographically defined risk factors. Occlusion of the opposite internal carotid artery, stenosis of the internal carotid artery in the siphon, extensive involvement of the vessel to be operated on with extension of the plaque greater than 3 cm. distally in the internal carotid artery or 5 cm. proximally in the common carotid artery; bifurcation of the carotid artery at the level of C-2 in conjunction with a short, thick neck and evidence of a soft thrombus extending from an ulcerative lesion.

Using these categories they showed that the patients at greatest risk were those with an unstabile neurological picture. However, they also showed, in contrast to the Joint Committee's report (1), that patients with unilateral carotid stenosis and contralateral carotid occlusion only had a morbidity rate of 2%, which is not much greater than for those with the least risk.

Strokes as complications of carotid endarterectomies can occur from both technical problems during surgery, as well as from systemic problems and from difficulties in management of the various physiological systems.

TECHNICAL INTRAOPERATIVE CAUSES

Embolization

Emboli may be dislodged from the ulcerated lesions during manipulation, dissection, or palpation of the carotid vessels. Dissection should be sharp with minimal manipulation. For this reason, it is best to occlude the internal carotid artery first.

Hypotension and Bradycardia

Hypotension and bradycardia from the carotid sinus reflex can be prevented by infiltration of the carotid wall with lidocaine. (However, I am unaware of any reports of cardiac arrest from carotid sinus manipulation during surgery.)

Inadequate Irrigation of the Artery

After the plaque has been dissected from the carotid wall, it is essential to irrigate all debris from the lumen of the vessel with heparinized saline so that none will act as emboli after the circulation is re-established. Before the final sutures are placed, the internal carotid should be unclamped to wash debris and air from the lumen. After the arteriotomy is closed, the vessels should be opened in a specific sequence. The flow is established in the external carotid system to wash any residual emboli into the external carotid before opening the internal carotid artery.

It has been suggested by both Sundt (7) and Fisher (3) that the hemorrhagic infarcts, which have been attributed to exposing infarcted brain to normal or elevated arterial pressures, are possibly due to embolization which has occurred during surgery.

Intimal Dissection Leading to Thrombosis of the Carotid Artery

If a loose tag of intima or plaque remains in the internal carotid artery, a dissection may occur. If there is any suspicion that this may occur, a 6–0 vertical suture can be used to secure the lining to prevent a dissection.

Carotid Occlusion from Inappropriate Closure

If the closure reduces the diameter of the lumen too much or if adventitia is tucked into the arterial lumen, thrombosis with resultant hemiplegia may be seen in the recovery room. If this develops, the patient should be returned to the operating room immediately for a re-exploration of the artery. Before closing this arteriotomy, an intraoperative angiogram with only a few milliliters of contrast agent may enable the surgeon to locate and remove a clot high in the carotid system before it beyond the siphon and is irretrievable.

SYSTEMIC CAUSES OF POSTOPERATIVE STROKE

Hypotension

In the presence of carotid stenosis, and certainly when one carotid system is occluded during endarterectomy, the cerebral blood flow is more dependent on systemic blood pressure. Not only should hypotension be avoided during any part of the procedure, but during occlusion of the carotid, systemic hypertension (20 to 30 mm. Hg above the patient's normal resting systolic blood pressure) should be maintained, and it should probably be maintained through the early postoperative period.

Hypotension must be avoided for several days following surgery and patients should be watched carefully when they first sit up to be sure postural hypotension does not develop.

Several authors have recommended that internal shunts be used routinely (5,7,8). Others have suggested that an internal carotid artery back pressure above 50 mm. Hg (and possibly above 25 mm. Hg) indicate that shunts are not necessary (4,6). This point and the routine use or avoidance of patch grafts to prevent postoperative occlusion have not been definitely established.

CONCLUSION

Most complications are related to difficulties in the *cervical* exposure *and embolization* from operative site and inadvertent hypotension during the procedure. The complication rate has been decreasing over the years with improved operative and anesthesia techniques. It is hoped that methods will be found in the future to reduce the risk of this surgery in the high risk patients.

REFERENCES

1. Bauer, R. B., Meyer, J. S., Fields, W. S., Remington, R., Macdonald, M. C., and Callen, P. Joint study of extracranial arterial occlusion. III. Progress report of controlled study of long-term survival in patients with and without operation. J.A.M.A., *208:* 508–518, 1969.
2. Fields, W. S., Crawford, E. S., and DeBakey, M. E. Surgical considerations in cerebral arterial insufficiency. Neurology (Minneap.), *8:* 801–808, 1958.
3. Fisher, C. M. Personal communication, 1974.
4. Hobson, R., Wright, C. B., Sublett, J. W., Fedde, C. W., and Rich, N. W. Carotid artery back pressure and endarterectomy under regional anesthesia. Arch. Surg., *109:* 682–687, 1974.
5. Howe, J. R., and Kindt, G. W. Cerebral protection during carotid endarterectomy. Stroke, *5:* 340–343, 1974.
6. Moore, W. S., Yee, J. M., and Hall, A. D. Collateral cerebral blood pressure; An index of tolerance to temporary carotid occlusion. Arch. Surg., *106:* 520–523, 1973.
7. Sundt, T. M. Jr., Sandok, B. A., and Whisnant, J. P. Carotid endarterectomy: complications and preoperative assessment and risk. Mayo Clin. Proc., *50:* 301–306, 1975.
8. Thompson, J. E. The development of carotid artery surgery. Arch. Surg., *107:* 643–648, 1973.
9. Toole, J. F., Truscott, B. L., Anderson, W. W., Aronson, P. R., Blarsdell, F. W., Dustan, H. P., Dyken, M. L., Foley, A. R., Halsey, J. H. Jr., Langfitt, T. W., Lawrence, M. S., and Mullan, J. F. Report of the joint committee for stroke facilities. VII. Medical and surgical management of stroke. Stroke, *4:* 269–320, 1973.
10. Wylie, E. J., and Ehrenfeld, W. K. *In* Extracranial Occlusive Cerebrovascular Disease; Diagnosis and Management, 231 pp. W. B. Saunders Co., Philadelphia, 1970.

CHAPTER

25

Complications of Aneurysm Surgery

KEMP CLARK, M.D.

Complications of aneurysm surgery might be best related to a system of events. These events include pre-existing diseases, complications of anesthesia, complications common to all surgical procedures, specifically neurosurgical complications, and unique complications of aneurysm surgery. The interaction of these many factors is often overlooked in defining complication rates for this type of surgery. Each will be considered independently in some detail. Exact incidence rates are hard to find; so much of information is not quantified. Additional information may be obtained from the references listed in the bibliography, many of these were chosen, not only for their primary interest, but also because of the quality of their bibliographic citations.

A number of pre-existing conditions may produce significant increase in operative risks which are independent of the operation *per se*. They are to be taken in account in determining the clinical grade of the patient (10). For instance, a diagnosis of arteriosclerotic heart disease increases the operation risk twofold (48). Certain cardiac arrhythmias, particularly conduction blocks, require attention. Prophylactic demand pacing prior to anesthesia may be required in certain patients (10, 57).

Evaluation of pulmonary function preoperatively is another important means of reducing operative mortality and morbidity. Postoperative pulmonary complications may be expected in about 5% of all operations (10, 85). If a patient smokes, the incidence is even higher. The most useful test in evaluating pulmonary function is the maximal expiratory flow rate (MEFR). The presence of CO_2 retention is a positive contraindiction to surgery (77, 85).

Age is certainly a pre-existing condition. Aneurysm surgery in the elderly has been the subject of very few specific reports. It would appear that the significant dimension is "physiological" age as opposed to "chronological" age. The problem is to measure the first and ignore the second. One report, specifically dealing with 41 individuals 60 years or older, reports a 24% mortality and a 7% morbidity rate for good risk patients (4). Pool speaks specifically to the problem in reporting eight patients over 50 with anterior communicating artery aneurysms (63). He had only four excellent results, two poor, and one death in the group.

As expected, aneurysm surgery in children is well tolerated. The incidence is low in this age group. Surgical experience indicates a mortality rate of 15%. In this series, reported by Matson, one operative patient had a hemiparesis, and two were retarded with anterior communicating aneurysms out of a total of 14 cases (47).

Another unique pre-existing condition is pregnancy. Here, two lives are at a risk, the mother's and the child's. It would appear that aneurysmal rupture is more likely to occur in the last 10 weeks of gestation and is associated with a lower fetal mortality than maternal subarachnoid hemorrhage from an arteriovenous malformation. Furthermore, patients with proven intracranial aneurysms have carried a child through gestation and labor with normal delivery and no recurrence of the hemorrhage. This says something about our knowledge of the precipitating and contributing factors to aneurysm rupture (67). Still, if rupture occurs during pregnancy, it seems clear that operative intervention is superior to conservative therapy, if possible to operate. Forty-seven per cent of mothers treated conservatively died, while none died in the operative group in two series in the literature (66, 67). Individual case reports support this (12).

Obviously, aneurysm surgery is done under anesthesia (46). This, in itself, carries a significant risk. This risk increases with the more complex types of anesthesia, for instance, profound hyperthermia with or without cardiac arrest (20, 49). Because of this problem, plus question of its real efficacy, hypothermia has fallen into disuse (25). The use of agents, like the fluorinated hydrocarbons (halothane), produce a rise in the intracranial pressure (34). These agents should be restricted to cases of normal intracranial pressure. Technical complications of anesthesia such as poorly placed endotrachial tubes, inadequate ventilation, reduction of cerebral blood flow by over vigorous hyperventilation, and infections about the sites of insertion of monitoring devices represent complications of the anesthesia. The use of arterial blood gas determinations will help avoid the more serious ones.

The use of hypotensive anesthesia has proven a great benefit to aneurysm patients (1, 29, 46). The ease and safety of manipulation of the aneurysm under these conditions is well known. Yet, in the face of profound hemorrhagic shock, this technique is dangerous. Only agents producing hypotension with short reversal times should be employed. Nitroprusside, given by a central venous catheter, is the optimal means of producing and maintaining hypotension (79). This technique allows rapid dispersion of the drug through the body, so that titration can be more safely done. Nitroprusside has a ratio of toxic to therapeutic dose of about 4:1, so this careful titration is very crucial. The maximal infusion rate should be 6 mg. per min. or 120 mg. per hr. to a maximal dose of 3 mg. per kg. Should resistance to the drug occur, or acidosis develop, the drug should be discontinued immediately (5).

Certain complications of aneurysm surgery, obviously, are the identical ones to any major surgical operation. Here, the problem of postoperative thrombophlebitis, and more ominously, pulmonary embolism (75), rests.

The incidence of deep venous thrombosis in neurosurgical cases has been studied and found to be 43%, if sophisticated means such as I^{125} labeled fibrogen technique is used. This is confirmed with the Doppler ultrasound method. In this series, only one patient out of ten showed the classic physical findings of calf tenderness and pedal edema (35).

Patients undergoing craniotomy are placed in a stressful state. As high as 7% of patients with intracranial pathology may develop stress ulceration (37). The mechanism and prevention still escapes us (9).

Problems of fluid and electrolyte balance must be recognized. The nutritional requirements of the surgical patients must be met (73).

Certain complications may reside in the "neurosurgical" part of the operation as opposed to that related to specifically dealing with the aneurysm. Infection of the scalp, bone flap, meninges, or brain, may occur. An incidence rate of from 0.1% to 9% has been reported. The age of the patient, the duration of surgery, and the requirement for reopening the wound clearly increase the rate. The use of ultraviolet light in the operating room reduces it. The use of postoperative or local antibiotics does not influence the rate (84).

Postoperative hemorrhage with hematoma formation is an infrequent, but feared, complication. The exact incidence is difficult to obtain (78). In our experience in aneurysm surgery, it is about 0.2%.

Dissection in and around the mesial sylvian fissure, or under the temporal lobe, may produce severe and lasting neurological deficits by interfering with blood flow through the lenticulostriate arteries (61). Overly vigorous retraction of the brain may occlude the arterial blood supply to a part of the brain. This may result in neurological deficit or it may enhance postoperative edema. Cranial nerves may be damaged in the dissection or exposure. The use of small bone flaps, placed low, and dissection in the subarachnoid space will help reduce this problem (40). Osmotic diuretic agents and hyperventilation anesthesia techniques to reduce brain bulk facilitate exposure.

The subarachnoid hemorrhage, itself, may produce complications which may not be apparent until the postsurgical period. Communicating hydrocephalus due to blood in the cerebrospinal fluid pathways may occur in as many as one-quarter of the cases (22, 74). The only complication in this group is either the failure to recognize, or to treat, the hydrocephalus.

Subarachnoid hemorrhage may, itself, produce cardiac arrhythmias. Rarely do these become troublesome, but it should be appreciated that treatment may be needed. Intravenous lidocaine by slow drip or procainamide hydrochloride by mouth should be used. Monitoring of the heart rhythm is needed when using these drugs.

Subarachnoid hemorrhage may produce changes in the patient's electrolyte balance. This is probably due to injury to the hypothalamic pituitary axis. Whether this is direct, or indirect, is not clear. Certainly, inappropriate antidiuretic hormone secretion has been reported as well as other less clearly defined abnormalities (36, 40, 41).

One final comment about the effects of the aneurysmal rupture on the ultimate end result seems in order. The jet of arterial blood produces a rise in intracranial pressure as well as focal damage to surrounding brain. Either may result in death or disability to the patient. We have learned, through evaluation of the clinical grade of the patient, to operate, or not, on certain patients. What we yet do not know is the effect the initial hemorrhage has on the ultimate quality of survival. Few studies have dealt with this problem directly. Two studies seem to indicate, that this, rather than operation, may be a major force in determining outcome (58, 71, 72). As discussion of specific aneurysms, in terms of operative morbidity occurs, this point must be kept in mind.

The specific complication of the surgery for the aneurysm deserves comment. This might be best divided into complication of timing of surgery, complication due to the surgical approach, and local complications at the aneurysm site.

There has been much discussion about the timing of aneurysm surgery (28, 30, 31, 37, 38, 44). Most authors seem to agree that the procedure is best done about 5 to 10 days after the hemorrhage. This waiting period is designed to allow resolution of cerebral swelling, to make exposure easier, and yet be short of the time of maximal rebleeding. Recently, the use of epsilon-amino caproic acid has been suggested as a way to lengthen this waiting time (54, 63, 64). Complications, including rebleeding, are associated by its use (76). The real question is, what is the waiting period for? The patient remains at risk of rebleeding: a preventable complication. If the clinical grade is I or better, and in certain lower grades with normal spinal fluid pressure, early operation is indicated (38).

Classification of patients by grade has proven a most worthwhile step in reducing mortality and morbidity in aneurysm surgery (67). The frequent mistake made is that of failure to grade the patient accurately. The surgeon must be extremely accurate in his clinical appraisal of the patient. Mistakes may mean a 4-fold increment in operative mortality alone (30, 31).

The surgeon's approach to an aneurysm may be another source of complication. Because of time and space limitations, plus a personal lack of experience, the more exotic forms of aneurysm surgery, such as stereotaxic coagulation, magnetically induced intravascular thrombosis, or piloinjection will be ignored (2, 23, 54–56). Nor will carotid ligation be considered, as it is an operation of predominately historic interest; useful only for the rare infraclinoid or ophthalmic artery aneurysm. Its complication rate is too high for routine use (26, 69, 82). Treatment of an aneurysm requires its obliteration from the circulation as the sole criterion of success.

However, a direct approach may produce specific complications. For instance, aneurysms lying at the tip of the basilar artery may be approached transtentorially. This approach has two prominent complications; one, hydrocephalus due to the arachnoidal adhesions produced, and two, damage to the IVth cranial nerve.

It is possible to operate on the wrong aneurysm. Identification of the proper, bleeding aneurysm is the major reason for careful cerebral angiography. When multiple aneurysms exist, it is usually the larger, the more ragged in appearance, with a definite teatlike projection, with spasm in the parent vessel, has a focal hematoma present, or has focal neurological deficit appropriate to its location, that has ruptured (83).

More specifically, once the bone flap is turned, problems of surgery for aneurysms arise during the dissection of the aneurysm. It may rupture or bleed. There is a difference. Rupture means a massive rent in the sac with violent and profuse hemorrhage. The exact incidence of this is hard to define, but it leads to significant mortality or morbidity (60). Control of a ruptured aneurysm during operation requires a cool head, a lot of suction, and careful application of a clip under direct vision. The surgeon, then, must make sure the aneurysm is secure and that no other vascular structure has been injured.

Bleeding from an aneurysm is a different matter. This results from a small hole made during dissection in the fundus. This is easily controlled by fibrin foam, oxycel gauze, a clip, or cottonoid patty. This happens, in our experience, in about 10% of the cases. The important point is not to panic and convert a bleed into a rupture, and then on to calamity. Hypotensive anesthesia, particularly with nitroprusside, has sharply reduced this complication.

Once dissection is complete, problems may still arise. The surgeon may place the clip or the ligature incompletely across the neck of the aneurysm (14), which may prove ineffectual (6, 19). The surgeon may place the clip across a parent or neighboring vessel resulting in neurological deficit, or even death.

Prevention or reduction of the incidence of both these complications is accomplished by two maneuvers. First, aneurysm surgery should be done using magnification provided by the operating microscope. The illumination and varying degrees of magnification provided render it superior to loupes and a headlight (88). Surgery for aneurysms without magnification, like elephant hunting with a black powder musket, is foolhardy.

The other tactic we recommend to avoid these complications is intraoperative angiography (42, 80, 81). This has virtually eliminated the inadvertent occlusion of a parent vessel or a failure to completely obliterate the aneurysm. We cannulate the superficial temporal artery during the craniotomy exposure. When the aneurysm is clipped, a single shot angiogram is made. The aneurysm site is visualized, and it is easy to determine the state of affairs. It requires about 5 minutes to place the catheter. This seems a reasonable period to prevent neurological deficit and to be sure the job is properly done while amends can still be made. It also reduces the need for postoperative angiography, as it correlates very well with later angiography (3).

Occasionally an aneurysm has no clippable neck. Here the surgeon is faced with one of two choices. The aneurysm may be wrapped with something: muslin, muscle, methylmethacrylate, and a variety of "glues" (7). Ethyl 2-cyanoacrylate seems to be the most popular, currently. It seems clear that muscle is the poorest choice of a material to invest the aneurysm (51). For the unwary, or inexperienced aneurysm surgeon, this maneuver requires extensive dissection of the entire aneurysm, a feat not easy to accomplish, and apposition of the materials to the entire aneurysm, also not an easy task. If the surgeon fails in either of the tasks, the aneurysm may rupture through the uncoated, untreated part at some time in the future. Failure rates ranging between 1% and 20% are reported with various agents (7).

An alternative is to make a neck by electrocoagulation of the aneurysm at the parent vessel with the bipolar cautery forceps. This produces a frightening change in the fundus of the aneurysm. It becomes redder and seems to swell. Rupture has occurred after coagulation, so the surgeon should proceed with the definitive application of a clip promptly after coagulation (88). Certain specific aneurysms have their own unique problems. Specific sites of aneurysms must be considered in a discussion of mortality and morbidity statistics. Because of the large number of cases documented in the Cooperative Study of Subarachnoid Hemorrhage and Aneurysms, these figures will be used as to the incidence, nonsurgical mortality and morbidity, and the operative result reported at that time. Other figures will be given from selected series in the literature.

Internal carotid artery aneurysms occurred in 38% of the series (69). The natural mortality and morbidity figures were 39% and 54% respectively with 12% of the conservatively treated patients severely handicapped. The surgical mortality was 38% over-all, 18% in good risk cases with a morbidity of 33%, of which 24% were severe. Lougheed and Marshall reported a surgical mortality of 9% in alert patients and 10% in good risk patients. Morbidity figures are 7% and 21% respectively (45). Peerless reported a 13.5% mortality rate and a 12% morbidity rate (62). Norlen reported a 2.8% operative death rate with an identical figure for disability (63).

The above figures are largely for posterior communicating artery aneurysms. All aneurysms on the carotid artery are not so simple. Three specific aneurysmal sites are much more prone to be troublesome. Carotid-ophthalmic artery aneurysms are the first in this troublesome group. The technical problem here is the limited space available for maneuver. The optic nerve, the anterior clinoid process, and the cavernous sinus are all in the way. The results indicate the problem. Drake and associates reported 11 cases, four of which were unruptured with three deaths after intracranial surgery. Four patients survived, treated by carotid ligation (17). Guidetti and La Torre reported surgery in 24 cases with only five deaths, and four complications (24). However, in 13 cases of aneurysmal neck occlusion were two of the deaths and two of the complications. In seven cases of intracranial trapping, three patients died, and two had complications. Our experience in five cases of this aneurysm is no better; two successfully ligated intracranially, one by carotid ligation, and two requiring coating. One patient died and one has some visual loss. Kothandaram and associates reported 19 cases, four of which were untreated, five treated with carotid ligation, and 10 by craniotomy. Of the four untreated cases, two had good results, one poor and died of hemorrhage 3 years later. Of the ten craniotomy patients, six had good results, two poor, and two died from the operation (39).

Carotid choroidal aneurysms are another challenge. Drake has reported seven cases, three of whom died after intracranial surgery, and only two had excellent results (18). We have treated one such aneurysm with an excellent result. The important thing is to recognize the exact origin and spare the choroidal artery.

The third is the carotid bifurcation aneurysm. The problem is to get enough exposure to define the usually broad necked aneurysm without

(1) producing a manipulation hemiplegia, and (2) get a clip across the aneurysm without involving a major vessel. We have dealt with four such aneurysms. One patient had an infected bone flap, the others did well. Sengupta and associates reported nine cases without mortality, but two cases developed complications (71).

Middle cerebral artery aneurysms have posed challenging problems to neurosurgeons. They comprise 21% of all aneurysms. The Cooperative Study indicates a "natural" mortality of 36% with an operation mortality of 20%. Morbidity figures are 80% of the survivals in the nonoperative group being disabled, 30% being very disabled. Operative statistics are 52% disabled and 34% severely so (69).

Krayenbuhl, Yasargil, Flamm, and Tew reported on 48 middle cerebral artery aneurysms; five died, eight had a poor result, and 35, a good outcome from surgery (40). Norlen reported 65 cases with an operative mortality of 3%, and 65% of the patients had full working capacity (58). Peerless found his experiences to have a 7% mortality and a 14% morbidity rate from intracranial approach to these aneurysms (62). Lougheed and Marshall reported 49 patients in excellent preoperative condition. Their results were three operative deaths, six fair results, and 40 excellent results. They contrasted this to 35 cases in fair condition. The results were three deaths, two bad results, nine fair, and 21 excellent. Thirty-one patients were classed as bad preoperatively by their criteria. Only five had an excellent result, a significant point for relating the grade of the patient preoperatively with the ultimate outcome (45). Robinson reported 55 Grade I patients with a mortality of 9.1% and a 69% good quality of survival. He also reported three patients who died of subsequent subarachnoid hemorrhage (SAH) after wrapping of the middle cerebral aneurysm with muscle (68).

Anterior communicating artery aneurysms present as a major surgical challenge. The anatomy of this complex makes it possible to occlude a variety of parent and adjacent vessels with devastating effects. The location of the anterior communicating artery makes exposure difficult and hazardous as indicated by the number of approaches to these lesions. These are bifrontal, through mesial frontal lobe, through the gyrus rectus, unilaterally with subarachnoid space, stereotaxically, and transsphenoidally (21, 27, 55, 63, 86, 88).

The Cooperative Study indicates an incidence of 30%, a natural mortality of 42%, and corresponding morbidity of 57% with 13% being severely handicapped. These figures support those of Sengupta and associates in pointing out the importance of the initial bleed in determining morbidity (69). In the Cooperative Study, a surgical mortality of 35% was reported but was 20% in good risk patients. A surgical morbidity was 40% with 30% severely handicapped (69).

Norlen reported 43 patients with occlusion of the "stalk of the aneurysm" by surgery. He had a 0% mortality and 77% of his patients returned to full employment. It must be remembered that most of these patients were operated more than 2 weeks after their hemorrhage. Still, this is a remarkable series (58, 59). Lougheed and Marshall reported on 158 ACA aneurysms operated upon with 19% mortality in all grades. Of more importance are the 71 cases in excellent condition, 52 of whom had an excellent result, seven died, and seven had a bad result. Of their 40 "bad" patients pre-operatively, only ten had an "excellent" result, while 15 had a bad result, and 12 died (45).

Pool, in 1961, reported on 23 cases with three deaths, and 16 excellent results (63). French and Ortiz-Suarez have reported 97 patients with anterior cerebral artery (ACA) aneurysms. Their over-all mortality for surgery in patients of all clinical grades was 14.4%. However, for patients in Grades I through III, the mortality rate fell to 10.6%. Of their patients, 75 in all, only seven were disabled (21). VanderArk, Kempe, and Smith reported on 100 patients operated through the gyrus rectus approach. Five patients died, 28 returned to full military duty, 46 with some restriction. Only 21 had to be retired for disability. More importantly, all 35 Grade I patients returned to duty (86). Krayenbuhl, Yasargil, Flamm, and Tew reported on 95 ACA aneurysms with an operative mortality of 3% and good results in 86% (40).

Tindall has summarized the use of proximal anterior cerebral artery ligation for this aneurysm. First popularized by Logue, a number of patients have been treated by this method (11, 43). It offers some theoretical advantages and is technically easier than direct surgery. However, the results are not good. Tindall summarized 282 cases from the literature; 66 patients died, and 14 of the survivors had suffered a recurrent SAH by the time of this report (80). We have one patient treated by this technique. He is mentally severely disturbed which he was not, prior to surgery.

Aneurysms of the distal anterior cerebral are rare but can be a challenge. We have had experience with five such cases, all had successful intracranial obliteration of the aneurysm without complication, save two. Here, the aneurysm was densely adherent to the falx and required coating with ethyl 2-cyanoacrylate. One aneurysm was treated by ligation of the neck. The patient had a stormy postoperative course, secondary to diffuse vasospasm.

Yasargil reported 13 pericallosal aneurysms with nine patients working and well, three patients have a hemiparesis severe enough to be disabled, and one of these patients developed hydrocephalus as well. He has had one death due to recurrent SAH (87).

Aneurysms of the vertebral basilar system are notoriously difficult. The incidence is 3% of all aneurysms. The Cooperative Study showed a mortality of 45% and a morbidity of 33% from such lesions (69). Jamieson's initial report of surgical treatment of 20 patients disclosed a surgical mortality of 10 patients, or 50%. Morbidity was also 50% in the survivors, one patient dying late, three patients had cranial nerve deficit, and one other, a hemiparesis severe enough to prevent full employment. Since he included four cases of posterior cerebral aneurysms (one death), eight basilar tip aneurysms (five deaths), three basilar trunk aneurysms (two deaths), and five vertebral aneurysms (two deaths), this early report covers the posterior fossa (32). He, subsequently, reported nine additional cases with two deaths, four patients returned to full employment, and one to partial employment (33). The deaths were in aneurysms of the basilar artery. Chou and Ortiz-Suarez reported 20 basilar bifurcation aneurysms with six deaths and six poor results. The other eight patients are in good to excellent condition. They also reported 13 other aneurysms in the posterior fossa. These included three on the posterior cerebral artery (one postoperative complication of hemiparesis), five basilar trunk aneurysms (one death, most of these aneurysms were treated by coating), and five vertebral artery aneurysms (two deaths) (8).

Drake has had extensive experience in dealing with these aneurysms. His earlier reports are less optimistic than his later ones (15, 16). In 1974, he summarized his experiences with these lesions. He has operated on 88 tip of the basilar artery aneurysms; seven are dead, 22 had a poor result; trunk of basilar aneurysms, 52, with four dead and nine poor results; vertebral artery aneurysms, 21, with three dead, and the rest, good results. This represents a total experience of 161 posterior fossa aneurysms with an operative mortality of 14 cases and a morbidity of 31 patients (13).

After a successful operation, even if all goes well, the patient still faces the most dreaded complication of all: vasospasm. Despite comments to the contrary, we don't doubt its existence or its significance (50). Reams of paper, hour on hour of prospective, retrospective, and laboratory research has been put on this problem. Everytime a light has been seen at the end of the tunnel, it has turned to be a barred window, and the tunnel continues on, dark and inscrutable as ever. This is not the place to review current theories on vasospasm (65). It is a real entity; it leads to cerebral infarction and death; it is unpredictable in time of occurrence; and it is unpreventable and untreatable. Of all the complications discussed, it alone is the major worry in discussing surgery with patients. It must relate to the initial rupture and be triggered by it in some way. To support that statement, a current review of our experience with 46 unruptured aneurysms showed no vasospasm occurred in any patient after intracranial clipping of the aneurysm (70). Others have noted identical experiences (51–53). Finally, be dissuaded from the concept that, if something goes wrong, it must be the surgeon's fault. That is not the point. Complications are not automatically an indication of a careless surgeon. In trying to apply the most efficacious and appropriate therapy, misadventures occur. We hail success but must acknowledge the contribution of failure. As Wilder Penfield so eloquently stated as a modern surgeon's addition to the Hippocratic oath, "I will faithfully record and analyze my failures in the care of the sick, seeking cause so that those who follow may be warned of danger." (61). This larger view is graphically represented by the topics discussed here.

REFERENCES

1. Aitken, R. R., and Drake, C. G. A technique of anesthesia with induced hypotension for surgical correction of intracranial aneurysms. Clin. Neurosurg., *21:* 107–114, 1974.
2. Alksne, J. F., and Rand, R. W. Current status of metallic thrombosis of intracranial aneurysms. *In* Progress in Neurological Surgery, edited by H. Krayenbuhl P. E. Maspes, and W. H. Sweet, Vol. 3 pp. 212–229, Year Book Medical Publishers, Chicago, 1969.
3. Allcock, J. M., and Drake, C. G. Postoperative angiography in cases of ruptured intracranial aneurysms. J. Neurosurg., *20:* 752–759, 1963.
4. Amacher, A. L., and Drake, C. G. Aneurysm surgery in the seventh decade. *In* Present Limits of Neurosurgery, edited by I. Fusch and Z. Kunc, pp. 263–266. Elsevier, Amsterdam, 1972.
5. Beyers, C. W. Personal Communication, 1975.
6. Bonnal, J., and Stevenaert, A. Thrombosis of intracranial aneurysms of the Circle of Willis after incomplete obliteration by clip or ligature across the neck. J. Neurosurg., *30:* 158–164, 1969.
7. Chou, S. N., and Ottiz-Suarez, H. J., and Brown, W. E. Technique and materials for coating aneurysms. Clin. Neurosurg., *21:* 182–193, 1974.
8. Chou, S. N., and Ortiz-Suarez, H. J. Surgical treatment of arterial aneurysms of the vertebrobasilar circulation. J. Neurosurg., *41:* 671–680, 1974.
9. Clark, K. Stress ulceration. Clin. Neurosurg., *18:* 426–440, 1971.
10. Clark, K. Pre- and post-operative care of the neurosurgical patient. *In* Advances in Neurology, edited by R. Thompson, and J. R. Green. Raven Press, New York, in press.
11. Cook, A. W., Dooley, D. M., and Browder, E. J. Anterior communicating aneurysms. Treatment by ligation of an anterior cerebral artery. J. Neurosurg., *23:* 371–374, 1965.
12. Davey, L. M., Fiorito, J. A., and Hehre, F. W. Intracranial aneurysm in late pregnancy. J. Neurosurg., *23:* 542–546 1965.
13. Drake, C. G. The surgical treatment of vertebrobasilar aneurysms. *In* Recent Progress in Neurological Surgery, edited by K. Sano, and S. Ishii, pp. 183–190. American Elsevier, New York, 1974.
14. Drake, C. G., and Allcock, J. M. Post-operative angiography and the "slipped" clip. J. Neurosurg., *39:* 683–689, 1973.

15. Drake, C. G. Management of aneurysms of posterior circulation. *In* Neurological Surgery, edited by J. R. Youmans, Chap. 34, W. B. Saunders Co., Philadelphia, 1973.
16. Drake, C. G. The surgical treatment of vertebrobasilar aneurysms. Clin. Neurosurg., *16:* 114–169, 1969.
17. Drake, C. G., Vanderlinden, R. G., and Amacher, A. L. Carotid ophthalamic aneurysms. J. Neurosurg., *29:* 24–31, 1968.
18. Drake, C. G., Vanderlinden, R. G., and Amacher, A. L. Carotid choroidal aneurysms. J. Neurosurg., *29:* 32–36, 1968.
19. Drake, C. G., and Vanderlinden, R. G. The late consequences of incomplete surgical treatment of cerebral aneurysms. J. Neurosurg., *27:* 226–238, 1967.
20. Drake, C. G., Barr, H. W. K., Coles, J. C., and Gergely, N. F. The use of extra corporeal circulation and profound hypothermia in the treatment of ruptured intracranial aneurysm. J. Neurosurg., *21:* 575–581, 1964.
21. French, L. A., and Ortiz-Suarez, H. J. Anterior communicating artery aneurysms: Technique of operation and results. Clin. Neurosurg., *21:* 115–119, 1974.
22. Foltz, E. L., and Ward, A. A., Jr. Communicating hydrocephalus from subarachnoid bleeding. J. Neurosurg., *13:* 546–566, 1956.
23. Gallagher, J. P. The closure of intracranial aneurysms by piloejection. *In* Intracranial Aneurysms and Subarachnoid Hemorrhage, edited by W. S. Fields, and A. L. Sahs, pp. 444–458, Charles C Thomas, Springfield, Ill. 1965.
24. Guidetti, B., and La Torre, E. Mangaement of carotid ophthalamic aneurysms. J. Neurosurg., *42:* 438–442, 1975.
25. Hamby, W. B. Intracranial surgery for aneurysm. Effect of hypothermia on survival. J. Neurosurg., *20:* 41–45, 1963.
26. Horwitz, N. H., and Rizzoli, H. V. Postoperative Complications in Neurosurgical Practice, 425 pp. Robert Krieger, Huntington, N.Y. 1973.
27. Hosobuchi, Y. Electro thromobosis of fistulas and aneurysms. Presented at the 8th Annual Meeting of the Forum of University Neurosurgeons. San Francisco, June 1972.
28. Hudson, C. H., and Raaf, J. Timing of angiography and operation in patients with ruptured intracranial aneurysms. J. Neurosurg., *29:* 37–41, 1968.
29. Hugosson, R., and Högström, S. Factors disposing to morbidity in surgery of intracranial aneurysms with special regard to deep controlled hypotension. J. Neurosurg., *38:* 561–567, 1973.
30. Hunt, W. E., and Hess, R. M. Surgical risk as related to time of intervention in the repair of intracranial aneurysms. J. Neurosurg., *28:* 14–20, 1968.
31. Hunt, W. E., and Kosnik, E. J. Timing and peri-operative care in intracranial aneurysm surgery. Clin. Neurosurg., *21:* 79–89, 1974.
32. Jamieson, K. G. Aneurysms of the vertebrobasilar system. Surgical intervention in 19 cases. J. Neurosurg., *21:* 781–797, 1964.
33. Jamieson, K. G. Aneurysms of the vertebrobasilar system; further experience with 9 cases. J. Neurosurg., *28:* 544–555, 1968.
34. Jennett, W. B., Barber, J., Fitch, W., and MacDowell, D. G. Effect of anaesthesia on intracranial pressure in patients with space occupying lesions. Lancet, *1:* 61–64, 1969.
35. Joffe, S. N. Incidence of postoperative deep vein thrombosis in neurosurgical patients. J. Neurosurg., *42:* 201–203, 1975.
36. Joynt, R. J., Afifi, A., and Harbison, J. Hyponatremia in subarachnoid hemorrhage, Arch. Neurol., *13:* 633–638, 1965.
37. Karch, S. B. Upper intestinal bleeding as a complication of intracranial disease. J. Neurosurg., *37:* 27–29, 1972.

38. Klafta, L. H., Jr., and Hamby, W. B. Significance of cerebrospinal fluid pressure in determining time for repair of intracranial aneurysm. J. Neurosurg., *31:* 217–219, 1969.

39. Kothandaram, P., Dawson, B. H., and Kruyt, R. C. Carotid-ophthalamic aneurysm. A study of 19 patients. J. Neurosurg., *34:* 544–548, 1971.

40. Krayenbuhl, H. A., Yasargil, M. G., Flamm, E. S., and Tew, J. M., Jr. Microsurgical treatment of intracranial saccular aneurysms. J. Neurosurg., *37:* 678–686, 1972.

41. Landolt, A. M., Yasargil, M. G., and Krayenbuhl, H. A. Distrubances of the serum electrolytes after surgery of intracranial arterial aneurysm. J. Neurosurg., *37:* 210–218, 1972.

42. Lazar, M. L., Watts, C. C., Kilgore, B., and Clark, K. Cerebral angiography during operation for intracranial aneurysms and arteriovenous malformations. J. Neurosurg., *34:* 706–708, 1971.

43. Logue, V. Surgery in spontaneous subarachnoid hemorrhage. Operative treatment of aneurysms in the anterior cerebral and anterior communicating artery. Br. Med. Jour., *1:* 473–479, 1956.

44. Lougheed, W. M. Selection, timing, and techniques of aneurysm surgery of the anterior Circle of Willis. Clin. Neurosurg., *16:* 95–113, 1969.

45. Lougheed, W. M., and Marshall, B. M. Management of aneurysms of the anterior circulation by intracranial procedures. *In* Neurosurgery, edited by J. R. Youmans, Chap. 32. W. B. Saunders Co., Philadelphia, 1973.

46. Marshall, B. M., Lougheed, W. M., and Gordon, R. A. Evaluation of the effect of anesthesia techniques on survival after intracranial surgery for ruptured aneurysms. Can. Anaesth. Soc. J., *15:* 227–231, 1968.

47. Matson, D. D. Intracranial aneurysms in childhood. J. Neurosurg., 23: 578–583, 1965.

48. Mauney, F. M., Ebert, P. A., and Sabiston, D. C., Jr. Postoperative myocardial infarction: A study of predisposing factors, diagnosis and mortality in a high risk group of surgical patients. Ann. Surg., *172:* 494–502, 1970.

49. McMurtry, J. G., III, Housepian, E. M., Bowman, F. D., and Matteo, R. S. Surgical treatment of basilar artery aneurysms. Elective circulatory arrest with thorocotomy in 12 cases. J. Neurosurg., *40:* 486–494, 1974.

50. Millikan, C. H. Cerebral vasospasm and ruptured intracranial aneurysm. Arch. Neurol., *32:* 433–449, 1975.

51. Mount, L. A., Antunes, J. L. Results of treatment of intracranial aneurysms by wrapping and coating. J. Neurosurg., *42:* 189–193, 1975.

52. Mount, L. A., and Brisman, R. Treatment of multiple aneurysms–Symptomatic and asymptomatic. Clin. Neurosurg., *21:* 166–170, 1974.

53. Moyes, P. D. Surgical treatment of multiple aneurysms and of incidentally discovered unruptured aneurysms. J. Neurosurg. *35:* 291–295, 1971.

54. Mullan, S., and Dawley, J. Antifibrinolytic therapy for intracranial aneurysms. J. Neurosurg., *28:* 21–23, 1968.

55. Mullan, S., Reyes, C., Dawley, J., and Dobben, G. Stereotaxic copper electric thrombosis of intracranial aneurysms. *In* Progress in Neurological Surgery, edited by H. Krayenbuhl, P. E. Maspes, and W. H. Sweet, Vol. 3, pp. 193–211. Year Book Medical Publisher, Chicago, 1969.

56. Mullan, S. Experiences with surgical thrombosis of intracranial berry aneurysms and carotid cavernous fistulas. J. Neurosurg., *41:* 657–670, 1974.

57. Mullins, C. B. Personal communication, 1975.

58. Norlen, G. Some aspects of the surgical treatment of intracranial aneurysms. Clin. Neurosurg., *9:* 214–221, 1961.

59. Paterson, A. Direct surgery in the treatment of posterior communicating aneurysms. Lancet, *2:* 808–811, 1968.
60. Paul, R. L., and Arnold, J. G. Operative factors influencing mortality in intracranial aneurysm surgery: Analysis of 186 operative cases. J. Neurosurg., *32:* 289–294, 1970.
61. Penfield, W., Lende, R. A., and Rasmusson, T. Manipulation hemiplegia. An untoward complication in the surgery of focal epilepsy. J. Neurosurg., *18:* 760–776, 1961.
62. Peerless, S. J. The surgical approach to middle cerebral and posterior communicating aneurysms. Clin. Neurosurg., *21:* 151–165, 1974.
63. Pool, J. L. Aneurysms of the anterior communicating. Bifrontal craniotomy and routine use of temporary clips. J. Neurosurg., *18:* 98–112, 1961.
64. Ransohoff, J., Goodgold, A., and Benjamin, M. V. Preoperative management of patients with ruptured intracranial aneurysms. J. Neurosurg., *36:* 525–530, 1972.
65. Robertson, J. T. Cerebral arterial vasospasm; current concepts. Clin. Neurosurg., *21:* 100–106, 1974.
66. Robinson, J. L. Treatment of subarachnoid hemorrhages in pregnancy. *In* Present Limits of Neurosurgery, edited by I. Fusch and Z. Kunc, pp. 263–266. Elsevier, Amsterdam, 1972.
67. Robinson, J. L., Hall, C. S., and Sedzimir, C. B. Arteriovenous malformations, aneurysms, and pregnancy. J. Neurosurg., *41:* 63–70, 1974.
68. Robinson, R. G. Ruptured aneurysms of the middle cerebral artery. J. Neurosurg., *35:* 25–33, 1971.
69. Sahs, A. L., Perret, G. E., Locksley, H. B., and Nishioka, H. Intracranial Aneurysms and Subarachnoid Hemorrhage, A Cooperative Study, 296, pp. J. B. Lippincott, Philadelphia, 1969.
70. Samson, D. S. Personal communication, 1975.
71. Sengupta, R. P., Lassman, L. P., de Moraes, A. A., and Garvan, N. Treatment of internal carotid bifurcation aneurysms by direct surgery. J. Neurosurg., *43:* 343–351, 1975.
72. Sengupta, R. P., Chiu, J. S. P., and Brierley, H. Quality of survival following direct surgery for anterior communicating artery aneurysms. J. Neurosurg., *43:* 58–64, 1975.
73. Shires, G. T., and Canazaro, P. C. Fluid, electrolyte, and nutritional management of the surgical patient. *In* Principles of Surgery, edited by S. I. Schwartz, Chap. 2. McGraw-Hill, New York, 1974.
74. Shulman, K., Martin, B. F., Popoff, N., and Ransohoff, J. Recognition and treatment of hydrocephalus following spontaneous subarachnoid hemorrhage. J. Neurosurg., *20:* 1040–1049, 1963.
75. Silver, D. Pulmonary embolism prevention, detection, and nonoperative management. Surg. Clin. North Am. *54:* 1089–1095, 1974.
76. Sonntag, V. K. H., and Stein, B. M. Arteriopathic complications of subarachnoid hemorrhage with epsilon-amino capron acid. J. Neurosurg., *40:* 480–485, 1974.
77. Stein, M., Koota, G. M., Simon, M., and Frank, H. A. Pulmonary evaluation of surgical patients. J.A.M.A., *181:* 765–770, 1962.
78. Stern, W. E. Preoperative Evaluation, Complications, Their Prevention and Treatment. *In* Neurological Surgery, edited by J. R. Youmans, Chap. 111. W. B. Saunders Co., Philadelphia, 1973.
79. Taylor, T. H., Stules, M., and Lamming, A. J., Sodium nitroprusside as a hypotensive agent in general anaesthesia. Br. J. Anaesth., *42:* 859–863, 1970.
80. Tindall, G. T. The treatment of anterior communicating aneurysms by proximal anterior cerebral artery ligation. Clin. Neurosurg., *21:* 134–150, 1974.
81. Turner, J. W., and Crossant, K. W. Angiography during surgery for aneurysm. *In*

Present Limits in Neurological Surgery, edited by I. Fusch, and Z. Kunc, pp. 281–286. Elsevier, Amsterdam, 1972.

82. Winn, H. R., Richardson, A. E., and Jane, J. A. Late mortality and morbidity of common carotid ligation for posterior communicating artery aneurysms: A comparison with conservative treatment. J. Neurol. Neurosurg. Psychiatry, *38:* 406, 1975.
83. Wood, E. H. Angiographic identification of the ruptured lesion in patients with multiple cerebral aneurysms. J. Neurosurg., *21:* 182–198, 1964.
84. Wright, R. L. Septic complications of intracranial surgery. *In* Cranial and Intracranial Suppuration, edited by E. S. Gurdjian, Chap. 6. Charles C Thomas, Springfield, Ill. 1969.
85. Wightman, J. A. K. A prospective study of the incidence of postoperative pulmonary complications. Br. J. Surg., *55:* 85–91, 1968.
86. VanderArk, G. D., Kempe, L. G., and Smith, D. R. Anterior communicating aneurysms; the gyrus rectus approach. Clin. Neurosurg., *21:* 120–133, 1974.
87. Yasargil, M. G., and Carter, P. L. Saccular aneurysms of the distal anterior cerebral artery. J. Neurosurg., *40:* 218–223, 1974.
88. Yasargil, M. G. Microsurgery Applied to Neurosurgery. Stuttgart, Geo. Thieme Verlag, 1969.

CHAPTER

26

Craniotomy Infections

SHELLEY N. CHOU, M.D., PH.D., AND DONALD L. ERICKSON, M.D.

Infections associated with craniotomy may be superficial, involving only the scalp, or more extensive, involving the subgaleal space and bone flap, or intradural such as meningitis and cerebritis. In this communication, neither superficial infection nor intradural infection will be further discussed but attention will be directed to subgaleal and epidural infections involving the bone flap.

The present day incidence of flap infection is difficult to ascertain. Wright's Review of 2146 "clean" craniotomies performed at the Massachusetts General Hospital from 1952 to 1962 revealed a 5.6% incidence of infection (9). In 1962 Odom (5) reviewed his experience at the Duke University Hospitals over a 17-year period from 1941 to 1958. In 2342 craniotomies performed under ultraviolet radiation, there were 16 infections representing 0.4%. Perhaps it should be mentioned that in 1916 Cushing (1) stated, "there has never been any infection, even of a stitch in the scalp, in something over 300 cranial operations in the writer's series".

We believe that there are several factors which influence the rate of craniotomy infections. We realize that some of the factors to be mentioned are more in the area of "scientific empiricism"; there has never been, to our knowledge, any publications on a controlled series regarding craniotomy infections. Other factors, however, seem to have some foundation for making a more definitive statement.

First, one must assess the patient or the host. It is generally recognized that debilitated patients, patients with certain metabolic diseases such as diabetes mellitus, hematological disorders such as coagulopathy, and patients who are on immunosuppressive medication are more susceptible to infection. In our early experience with transcranial hypophysectomy and pituitary stalk section for diabetic retinopathy, we encountered a 20% infection. The condition of the scalp is an important factor. It is known that patients with multiple craniotomies, particularly in short order, have a higher incidence of craniotomy infection. Those patients that have multiple incisions will most likely have impairment of blood supply of the scalp, and therefore higher incidence of craniotomy infection. Likewise, patients with dermatological problems involving the scalp may be more susceptible to infection. We have observed that patients who had been on long term anticonvulsant therapy, particularly Dilantin, have a tendency to ooze from the scalp incision and they seem to have a relatively higher incidence of scalp flap infection. Such patients, of course, often undergo electrocorticography for resection of epileptogenic foci which increases the duration of the operation and in that manner may favor flap infection.

Secondly, the nature of the surgical procedure and the technique are obviously important factors with regard to flap infection. The length of operating time is definitely a factor as shown by Wright(9). The use of hemostatic clips if too tight in a relatively long procedure may tend to cause ischemic necrosis of the scalp, thus delaying healing and favoring infection. Once it was said that a free bone flap was more conducive to infection (6), but we are not certain this is true. If the incision and the flap are such that the frontal sinus has been entered, there is an increased risk of infection, although according to Ray, with the proper technique of covering the sinus with pericranium, the infection rate was, at least in his experience, minimal (7).

Finally, the use of foreign body in the wound, such as tantalum or plastic buttons for covering the burr holes, particularly if placed close to the frontal sinus, will increase the risk of infection. Obviously, gentle handling of the tissue and perfect hemostasis is one of the best preventive measures against postoperative infection of the craniotomy flap.

Third, the operating room situation is another important factor. In our institution, bacteriological studies have been done in the different operating suites (3). Multiple entering and exiting of personnel will significantly increase the bacterial count. Dry shaving of the hair in the operating room similarly can increase the bacterial count. It is superfluous to mention proper aseptic techniques and the necessity to detect personnel who may chronically harbor or carry certain types of bacteria.

In the postoperative period a number of factors may influence the incidence of infection. Generally, the use of a drain will increase the infection rate (4, 8). The application of a tight bandage may interfere with blood supply of the scalp, thus impeding healing process and favoring infection. Prophylactic use of antibiotics remains controversial. In Wright's analysis it does not seem to be a factor (8). It is a fair statement that the less number of personnel with whom the patient comes into contact from the preoperative period through intraoperative period and postoperatively, the less likely the patient will develop an infection. This has been the experience of both of the authors who have had several years of clinical practice outside of teaching institutions. We were involved in the preoperative care, positioning the patient, shaving the head, draping, handling the entire operative procedure, and the postoperative care with the least degree of assistance. Cumulatively, we have had 7 years of surgical experience under these circumstances and have had only twc craniotomy infections. At the present time, the craniotomy infection rate at the University of Minnesotal Hospitals runs about 3%. We have not found short term use of steroids to be a factor.

Insofar as the treatment of flap infection is concerned, obviously, early detection is important. The infection will begin to manifest in the 1st or 2nd week postoperatively. Occasionally it may even be several months later when signs of infection appear. Inspection of the wound would reveal induration, redness, and the presence of edema. The area is usually tender and fluctuance may be present.

We believe that it is important at this time to try to aspirate for culture. The patient then is put on broad spectrum antibiotics preferably chloramphenicol and penicillin or sodium cephalothin (Keflin, Lilly, Indianapolis, Ind.). After the organism is identified which is in most instances a *Staphylococcus aureus*, and the sensitivity studies have been

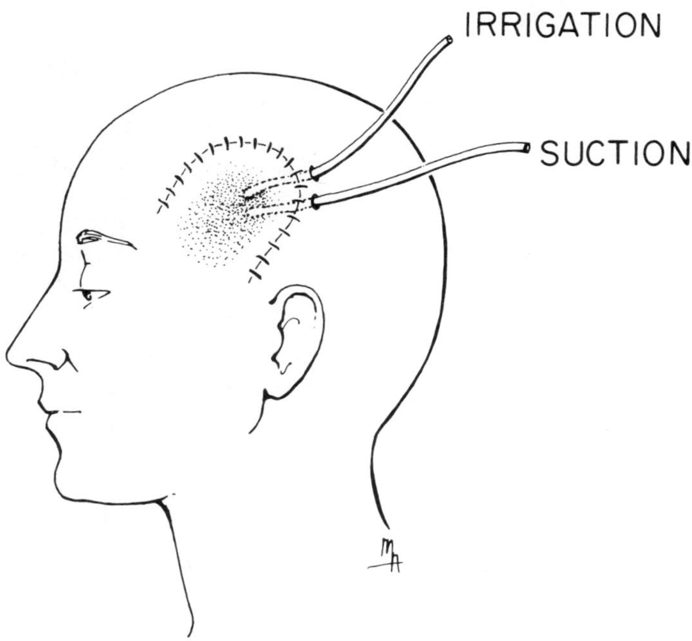

FIG. 26.1. Placement of irrigation and suction tubes.

done, the antibiotics should obviously be switched to the most effective one.

Once the flap infection is definitely present, we have had fairly good results with suction-irrigation treatment (2). Briefly, the technique involves the reopening of the wound, removal of all visible suture material with exception of wire, and removal of all purulent and necrotic material by mechanical debridement and irrigation. The bone flap is left in place. Two medium size Hemovac drains are then inserted through the adjacent scalp into the subgaleal space over the bone flap as indicated in Figure 26.1. Should purulent material be present in the epidural space, a second set of Hemovac drains can be inserted under the bone flap as well. The scalp is then closed in a single layer with interrupted wire sutures

TABLE 26.1
Patients Tested with Irrigation–Suction Procedure

Case	Diagnosis	No. of Days Postoperative	Culture	Result
1	Epidural hematoma	10	Negative	Healed
2	Meningioma	21	Coag. + staph	Healed
3	Carotid-cavernous fistula	200	Coag. + staph	Healed
4	A-V malformation	60	Coag. − staph	Healed
5	Glioma	9	Coag. − staph	Healed
6	Glioma	7	Coag. + staph	Draining 7 mos. later
7	Glioma	19	Coag. + staph	Healed
8	Aneurysm	8	Negative	Healed
9	Glioma	26	Staph epidermis	Healed
10	Ca-ethmoid	90	Coag. + staph entero-bacteria	Bone flap removed
11	Glioma	21	Coag. + staph	Slight drainage 8 mos. later
12	A-V malformation	16	Coag. + staph	Draining
13	Glioma	54	Gm. + rods anaerobic	Flap removed
14	Hamartoma	30	Proteins, anaerobic diphtheroids	Flap removed
15	Aneurysm	14	Coag. + staph	Healed
16	Pituitary tumor	9	Negative	Healed
17	Meningioma	17	Coag. + staph	Draining
18	Aneurysm	7	Gm. + cocci	Healed
19	Ca-maxillary sinus	23	Staph + strep	Flap removed
20	Glioma	15	Staph	Healed
21	Glioma	8	Staph	Healed
22	Infarction	6	Staph	Healed
23	Glioma	7	Staph	Healed
24	Infected cranioplasty	27	Staph	Flap removed
25	Infected cranioplasty	35	Staph	Flap removed

and the Hemovac drains are fixed in place. One limb of the drain is connected to an intravenous tube and a liter of saline-antibiotic mixture is prepared as an irrigation solution. Generally we use 1 gm. Keflin per liter unless the sensitivity tests indicate that some other antibiotic is more desirable. The second limb of the Hemovac tubing is connected to a suction system. If two pairs of Hemovac drains are used, each should be connected with separate irrigation and suction systems. The irrigation solution is infused at the rate of 1 to 2 liters per 24 hours. This procedure is continued for 5 to 7 days. Meticulous attention must be paid to assure that the volume of output is equivalent to that of the irrigation input to avoid building up of subgaleal or epidural pressure. During this period of time, systemic antibiotics are continued. After the desired period of treatment, 5 to 7 days, the tubes are removed and a simple dressing placed over the drainage sites.

We have had up to this time a total of 25 patients who were subjected to the irrigation-suction procedure. These patients were cared for over a period of 3 years. The results of the treatment are shown in Table 26.1. It is clear that 15 patients did not lose their flap. It should be pointed out that two patients who did lose their bone flaps with this treatment had combined ear, nose, and throat, and neurosurgical procedures to remove carcinomas of the antrum and ethmoids. The other two who likewise lost their bone flaps following this treatment were subjected to their reoperation after initial postoperative radiation therapy. Two infected cranioplasty cases failed completely. The flaps had to be removed to eradicate infection. We think that this simple procedure is helpful and even with 50% success rate is still very worthwhile. We would like to point out that the concept of this technique is not new. Our orthopedic colleagues have used it successfully for infected wounds with prosthetic metal devices. It is important to start the treatment early in the course of the infection to avoid osteomyelitis which would be unlikely to resolve even with this procedure. A summary of our results is presented in Table 26.2.

If infection persists, the standard surgical removal of the bone flap and necrotic tissues and generous irrigation of the wound becomes necessary.

TABLE 26.2
Results of Treatment by Irrigation and Suction

Condition	No. of Patients
Healed	15
Flap removed	6
Slight drainage	4
Total	25*

* Average follow-up time = 18 months.

The wound can be closed without a drain. Appropriate systemic antibiotics should be continued for 2 weeks. Cranioplasty can be done preferably a year later.

In summary, we have reviewed the factors in the occurrence of cranioplasty infections. We recommend using the irrigation and suction procedure to eradicate the infection. We suggest that if infection is detected and treatment started early, at least 50% of the bone flaps may be saved.

REFERENCES

1. Cushing, H. Surgery of the Head, *In* Surgery, Its Principles and Practice, edited by W. W. Keen. pp. 17–276. W. B. Saunders, Philadelphia, 1916.
2. Erickson, D. L., Seljeskog, E. S., and Chou, S. N. Suction irrigation treatment of craniotomy infections. J. Neurosurg., *41:* 265–276, 1974.
3. Greene, V. W. Personal communication, 1973.
4. Meleny, F. L. Infection in clean operative wounds, A nine years study. Surg. Gynecol. Obstet., *60:* 264–276, 1935.
5. Odom, G., Hart, D., Johnson, P., Smith, W., and Brown, I. Neurosurgical operative infections. A seventeen year survey of the use of ultraviolet radiation. Presented at the 24th meeting of the American Academy of Neurological Surgeons, New Orleans, La, November 1962.
6. Olivecrona, H. Die Parasagittalen Meningeome, 114 pp. Georg Thieme Verleg, Leipzig, 1937.
7. Ray, B. S., and Horwith, M. Surgical treatment of acromegaly. Clin. Neurosurg., *10:* 31–59, 1964.
8. Williams, R. E. O. Incidence of surgical wound infections in England and Wales. Lancet, *2:* 659–663, 1960.
9. Wright, R. L. Postoperative Craniotomy Infections, 166 pp. Charles C Thomas, Springfield, Ill., 1966.

CHAPTER

27

Spinal Fluid Fistulae

AYUB KHAN OMMAYA, M.D.

Leakage of cerebrospinal fluid (CSF) from nose or ear is a symptom of failure in containment of this fluid to its normal compartments around the central nervous system. Just as the exact explanation of any neurological symptom must precede its adequate treatment, the correct management of spinal fluid fistulae demands a clear understanding of their etiology and pathogenesis. The great majority of such leaks occur at the base of the skull, a fact undoubtedly related to the particular anatomy of the area and its relative fragility. Moreover, CSF leaks elsewhere are easy to detect and easy to repair. The fundamental cause of leakage is a break in the meningeal continuity combined with impaired healing of tissues at the site of rupture. The meningeal rupture may be caused by a number of factors of which trauma is the commonest and impaired tissue repair may be due to lack of proper closure, inadequate support of weak healing tissues, and poor healing of the tissue due to infection, metabolic disorders, or other chronic diseases. Persistence of leakage is facilitated when intracranial pressure (ICP) is increased either continuously or periodically due to any cause. This review will attempt to cover our present understanding of the subject from the etiological, diagnostic, and therapeutic aspect with special attention to surgical aspects and the problem of recurrent meningitis.

HISTORICAL ASPECTS

It is of interest to note that although traumatic leakage of CSF is more common, the first published case of CSF rhinorrhea was of the nontraumatic "high pressure" type due to hydrocephalus (43). This report by Miller in 1826 was followed by that of King in 1834 (33), and the monograph on "spontaneous" rhinorrhea by St. Clair Thomson in 1899 admirably summarized knowledge to the end of the 19th century (57). It was not until 1923, however, that Grant (25) and later Dandy (in 1926) proposed neurosurgical treatment for CSF rhinorrhea (13). Cushing, in 1927, published three cases of traumatic leakage treated surgically (12). The first series of cases treated by the Grant-Dandy technique of transcranial extradural repair using fascia lata was published by Hugh

Cairns in 1937 (7). Transnasal approach to this problem until 1948 was limited to cauterization; in that year Dohlman described an intranasal (transethmoidal) approach which could seal off leaks through the cribriform plate with a septal and middle turbinate flap (17). The intradural repair technique which is currently the most widely used method was first used by Taylor, as reported by Eden in 1941 (20). The evolution of the modern approach to therapy has indeed been the result of the discoveries and experience occurring within the past 30 years.

CLASSIFICATION

An etiological classification which was developed some years ago and has since been generally accepted is shown in Figure 27.1 (10, 47, 49). Note that these classes are to some extent artificial and not mutually exclusive insofar as the mechanism of leakage is concerned. Thus certain cases of delayed onset traumatic CSF rhinorrhea have signs and symptoms identical to nontraumatic cases and the actual precipitating cause of the leak may be identical. Thus Voena has described patients with delayed onset traumatic CSF rhinorrhea in whom a congenital anomaly was found, *e.g.*, persistence of the basioccipital canal (60).

Similarly, onset of CSF rhinorrhea in certain cases of pituitary tumor treated with x-irradiation alone also suggests atrophy of tissues (? on ischemic basis) possibly analogous to that found in delayed onset traumatic leaks. Moreover, their presentation, complications, and role of raised ICP in the traumatic and nontraumatic groups are significantly different. The nontraumatic leak is much rarer, insidious rather than

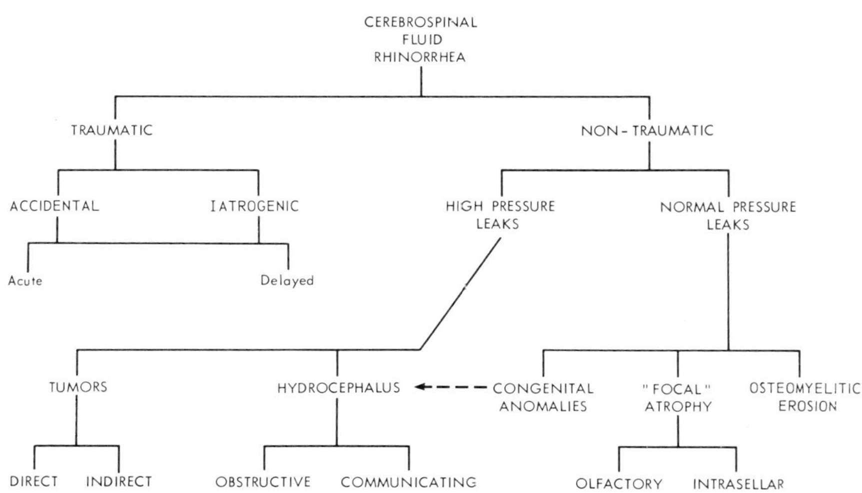

FIG. 27.1. Classification of CSF leaks. Description in text.

abrupt in onset, and may last for years. In 50% of the traumatic cases, rhinorrhea stops within 1 week and in most within 6 months. Flow of CSF is more profuse in the nontraumatic type, the side affected is not constant, aeroceles rarely develop intracranially, and anosmia, found in 78% of traumatic cases, is rare. Headache is common in nontraumatic cases and, whereas traumatic rhinorrhea bears no relationship to age or sex, the nontraumatic variety affects adults mainly over 30 and females twice as often as males. Meningitis, the main danger in traumatic cases, is rare. These and other contrasts between the two major subdivisions of CSF fistula are given in Table 27.1.

There is a certain degree of confusion in the literature concerning nasal leakage of CSF when trauma is not the cause. The term "spontaneous CSF rhinorrhea" has been used more or less consistently to describe such cases since 1899. Although isolated observations had been made earlier, it was the monograph by St. Clair Thomson (1899) (57) that first clearly described and attempted to define spontaneous CSF rhinorrhea as a clinical entity. Other authors have since essayed to subdivide this condition into "primary spontaneous" or "idiopathic" rhinorrhea when a precipitating cause could not be found and "secondary spontaneous" rhinorrhea when a cause, usually a tumor, was discovered (48). Quite apart from the nosological adequacy of such a subdivision, the term "spontaneous" CSF rhinorrhea itself would appear to be inexact, bearing no relationship to either the pathogenesis or natural history of the disease. The word "spontaneous" means "arising from natural impulse, without external stimulant, or having a self-contained cause or origin, or arising from or entirely determined by the internal operative or directive forces of the organism" (Shorter Oxford English Dictionary, 1962). It is our thesis that a careful study of the natural history of patients suffering such rhinorrhea reveals no actual case which can fit such a definition—that is, in being truly "spontaneous." It would therefore be more accurate to describe all such cases, hitherto labeled spontaneous, by the more general term of nontraumatic CSF rhinorrhea. It is then possible to subdivide this category etiologically on the basis of facts that emerge from a study of such patients and assign each case according to the causative lesion. Quite apart from clarifying our understanding, this approach avoids what is essentially a "wastebasket" category of "primary spontaneous" rhinorrhea, for those cases in which the true diagnosis has often not been discovered, as well as dispensing with the logically impossible phrase "secondary spontaneous rhinorrhea."

It will be made apparent from this etiological classification that the subdivisions of rhinorrhea are closely related in terms of the mechanism of the leakage. The nontraumatic group is subdivided into "high

TABLE 27.1

Features of Traumatic and Nontraumatic CSF Rhinorrhea

Type	Incidence	Age and Sex	Onset	Duration of Leakage	Amount of Leakage	Laterality	Aerocele and Intracranial Air	Anosmia	Headache	Risk of Infection
Traumatic	Approx. 2% of unselected head injuries, relatively common condition	Irrespective of age, sex	Usually within 48 hr. of trauma; occasionally after a few wks., rarely after mos.; longest interval reported is 4½ yr.; onset is always abrupt	Over 70% cease within 1 wk., 20–30% may continue for mos.; it is very unusual for flow to persist for yrs.; nearly all stop within 6 mos.; recurrent leak is very rare	From few drops to few ounces daily; profuse leakage extremely unusual	Usually unilateral and this often indicates side of fistula, but side of fracture is better index	Found in about 20% of cases	Present in 78% of cases	Relatively uncommon; in about 10% of cases, usually when marked aerocele or profuse flow present; this headache not relieved by flow	High, being from 25% to 50% of untreated cases
Nontraumatic	Rare condition; Only 82 cases in literature have been found	Usually in mature adults (over 28); average age 43; females predominate, ratio being nearly 2:1	Insidious onset of leakage; often mistaken for allergic rhinitis; later becomes profuse flow; in few cases, after bout of headache, sneezing	Untreated, leak usually persists for years; in about 1/3 of cases spontaneous arrest occurs; flow is characteristically intermittent; recurrent leak after long stoppage is common	Usually profuse flow; varies from few ounces to over 30 ounces daily	Variable, bears no relation to side of fistula	Unusual	Smell sense usually preserved	Fairly common; characteristically, cessation of flow associated with headache; then relieved by onset of flow	Lower when factor of longer duration taken into consideration; appears to be especially true of those cases due to intracranial tumors—that is, high pressure leaks

pressure" and "normal pressure" categories. This reflects an important difference. In the high pressure category the leakage of cerebrospinal fluid is usually acting as a real safety valve, closure of which will invariably worsen the patient's condition if the causative lesion is not treated. Each of these categories is then subdivided into certain etiological groups under which the mechanism of the rhinorrhea may be better understood. The classification will be analyzed in detail below where the concept of "focal atrophy" will also be presented in the course of a discussion of nontraumatic leaks.

DIAGNOSIS

This includes identification of CSF as the constituent of the rhinorrhea, demonstration of the cause whenever possible, as well as localization of the fistula itself. Identification of CSF is usually easy except in a few cases of "vasomotor rhinorrhea" or allergic rhinitis where a faulty initial diagnosis can be misleading. However, persistence of a clear nonsticky nasal discharge should immediately rouse suspicion and lead to further investigations. Biochemical tests on the collected fluid, particularly the often quoted use of glucose-oxidase test papers, are not fully reliable. The latter method has been shown to have a 45 to 75% chance of positive results with normal nasal secretions. If sufficient clear fluid can be collected to perform quantitative testing for glucose, a value greater than 30 mg. per ml. is confirmatory for CSF (23). Positive identification of CSF necessitates introduction of suitable tracers into the CSF cavities and their recovery in the nasal discharge (40). These techniques are part of fistula localization and will be considered below.

Concerning demonstration of the cause of the leakage, it should be remembered that over half the cases of nontraumatic rhinorrhea are high pressure leaks due to tumors, and the diagnostic approach to such patients should therefore be the same as that to patients with epilepsy of late onset. However, it is not enough to display the causative space-taking lesion; the fistula must also be localized. Naturally, such localization takes precedence when a normal pressure leak is present.

It cannot be sufficiently emphasized that the assessment of the location of the leakage is often a difficult and always a challenging diagnostic problem. This is due to the fact that the possible leaking sites are quite numerous and may occur in the anterior, middle, and posterior fossae. Most frequently the CSF reaches the nasal cavity through the frontal sinus, the lamina cribosa, the sphenoidal roof, or the petrous bone *via* the middle ear and the Eustachian tube (Fig. 27.2). The fact that the leak may be found on the side opposite to the dripping nostril and the possible multiplicity of fistulae further complicate the matter. Consider-

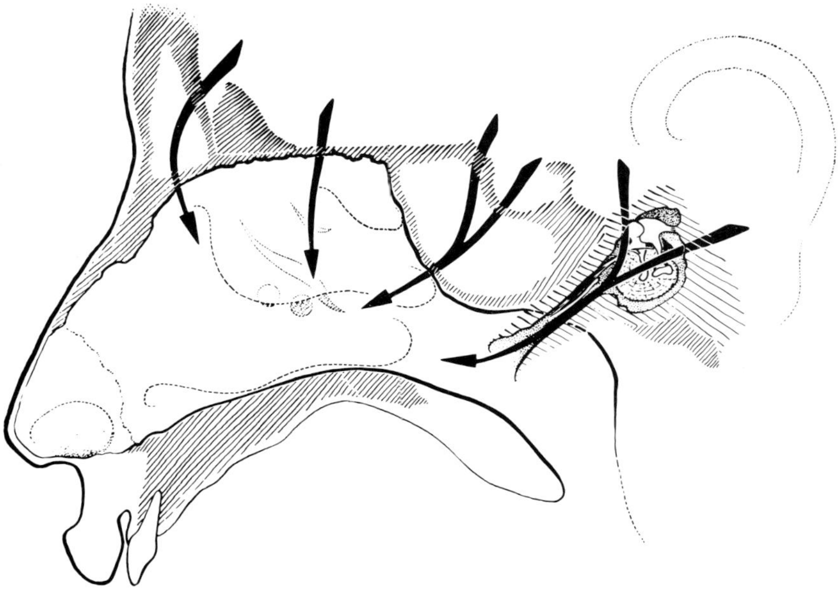

FIG. 27.2. Diagrammatic summary of common sites of CSF leakage.

ing that if the fistula does not heal spontaneously the patient is in serious danger of recurrent meningitis and that the mandatory corrective surgery will be successful only if the actual leaking site is exposed at operation, the importance of a diagnostic localizing method is obvious.

To localize the fistula responsible for the CSF loss, one can use dyes, fluorescent substances, radiography, or radioactive tracers (Table 27.2). Dyes (methylene blue, phenolsulfonphthalein, indigo carmine) have been introduced before or during surgery within the subarachnoidal spaces or intranasally for visual localization of the fistula. Fluorescein has also been used. Most of these dyes and particularly methylene blue can, however, cause significant morbidity (63). Tomography, pneumoencephalography, and subdural pneumography frequently provide help for the localization of the leaking break. Various attempts have been made to localize the fistula by Pantopaque injected into the subarachnoidal space (53) as well as the ventricular system, a pneumocephalic cavity, and intranasally (55). After the injection of Pantopaque, the passage of the opaque material is observed with fluoroscopy and radiography. However, this contrast medium causes meningeal irritation. The recent introduction of less irritant water-soluble positive contrast media in neuroradiology suggests their possible use as leak detectors but the short time period for x-ray visibility for these agents may preclude such use. A combination of such agents and computerized tomography may, however, be feasible to detect "pooling" of the agent at the base of the skull in selected cases. It would be of interest to pursue this idea. In 1956 the use of radioactive sodium (^{24}Na) was suggested by Crow and associates (11). This tracer was injected into the cisterna magna, and cotton pledgets conveniently distributed in the walls and roof of the nose and nasopharynx and upon the openings of the Eustachian tubes were afterward examined with a counter. The cotton pledget showing the highest radioactivity indicated the site of leakage. A similar isotope-counting technique has been reported employing radioiodinated serum albumin (RISA). Isotope cisternography was introduced by Di Chiro, working in our Institute, and has been used successfully to visualize the fistula in many cases of traumatic and nontraumatic CSF rhinorrhea. The technique and results have been previously reported (14, 16, 49). Figures 27.3 and 27.4 show examples of the visualization of CSF leaks through the cribriform plate and sphenoid sinus by this method. A recent review of the use of isotopes in the assessment of CSF pathways is given by Holman and Davis (27). Plain radiographs may demonstrate air-fluid levels within the sphenoidal sinus as well as reveal an enlarged sella turcica. With tomography a bone defect may be demonstrated (Fig. 27.5). At pneumoencephalography a dilated intrasellar subarachnoid space may be put in evidence. The intrasellar subarachnoid pocket,

TABLE 27.2
Diagnostic Procedures for CSF Fistula Localization

Modality	Agent	Comment
Dyes	a) PSP b) Indigo carmine	Not needed unless radioisotopes are not available
Photoluminescence	Fluorescin	Do
Radiography with x-rays	a) Conventional films of skull base	All useful procedures; provisos are: a) Must show paranasal sinuses
	b) Tomography (pluridirectional)	b) Is particularly of value in traumatic leaks and in high pressure nontraumatic leaks
	c) Pneumoencephalography	c) Useful mainly for anterior leaks communicating with ventricles
	d) Subdural pneumography	d) Applicable only to frontal traumatic leaks
	e) Positive contrast radiography	e) Especially of value in posterior fossa leaks
Radioisotopic assessment	a) ^{99m}Tc-albumin b) Chelated ^{169}Yb-diphosphothiamine	Fistula track only seen if leak is profuse and track large. Accumulation of nuclide in sinus also helps localization

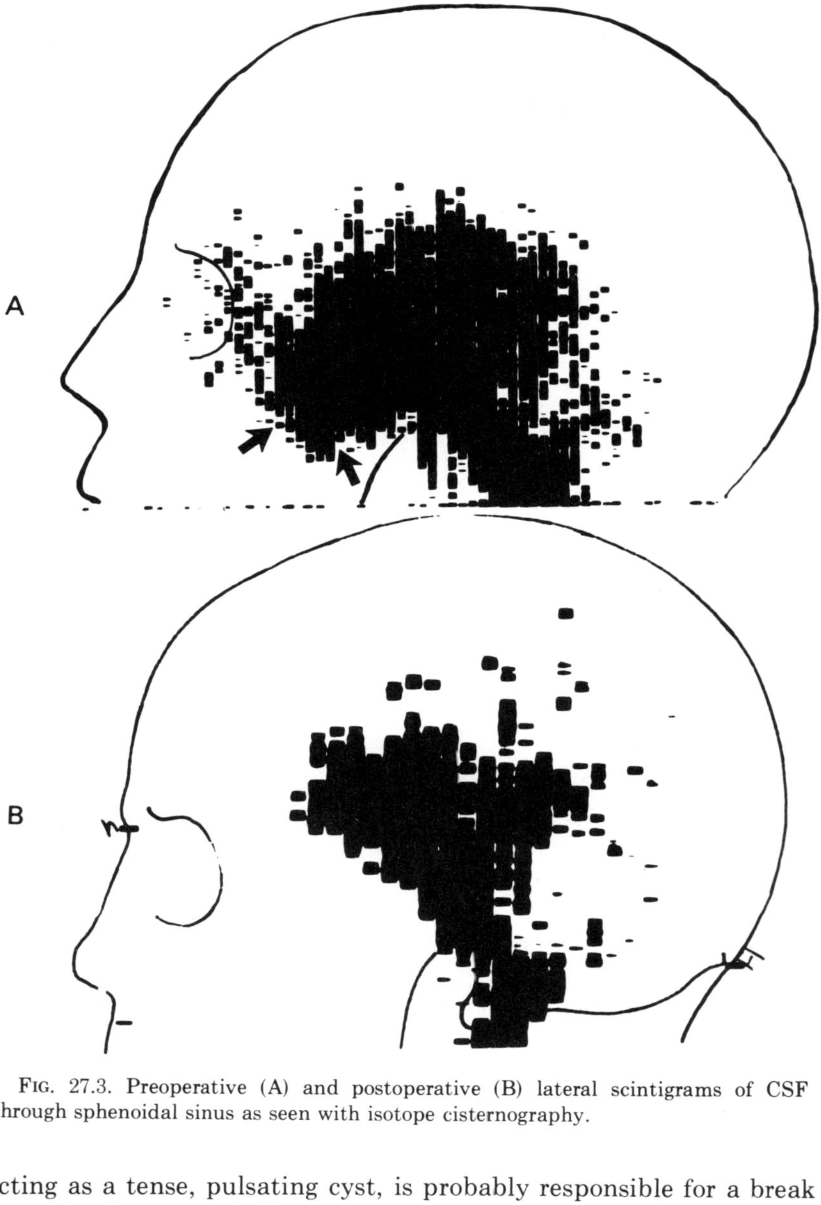

FIG. 27.3. Preoperative (A) and postoperative (B) lateral scintigrams of CSF leak through sphenoidal sinus as seen with isotope cisternography.

acting as a tense, pulsating cyst, is probably responsible for a break in the sellar floor (6, 21). The pneumoencephalogram is essential to decide between such a cyst and a pituitary adenoma. Subdural pneumography is a useful adjunct in traumatic cases with leaks through the anterior cranial fossa (Fig. 27.6). In addition, air studies permitted us in one of

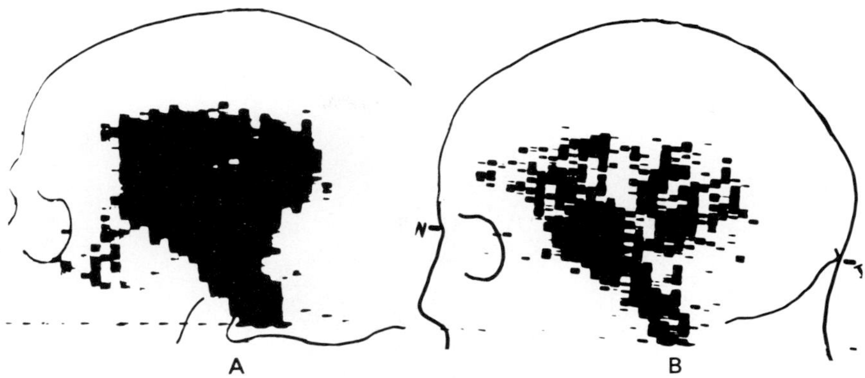

FIG. 27.4. Preoperative (A) and postoperative (B) lateral scintigrams of patient with CSF leak through cribriform plate (posterior) as seen with isotope cisternography.

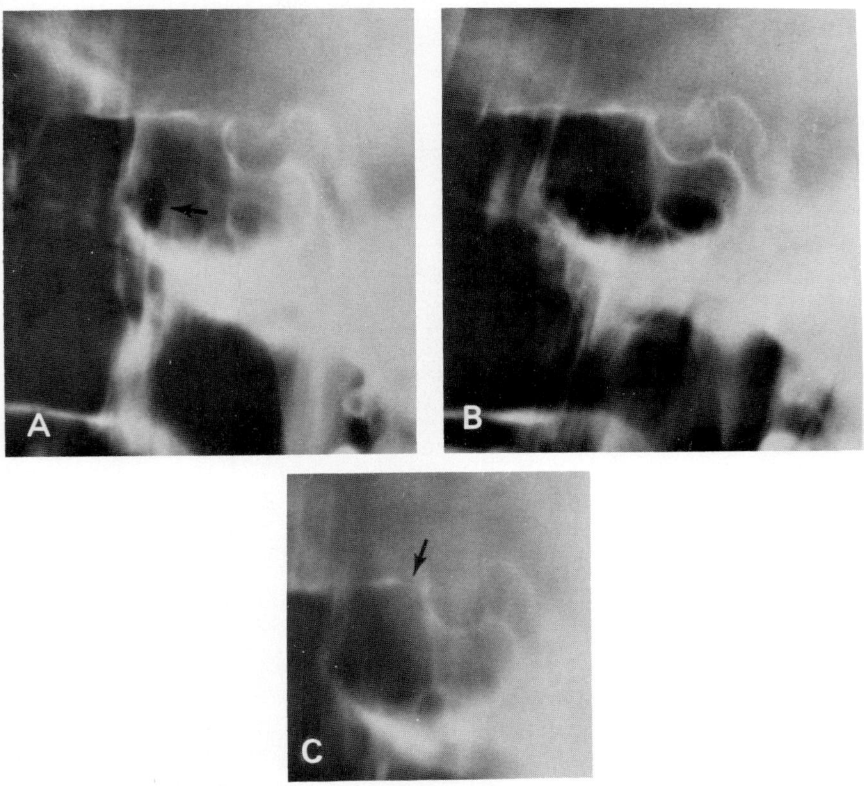

FIG. 27.5. Lateral tomograms through sellar region in patient with CSF leak through sphenoid sinus. Note changing air fluid level as patient is moved from brow up (A) to hanging head (B) position. The bony defect itself is partly shown in (C).

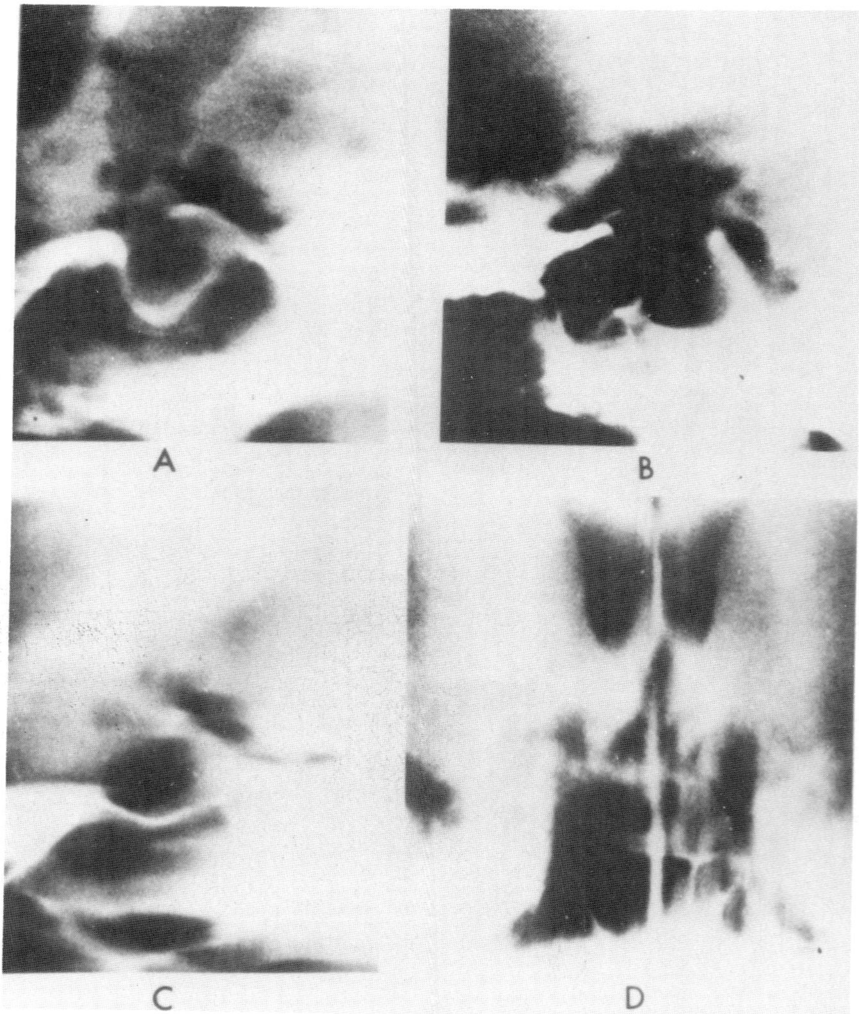

FIG. 27.6. Pneumoencephalogram in patient with CSF leak showing fistula from 3rd ventricle through empty sella into sphenoid sinus. (Patient No. 15 in Table 27.5.)

our cases to make the tentative diagnosis of direct third ventricle-cisternal-sphenoidal sinus communication (Fig. 27.7). Specific diagnostic aspects for each of the two main categories of CSF leakage will be considered below. It should be noted, however, that the dictum of Dandy in 1944 that visualization of the fistula may on occasion be impossible is still true today.

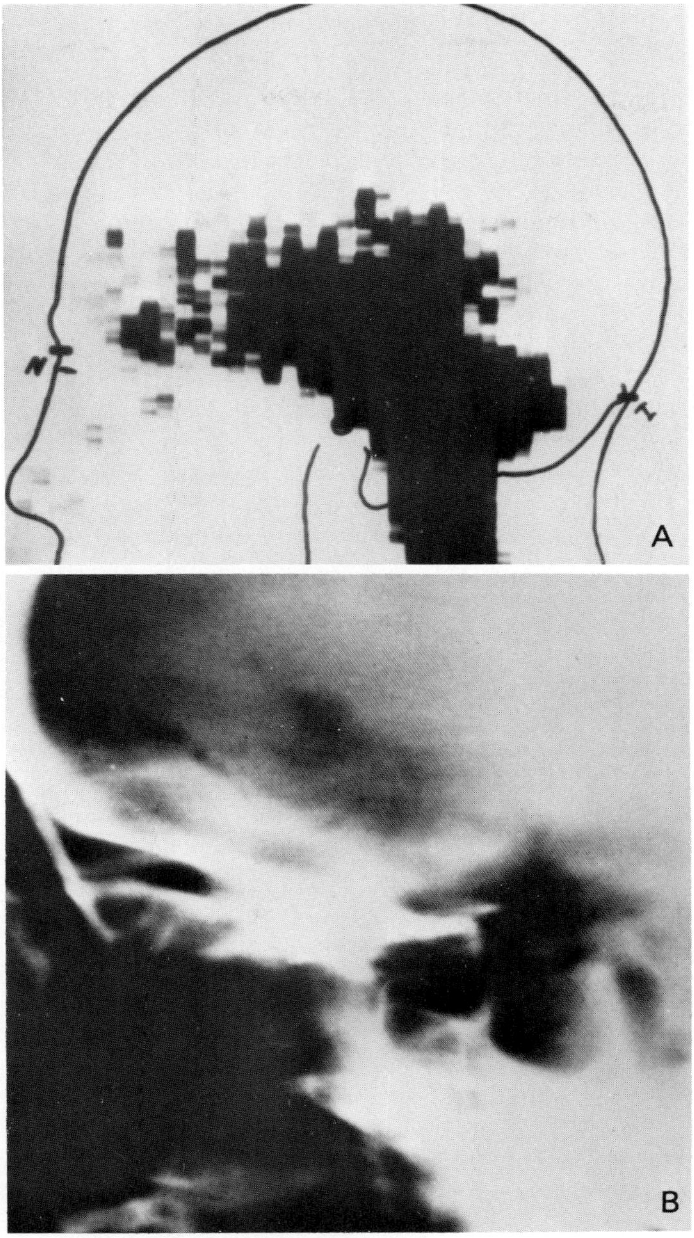

FIG. 27.7. Isotope cisternography (A) and subdural pneumography (B) in a child with traumatic CSF rhinorrhea show precise correspondence for site of fistula and herniation of frontal lobe.

Traumatic Leaks

DIAGNOSIS

The overriding significance of CSF leaks after trauma concerns the hazard of meningitis which may on occasion be fulminant in onset. Lewin has reported the case of a patient who died within 36 hours after head injury causing CSF rhinorrhea through a fracture involving the frontal sinus. Pyogenic meningitis followed and the patient died in spite of antibiotics started within a few hours of the injury (36). Wehrle and associates reported 21% incidence of meningitis after traumatic leaks, (62). Lewin, summarizing his extensive experience with traumatic leaks, noted that two-thirds of his cases leaked within 48 hours of the trauma with the majority of the remainder presenting as delayed leaks up to 3 months from head injury. In a few cases the onset was delayed by many months or even years; the longest delay being 9 years in this series. The longest published delayed onset of CSF rhinorrhea was 14 years (37). Because spontaneous closure of such fistulae occurs by adhesions or herniations of brain into bony crevices or by granulation tissue resulting from local meningitis, the quality of closure is poor and the risk of meningitis remains in some cases of spontaneous closure. Therefore, it is imperative to search for evidence of CSF leakage in all patients with head injury, particularly those with fractures of the skull base passing either through the frontal or ethmoidal sinuses or in patients having the common middle fossa fracture which passes parallel to the long axis of the petrous bone. This type of fracture almost always involves the middle ear, and if the tympanic membrane is torn, CSF otorrhea is evident. If the membrane is not torn, fluid will be visible through the tympanic membrane in the middle ear. Transverse temporal bone fractures pass at right angles to the petrous and thus damage the membranous labyrinth but rarely tear the tympanic membrane. Meningitis is usually of delayed onset in such cases and it has been suggested that many cases of meningitis may be due to undiagnosed transverse temporal fracture—healing of endochondral bone being notoriously poor. An episode of otitis media at any time following such a fracture is capable of causing meningitis because of the communication between middle ear and subarachnoid space (31).

Acute traumatic leaks are invariably bloody initially and then become clear. Delayed leaks may present with a fairly sudden copious gush or as an attack of meningitis without obvious leak. The rate and constancy of the leakage are probably the key factors in determining the onset of meningitis. Thus a copious, continuous leakage is less likely to be associated with meningitis as compared to a scanty, "stop-and-go" type of leak.

In the Lewin series of 100 unselected patients with head injury, 7% had basal skull fractures of which one-third or 2% of the total had CSF leaks. One quarter of these patients, *i.e.*, 0.5% of the total, developed meningitis (36). McGee and associates reported a lower incidence of 0.25% of head injuries in their series (39).

In addition to the clinical search for evidence of leak or meningitis, the skull radiographs should also be carefully examined for presence of fluid levels in the sinuses (49) and intracranial air. In Lewin's series air was present intracranially in one-third of patients with CSF leakage (36). Marc and Schecter have described an interesting pneumoencephalographic technique which by positioning the patient with a leak can create an air-fluid level in the sphenoid sinus if that is the site of the fistula (38). Occasionally, other clinical evidence may alert one to the possibility of a fractured sinus and thus the risk of CSF leak and meningitis. Thus CSF escaping *via* the ethmoidal sinuses may collect in the periorbital tissues to cause local edema. In 50% of cases with fractures involving the sphenoid sinus, nearby structures are damaged and form the presenting neurological deficit, *e.g.*, visual defects due to chiasmatic injury and evidence of trauma to the hypothalamus or internal carotid artery. However, one-third of patients with fractures involving the sinuses but with no obvious leak will be found to have no dural tear on intracranial exploration of the sinus fracture.

Radioisotope Techniques

Although it is true that gamma scintigraphic display of the site of CSF leak is eminently desirable, there is still a place for the simpler method of Crow and associates in cases of CSF rhinorrhea, particularly when the plain x-ray shows a fracture passing through the cribriform plate and a gamma camera is not available (11, 30). A quantitative variant of this technique using chelated ^{111}In-DTPA has also been published (46).

A detailed analysis of the use of isotope cisternography in CSF rhinorrhea by Oberson provides a useful listing of "radioisotope signs" and their incidence in this condition is given below in Table 27.3. There were a total of 71 patients referred with a clinical suspicion of CSF rhinorrhea (38). It is of interest to note that 7 of 11 large and 10 of 18 slight fistulae were seen only on the 24-hour scan. A basal cisternal pouch was not thought to be diagnostic unless it was retained on the 24-hour scan. Lateralization of the leak, a key need for the surgeon, was possible in only one-third of cases, an experience in keeping with our own (15). Contamination of the nasopharynx was variable and did not correspond to the side of the fistula in 10% of cases. The 34 patients who had negative radioisotope signs in spite of a clinical suspicion of CSF

TABLE 27.3
Radioisotope Signs and Incidence in CSF Rhinorrhea

Sign	No. of Cases	Time of Positive Scan (No. of Cases)	
		On 1st day	On 2nd day
No visible fistula	34	0	0
Large fistula	11	4	11
Slight fistula	18	6	16
Basal cisternal pouch	22	13	20
Rhinopharyngeal contamination	19	6	17
Radioactive handkerchieves	29	15	29
Rinsings from nostrils	8	—	8

rhinorrhea or otorrhea had no subsequent evidence of a leak in their clinical course and none developed meningitis. All patients with a positive scan had radioactive handkerchieves. Washing of the nostrils with physiological water demonstrated contamination of the mucosa in eight cases of CSF fistula without evidence of a rhinorrhea. In cases where the handkerchieves were equivocal, radioactivity in the saliva was compared to the activity of the rinsing water. The test is considered positive only if the radioactivity of the handkerchief is superior to that of the saliva. The saliva is always somewhat radioactive because the resorption of radioiodine varies from one solution to another depending on the stability of the preparation.

Alazraki and associates have recommended the use of 10% dextrose in water as a vehicle for the radioisotope in order to provide a hyperbaric medium which apparently results in fewer scan failures, higher count efficiency, and decreased radiation exposure (2).

Positive Contrast Myeloencephalography and Ventriculography

In difficult cases where the side and site of the fistula is not obvious and particularly in cases of CSF otorrhea where it is not clear whether the leak is *via* the middle fossa or posterior fossa, these techniques are recommended. Special care must be taken to use small amounts of dye and careful x-ray techniques as described in two recent reports on this method (3, 18). The technique is successful usually only with large fistulae causing copious CSF leakage and the risk of meningeal inflammation must always be kept in mind.

IATROGENIC TRAUMATIC FISTULAE

CSF leakage through the nose after pituitary surgery and through the ear after surgery in the cerebellopontine angle has been much more common in the past. With the introduction of the surgical microscope this complication has been markedly reduced. Thus in recent series, CSF leakage has been reported in only 5 to 10% of cases of acoustic neuroma (29, 64) and in 3 to 6% of patients undergoing microneurosurgical pituitary surgery (9, 59). The routine use of fascial and muscle stamps to close any fistula created at the time of surgery has virtually eliminated this complication in contemporary practice.

TREATMENT OF TRAUMATIC LEAKS

The surgical attitude to traumatic leaks ranges from the extremely vigorous one of Cairns and Lewin who recommended exploration and repair of all leaks as soon as the patient is fit for surgery to the more moderate approach of waiting to see if spontaneous arrest would occur. There is very little firm evidence that surgery is essential in every case, although the special case of fractures involving the frontal sinus is one of which to be aware. There are basically six areas of controversy which do require further comment. These are as follows.

1. Duration of Conservative Management before Surgery Is Recommended. Because many leaks stop spontaneously and a significant number do not develop complications and, also, because no surgical repair guarantees closure of all possible leaks, it is reasonable to wait for the general condition of the patient to stabilize after the head injury. During the 1st week to 2 weeks, the indications for surgery are: (a) no decrease in rate of flow over 6 to 8 days, (b) initial decrease of flow followed by continuation of flow for more than 10 to 12 days, (c) the presence of intracranial air on x-ray examination, (d) meningitis (surgery to follow medical control and recovery from meningitis), (e) special cases, *e.g.*, very extensive skull fracture involving the sinuses, especially frontal, and, if in the course of surgery for a compound skull fracture, a dural tear is discovered.

2. Use of Antibiotics. Nose and throat cultures should be taken immediately assuming the absence of a positive culture of CSF taken if meningitis occurs. All patients with CSF leaks should be placed on antibiotics immediately after taking the cultures. The antibiotics should be changed to cover the culture results as they are discovered. Postoperative antibiotics are required only for 3 to 5 days. Broad spectrum antibiotics are not recommended and all cultures must be repeated at 48-hour intervals in the 1st week.

3. Timing of Sinus Repair. It is not necessary to have the local sinus repair precede the fistula repair. Cairns showed that sinusitis rarely follows sinus injury whereas meningitis was a real risk. The only exception to this advice is in the case of mastoid sinus injuries. Repair of the mastoid sinuses should precede closure of a related CSF fistula (7, 8).

4. CSF Drainage. This should not be used because of the high risk of reversing the flow gradient and inducing infection.

5. Timing of Reduction of Facial Fractures in Association with CSF Rhinorrhea. Collins has reviewed 19 patients of this type and strongly recommends early reduction (within 48 hours) of the facial fracture, delay only serving to increase the risk of infection with hospital germs and reduce the chance of the more efficient primary healing of fractures. Collins emphasizes the greater difficulty in reducing partly healed fractures and the supportive advantage of a reconstituted bony support structure at the time of surgical closure of the CSF fistula.

Conservative management while waiting the surgical decision should consist of total bed rest, 15 to 20% elevation of the head to decrease ventricular pressure, cultures of the nose and throat, and penicillin, 1 to 2 million units per day. In children, ampicillin is of value because of the risk of H. influenza infection. Traumatic otorrhea stops spontaneously more frequently than traumatic rhinorrhea and, if persistent, is suggestive of raised intracranial pressure.

Nontraumatic CSF Leaks

DIAGNOSIS

As described earlier, the clinical presentation of the nontraumatic leak is clearly different. Patients may present either with a leak as part of a neurological picture describing a space occupying lesion (*i.e.*, a high pressure leak), as a simple "leaky nose" often mistaken to be a "rhinitis" or as recurrent meningitis without an obvious leak. Flow of CSF is usually more copious than the traumatic leak and often heavier on rising in the mornings. This class of CSF leakage seldom stops spontaneously and thus the first aim in diagnosis is to determine whether a "high pressure" or "normal pressure" type of mechanism is causative. Our experience with 18 cases of nontraumatic leaks in these two major subcategories is summarized in Tables 27.4 and 27.5. Each of the etiological factors in the two categories will now be reviewed in turn. Leakage caused by tumors is subdivided in our classification into "direct" and "indirect" types. This indicates the two ways in which the fistula may be created by the tumor—that is, either directly by erosion of meninges and bone (Cases 9 to 15 in Table 27.5) or indirectly *via* pressure erosion of anatomically fragile areas of the skull base (Cases 16, 17, and 18 in Table 27.5). It is significant that in all three of these indirect rhinorrheas the fistula was in the cribriform plate, an indication of the fragility of this area. Previous reports on tumor-induced CSF rhinorrhea (24, 51, 56) have emphasized that pituitary tumors are the commonest lesion and in our series of 10 patients with high pressure leaks there were

TABLE 27.4
Summary of Case Material—Normal Pressure Leaks

No.	Lesion	Surgery for Lesion	Surgery for Rhinorrhea	Result for Lesion	Result for Rhinorrhea	Follow-up Results
1	Hole in cribriform plate with arachnoid hernia, age 54, C.S.	Yes (Same operation)	Yes	Recurred	Recurred	Leak persists minimally *10 yr.* after surgery with no attacks of meningitis
2	Arachnoid hernia into enlarged "empty sella," age 58, R.F.J.	Yes (Same operation)	Yes	Cured	Cured	No further leak *3 yr.* after surgery; patient well
3	Hole in cribriform plate with meningeal hernia, age 32, E.P.	Yes (Same operation)	Yes	Cured	Cured	No further leak *25 yr.* after surgery; patient well
4	Nasal encephalocele, age 4, B.D.	Yes (Same operation)	Yes	Cured	Cured	No further leak *13 yr.* after surgery; patient well
5	Hole in cribriform plate with brain and meningeal hernia, age 24, K. P.	Yes (Same operation)	Yes	Cured	Cured	No further leak *10 yr.* after surgery; patient well
6	Hole in anterior cranial fossa with meningeal hernia, age 52, B.B.	Yes (5 operations)	Yes	Recurred	Recurred	Leak persisted till death *11 yr.* after 1st operation; p.m. confirmed congenital hole; no evidence of tumor
7	Hole in front of sella turcica, age 50, J.Y.	Yes (Same operation)	Yes	Cured	Cured	No further leak *8 mos.* after surgery; patient well
8	Hole in floor of sella with arachnoid hernia into sella, age 48, B.P.	Yes (Same operation)	Yes	Cured	Cured	No further leak *3 mos.* after surgery; patient well

TABLE 27.5
Summary of Case Material—High Pressure Leaks

No.	Lesion	Surgery for Lesion	Surgery for Rhinorrhea	Result for Lesion	Result for Rhinorrhea	Follow-up Results
9	Pituitary adenoma; leak *via* sellar floor, N.W.	Yes (1)*	Yes (2)	Cured	Recurred	Leak persists *6 yr.* after surgery; on replacement therapy and penicillin
10	Acoustic neurinoma; leak *via* eustachian tube? E.K.	Yes (1)	No	Cured	Cured	No leak for *6 yr.*
11	Acoustic neurinoma; leak *via* eustachian tube? J.D.	Yes (2)	No	Cured	Cured	No leak for *9 yr.*
12	Nasopharyngeal carcinoma, A.H.	Yes (1)	No	Persisted	Stopped	Died *1 yr*; No P.M.
13	Pituitary adenoma, E.R.	Yes (1) +DXr‡	No	Persists	Stopped	No leak *5 yr.* later
14	Pituitary tumor, Q.J.	No DXr only	No	? Cured	Persists	Minimal leak persists; patient refuses surgery; *6 yr.*
15	Pituitary adenocarconoma; leak *via* sellar floor, F.K.	Yes (2) +DXr	Yes	? Cured	Cured	Massive tumor regressed after radiation; no tumor recurrence for *3 yr.* leak arrested
16	3rd ventricle tumor; leak in cribriform plate, P.M.	No	Yes (shunt)	Persists	Cured	No leak *11 yr.*
17	Cerebellar glioma; leak *via* cribriform plate, B.L.	Yes (3)	Yes (1)	? Cured	Cured	No leak or tumor recurrence *6 yr.*
18	Cerebellar glioma; leak *via* cribriform plate, N.L.	Yes (3)	Yes (2)	? Cured	Persisted	Died after 2nd leak surgery from pulmonary embolism

* Numbers in parentheses refer to number of operations.
‡ DXr = Deep x-ray therapy.

four cases (Cases 9, 13, 14 and 15 in Table 27.5). It should be stressed that CSF rhinorrhea is an extremely rare complication of such tumors.

Hydrocephalus. This is a much rarer cause of CSF rhinorrhea. The earliest report of a case due to communicating hydrocephalus is by Miller and little can be added to that account (43). Occasionally hydrocephalus is associated with a congenital anomaly as the cause of a high pressure CSF leak and such an association has been reported with Crouzon's disease and Albers-Schoenberg disease (osteopetrosis). In the majority of cases, however, congenital anomalies are etiologically more important for normal pressure leakages. Here nasal encephalocele is the usual lesion discovered (Case 4 in Table 27.5) and such patients are the usual examples of normal pressure leakages occurring in childhood.

Focal Atrophy. Congenital anomalies may also play a role in the next category of our classification, namely "focal atrophy." This is a speculative idea suggesting that the normal contents of the cribriform plate or sella turcica areas are reduced in bulk. This atrophy may be due to ischemia. The empty space thus created is filled with a CSF arachnoidal pouch which is an enlargement of the normal arachnoidal space extensions. This pouch enables the normal CSF pressure pulse to exert a focal and continually erosive effect analogous to the creation of cranial vault excavations by the arachnoidal granulations. This concept of focal atrophy was developed to explain the mechanism of CSF rhinorrhea in three of our patients with sellar leaks (Cases 2, 7, and 8 in Table 27.4). But it may be invoked to explain normal pressure CSF leakage from any site in adults. Thus it agrees quite well with the hypothesis advanced by O'Connell. He described in two patients a combination of an excavated lamina cribrosa plus a shrunken olfactory bulb enabling the development of a pulsating pocket of CSF over the fistula (48). In our series, Case 1 in Table 27.4 appeared to have a similar lesion. A recent report by Front and Penning from Groningen described three cases of recurrent meningitis without obvious rhinorrhea in whom a pouch of arachnoid bulged through the floor of the anterior cranial fossa into the nasal cavity (22).

Recently Leclerc, Hardy, Vezina, and Mercky reviewed the "empty sella" syndrome and presented arguments indicating that a more suitable name for this example of "focal atrophy" would be intrasellar arachnoidocele (35). They argued that the sella is filled with a fluid pouch of arachnoid overlying a normal though shrunken pituitary gland. The syndrome is relatively benign as noted earlier by others (5, 19, 26, 32, 42). These authors would reserve the term "empty sella" for the sella "emptied" by surgery—a most logical recommendation, but the "empty sella syndrome" is perhaps too well established to be considered a misnomer!

Drolet, Bouche and Belanger reported one additional case of empty sella with CSF leak which illustrates important points in the diagnosis and treatment of such lesions. Because of the posterolateral posture of the fistula, it required three operations to stop the leak. The third successful operation was the only one that could truly inspect the site of the fistula—*i.e.*, when it was approached *via* the transnasal transsphenoidal route (19).

The anatomy of the sphenoid bone in relation to CSF leaks has been carefully studied by A. C. Hooper. In 138 adult sphenoids, 27 defects were found which could cause CSF rhinorrhea. Fourteen holes were located at the site of the superior opening of the transient lateral craniopharyngeal canal. The remaining 13 were along the pathway of the internal carotid artery. Hooper concluded that the gross and microscopic appearances of these defects were consistent with their production by a process of "focal atrophy" as suggested by us in 1968 (28).

Minor degrees of congenital meningeal and meningocerebral hernia can also act as actual or potential pathways in the anterior skull base and present in adult life with CSF rhinorrhea—for example, Cases 3, 5, and 6 in Table 27.4. The majority of case reports of "primary spontaneous" rhinorrhea are explicable by the etiology. The genesis of such a leak,

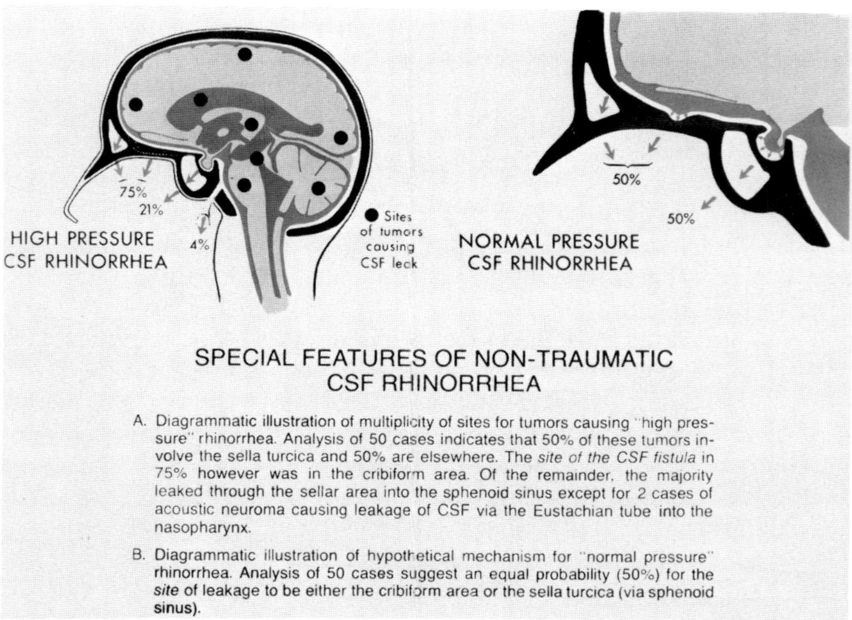

FIG. 27.8. Summary of special feature of nontraumatic rhinorrhea.

I. TRAUMATIC RHINORRHEA.

A. *Intradural surgical repair* of the dural laceration is recommended for *all* cases of proven CSF rhinorrhea as prophylaxis against infection.

B. *Timing of Surgery:* 10-14 days after trauma for *acute* leaks and as soon as possible after onset of *delayed* CSF rhinorrhea.

C. *Conservative management:* Reserved for older and poor risk patients only.

(c.f. Lewin, W., CSF rhinorrhea in non-missile head injuries, Clin. Neurosurg., Vol. 12, p. 237, 1966)

I. NON-TRAUMATIC RHINORRHEA.

A. *High Pressure Leaks:* Treat the cause, e.g. removal of tumor or CSF shunt surgery for hydrocephalus. Only if leak persists after cause is treated should fistula be localized and surgically closed.

B. *Normal Pressure Leaks:* The fistula will be found either in the anterior fossa (usually via cribiform area) or in the middle fossa (usually via the sellar or parasellar area & sphenoid sinus). Localize & close either by intradural or trans-sphenoidal method.

(c.f. Ommaya et al. Non-traumatic CSF rhinorrhea. J. Neurol. Neurosurg. Psychiat., 1968, 31: 214-225).

FIG. 27.9. Summary of principles of treatment of CSF leaks.

aside from the role of focal atrophy, is probably related to the attainment of the maximal CSF pressure in adults, which is almost three times that of infants, as well as in association with factors such as sneezing, coughing, or other causes of normal fluctuations in CSF pressure (48).

Osteomyelitic Erosion. The final etiological category is of osteomyelitic erosion. This is a very rare cause (44) and we have not had a single patient with this condition. The special features of nontraumatic rhinorrhea are summarized in Figure 27.8.

Nontraumatic Otorrhea

CSF fistulae of the temporal bone are rare. They usually present as otorrhea but just like the traumatic fistulae may present as rhinorrhea *via* the Eustachian tube. Otorrhea is often unrecognized, especially if the tympanic membrane is intact. The presentation can then be unusual and Kramer and associates have reported one case of CSF otorrhea due to a congenital defect in the temporal bone which simulated serous otitis media. Tomography showed the bony defect clearly (34).

Treatment of CSF Leaks

This is primarily surgical, although nonsurgical measures have resulted in successful management of such patients on rare occasions. The principles of treatment of both traumatic and nontraumatic leaks is

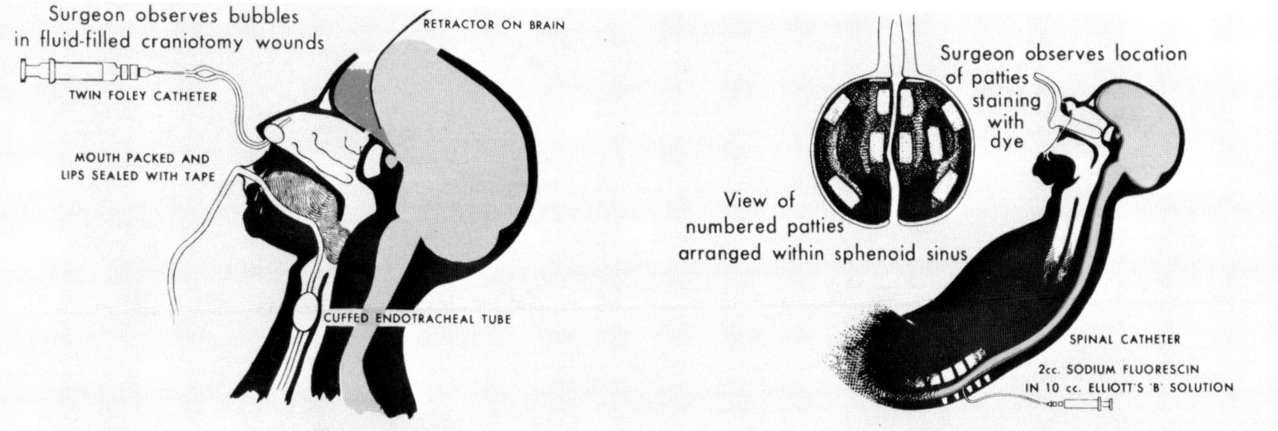

Methods for Visualizing Fistulae During Surgery

A. *During Craniotomy*

Anesthesiologist injects air via syringe into nasopharynx. Escape of air is allowed only via fistula by occluding mouth & nostrils. Surgeon observes bubbles emerging from fistula & entering operative field flooded with clear irrigating fluid.

Indication In the rare patient with profuse rhinorrhea when all pre-operative localization methods do not succeed.

B. *During Sphenoidotomy*

2 cc of 1% Sodium Fluorescein in 10 cc of Elliot's B (mock CSF) solution injected via spinal catheter into CSF

Surgeon observes staining of pre-arranged patties at various locations in the sinus with the U-V light.

Indication In patient selected for trans-sphenoidal closure & in whom site of fistula into sphenoid sinus is not known.

FIG. 27.10. Intraoperative diagnostic techniques for site of fistula in course of their treatment.

summarized in Figure 27.9. Two methods of intraoperative diagnosis of the site of leakage are shown in Figure 27.10, but with careful attention to the details of diagnostic techniques as given above, these are infrequently necessary. Remission of leakage, rarely permanent, may follow lumbar puncture, meningitis, or dye injection. Long term medical management with antibiotics has been reported to be possible (4), but with the increasing number of resistant organisms, this conservative therapy becomes hard to justify. Repeated lumbar punctures have been tried and recommended but may now be considered an obsolete method and as indicated above, liable to precipitate meningitis. Similarly, x-ray therapy to the site of the fistula is of no value. Instillation of substances nasally to promote closure of the fistula from below—for example, silver nitrate—has not been routinely successful, but a recent cure of a CSF rhinorrhea has been reported following the application of Eastman 9–10 glue to the roof of the ethmoid sinus (24). It is often recommended that following the identification of CSF in a rhinorrhea, expectant treatment, including nursing in a semi-Fowler position, discouragement of nose blowing, sneezing and straining, and antibiotic administration be tried for 6 to 8 weeks before surgery is considered. While it is true that the majority of cases of CSF rhinorrhea, particularly the traumatic variety, will stop leaking, it would be risky to suggest that this conservative therapy be adopted routinely. Indeed, the occurrence of repeated attacks of meningitis after spontaneous closure of such fistulae, even in the

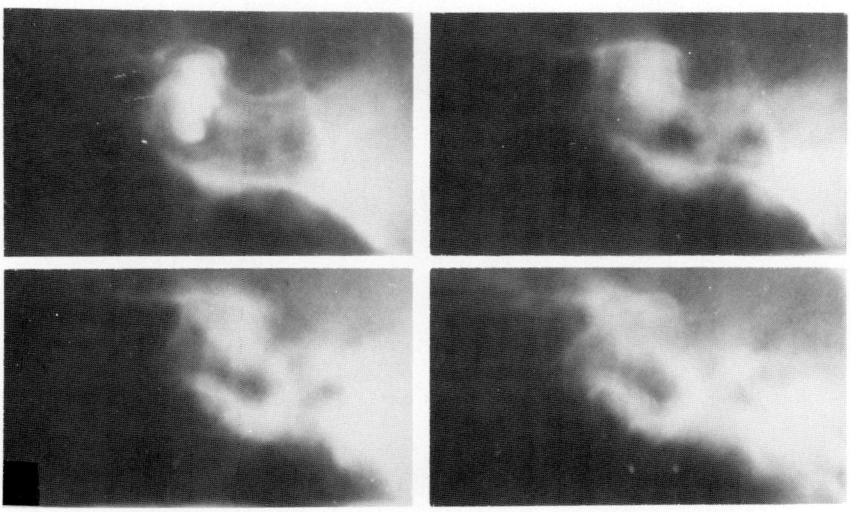

FIG. 27.11. Lateral tomograms of patient with persistent sellar leak (3 frontal craniotomies) after transnasal "plugging" of sphenoid sinus on affected site with radiopaque methyl methacrylate (tantalum powder impregnation of polymer).

absence of obvious leakage of fluid (54), would support a more active approach to some of these patients. Thus in nontraumatic CSF rhinorrhea, a conservative attitude is probably justifiable only in those patients with high pressure leaks in whom the causal lesion cannot be removed. This was the initial management of our Case 15 in Table 27.5. However, after apparently complete regression of her adenocarcinoma following deep x-ray therapy, her fistula was closed intracranially to prevent recurrent meningitis. In normal pressure leaks, surgical repair of the fistula is usually easy and is to be recommended as soon as the diagnosis is established.

ANESTHESIA

Positive pressure respiration at induction must be carefully avoided to protect against risk of infection. Thus tracheal intubation while awake is recommended.

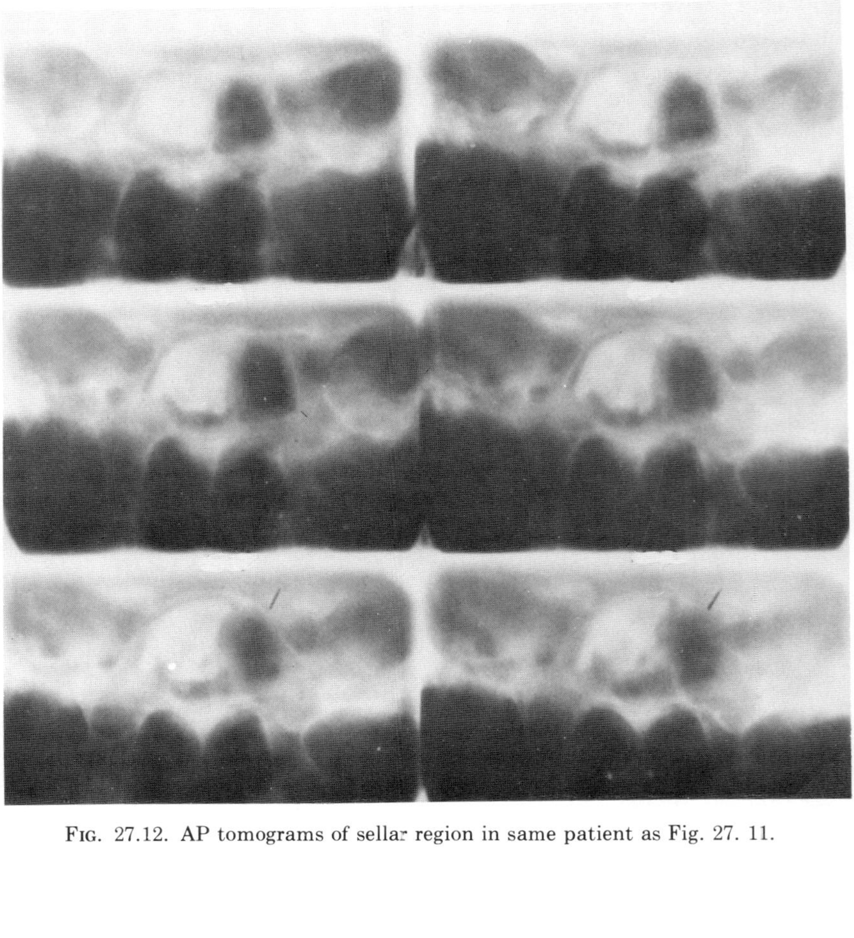

FIG. 27.12. AP tomograms of sellar region in same patient as Fig. 27. 11.

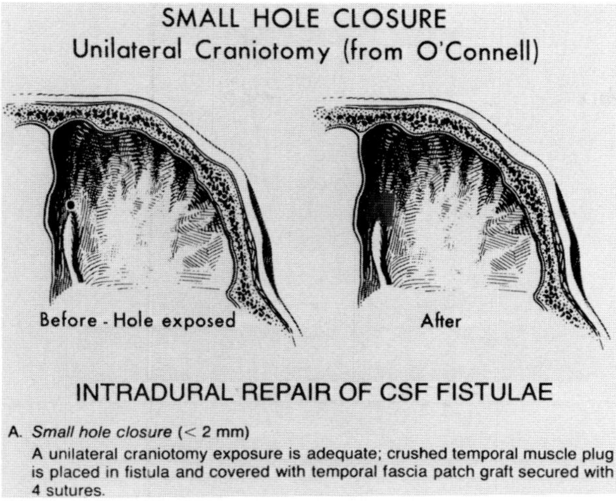

FIG. 27.13. Technique for repair of small fistula in anterior cranial fossa.

USE OF SYNTHETIC ADHESIVES

This has been recently reviewed by VanderArk and associates and should be considered in the difficult case not responding to the more routine methods described above (58). Nystrom (45) and Probst and Rahn (50) have used a combination of adhesive (Biobond) and fascia to achieve good results.

Surgical techniques to repair such fistulae are numerous but may be considered briefly under two heads. First, the extracranial, usually transnasal, approach, and, secondly, the intracranial approach. The extracranial, extranasal approach to fistulae through the frontal and ethmoidal sinuses has been recently recommended by Aboulker, Le Beau, Sterkers, and Elbaz (1). Mennig has described a transethmoidal trans-sphenoidal approach to repair a fistula through the floor of the sella turcica which was successful after an intracranial attempt at closing the leak had failed (41). A recent review of such extracranial techniques is by Vrabec and Hallbeg (61). In our opinion, such extracranial techniques should be reserved for sellar and parasellar leaks, and in the carefully selected patient in whom the etiology of the leakage has been clearly understood, the fistula track demonstrated, and in whom the intracranial methods cannot be undertaken for definite reasons. The rationale for this opinion is that CSF rhinorrhea is not simply a matter of closure of the bony defect but, more importantly, necessitates repair of the meningeal defects. Such meningeal repairs are best conducted after adequate inspection intradurally, and rhinological procedures seldom provide an adequate view within the dura mater. On the other hand, leaks through the sella turcica and sphenoid sinus are best approached *via* the microneurosurgical trans-spenoidal route. In one case we were able to stop a trans-sphenoidal leak using tantalum-impregnated methacrylate after three prior craniotomies had failed to stop the flow (Figs. 27.11 and 27.12).

The intracranial procedures have been adequately described by Dandy (13), and only a few comments are necessary. As stated before, the crucial factor in adequate surgical treatment is closure of the meningeal defect. This is often quite small in nontraumatic leaks and easy to overlook. Some neurosurgeons have resorted to filling the craniotomy site with saline and with the help of the anesthesiologist obtain a visual demonstration of the hole by forcing air from the nasopharynx into the exposure area where the escape of bubbles may be seen (92) (Fig. 27.10). However, with accurate preoperative diagnosis, this maneuver with its attendant risk of sepsis may be avoided. After demonstration of the meningeal defect, the patient's own fascia, pericranium, muscle, or strips of Gelfoam may be used to provide the intradural repair, with fascia being the most satisfactory. It is not essential to strip the dura and display small bony defects and attempt to seal them with bone wax, acrylic cements, or other substances. This is necessary only where the bony defect is large enough to necessitate support of the intradural graft.

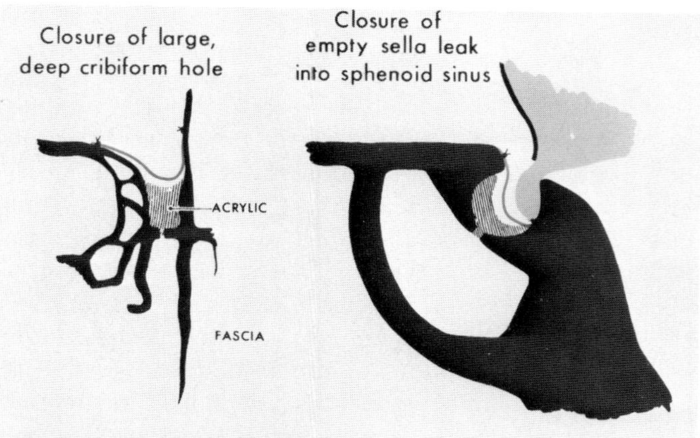

B. *Large hole closure* (> 2 mm)

Unilateral exposure usually adequate but bilateral craniotomy occasionally needed. Defect in skull base is filled with plug of methyl methacrylate & made to lie flush with bone. A large temporal fascia or fascia lata graft is then placed over the defect so that a minimum of 2 cm of graft exceeds all dimensions of the defect.

FIG. 27.14. Technique for repair of large fistulae in anterior fossa and sellar region.

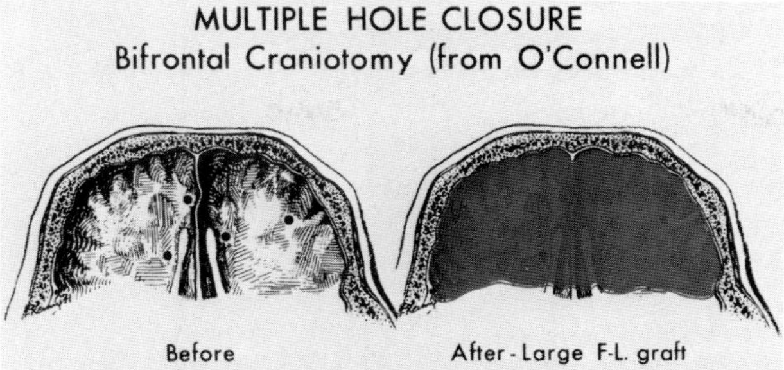

C. *Closure for multiple fistulae* or for the "occult" case (usually) due to small fistulae in one or both cribiform fossae). A bilateral frontal craniotomy allows placement of a large fascia lata graft fashioned to cover both anterior cranial fossae. Middle fossa leaks are repaired separately via temporal craniotomies with similar large fascia lata grafts. No sutures are required for such grafts.

FIG. 27.15. Technique for closure of multiple deficits.

In such cases methyl methacrylate is a satisfactory caulking material. The methods for closure of small, large, and multiple holes are shown in Figures 27.13–27.15.

In summary, the intracranial, intradural approach is recommended for most traumatic and nontraumatic cerebrospinal fistulae with careful "patching" of the fistula site, preferably using the patient's own tissues as free grafts. Sealing of subjacent bony defects is required only when the hole is of significant size—for example, greater than 2 mm. in diameter. In high pressure leaks, removal or bypass of the tumor or obstruction should always precede repair of the fistula which should be carried out only where it is positively established that a "safety valve" function is no longer required. In normal pressure leaks, obliteration of the arachnoid hernia should accompany careful intradural repair of the fistula. It is hoped that optimal management for every case of nontraumatic CSF rhinorrhea may be achieved by consideration of these facts.

REFERENCES

1. Aboulker, P., Le Beau, J., Sterkers, J. M., and Elbaz, P. Traitement des fistules méningees ethmoïdo-frontales. A propos de 15 cas opérés avec succès par voie exocránienne. Ann. Otolaryngol. (PARIS), *83:* 27–32, 1966.
2. Alazraki, N. P., Halpern, S. E., Ashburn, W. L., and Coel, M. Hyberbaric cisternography: Experience in humans. J. Nucl. Med., *14:* 226–229, 1973.
3. Allen, M. B., El Gammal, T., Ihnen, M., and Cowan, M. A. Fistula detection in cerebrospinal fluid leakage. J. Neurol. Neurosurg. Psychiatry, *35:* 664–668, 1972.
4. Anderson, W. M., Schwarz, G. A., and Gammon, G. D. Chronic spontaneous cerebrospinal rhinorrhea. Arch. Intern. Med., *107:* 723–731, 1961.

5. Bernasconi, V., Giovanelli, M. A., and Papo, I. Primary empty sella. J. Neurosurg., *36:* 157–161, 1972.
6. Busch, W. Die Morphologie der Sella turcica and ihre Beziehungen zur hypophyse. Virchows Arch. (Pathol. Anat.), *320:* 437–458, 1951.
7. Cairns, H. Injuries of the frontal and ethmoidal sinuses with special reference to cerebrospinal fluid rhinorrhea and aeroceles. J. Laryngol. Otol., *52:* 589–623, 1937.
8. Cairns, H. Discussion on injuries of the frontal and ethmoidal sinuses. Proc. R. Soc. Med., *35:* 809–810, 1942.
9. Cirić, I. S., and Tarkington, J. Transsphenoidal microsurgery. Surg. Neurol., *2:* 207–212, 1974.
10. Collins, W. F. Dural fistulae and their repair. *In* Neurological Surgery, edited by J. R. Youmans, Vol. 2, Chap. 50. W. B. Saunders, Philadelphia, 1973.
11. Crow, H. J., Keogh, C., and Northfield, D. W. C. The localisation of cerebrospinal-fluid fistulae. Lancet, *2:* 325–327, 1956.
12. Cushing, H. Experiences with orbito-ethmoidal osteomata having intracranial complications. Surg. Gynecol. Obstet., *44:* 721–742, 1927.
13. Dandy, W. E. Pneumocephalus (intracranial pneumatocele or aerocele). Arch. Surg., *12:* 949–982, 1926.
14. Di Chiro, G., and Grove, A. S., Jr. Evaluation of surgical and spontaneous cerebrospinal fluid shunts by isotope scanning. J. Neurosurg., *24:* 743–748, 1966.
15. Di Chiro, G., Ommaya, A. K., Briner, W., and Ashburn, W. Isotope cisternography in the diagnosis and follow-up of cerebrospinal fluid rhinorrhea. J. Neurosurg., *28:* 522–529, 1968.
16. Di Chiro, G., Reames, P. M., and Matthews, W. B., Jr. RISA-ventriculography and RISA-cisternography. Neurology (Minneap.), *14:* 185–191, 1964.
17. Dohlman, G. Spontaneous cerebrospinal rhinorrhoea: Case operated by rhinologic methods. Acta Otolaryngol. (Stockh.) (Suppl.), *67:* 20–23, 1948.
18. Doron, Y., Simon, J., and Peyser, E. Positive contrast myeloencephalography for visualization of cerebrospinal fluid fistula. Neuroradiology, *3:* 228–230, 1972.
19. Drolet, M., Bouche, B., and Belánger, C. Syndrome de la grosse selle turcique vide et de la rhinorrhée du liquide céphalo-rachidien. CMA J., *107:* 1199–1202, 1972.
20. Eden, K. Traumatic cerebrospinal rhinorrhoea. Repair of the fistula by a transfrontal intradural operation. Br. J. Surg., *29:* 299–303, 1941.
21. Engels, E. P. Roentgenographic demonstration of a hypophysical subarachnoid space. Am. J. Roentgenol., *80:* 1001–1004, 1958.
22. Front, D., and Penning, L. Occult spontaneous cerebrospinal fluid rhinorrhea diagnosed by isotope cisternography. Neuroradiology, *2:* 167–169, 1971.
23. Gadeholt, H. The reaction of glucose-oxidase test paper in normal nasal secretion. Acta Otolaryngol. (Stockh.), *58:* 271–272, 1964.
24. Gotham, J. E., Meyer, J. S., Gilroy, J., and Bauer, R. B. Observations on cerebrospinal fluid rhinorrhea and pneumocephalus. Ann. Otol. Rhinol. Laryngol., *74:* 215–233, 1965.
25. Grant, F. C. Intracranial aerocele following fracture of the skull. Report of a case with review of the literature. Surg. Gynecol. Obstet., *36:* 251–255, 1923.
26. Hodgson, S. F., Randall, R. V., Holman, C. B., and MacCarty, C. S. Empty sella syndrome. Med. Clin. North Am., *56:* 897–907, 1972.
27. Holman, B. L., and Davis, D. O. Radioisotopic assessment of cerebrospinal fluid pathways. Prog. Nucl. Med., *1:* 359–375, 1972.
28. Hooper, A. C. Sphenoidal defects—a possible cause of cerebrospinal fluid rhinorrhoea. J. Neurol. Neurosurg. Psychiatry, *34:* 739–742, 1971.

29. House, W. F., and Hitselberger, W. E. Surgical complications of acoustic tumor surgery. Arch. Otolaryngol., *88:* 659–667, 1968.
30. Jacobson, I., and Maran, A. G. Localization of cerebrospinal fluid rhinorrhea. Arch. Otolaryngol., *93:* 79–80, 1971.
31. Jones, H. M. The problem of recurrent meningitis. Proc. R. Soc. Med., *67:* 1141–1147, 1974.
32. Keravel, Y. Contribution au diagnostic et au traitement chirurgical de la selle turcique 'vide.' Thèse de Doctorat en Médecine, Paris, 1973.
33. King, D. Report to Westminster Medical Society. London Med. Surg. J. *4:* 823–825, 1834.
34. Kramer, S. A., Yanagisawa, E., and Smith, H. W. Spontaneous cerebrospinal fluid otorrhea simulating serous otitis media. Laryngoscope, *81:* 1083–1089, 1971.
35. Leclercq, T. A., Hardy, J., Vezina, J. L., and Mercky, F. Intrasellar arachnoidocele and the so-called empty sella syndrome. Surg. Neurol., *2:* 295–299, 1974.
36. Lewin, W. Cerebrospinal fluid rhinorrhea in nonmissile head injuries. Clin. Neurosurg., *12:* 237–252, 1966.
37. Linell, E. A., and Robinson, W. L. Head injuries and meningitis. J. Neurol. Neurosurg. Psychiatry, *4:* 23–31, 1941.
38. Marc, J. A., and Schecter, M. M. The significance of fluid-gas displacement in the sphenoid sinus in post-traumatic cerebrospinal fluid rhinorrhea. Radiology, *108:* 603–606, 1973.
39. MacGee, E. E., Cauthen, J. C., and Brackett, C. E. Meningitis following acute traumatic cerebrospinal fistula. J. Neurosurg., *33:* 312–316, 1970.
40. McKusick, K. A., Malmud, L. S., Kordela, P. A., and Wagner, H. N., Jr. Radionuclide cisternography: Normal values for nasal secretion of intrathecally injected ^{111}In-DTPA. J. Nucl. Med., *14:* 933–934, 1973.
41. Mennig, H. Heilung einer schwierigen Liquorfistel durch rhinochirurgisches Vorgehen. Z. Laryngol. Rhinol. Otol. *43:* 412–419, 1964.
42. Metzger, J., Helias, A., Messimy, R., and Fischgold, H.: Nouveaux cas de selles turciques dites vides avec signes neuro-ophtalmologiques ou rhinorrhée. Rev. Neurol. (Paris), *123:* 435–442, 1970.
43. Miller, C. Case of hydrocephalus chronicus with some unusual symptoms and appearances on dissection. Trans. Med. Chir. Soc. Edinb., *2:* 243–248, 1826.
44. Nori, A., and Carteri, A. Rinoliquorrea: Trattamento e risultati a distanza. Chir. Ital., *16:* 161–165, 1964.
45. Nyström, S. H. M. On the use of biobond in the treatment of cerebrospinal rhinorrhea and frontobasal fistula. G. Int. Coll. Surg., *54:* 332–340, 1970.
46. Oberson, R. Radioisotope diagnosis of rhinorrhea. Radiol. Clin. Biol. *41:* 28–35, 1972.
47. Obrador, S. Primary non-traumatic spontaneous cerebro-spinal fluid rhinorrhea with normal cerebro-spinal fluid pressure. Schweiz Arch. Neurol. Neurochir. Psychiatr. *111:* 369–376, 1972.
48. O'Connell, J. E. A. Primary spontaneous cerebrospinal fluid rhinorrhea. J. Neurol. Neurosurg. Psychiatry, *27:* 241–246, 1964.
49. Ommaya, A. K., Di Chiro, G., Baldwin, M., and Pennybacker, J. B., Non-traumatic cerebrospinal fluid rhinorrhea. J. Neurol. Neurosurg. Psychiatry, *31:* 214–255, 1968.
50. Probst, C., and Rahn, B. A. La fermeture plastique des fistules frontobasales au moyen de Biobond-Tabotamp. Expériences cliniques et expérimentales. Neurochirurgie, *18:* 203–212, 1972.
51. Raskind, R. Cerebrospinal fluid rhinorrhea and otorrhea: Diagnosis and treatment in 35 cases. G. Int. Coll. Surg., *43:* 141–154, 1965.

52. Ray, B. S., and Bergland, R. M. Cerebrospinal fluid fistula: Clinical aspects, techniques of localization, and methods of closure. J. Neurosurg., *30:* 399–405, 1969.
53. Rockett, F. X., Wittenborg, M. H., Shillito, J., Jr., and Matson, D. D. Pantopaque visualization of a congenital dural defect of the internal auditory meatus causing rhinorrhea; report of a case. Am. J. Roentgenol. *91:* 640–646, 1964.
54. Schneider, R. C., and Thompson, J. M. Chronic and delayed traumatic cerebrospinal rhinorrhea as a source of recurrent attacks of meningitis. Ann. Surg., *145:* 517–529, 1957.
55. Teng, P., and Edalatpour, N. Cerebrospinal fluid rhinorrhea with demonstration of cranionasal fistula with Pantopaque. Radiology, *81:* 802–806, 1963.
56. Teng, P., and Papatheodorou, C. Cerebrospinal rhinorrhea and otorrhea. Arch. Otolaryngol., *82:* 56–61, 1965.
57. Thomson, St. C. The Cerebrospinal Fluid; Its Spontaneous Escape from the Nose, 144p.p. Cassell & Co Ltd., London, 1899.
58. VanderArk, G. D., Pitkethly, D. T., Ducker, T. B., and Kempe, L. G. Repair of CSF fistula using tissue adhesions. J. Neurosurg., *33:* 151–155, 1970.
59. VanGilder, J. C., and Goldenberg, I. S. Hypophysectomy in metastatic breast cancer. Arch. Surg., *110:* 293–295, 1975.
60. Voena, G. Considerazioni su un caso di grave cranio-rino-liquorrea da persistenza del canale basi-occipitale. Arch. Ital. Otol., *70:* 212–222, 1959.
61. Vrabec, D. P., and Hallberg, O. E. Cerebrospinal fluid rhinorrhea. Arch. Otolaryngol., *80:* 218–229, 1964.
62. Wehrle, P. F., Mathies, A. W., Jr., and Leedom, J. M. Management of bacterial meningitis. Clin. Neurosurg., *14:* 72–85, 1967.
63. Wolman, L. The neuropathological effects resulting from the intrathecal injection of chemical substances. Paraplegia, *4:* 97–115, 1966.
64. Yasargil, M. G., and Fox, J. L. The microsurgical approach to acoustic neurinomas. Surg. Neurol., *2:* 393–398, 1974.

CHAPTER

28

Shunt Complications

MARTIN P. SAYERS, M.D.

One speaks of complications with humility, wishing for the opportunity for a replay. We can and do learn from experience, and I appreciate this opportunity to pass on to you, my friends in the Congress, this crystallization of a great many of my shunt experiences.

In fact, one cannot entirely separate the inter-relationships of the patient's primary disease, hydrocephalus, growth from the shunt, and its follow-up care. So it is that an obstructed shunt is often really a complication of the five inter-related factors rather than of the shunt alone. The proper selection of patients for shunting proves to be as important as the procedure itself. The decision not to repair or to delay surgery for a child with myelomeningocele can exclude a number of complications and a mortality (Table 28.1).

The statistical data are based on a consecutive series of shunts done by or supervised by the author between 1957 and 1974 inclusive. Patients initially shunted elsewhere are excluded. We have resisted the temptation to shunt because the ventricles and/or the head are large and have treated only documented progressive hydrocephalus (Table 28.2).

Forty-six percent of the series have required at least one shunt revision, and the neurosurgeons have performed 1390 procedures on the 730 cases excluding myelomeningocele repair in the course of the 18-year period. Many have had additional operations in the hands of other surgical disciplines and six have died from the complications of those procedures (Table 28.3).

Complications and mortality are unquestionably related to errors in management and diagnosis. We missed small tumors in the periaqueductal gray matter and in the low basal ganglia and midbrain, labeling them aqueduct stenosis.

Early in the series arachnoid cysts in the cisterna magna were called basal arachnoiditis and a cyst developing in the 3rd ventricle was ignored in the face of progressive optic atrophy because the shunt was still functioning. Another of our early "aqueduct stenosis" cases bled from her aneurysm of the vein of Galen at age 8 years (Table 28.4).

TABLE 28.1
Myelomeningocele—Patient Selection (1957–1974)

Repaired	522	
Not repaired	133	
	655	Total cases
Shunted	373	57% of total
		71% of repaired

TABLE 28.2
Hydrocephalus (1957–1974)—Shunted

Myelomeningocele	373	
Hydrocephalus (other)	357	
Total cases	730	
Mortality (1974)	82	(11%)

TABLE 28.3
Hydrocephalus (1957–1974)—Status (Jan. 1975)

Shunted cases	730	
Required revision	335	(46%)
Additional revisions, etc.	209	
Third ventriculostomy	86	(12%)
Arnold-Chiari (operated)	30	
Total procedure (neurosurgery (excluding myelomeningocele repair)	1390	
Mortality	82	(11%)

TABLE 28.4
Shunt Complications—Incorrect Diagnosis

Unrecognized neoplasm	
Obstructing	3
Choroid plexus	1
Arachnoid cyst	
Posterior fossa	2
Third ventricle (secondary)	2
Aneurysm of vein of Galen	1
Compensated hydrocephalus	?

Although the frustrated statistician encounters 839 complications in the chronological course of these 730 patients, more than half of the group encountered only very brief intervals of discomfort and additional hospitalization with mechanical problems related to growth, foreign body reaction, and operative techniques. A careful follow-up and good physician-patient relations prevented potentially severe morbidity (Table 28.5).

Many of these incidents occurred more frequently in our early years of shunting. The distal foreign body reaction was greatly reduced by cutting the mass of our tubing to less than one-third that of the earlier apparatus. Junctional separation was discouraged by reinforcement, ventricular catheter obstruction by careful placement with a stiffer plastic, and migration was halted immediately by a swedged on segment of larger catheter just below each shunt connection. Common errors in operative technique are listed in Table 28.6.

The house staff rarely misses a chance to watch me vibrate by reminding me that it is said that "after all, a shunt is just a 'burr hole' connected

TABLE 28.5
Shunt Complications (1390 Procedures)—Mechanical

Thoracic occlusion	351
Ventricular occlusion	83
Shunt separation	33
Kinked tubing	28
CSF fistula	16
Migrating catheter–ventricular	15
Migrating catheter–distal	3
Subdural hemorrhage	10
Surfacing shunt	8
Ventricular hemorrhage (gross)	6
	553

TABLE 28.6
Shunt Complications—Errors in Technique

1. Failure to cover foreign materials with pericranium
2. Placement of tubing superficially under parallel incision
3. Use of unclean or contaminated apparatus
4. Improper selection of shunt apparatus
5. Poorly located shunts
6. Excessive buried foreign material
7. Overtight ligatures
8. Failure to excise scar
9. Inadequate or excessive surgical exposure
10. Overlarge dural opening
11. Excessive ventricular drainage at surgery
12. Improper placement of catheters
13. Failure of shunt fixation
14. Misplaced distal catheters
15. Flexibility of shunt system
16. Failure to allow for motion and growth

to a 'cutdown'." Yet if the unsuspecting surgeon places his tube directly under a parallel incision and fails adequately to cover it with pericranium or to countersink a bulky part under thin scalp, the foreign material will tend to surface and one or several new complications may appear on our charts.

In 1957, 20% of the patients came down with septicemia. Other infections either predisposed or resulted from the blood stream infection. We countered by soaking "mini" tubes in Bacitracin–Neomycin solution and by timing our procedures to minimize the possibility of bacteremia at the moment of the shunt (Table 28.7).

Remote and systemic infections are treated intensively as most shunt infections are metastatic and seat on or near the foreign shunt material (Table 28.8). Routine prophylactic antibiotics in an individual who will carry the predisposing shunt for many years has never caught on with us.

In the postoperative period we start with the patient face down on a

TABLE 28.7
Shunt Complications (1390 Procedures)—Infections

Septicemia	46	(6%)
Pneumonia	35	
Wound infection	27	
Ventriculitis	28	
Meningitis	5	
Chronic basal arachnoiditis	6	
Pylephlebitis	1	
Peritonitis	1	
	149	

TABLE 28.8
Shunt Complications—Timing

Wait awhile before shunt
Related to:
- Ventricular drainage
- Fractional ventriculography
- Meningocele repair
- CSF fistula
- Systemic infection
- Wound healing
- Weeping meningocele
- Debilitated patient
- Undiagnosed fever
- Septicemia
- Electrolyte imbalance
- "Pallid asphyxia" or shock

frame to avoid decubitus, contamination, and excessive or obstructed drainage which can predispose subdural hemorrhage or fistula along the ventricular catheter. We pump only to test during this period of floating detritus and shunt establishment. Very rapid reduction in ventricle size is not desirable. The parents are furnished an instruction sheet and requested specifically never to pump the shunt unless so instructed. Probably this is an important factor in avoiding ventricular catheter obstruction.

It is probable that many children and adults have undergone shunt revisions because of very painful low pressure or vascular headaches not related to increased intracranial pressure. I have felt the temptation but have temporized with a rather routine program of observation and medication with Diamox 15 to 25 mg./kg. per day on week days skipping Saturday and Sunday until the pattern becomes clear. Often there is a family history of migraine, and occasionally photophobia, scotomata, and other typical clinical signs help the physician to recognize a vascular headache pattern.

Of course, severe headaches can be dangerous, and even with ventricular pressure measurements one must sort out the acute symptomatic Arnold-Chiari syndrome which has been fatal in several instances in our patients. Head retraction is a giveaway and x-rays of the foramen magnum may serve to confirm the dangerous acute Arnold-Chiari brain stem impaction.

Two have died from, and four experienced recognizable pulmonary embolus. The incidence of direct micro emboli to the lung and paradoxical to the kidney has become minimal with the use of the very fine or low mass thoracic catheter (Table 28.9).

Careful follow-up cannot be overstressed, and loss of follow-up without orderly transfer to another reliable physician is a catastrophe! The families' report of sudden change of behavior or dulled intellect continues to be a most important indicator to me. In the younger children, the

TABLE 28.9
Shunt Complications (1390 Procedures)—Late

Low pressure headaches	36
Optic atrophy—progressive	35
Central visual loss—unilateral	2
Blindness	4
Arnold-Chiari—symptomatic	30
Pulmonary hypertension	6
Pulmonary embolus (gross)	4
Embolic renal hypertension	3
Loss of follow-up	23

fontanel and head measurements are reliable. Suture separation by percussion and x-ray is a strong and reproducible indicator in the intermediate ages. A single CAT scan showing moderately enlarged ventricles is not, in my opinion, cause for immediate shunt revision even though it is well known that the shunt has not functioned for some years. I believe that one should follow clinically, carefully evaluate intellectual performance, and watch for significant change before tilting the balance in a borderline compensated patient. Probably a moderate hydrocephalus is not always a bad thing, and it may be greatly superior to shunt dependency with some of its potential problems (Table 28.10).

On the other hand, careful funduscopic follow-up (preferably by the same observer) and documented progressive optic atrophy requires a full workup and possibly a new shunt. As we all well know but need to be reminded, the problem is not always chronic CSF pressure. We must be careful not to be trapped into senseless reshunting without a full understanding of the cause of progressive loss of vision. Too often the ophthalmologist goes down with us (Table 28.11).

A look at mortality statistics tends to be a little discouraging in that many of the causes of death are closely related to the primary disease, but the rate is falling with experience and careful selection (Table 28.12). Many deaths in this series are obviously preventable. Septicemia now seems to be fatal only in the very weak individuals. It tends to be a

TABLE 28.10
Shunt Complications—Follow-up Monitoring

Family report
Fontanel
Head measurements
Behavior and intellect
Optic fundi—edema or atrophy
Percussion of head
Skull x-rays
Computerized axial tomography (CAT) scan
Loss of follow-up is a catastrophe

TABLE 28.11
Shunt Complications—Optic Atrophy (Often Congenital)

If progressive, can denote:
1. Chronic excessive pressure–even with functioning shunt
2. cyst in 3rd ventricle or chiasmatic cistern
3. missed neoplasm
4. basal arachnoiditis

TABLE 28.12
Shunt Complications—Shunt Mortality (730 Cases)

Septicemia	21	
Acute pressure	11	
Neoplasm	8	
Pyelonephritis	6	
Ventriculitis	5	
Arnold-Chiari malformation	5	
Spine ostectomy	4	
Pneumonia	3	
Laryngeal obstruction	2	
Wound complications	2	
Pulmonary embolus	2	
Third ventriculostomy	2	
Ileal conduit	2	
Operative hemorrhage	1	
Pulmonary hypertension	1	
Vascular anomaly	1	
Pylephlebitis	1	
Malignancy	1	
Accident	1	
Unknown causes	3	
Total	82	(11%)

TABLE 28.13
Hydrocephalus (1957–1974)—Status 1974 (18 Years) (Author's Estimate)

Shunt survivors		648	
"Compensated"*	168		
Functioning 3rd ventriculostomy	83		
"Probably compensated"‡	90		
		341	
Still shunt dependent		307	(47%)

* Criteria for "compensated": (1) no shunt for 8 years and/or (2) shunt demonstrated nonfunctioning.

‡ "Probably compensated": 25% of survivors last 8 years.

terminal event in a downhill course. We can and usually do defeat it in a child with reasonable intellectual potential.

Eleven deaths due to acute intracranial pressure can certainly be improved. This statistic points up poor communications, unfavorable home circumstances, lapses in follow-up and staff procrastination. Unfortunately it can and does happen on well organized teaching services—reminding us that we are dealing with a very dangerous disease.

The Arnold-Chiari malformation and its dangers, chronic and acute, are subject for a separate treatise.

SUMMARY

To some extent our greatest problem is the philosophic answer to the question, "who shall be treated, how intensely and to what expense?" The cost of care is almost always greatest in the child who is borderline in selection and least likely to survive. Over half of the children shunted after application of searching criteria appear to this author to be compensated (Table 28.13).

CHAPTER

29

Complications of Trans-sphenoidal Surgery

EDWARD R. LAWS, JR, M.D., AND EUGENE B. KERN, M.D.

The first report of a complication of the trans-sphenoidal approach for the treatment of pituitary tumors was published in 1910 (15, 26). A paper by A. E. Halstead (15) described two patients on whom he operated utilizing the sublabial trans-septal approach. One of the two patients died after the operation with a clinical course suggestive of hypothalamic damage. This patient had been operated on in 1909, the same year that Harvey Cushing first removed a pituitary tumor from an acromegalic patient (5) referred to him by Dr. C. H. Mayo. Between 1909 and 1928, Harvey Cushing performed 242 trans-sphenoidal procedures on 238 patients (5–8, 11, 21). Whereas his mortality figures were acceptable for the era before the development of steroid replacement and antibiotic therapy, he abandoned the trans-sphenoidal approach for the transcranial. In 1910, Oskar Hirsch began a long career with the trans-sphenoidal management of pituitary lesions which lasted until 1962 and included some 425 procedures (17, 22–24). Hirsch remained a faithful and vigorous exponent of the method. Norman Dott of Edinburgh learned the trans-sphenoidal approach when he worked and trained with Cushing and also remained faithful to this method of treatment of pituitary tumors, reporting on some 177 procedures in 162 patients (10). It was Dott who introduced Gerard Guiot (12–14, 30) of France to the trans-sphenoidal approach and he, in turn, was the major influence in the extensive current work of Jules Hardy of Montreal (18–20). These men have been the major contributors to the field, and their experience covers a period measured not only in years but also in scientific and technological developments that have altered both the indications and the risks related to the trans-sphenoidal approach.

Cushing, Hirsch, and Dott all began their work at a time when there was no steroid replacement therapy available and when antibiotics were not in use. For them, the trans-sphenoidal approach represented a decompressive procedure, and the level of success they attained is a tribute to their skill and to the fact that some normal functioning pituitary tissue was usually left intact. Guiot's series has the advantage of routine use of steroids and antibiotics, and both Guiot and Hardy's series reflect the use of the operating microscope and the x-ray image intensifier. These advances were introduced by Hardy and have allowed extension of the technique to definitive microsurgery of a variety of pituitary disorders (18–20). The mortality figures shown in Table 29.1 reflect these changes in management and technique. Many other smaller series of surgical cases have been reported (1, 3, 4, 9, 16, 21, 25, 28, 32, 33, 35), and the complications that developed will be included in this review. It should be recognized, however, that some series are heavily weighted toward hypophysectomy rather than toward pituitary tumor, and the proportions of patients in each category influence to some extent the incidence and nature of the complications.

The complications of trans-sphenoidal surgery may be divided into a number of categories, based both on anatomic structures and on systems that may be involved.

CATEGORIES

Intracranial complications are probably the most devastating and have frequently been reported as the cause of fatalities. Hypothalamic injury may be caused both by direct trauma and by secondary vascular effects. The clinical course, marked by high fever and coma, is characteristic and usually is not reversible. Direct intracranial hemorrhage may occur, and subarachnoid bleeding or organized intracranial hematoma may be the cause of complications or death. Branches of the circle of Willis may be torn or injured. Meningitis may result from the introduction of organisms into the intracranial space at operation or later when cerebrospinal rhinorrhea is present. One of the contraindications to the trans-sphenoidal approach is extension of the tumor into the anterior or middle cranial fossae. When unusually large intracranial tumor extensions are present, trans-sphenoidal surgery frequently results in complications related to the tumor which is not accessible by the approach selected (Fig. 29.1).

Carotid artery complications are equally devastating and commonly result in death or serious disability. Arterial hemorrhage may occur when the carotid artery, as it lies in the cavernous sinus, is lacerated,

TABLE 29.1
Mortality from Trans-sphenoidal Surgery (Major Series)

Surgeon	Dates	No. of Procedures	Mortality
			%
Cushing	1909–1928	242 (238 patients)	5.4
Dott	1925	177 (162 patients)	8.6
Hirsch	1910–1962	425	≈4.7
Guiot	1957–1974	582	≈1.24
Hardy	1962–1975	434	≈2.0

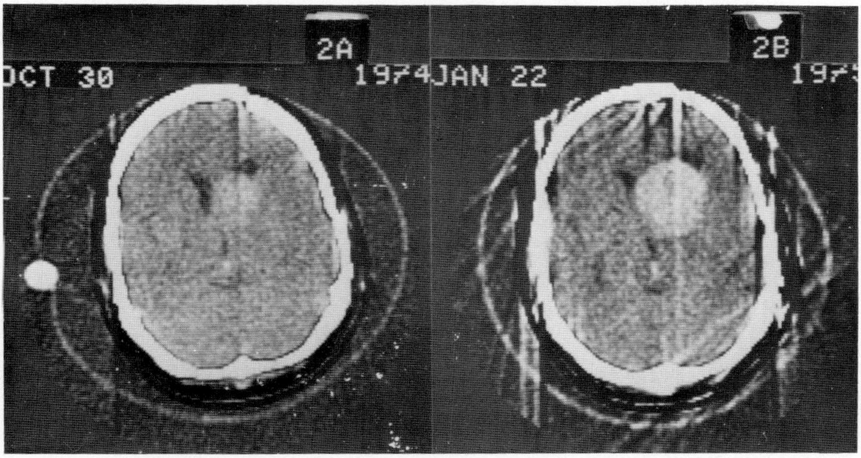

FIG. 29.1. Nonfunctioning pituitary adenoma. Computerized tomographic scan before and after trans-sphenoidal surgery. Note incomplete removal of intracranial extension.

perforated, or avulsed. Hemorrhage may be difficult to control without interrupting distal flow to the brain. Occlusion of a more spontaneous nature has been reported to follow procedures that were otherwise uncomplicated. The cavernous carotid artery may go into spasm as a result of manipulation within the sella turcica, and thrombosis and distal embolism also have been encountered (Fig. 29.2). A few patients have tortuous or redundant carotid arteries that may be visible within the sella and may be so close together as to occlude the sella, making the trans-sphenoidal approach impractical. Intrasellar aneurysms may simulate or coexist with pituitary lesions (34), but their presence should be recognized if preoperative angiography is to be performed. False aneurysms may occur after injury to the carotid artery and presumed satisfactory control; under the same circumstances, a carotid cavernous fistula might also be provoked.

Complications involving the visual system are rarely fatal but obviously they are capable of causing severe disability. Direct damage to the optic nerves or chiasm may occur while a tumor is being removed from the sella or from the suprasellar space. Such damage is more likely to happen when the capsule of the tumor is disrupted or when the capsule is adherent to the visual apparatus. Dissection and removal of pituitary tumors may interfere with the blood supply to the optic nerve or chiasm and may produce visual deficit related to ischemia. Loss of vision has developed after removal of a pituitary tumor when the chiasm has been compressed by the muscle plug commonly used to obliterate the empty sella (Fig. 29.3). One of the reasons for using such a muscle plug was the report of visual loss caused by postoperative prolapse of the optic nerves

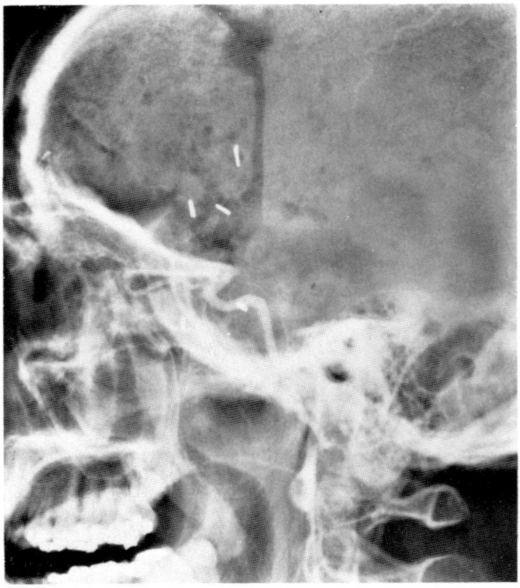

FIG. 29.2. Nonfunctioning pituitary adenoma. Previous craniotomy elsewhere. Left carotid angiogram after trans-sphenoidal surgery. Note occlusion of left internal carotid artery as it exits from cavernous sinus.

and chiasm into an empty sella after removal of a tumor. The optic nerves have been damaged by fractures of the optic foramen and orbit (27) produced by the retractors used for the trans-sphenoidal approach.

The cavernous sinus together with its contents other than the carotid artery also serves as a source for complications, during trans-sphenoidal surgery. Venous hemorrhage may occur from it or from anomalies of connections between the two cavernous sinuses (29). Laceration or disruption of these venous structures may be accompanied by venous bleeding. In addition, the removal of a tumor or a normal pituitary gland from the lateral wall of the sella may be associated with damage to the cranial nerves that run within the cavernous sinus, and involvement of the IIIrd, IVth, Vth, and VIth cranial nerves subsequent to operation has developed as either an immediate or a more delayed complication. These cranial nerve injuries usually are produced by trauma or stretching and are almost always transient.

The sella turcica itself may be the source of complications. The anatomy of the sella and its relation to the sphenoid sinus are of primary importance (2). In patients with a shallow sella and a poorly pneumatized sphenoid sinus (Fig. 29.4), trans-sphenoidal approach may require excavation of bone with a drill which may be so difficult technically as to

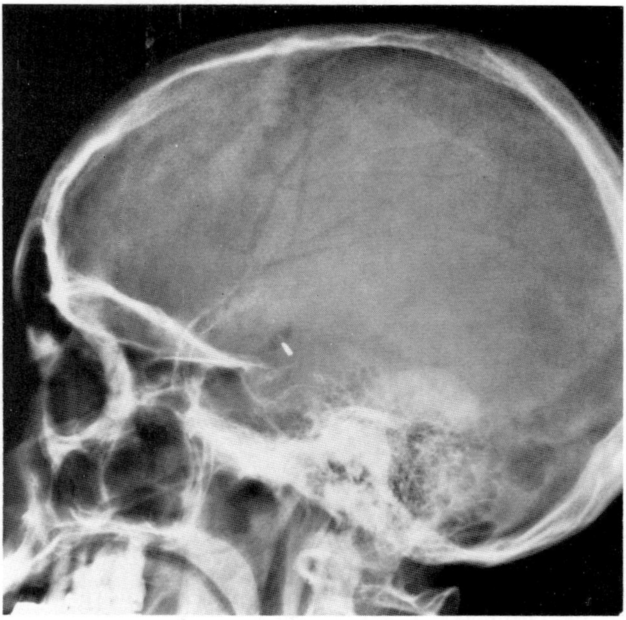

FIG. 29.3. Nonfunctioning pituitary adenoma. Lateral skull film after trans-sphenoidal surgery. Tantalum clip attached to muscle plug indicates incorrect intracranial placement of muscle.

be a contraindication to the approach. Postoperative cerebrospinal rhinorrhea most commonly occurs through the sella and its diaphragm, either because of iatrogenic injury to the roof of the sella or because of anatomic variations such as prolapse of the arachnoid into the sella or unusually large infundibular apertures in the diaphragm. Excessive enlargement or erosion of the sella from a very large intrasellar lesion has been recognized as a predisposing factor to complications (9, 32), generally of a hemorrhagic nature.

Sphenoid sinus and nasofacial complications are rarely fatal but can be troublesome and may persist for some time after surgery. Imprudent use of the retractor may result in diastasis or fracture of the hard palate. Injury to or fracture of the cribriform plate may cause cerebrospinal rhinorrhea. In the postoperative period, the mucosa of the sphenoid sinus may produce symptomatic sinusitis and eventual development of a mucocele (31). Technical errors in handling the nasal mucosa and the nasal septum may result in postoperative nasoseptal perforation, epistaxis, or postoperative external nasal deformity (Fig. 29.5). Inadequate control of bleeding from the nasal portion of the procedure may lead to superficial wound hemorrhage and swelling.

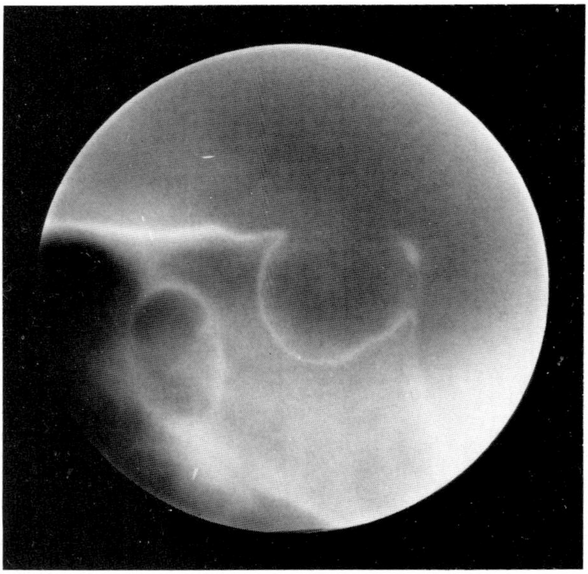

FIG. 29.4. Pituitary adenoma. Lateral tomogram of sella turcica. The sphenoid sinus is poorly pneumatized, making the trans-sphenoidal approach technically difficult.

Finally, endocrinological complications that are related both to the preoperative endocrine state of the patient and to the postoperative alteration in endocrine activity may occur. Most common of these is hypopituitarism which should be quickly recognized and rapidly corrected with the use of appropriate steroid medication. Diabetes insipidus may develop because of damage to the posterior pituitary gland or the infundibulum; water and electrolyte imbalance may follow and may be life threatening if unrecognized or inappropriately treated. In patients who present for operation with pituitary tumors producing endocrine hyperactivity, persistence of such hyperactivity subsequent to surgery must be regarded as an unsatisfactory result.

After establishing these categories by analysis of the published experience with trans-sphenoidal surgery, the Mayo Clinic experience was reviewed.

MAYO CLINIC EXPERIENCE

Between September 1972 and September 1975, 193 trans-sphenoidal procedures were performed on 185 patients at this clinic. A modification of the sublabial, trans-septal approach utilized by Cushing, Guiot, and Hardy was used for all but three of these 193 procedures. The pathological findings are presented in Table 29.2.

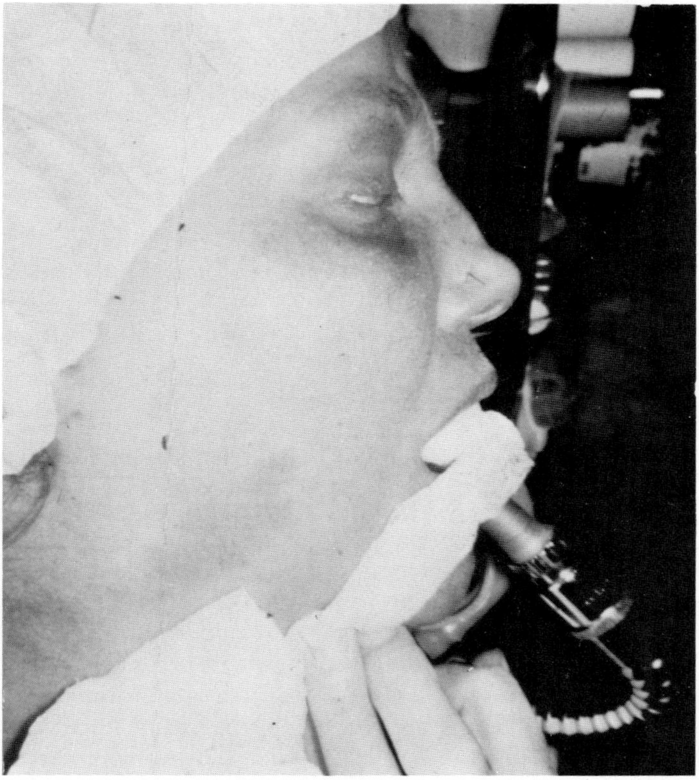

FIG. 29.5. Pituitary adenoma, Nelson-Salassa syndrome. Previous trans-sphenoidal surgery elsewhere. Postoperative saddle-nose deformity.

Pituitary adenomas accounted for 139 procedures in 137 patients. Fifty tumors were nonfunctioning or chromophobe adenomas; 37 of the 50 tumors had suprasellar extensions and two were "microadenomas" (<10 mm. in diameter). Four of the 50 tumors were cystic and six were "fibrous." Nine patients had been operated on previously, one by the trans-sphenoidal approach. Among the patients with chromophobe adenomas, there was one fatality—a patient who had undergone previous craniotomy. Death was attributed to a hypothalamic injury, although no definite cause could be discovered at autopsy. The patient never awoke from anesthesia and had unstable blood pressure and temperature regulation during the 3 days that he survived after surgery. No evidence of either hemorrhage or infarct could be found at autopsy. Two patients having chromophobe adenomas suffered postoperative strokes, thought to be the result of vascular occlusion in the carotid system. One of these

TABLE 29.2
Trans-sphenoidal Surgery—Mayo Clinic Series (1972–1975; 193 Procedures, 185 Patients)

Pathological Findings	Procedures	
Pituitary adenoma		139
Nonfunctioning adenoma	50	
Acromegaly	44	
Forbes-Albright syndrome	18	
Nelson-Salassa syndrome	14	
Cushing's disease (primary)	11	
Male galactorrhea	1	
Malignant chromophobe	1	
Craniopharyngioma		15
Empty sella–arachnoid cyst		6
Hypophysectomy		13
Sphenoidal pathology		6
Chordoma		5
Cerebrospinal rhinorrhea		5
Miscellaneous		4

patients had previously undergone craniotomy and during the postoperative period had had several episodes of transient right-sided paresis with aphasia. Angiography (Fig. 29.2) revealed multiple focal occlusive disease in the intracranial carotid system, and despite anticoagulant therapy, a permanent deficit developed. In the second patient, mild right hemiparesis and dysphasia developed soon after operation but cleared over a 10-day period. The patient refused postoperative angiography and an EMI scan was performed; no definite evidence of ischemia or infarction was revealed. In three patients with preoperative visual field defects, the vision was worse in the postoperative period. The deficit remained in one of the three patients but was transient in the other two and their vision eventually improved. These complications were related to direct pressure on the chiasm from the muscle plug in one patient (Fig. 29.3), to a residual intracranial tumor that was not accessible in one, and to a vascular injury in the third patient (the previously described patient who suffered a stroke). In the group with nonfunctioning adenoma, two patients had transient cranial nerve palsies—one of the IIIrd nerve and one of the VIth nerve. Permanent postoperative diabetes insipidus developed in one patient and symptomatic nasoseptal perforation in another.

The acromegalics were the second largest group among the patients having pituitary tumors, totaling 43 with 44 procedures. Their tumors were largely chromophobe adenomas, and in seven patients the tumor extended above the diaphragm. Ten patients had microadenomas and three had cystic adenomas. Four had undergone operation previously: two *via* the radio frequency stereotactic approach, one *via* craniotomy, and one by the trans-sphenoidal approach. There were no fatalities in this group. In one instance an unusually large intercavernous sinus presented, and the hemorrhage from this structure led us to abandon the procedure; the patient subsequently underwent proton-beam therapy. In two of these 43 patients, we were unsuccessful in controlling the signs and symptoms of acromegaly; one patient required craniotomy and the other, a second trans-sphenoidal procedure. One patient in this group had a symptomatic nasoseptal perforation.

Eighteen women in the pituitary adenoma group had the Forbes-Albright syndrome of amenorrhea and galactorrhea. Three of these 18 patients had tumors with suprasellar extension, 11 had microadenomas, and three had cystic tumors; none had been operated on previously. There were no fatalities among the 18. Complications included persistent galactorrhea in one patient, permanent postoperative diabetes insipidus in one patient, and symptomatic nasoseptal perforations in two patients.

The Nelson-Salassa syndrome with hypersecretion of corticotropin (ACTH) and melanocyte-stimulating hormone (MSH) after adrenalectomy for Cushing's syndrome was present in 13 patients who underwent 14 surgical procedures. All 13 patients had hyperpigmentation; two had suprasellar extensions of their tumors, nine had microadenomas, and one had a cystic tumor. Three had undergone previous pituitary surgery; one a craniotomy, one a trans-sphenoidal procedure, and one both a craniotomy and a trans-sphenoidal approach. The complications in this group consisted of early recurrence of a tumor in one patient on whom we reoperated, and symptomatic nasoseptal perforation in another. It is probably true that a number of patients have not achieved totally satisfactory control of their disease, though endocrine measurements have not been performed in every case.

A total of 11 patients had primary Cushing's disease, seven of whom had microadenomas; none had been operated on previously. In this group the only complication was persistent hypercortisolism in one patient.

Among the miscellaneous pituitary adenomas, we encountered a malignant chromophobe adenoma in one patient and galactorrhea in a man who had a microadenoma. Neither of these patients had any complications.

The next large group consisted of 14 patients with craniopharyngioma on whom a total of 15 procedures was performed. Eleven patients had suprasellar extensions of their tumors and 10 of these had visual field defects. Six of the patients had undergone previous surgery—five, craniotomy and one, both craniotomy and trans-sphenoidal decompression. "Total" removal of a primarily intrasellar craniopharyngioma was thought to have been accomplished in seven patients, though one was a fatality. This patient was a young girl with a calcified intrasellar craniopharyngioma with a small suprasellar extension (Fig. 29.6). The lesion was solid and extremely difficult to deal with surgically; however, total removal was accomplished. In the postoperative period the patient had a left-sided hemiparesis, and, over the course of 24 hours, suffered progressive occlusion of all of the vessels of the circle of Willis (Fig. 29.7). There were no other fatalities. The vision of one patient was transiently worse after surgery. This woman had a huge solid calcified intracranial tumor (Fig. 29.8), and we had hoped to decompress a cystic component. Surgery was essentially unsuccessful and the worsening in her visual field defect was undoubtedly the result of manipulation of the large tumor. Two of the 15 trans-sphenoidal procedures for craniopharyngioma were followed by cerebrospinal rhinorrhea; both patients required reoperation which successfully controlled the spinal fluid leak. In one case, vigorous opening of the trans-sphenoidal retractor resulted in diastasis of the hard palate which healed spontaneously. In five cases permanent postoperative diabetes insipidus developed; it was managed with appropriate vasopressin (Pitressin) therapy.

Six patients had primary empty sella or intrasellar arachnoid cysts. One of the six presented with a visual field defect and one, with preoperative cerebrospinal rhinorrhea. One patient who did not have an obvious cerebrospinal fluid leak died from postoperative Klebsiella

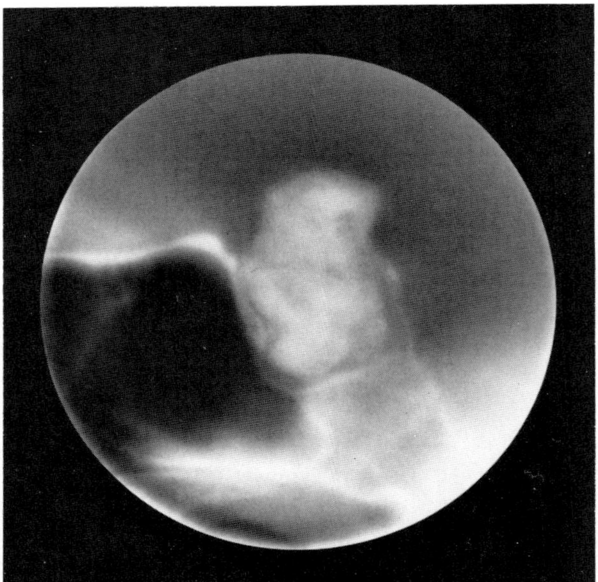

FIG. 29.6. Craniopharyngioma. Lateral tomogram of sella turcica. Calcified intrasellar tumor with small suprasellar extension.

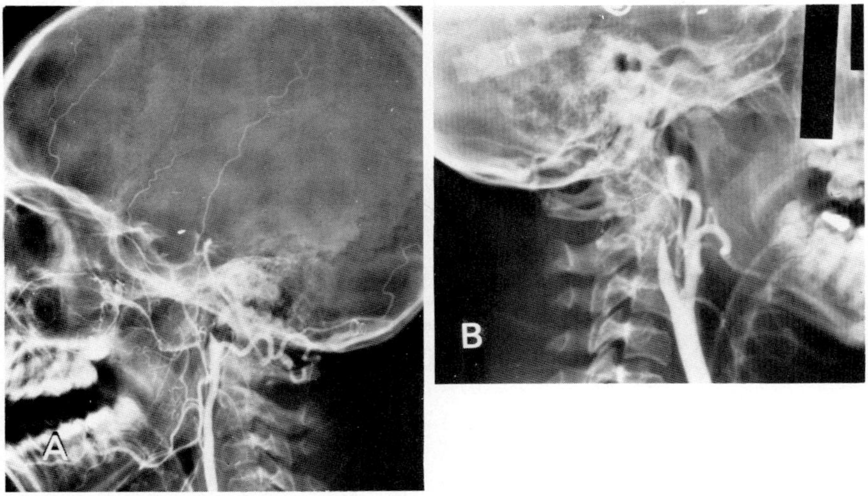

FIG. 29.7. Craniopharyngioma. Postoperative left (A) and right (B) carotid angiograms (same case as Fig. 29.6). Bilateral internal carotid artery occlusion. Collateral flow from the left occipital artery to the vertebrobasilar system suggests vertebral occlusion or incompetence as well.

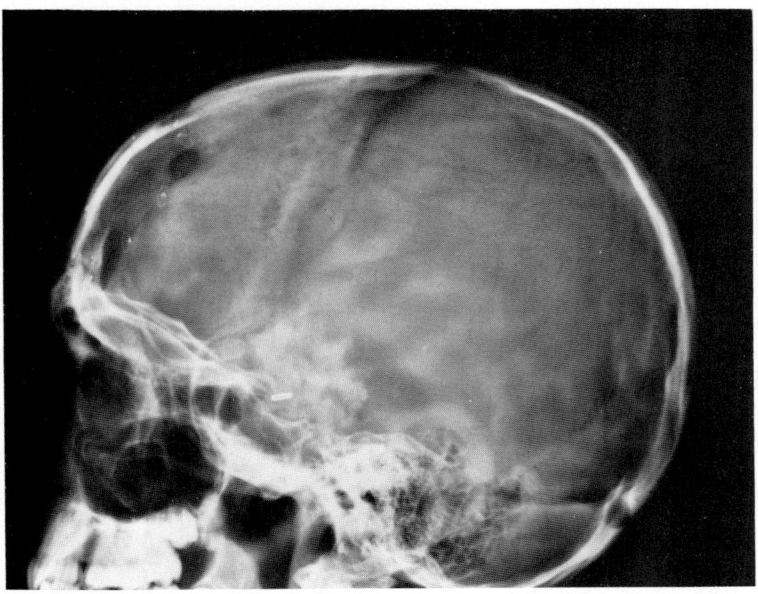

FIG. 29.8. Craniopharyngioma. Lateral view of skull after trans-sphenoidal exploration. Large solid calcified intracranial tumor incapable of removal *via* the trans-sphenoidal approach.

meningitis. Fulminant meningitis developed 6 days after operation and the patient did not respond to what seemed to be appropriate antibiotic therapy. Autopsy failed to reveal the source of the infection. A preoperative nasopharyngeal culture had not shown the presence of Klebsiella as part of the nasal flora. Two other patients having empty sella had postoperative cerebrospinal rhinorrhea. This resolved spontaneously in one patient, and in the second, reexploration with successful packing of the sella was accomplished. Symptomatic nasoseptal perforation also occurred in one of these patients. Three patients had a secondary empty sella resulting from previous surgery done for craniopharyngioma, nonfunctioning pituitary adenoma, and acromegaly, respectively. One of the three patients had a visual field deficit from the empty sella. No postoperative complications were encountered in this group.

There were no complications in a series of five patients with chordoma of the clivus.

Six patients presented with primary sphenoidal pathology. Two of the six patients had sphenoid carcinomas, one primary and one metastatic. One patient had a primary cyst of the sphenoid sinus, two patients had nasal gliomas, and one patient had a sphenoidal meningioma associated with a pyocele of the sphenoid sinus. One of these patients suffered diastasis of the hard palate that healed spontaneously, and one had symptomatic nasoseptal perforation.

Four patients had miscellaneous sellar and parasellar pathology, consisting of ectopic pinealoma in one, fibrous dysplasia in one, cavernous hemangioma in one, and intrasellar myeloma that appeared as a calcified lesion in one. This last case was complicated by cerebrospinal rhinorrhea, which required reexploration and was successfully obliterated. There were no other complications in this group.

In our series, 13 patients underwent hypophysectomy. Nine of the 13 operations were for metastatic carcinoma of the prostate. One of these developed cerebrospinal rhinorrhea requiring reexploration and packing, and another, a transient IIIrd cranial nerve palsy. One moribund patient had metastatic hypernephroma; subsequent to operation, cerebrospinal rhinorrhea and fatal meningitis developed. Three patients had diabetic retinopathy with no complications. Permanent diabetes insipidus developed after hypophysectomy in one of the 13 patients in this group.

Eight patients were operated on for cerebrospinal rhinorrhea. One patient had spontaneous rhinorrhea associated with an empty sella syndrome and seven had reoperations after previous trans-sphenoidal surgery. In this group there were no complications other than uncontrolled rhinorrhea in three patients, one of whom subsequently died of meningitis (the man with metastatic hypernephroma).

COMMENT

A recapitulation of the complications in the Mayo Clinic series of 193 procedures in 185 patients is seen in Table 29.3. There were four fatalities, giving a mortality rate of 2%. There were three cases of postoperative meningitis, six cases of postoperative cerebrospinal rhinorrhea, three cases of vascular occlusion, and one hypothalamic injury. Permanent worsening of a visual field defect occurred in two of the 50 patients who had preoperative visual loss for an incidence of 4%. Four patients had cranial nerve palsy which was transient in all instances. Seven patients had permanent postoperative diabetes insipidus. We were unsuccessful in controlling a hypersecreting form of endocrinopathy in six of 137 patients presenting with such a condition for an incidence of 4.7%. Symptomatic nasoseptal perforations developed in six patients; two patients suffered diastasis of the palatal suture, and in one patient, hemorrhage from the intercavernous sinus resulted in abandonment of the trans-sphenoidal procedure. Both the nature and the incidence of these complications are compatible with other large series of trans-sphenoidal procedures

While some complications may be anticipated and avoided, others must be recognized promptly and treated appropriately. A review of our experience would indicate that the patients most likely to suffer serious complications are those who have been subjected to previous craniotomy.

TABLE 29.3
Trans-sphenoidal Surgery—Mayo Clinic Series (1972–1975; 193 Procedures, 185 Patients)

Complication	No. of patients	Incidence
		%
Mortality	4	2
Meningitis	3*	1.6
CSF rhinorrhea	6	3.1
Vascular occlusion	3*	1.6
Hypothalamic injury	1*	0.5
Permanent worsening of visual field defect	2/50	4
Cranial nerve palsy	4 (all transient)	2
Permanent postop diabetes insipidus	7/177	4
Failure to control endocrinopathy	6/137	4.4
Nasal septal perforation	6	3.1
Palatal diastasis	2	1
Hemorrhage	1	0.5

* Deaths: 2 patients with meningitis, 1 patient with vascular occlusion, 1 patient with hypothalamic injury.

Additional factors that increase risk include excessive enlargement of the sella, erosion of parasellar bony structures, very large suprasellar extensions of pituitary tumors, and poor general medical condition because of other disease factors. The nasoseptal perforations were more common in patients operated on without the assistance of an otorhinolaryngologist. Participation by ear, nose, and throat specialists in the trans-sphenoidal procedure has been a major factor in reducing postoperative nasal complications.

Diligent preoperative assessment of the anatomy is essential and should be accomplished in each case with the utilization of tomograms of the sella and sphenoid sinus in both the lateral and anteroposterior projections. It is our belief that bilateral carotid angiography and, in some cases, vertebral angiography is also essential. Antibiotic therapy is routinely employed and may be guided when necessary by the results of preoperative nasopharyngeal cultures. Pneumoencephalography is performed whenever the possibility of an empty sella or primary arachnoidal cyst exists and when angiography is not totally satisfactory in outlining the suprasellar extension of large pituitary tumors.

Undoubtedly the nature of complications of trans-sphenoidal surgery will continue to change as the approach is utilized for the treatment of new conditions, and it is our hope that in the future this procedure may be applied even more effectively and with greater safety than it is at present.

REFERENCES

1. Atkinson, R. L., Becker, D. P., Martins, A. N., Schaaf, M., Dimond, R. C., Wartofsky, L., and Earll, J. M. Acromegaly: treatment by transsphenoidal microsurgery. J.A.M.A., *233:* 1279–1283, 1975.
2. Bergland, R. M., Ray, B. S., and Thorac, R. M. Anatomical variations in the pituitary gland and adjacent structures in 225 human autopsy cases. J. Neurosurg., *28:* 93–99, 1968.
3. Cirić, I. S., and Tarkington, J. Transsphenoidal microsurgery. Surg. Neurol., *2:* 207–212, 1974.
4. Collins, W. F. Hypophysectomy: historical and personal perspective. Clin. Neurosurg., *21:* 68–78, 1974.
5. Cushing, H. Partial hypophysectomy for acromegaly: with remarks on the function of the hypophysis. Ann. Surg., *50:* 1002–1017, 1909.
6. Cushing, H. Operative experiences with lesions of the pituitary body. Trans. Am. Surg. Assoc., *31:* 467–468, 1913.
7. Cushing, H. Surgical experiences with pituitary disorders. J.A.M.A., *63:* 1515–1525, 1914.
8. Cushing, H. Intracranial Tumors, 150 pp. (c.f. p. 69) Charles C Thomas, Springfield, Ill., 1932.
9. Deborsu, F. L. Difficultés de la voïe transphénoïdale de l'opération de l'adénome de l'hypophyse. Neurochirurgia (Stuttg.), *1:* 209–215, 1959.

10. Dott, N. M., and Bailey, D. A consideration of the hypophysial adenomata. Br. J. Surg., *13:* 314–366, 1925.
11. German, W. J., and Flanigan, S. Pituitary adenomas: a follow-up study of the Cushing series. Clin. Neurosurg., *10:* 72–81, 1964.
12. Guiot, G. Transsphenoidal approach in surgical treatment of pituitary adenomas: general principles and indications in non-functioning adenomas. Excerpta Medica International Congress Series No. 303, pp. 159–178, 1973.
13. Guiot, G., and Cheibani, G. Risques et problèmes de l'exérèse trans-sphénoïdale des adénomes hypophysaires. Nouv. Presse Med., *1:* 2117–2119, 1972.
14. Guiot, G., Derome, P., Demailly, P., and Hertzog, E. Complication inattendue de l'exérèse complète de volumineux adénomes hypophysaires. Rev. Neurol. (Paris), *118:* 164–167, 1968.
15. Halstead, A. E. Remarks on the operative treatment of tumors of the hypophysis. Surg. Gynecol. Obstet., *10:* 494–502, 1910.
16. Hamberger, C. A., Hammer, G., Norlén, G., and Sjögren, B. Hypophysectomy in acromegaly (letter to the editor). J. Clin. Endocrinol., *19:* 1500–1502, 1959.
17. Hamlin, H. The case for transsphenoidal approach to hypophysial tumors. J. Neurosurg., *19:* 1000–1003, 1962.
18. Hardy, J. Transsphenoidal microsurgery of the normal and pathological pituitary. Clin. Neurosurg., *16:* 185–217, 1969.
19. Hardy, J. Traitement chirurgical de l'adénome hypophysaire. Neurochirurgie, *19* (Suppl. 2): 75–99, 1973.
20. Hardy, J. Transsphenoidal surgery of hypersecreting pituitary tumors. Excerpta Medica International Congress Series No. 303, pp. 179–194, 1973.
21. Henderson, W. R. Pituitary adenomata: a follow-up study of surgical results in 338 cases (Dr. Harvey Cushing's series). Br. J. Surg., *26:* 811–921, 1939.
22. Hirsch, O. Endonasal method of removal of hypophyseal tumors: with report of two successful cases. J.A.M.A., *55:* 772–774, 1910.
23. Hirsch, O. Ueber Hypophysentumoren und deren Behandlung. Klin. Monatsbl. Augenheilkd., *85:* 609–640, 1930.
24. Hirsch, O. Life-long cures and improvements after trans-sphenoidal operation of pituitary tumors. Acta Opthalmol. (Suppl.) (Kbh.), *56:* 1–60, 1959.
25. Horwitz, N. H., and Rizzoli, H. V. Postoperative Complications in Neurosurgical Practice: Recognition, Prevention, and Management, 427 pp. Williams & Wilkins Co., Baltimore, 1967.
26. Johnson, H. C. Surgery of the hypophysis. *In* A History of Neurological Surgery, edited by A. E. Walker, pp. 152–177, Williams & Wilkins Co., Baltimore, 1951.
27. Kirchner, J. A., and VanGilder, J. C. Transethmoidal hypophysectomy: some surgical landmarks. Trans. Am. Acad. Opthalmol. Otolaryngol., *80:* 391–396, 1975.
28. Nicola, G. C., and Giovanelli, M. Il decorso postoperatorio nella chirurgia dell'ipofici: confronto tra la via transfrontale e la via transnasosfenoidale. Minerva Neurochir., *14:* 89–91, 1970.
29. Renn, W. H., and Rhoton, A. L., Jr. Microsurgical Anatomy of the sellar region. J. Neurosurg., *43:* 288–298, 1975.
30. Reyes-Oliveros, M. F. Considérations sur la chirurgie trans-sphénoïdale de l'hypophyse: d'après une statistique de 401 cas. Neurochirurgie, *17:* 209–215, 1971.
31. Schoen, D. Mukozele des Keilbeines nach Hypophysektomie. Fortschr. Geb. Roentgenstr. Nuklearmed., *112:* 114–116, 1970.
32. Svien, H. J., Kennedy, W. C., and Kearns, T. P. Results of surgical treatment of pituitary adenoma. The factor of the excessively enlarged sella. J. Neurosurg., *20:* 669–674, 1963.

33. Svien, H. J., and Litzow, T. J. Removal of certain hypophyseal tumors by the transantral-sphenoid route. J. Neurosurg., *23:* 603–611, 1965.
34. White, J. C., and Ballantine, H. T., Jr. Intrasellar aneurysms simulating hypophyseal tumors. J. Neurosurg., *18:* 34–50, 1961.
35. Williams, R. A., Jacobs, H. S., Kurtz, A. B., Millar, J. G. B., Oakley, N. W., Spathis, G. S., Sulway, M. -J., and Nabarro, J. D. N. The treatment of acromegaly with special reference to trans-sphenoidal hypophysectomy. Q. J. Med., *44:* 79–98, 1975.

CHAPTER

30

Neurosurgical Complications: Fluid and Electrolyte Imbalance

WILLIAM F. COLLINS, M.D.

Fluid and electrolyte imbalance in neurosurgery is commonly more fluid than electrolyte, for the most frequent complications of fluid management of neurosurgical patients are concerned with water and their resolution relates to control of intake and output of water. This is in contrast to the problems of fluid management of surgical patients in general that relate to blood volume and electrolyte availability to correct variation in electrolyte concentration. The neurosurgical patient, however, is a surgical patient and blood volume and electrolyte balance are important. Perhaps the reason they are not frequent problems in the neurosurgical patient is that loss of fluids containing electrolytes either from the body or into areas of surgical injury is relatively small, physicians are familiar with measurements indicating need for and the method of blood and electrolyte replacement and the major stress in medical school, in surgical internship, and other postgraduate surgical education is on replacement of blood and electrolytes (6). The importance of this was marked in my training, and electrolyte imbalance was treated by correcting the deficit with a solution of the deficient electrolyte *e.g.*, low sodium was treated with normal or hypertonic saline, and water was considered necessary only to replace insensible water loss, obligatory urinary water excretion, or to decrease the elevated concentration of electrolytes. Another aspect is that our standard laboratory determinations are measures of concentration of solutes *e.g.*, mEq. per liter of sodium or other electrolytes, while measure of the solvent water is not only difficult, but inaccurate at best.

Water is a major component of the human body (Table 30.1). In the infant it is approximately 75% of body weight and with age it gradually decreases to 50% or 60%. Males with less subcutaneous tissue than females have a larger percentage of their body weight made up of water. Intravascular water and extracellular water constitute about 20% of the body weight, while intracellular water is between 30% and 40% (7).

Water freely permeates cell membranes, and its volume in each compartment relates to relative concentration of electrolytes and other osmotically active solutes. The concept that electrolytes are necessary for the retention of water in the body is correct if there is no malfunction of the excretion of water by the kidney and therefore no aberrant retention or loss of the dilutant water. The concept that electrolytes are necessary for retention of fluid led in my early years of neurosurgical practice to the use of 5% glucose in water and no electrolytes in order to control possible cerebral edema. This practice of having the preoperative and intraoperative fluid be a solution without electrolytes and I admit other factors, led to the use of a sucker on opening the dura so that the hemisphere would not rupture. It is not the absolute concentration of electrolytes that determines the shift of water from vascular to extravascular to intracellular compartments, but the relative concentration. Excess solvent in the intravascular compartment will certainly lead to excess solvent in the intracellular compartment or a loss of intracellular electrolyte.

The commonest problems in the neurosurgical patient concerned with water are at both extremes of water balance, excess retention, and loss. While the syndromes can be called water intoxication and water deprivation, they are more commonly called hyponatremia, a carry-over from the concentration concept, and diabetes insipidus, a common but not exclusive cause of excess water loss. Hyponatremia occurs as a result of either dilution or depletion of body sodium, but in neurosurgical patients it is almost always secondary to dilution from water retention. The apparent sodium deficit in a patient with hyponatremia can be calculated by assuming water volume to be approximately 50% of body weight and multiplying the number of liters by the mEq. deficit as measured by the sodium concentration (Table 30.2). Thus in the 70-kg patient, there would be 35 liters of water and with 20 mEq. of sodium per liter deficit in a patient with a sodium of 120 mEq. per liter, there would be approximately 700 mEq. deficit of sodium. The common parenteral fluids utilized to replace this as compared to extracellular fluid are seen in Table 30.3 and the rule is to replace approximately half the deficit in a brief period of time, that is in terms of hours, and thus almost 2 liters of

TABLE 30.1
Body Water as Percentage of Body Weight

Males	60%
Females	50%
Infants	75–85%
Intravascular	5%
Extracellular	15%
Intracellular	30–40%

normal saline could be used or 500 or 600 ml. of 3% saline. When this is infused in neurosurgical patients and the resulting serum sodium later measured, it usually is not 130 mEq. per liter as might have been expected with half of the sodium deficit replaced but is found to be even lower because of water retention and further dilution. The intravenously administered sodium is excreted and the water is retained. If, however, instead of calculating the sodium deficit, the water necessary to dilute the concentration of sodium from 140 mEq. per liter to 120 mEq. per liter is calculated, the answer of approximately 5 liters of excess water is arrived at (Table 30.4). The treatment for this situation of course is either restriction of water intake, increase in obligatory urinary excretion of water, or a combination of these. I remember attempting to correct hyponatremia in a patient with a head injury and measuring both the sodium intake and output. Despite giving 1200 mEq. of sodium intravenously during one 24-hour period, the patient not only maintained a slightly negative sodium balance but also lowered his serum sodium concentration even more than the negative balance would have indicated

TABLE 30.2
Hyponatremia

Weight	= 70 kg.
Serum Na	= 120 mEq./kg.
Total body water	= 35 liters
Na deficit	= 20 mEq. × 35 = 700 mEq.

TABLE 30.3
Parenteral Fluids

Solutions	Electrolyte Content (mEq./liter)							
	Cations					Anions		
	Na	K	Ca	Mg	NH_4	Cl	HCO_3	HPO_4
Extracellular	142	4	5	3	3	103	27	3
½ Normal saline	77	—	—	—	—	77	—	—
Normal saline	154	—	—	—	—	154	—	—
Lactated Ringers	130	4	2.7	—	—	109	28	—
3% NaCl	513	—	—	—	—	513	—	—
M/6 Na lactate	167	—	—	—	—	—	167	—

TABLE 30.4
Hyponatremia

120 mEq./liter Na × 35 liters = 140 mEq./kg. × X(liters)
X = 30 liters
Water excess = 5 liters

(4). My stupidity in not recognizing what was happening in this patient and others we studied was even more difficult to bear when the suggestion was made in the literature that water retention was the problem, for the evidence to support this hypothesis was present in my study and I failed to recognize it (5). That the problem relates to inappropriate secretion of antidiuretic hormone is now accepted, even though no direct measures of antidiuretic hormone are available. I commend to you Bartter and Schwartz's article (published in the *American Journal of Medicine* in 1967) summarizing this evidence (1). The problems of prevention, recognition and appropriate treatment of the syndrome remain.

We have had at various times epidemics of hyponatremia or more accurately, water retention, on my service and they were difficult to understand for they did not seem to relate to changes in the type or severity of the lesions that were being treated. The answer, however, came with study of the preoperative, intraoperative and postoperative water balance, for it became apparent that craniotomy and other head-injured patients not only almost routinely retained water, but that the retention was enhanced if it was not recognized early in the postoperative period. Retention of water was in itself a stimulus for the paradoxical secretion of antidiuretic hormone and the resulting increased intravascular volume almost certainly enhanced the excretion of infused sodium *via* the aldosterone mechanism. Thus in the late intraoperative period and early postoperative period a relatively small, that is a liter or more of retained water exacerbated a problem that was present. Since our neurosurgeons and neuroanesthesiologists have recognized this, the problem of control of patients with inappropriate secretion of antidiuretic hormone has become rare and the diagnosis is usually evident only with careful laboratory studies rather than clinical findings.

Increase in body weight has been mentioned as a method for determining that retention of water is occurring in the neurosurgical patient. When I read this in a text, I am certain that the writer has never worked in any hospital I have worked in, for the difficulties and errors in the determination of change in body weight are formidable when the critically ill neurosurgical patient with tubes, respirators, electrodes, and dressings is placed on the usually inaccurate scales available to weigh the unconscious patient. The syndrome is present whenever the urine is not dilute at the time when the serum is hypotonic. Since almost the entire effective osmotic pressure of the extracellular fluid normally relates to sodium chloride concentration, with only small amounts of osmotic pressure from other electrolytes, glucose, and colloid substances, a decrease in sodium concentration and a concentrated urine suggest the diagnosis, and the presence of any significant excretion of sodium in the urine with decreased concentration of serum sodium confirms it.

The clinical signs of the hypo-osmolar syndrome in the postoperative patient can be confusing for they may mimic an extra or intracerebral mass causing increasing intracranial pressure and/or focal or general central nervous system dysfunction. The reason for these symptoms is not just increased intracranial pressure, for although rapid shifts in osmolarity of the serum can acutely increase or decrease brain water and intracranial pressure, in more chronic states, that is after a number of hours, experimentally cerebral edema is not enhanced by hypo-osmolarity and decrease in the intracellular concentration of potassium appears to be the cause of the central nervous system dysfunction (2, 3). Thus the patient with hypo-osmolarity may have either increased intracranial pressure or relatively normal pressure with progressive neurological dysfunction.

In the less severe cases, water restriction is adequate therapy. The restriction should be replacement of urinary output which will allow a decrease in body water equivalent to the insensible water loss minus the water gained from endogenous metabolism. At normal body temperature this will be approximately 700 to 900 ml. per day. It must, however, be borne in mind that with prolonged low caloric intake and low solute load, endogenous metabolic water may approximate or even exceed insensible water loss and failure to correct hypo-osmolarity may result. In the severe case, that is in life-endangering neurological dysfunction or increased intracranial pressure, increase in obligatory urinary excretion of water by the use of solute diuretics is indicated, but it must be administered slowly since intravascular volume is high and cardiac function may be impaired by an acute increase in intravascular volume. Generally, 200 to 300 mg. of manitol per kg. is a safe initial dose if administered over a number of hours and can be repeated until the hypo-osmolarity as measured by sodium concentration is corrected.

Hyperosmolarity is the opposite aspect of fluid balance problems in neurological surgery. It is usually secondary to a deficiency of antidiuretic hormone and is most commonly seen in lesions of the hypothalamic-pituitary axis but may occur as an isolated lesion of the hypothalamus or in conjunction with diffuse injury to the intracranial contents. The diagnosis of deficiency of antidiuretic hormone is made by the observance of continued output of dilute urine in the face of increasing serum osmolarity. Loss of electrolytes in the usually large urine output is minimal and the treatment required is replacement of water and antidiuretic hormone. Failure of the kidney to respond to parenteral administration of the anterior pituitary extract Pitressin may be secondary to a lack of antidiuretic hormone activity in the preparation used. This is most frequently seen with the preparation Pitressin tannate in oil but can be seen with the aqueous preparation. The use of an ampule from a different preparation lot, identified by the preparation number, is indicated. A dry syringe when using the tannate preparation as well as warming the solution and shaking it well is necessary if prolonged antidiuretic action is to be expected.

Diabetes insipidus, however, is not the only reason for the development of hyperosmolarity in the postoperative or post-traumatic neurosurgical patient and other causes must be considered; failure to replace insensible water loss over a number of days, most commonly seen when insensible water loss has been underestimated in the patient with prolonged fever and/or tracheostomy without humidified air; excessive solute loading with tube feedings where the high solute load causes an increase in obligatory excretion of water by the kidneys and the ingested fluids are inadequate; high output renal failure seen after a renal injury that is usually less severe than that producing oliguric renal dysfunction, which can occur following hypotension of a moderate level in surgery; and pre-existing renal disease not recognized before surgery or injury are some of the conditions. A rising nonprotein nitrogen and/or serum potassium as well as creatinine can be seen in all of the hyperosmolar states, although they are more frequently severe in those conditions secondary to renal dysfunction. The neural dysfunction of altered consciousness and seizures can be marked and life-threatening at moderate levels of serum osmolarity, such as 340 or 350 milliosmoles per liter, depending on the rate at which the hyperosmolar state has been attained. The neural dysfunction is reversible in adults, but in infants such levels of hyperosmolarity can cause venous and arteriolar occlusions, with hemorrhagic infarcts and/or subdural hematomas. The mortality in infants is extremely high unless recognition and treatment of the syndrome is prompt.

Hyperosmolarity can also occur from increased serum concentrations of osmotically active substances other than electrolytes, such as glucose. Determination of total serum osmolarity is indicated when hyperosmolarity is suspected as a cause of neural dysfunction. Increase in blood glucose to 800 or 1000 mg per 100 ml. can cause hyperosmolar coma and occurs in the diabetic whose growth hormone is absent or suppressed from a pituitary tumor or after pituitary ablation. The lack of ability to metabolize fat and and the resulting acidosis makes the condition difficult to recognize, for the alterations in respiration and presence of urinary acetone are absent. Treatment consists of insulin and fluids to reduce the hyperglycemia and replace the fluid loss.

Chronic hypernatremia is seen with hypothalamic lesions, in general lateral hypothalamic lesions but is rare, and more often the causes listed above are operative in the critically ill patient and altered thirst mechanisms in the awake patient. Evidence of normal thirst mechanisms is important in the awake patient with a suspected hypothalamic or pituitary lesion, and careful water balance is necessary in the confused or unconscious patient in order to prevent iatrogenic hypo-osmolarity during the treatment of hypernatremia.

The reasons for emphasis on water balance in the complication of fluid management in neurosurgical patients is not to de-emphasize the fact that abnormalities in the concentration of electrolytes or blood volume arise in neurosurgical patients but only to correct the stress that is made in surgery in general in the discussion of the fluid management of the surgical patient in most surgical texts. If the emphasis allows the reader to feel that the principles of fluid and electrolyte management of the surgical patient in general are not important, the point of the presentation will be missed, for the neurosurgeon has within his ken all the problems of surgery plus those special aspects that occur when the protective mechanisms of the central nervous system are altered.

REFERENCES

1. Bartter, F. C., and Schwartz, W. B. The syndrome of inappropriate secretion of antidiuretic hormone. Am J. Med., *42:* 790–806, 1967.
2. Dodge, P. R., Crawford, J. D., and Probst, J. H. Studies in experimental water intoxication. Arch. Neurol. *3:* 513–529, 1960.
3. Katzman, R., and Pappius, H. M. Brain Electrolytes and Fluid Metabolism, 419 pp. Williams & Wilkins Co., Baltimore, 1973.
4. Peters, J. P., Welt, L. G., Orloff, E. A. H., and Needham, J. A. Salt wasting syndrome associated with cerebral disease. Trans. Assos. Am. Physicians, *63:* 57–66, 1950.
5. Rapoport, S., West, C. D., and Brodsky, W. A. Salt-losing conditions; the renal deficit in tuberculous meningitis. J. Lab. Clin. Med., *37:* 550–561, 1951.
6. Shires, G. T., and Canizaro, P. C. Fluid, electrolyte, and nutritional management of the surgical patient. *In* Principles of Surgery, edited by S. I. Schwartz, Chap. 2, pp. 65–96. McGraw Hill, New York, 1974.
7. Wise, B. L. Fluids and Electrolytes in Neurological Surgery, 117 pp. Charles C Thomas, Springfield, Ill., 1965.

CHAPTER

31

Complications of Surgery of the Anterior Cervical Spine

JOHN McLELLAN TEW, JR., M.D., F.A.C.S., AND
FRANK H. MAYFIELD, M.D., F.A.C.S.

The original development of an anterior surgical approach to the vertebral bodies was an outgrowth of the need to reach the seat of infection in Pott's disease (16, 37). Early reports encouraged others to introduce a new phase in the surgery for spinal fusion. Orthopedists, first in Britain (17, 20), and later in the United States (31), recognized the advantages of the anterior approach for interbody fusion and quickly moved to apply this technique in dislocations of the lumbar spine. Nearly 20 years passed, however, before the anterior approach to the cervical spine for fusion was described by Wiltberger in 1952 (38) and Hodgson, in 1956 (14). The first report of anterior cervical fusion for disc degeneration was by Robinson and Smith in 1955 (27). Cloward, in 1958 (3), reported an anterior approach which utilized a dowel graft for interbody fusion. During the ensuing 20 years, thousands of patients have been operated by the anterior cervical approach for a variety of disorders including acute herniated disc, chronic spondylotic deformity, fracture dislocation, and collapse of the spine due to neoplasia and infection. The two original procedures have been modified by many surgeons but the basic aspects remain essentially unchanged.

The complications which follow the anterior approach are varied due to the diversity of anatomic structures encountered during their exposure and subsequent spinal procedure. Interbody fusion, a standard feature of the anterior approach to the cervical spinal procedure, adds yet another area for possible complications.

The purpose of this presentation is to review the specific problems related to the surgery of the anterior cervical spine as reported in the literature and gathered from discussion with colleagues. In addition, we will consider 500 cases that have been treated and observed by the authors. This group will serve as a statistical reference and base for enumeration of specific problems. Throughout the discussion, certain recommendations will be suggested which have been beneficial in preventing complications or alleviating those which could not be avoided. Since our total involvement has been with the interbody approach as modified after Robinson and Smith (28, 30), we will not report any direct observations from the technique advocated by Cloward (3, 4).

In addition, a series of patients have been studied who were suffering from acute disc herniation and who were all treated by discectomy without fusion (34) as originally suggested by Hirsch (12) and others (10, 21, 32). This technique has eliminated the problems specifically related to the bone graft and the graft donor site. Finally, the anterior approach for the treatment of fractures and fracture dislocation of the cervical spine will be discussed. The keystone technique of anterior cervical fusion as described by Bailey and Badgley (2) has been infrequently used in neurosurgical centers and is included only because a variation of the procedure is useful in vertebral replacement fusion which may be required in certain cases of compression fractures of the vertebral bodies.

Discussion of specific problems related to surgery of the anterior cervical spine can be best elucidated by dividing them into three types: (1) exposure injuries, (2) spinal cord or nerve root injuries, (3) problems related to bone fusion (Table 31.1).

EXPOSURE INJURIES

In the course of exposure of the cervical vertebrae from the anterior approach, a number of important soft tissue structures are encountered

TABLE 31.1
Complications—Surgery Anterior Cervical Spine

Soft tissue injuries (exposure):
Perforation of esophagus and trachea
Edema
Recurrent laryngeal palsy
Vertebral artery injury
Pneumothorax
CSF fistula
Horner's syndrome
Carotid artery or jugular vein injury
Hematoma
Wound infection
Neurologic injuries:
Nerve root
Spinal cord
Bone graft and donor site problems:
Failure of fusion
Angulation deformity
Aseptic necrosis and discitis
Extrusion of bone graft
Infection, seroma, hematoma
Painful hip

which must be recognized, spared and/or retracted. Injury to nearly all of the structures has been reported either in the literature or in personal communication. The more frequent and serious problems include the following (Fig. 31.1).

Perforation of the Pharynx, Esophagus, and/or Trachea

Perforation of the pharynx (30), esophagus (5) and/or trachea or other soft tissue structures is in most circumstances related to penetration by the sharp blades of a spreading retractor. For this reason, it is recommended that blunt retraction be used in all stages of the exposure until the longus colli muscles are exposed and that each muscle then be separated from its attachment to the vertebrae and the blades of the retractor placed securely beneath the muscle belly (Fig 31.2). Not only does this maneuver prevent perforation of soft tissue by the retractor blades but undue pressure on the trachea is limited. Precautions have also been taken to file the tips of the retraction blades to a blunt point. Temporary dysphagia and hoarseness (35) resulting from edema of these structures produced by retraction against the resisting force of an endotracheal tube is a feature associated with almost all cases to some degree (19). Serious edema must be recognized early as tracheal obstruction may lead to asphyxia and death. Respiratory insufficiency is a particularly menacing problem in cord injury due to acute fractures of the spine.

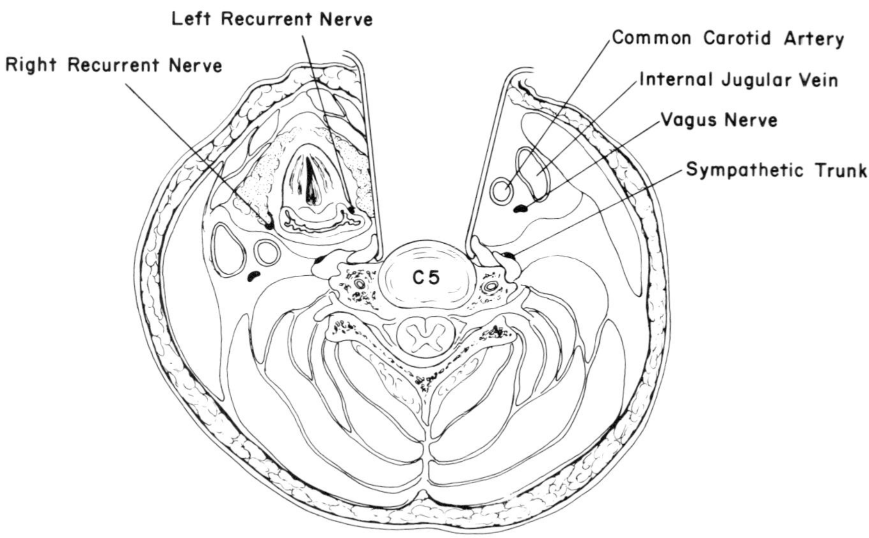

FIG. 31.1. Anatomy of the midcervical region.

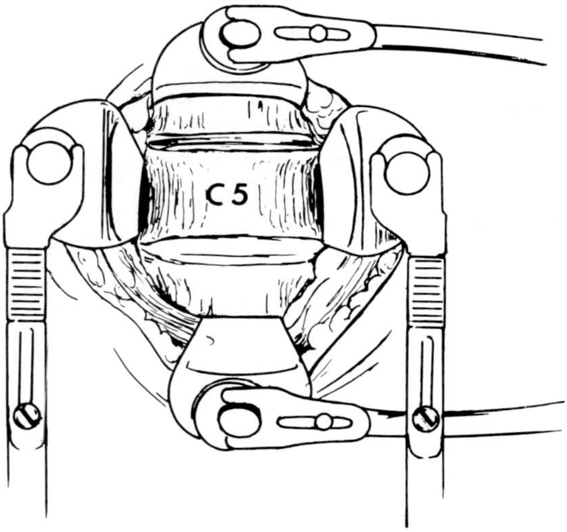

FIG. 31.2. Illustration of proper placement of retractor blades beneath the longus colli muscles.

Vocal Cord Paresis

Vocal cord paresis due to injury to the recurrent laryngeal or vagus nerve has been reported in most series (9, 19, 28). In most instances the hoarseness has been temporary with only a few reporting permanent difficulty. In a protracted follow-up of 85 cases, Heeneman (11) found that 11% show postoperative voice changes, 3 cases of which had permanent vocal cord paralysis.

It is unlikely that the vagus or recurrent laryngeal nerve is divided or cauterized during exposure of the anterior cervical spine particularly if one remains in the fascial plane and avoids sharp dissection in the paratracheal muscles. Overstretching or contusion of the nerve may be less likely on the left side as the nerve has a longer course and lies in a more protected position in the tracheoesophageal groove. Prolonged pressure against the trachea seems to be the most likely cause (22) of paralysis in operative approaches.

Vertebral Artery Injury

Vertebral artery injury has been mentioned by several surgeons in communication. One case of vertebral thrombosis resulting in lateral medullary thrombosis has been reported. Bleeding from tears in the vertebral artery has been encountered according to several reports. This complication is seldom a problem if, rather than attempting to control hemorrhage by packing the intervertebral space, the vertebral artery is exposed at the foramen transversarium where the rent can be repaired directly.

Pneumothorax

Pneumothorax is an infrequent occurrence and does not pose a problem if treated by aspiration and temporary pleural drainage (5, 6).

Cerebrospinal Fluid Fistula

Cerebrospinal fluid fistula is usually related to laceration of the dura and arachnoid over the nerve root by the high speed air drill. The defect cannot be closed directly, but the placement of fascial graft beneath the bone plug has prevented delayed leak in all cases observed.

Horner's Syndrome

Horner's syndrome, injury to the sympathetic trunk, occurs when dissection extends lateral to the longus colli muscles and is usually temporary or of little clinical significance.

Carotid Artery or Jugular Vein Injury

Carotid artery or jugular vein injury is an uncommon occurrence mentioned in an occasional report (25). This complication is due to penetration of the vessel by the misplacement of a sharp toothed retractor. However, thrombosis of the carotid artery or cerebral ischemia may occur as a result of prolonged pressure against the carotid artery.

Postoperative Hematoma

Postoperative hematoma, seldom a serious problem, may develop if unrecognized during the early postoperative course. The standard practice of applying a cervical collar in the operating room was abolished on our Service due to this occurrence in one case. A rapidly enlarging hematoma was unrecognized until respiratory arrest due to tracheal compression occurred. The collar was quickly removed and the clot evacuated. Subsequently collars have not been applied until the patient is erect.

Wound Infections

Wound infections generally occur in less than 1% of patients. Rejection of the bone graft requiring sequestrectomy has not occurred in our experience. Infections are drained early, irrigated with local antibiotics, and systemic antibiotics are administered.

SPINAL CORD OR NERVE ROOT INJURIES

Injury to the nervous system was reported with considerable frequency in the early years of anterior spinal surgery. The increased incidence of cord injury in cases operated by the dowel technique is possibly related to the fact that Smith and Robinson did not recommend total excision of the osteophyte and subsequent removal of the intraspinal projection. Subsequently, neurosurgeons who have adopted the interbody technique seek total osteophyte resection by the use of high speed drill and punch. Patients with myelopathy due to a constricted canal are particularly prone to operative injury despite decompression by the most careful technique. Penetration of the osteophyte at the most lateral margin of the interspace has virtually eliminated this problem in our cases; however, the risk of injury to the underlying nerve root is enhanced.

Another source of possible cord injury is related to tracheal intubation. Hyperextension of the neck in the narcotized patient may lead to acute cord compression. Because of this potential problem, anesthesia colleagues have been instructed to establish the maximal tolerance of neck extension appropriate for the patient prior to his induction for surgery. This level of tolerance is not exceeded subsequently.

Adequate operative illumination and vision are essential to a complete removal of the intraspinal osteophyte, thickened annulus, and posterior longitudinal ligament. It is suggested that the superior illumination and magnified vision provided by the operating microscope may greatly facilitate this maneuver (1, 34). Even with minimal resection of the vertebral body, binocular vision and depth perception are provided.

Finally, care must be exercised in placement of the bone graft. The graft must be shorter than the length of the interspace and restraint must be exercised in tapping the graft into place. Concussion of the cord, indicated by jerking of the limbs, may result in postoperative increase in spastic paresis if residual osteophytes are driven against the spinal cord (25). A rare complication, sleep-induced apnea, has been reported in patients operated at the C_3-C_4 level (18, 24) and in some cases with spinal cord trauma (23). Orthostatic hypotension, bradycardia, and cardiorespiratory instability are also features of this condition. While usually self-limiting, prompt recognition and treatment are necessary to prevent death.

PROBLEMS RELATED TO BONE FUSION

At least four methods of anterior cervical fusion have been described: the interbody methods of Smith-Robinson (29), the dowel technique of Cloward (3), the keystone technique of Bailey and Badgley (2) and finally, the interbody approach without fusion of Hirsch (12). Each method has many advocates and similar long term results have been reported with each technique (Fig. 31.3).

Failure of fusion or nonunion appears to be higher in the dowel technique (5, 6). The incidence varies from 2 to 20%. With the interbody

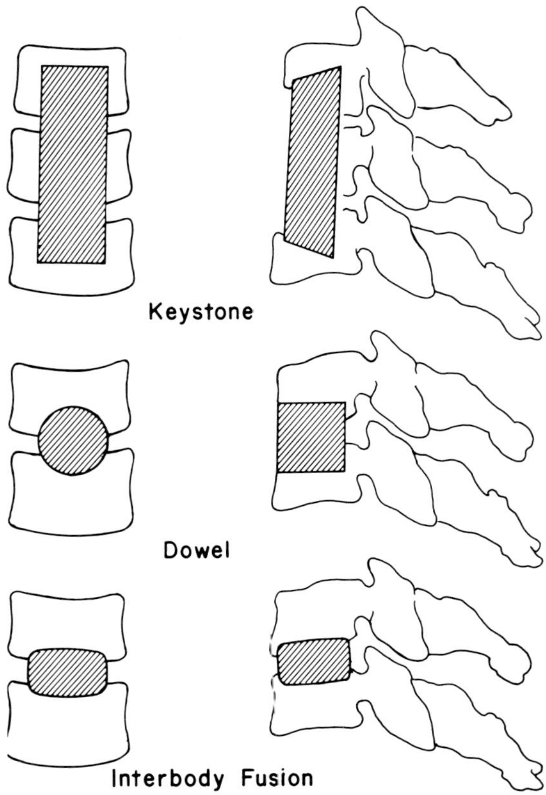

FIG. 31.3. Types of anterior spinal fusion.

approach, the incidence of pseudoarthrosis has been near 10% in most series (1, 7, 9, 19, 20, 28). Simmons and Bhalla (29) reported no cases of nonunion in the 68 patients fused with the keystone technique. Bony fusion or fibrous union as indicated by early absence of movement and subsequent lack of osteophyte formation has been reported in nearly all cases operated by the interbody technique of Hirsch (13, 34). Finally, there is not a clear relationship between adequacy of fusion and the clinical result in the opinion of several authors. Long term follow-up will be required to determine if fibrous union, frequently seen in simple disc resection, is as satisfactory as solid bony fusion seen in the other techniques.

Anterior angulation deformity may be a serious consequence of anterior approaches using the dowel technique, particularly when multiple resections have been performed. Kempe reported 60% incidence in his first 100 cases; 10% developed delayed myelopathy. He advised prolonged immobilization of the spine by plaster jacket to eliminate this problem (15). A similar angulation deformity may develop in the Hirsch technique if resection of the margins of adjacent bone has been excessive. Aseptic necrosis or resorption of the bone plug has been frequently cited as the factor responsible for angulation deformity. Cloward (4) insists that this problem is reduced by the use of cadaveric bone grafts while others prefer fresh autogenous graft or Kiel bone (33).

Extrusion of the graft has been reported in approximately 2% in most series (9, 19, 26, 36). However, graft extrusion rarely requires reoperation unless mechanical compression of the esophagus or trachea is produced. Subsequent fusion usually occurs although a significant delay may be expected.

TABLE 31.2
500 Operations by the Anterior Cervical Approach (1967–1975)

Anterior interbody fusion	439
Anterior discectomy without fusion	40
Vertebral body replacement—fracture	21
	500

TABLE 31.3
Complications of 500 Operations by the Anterior Cervical Approach

Soft tissue injuries:	
Laceration of the pharynx (primary closure)	1
Recurrent laryngeal palsy—1 permanent	4
Infection	1
Hematoma (required tracheostomy)	1
Horner's syndrome	1
Nervous system injury:	
Root injury (temporary)	1
Cord injury (spinothalamic tract lesion)	1
Bone graft and donor site problems:	
Failure of fusion	? ACDF*
	0 Fracture
	0 ACD†
Extrusion bone graft (fracture)	2
Angulation deformity	1
Infection	4
Seroma (required drainage)	2
Persistent pain (fractured spine)	3
	22 (4.4%)

* Anterior cervical disectomy and fusion.
† Anterior cervical disectomy.

Problems related to the iliac donor site are seldom serious but at times cause a significant aggravation in the postoperative period and delay in convalescence (8). The problems include hematoma, seroma, infection, and persistent pain due to eschar, fracture of the anterior superior iliac spine, and entrapment of the lateral femoral cutaneous nerve. The magnitude of the hip pain is such that it has led some surgeons to eliminate fusion or to seek other sources of bone graft.

As a statistical reference prior to reporting this subject, 500 cases operated by the authors since 1967 were reviewed (Table 31.2). Complications are as listed in Table 31.3. There were no deaths.

CONCLUSIONS

Complications of anterior cervical spine surgery are varied and related to soft tissue injuries encountered during exposure. Nervous system injuries are infrequent but may be quite serious in the patient with a spinal cord which is compromised by a shallow spinal canal. Problems related to the bone graft and donor site are most common, are usually minor in nature, and can be avoided or treated with early resolution.

It is the opinion of the authors that the anterior approach has less risk of over-all complications than the posterior approach when considered as a broad approach to degenerative and traumatic disorders of the cervical spine.

REFERENCES

1. Aronson, N. I., Bagan, M., and Filtzer, D. L. Results of using the Smith-Robinson approach for herniated and extruded cervical discs. Technical note. J. Neurosurg., *32:* 721–722, 1970.
2. Bailey, R. W., and Badgley, C. E. Stabilization of the cervical spine by anterior fusion. J. Bone Joint Surg., *42A:* 565–594, 1960.
3. Cloward, R. B. The anterior approach for removal of ruptured cervical discs. J. Neurosurg., *15:* 602–617, 1958.
4. Cloward, R. B. Lesions of the intervertebral discs and their treatment by interbody fusion methods: the painful disc. Clin. Orthop., *27:* 51–77, 1963.
5. Cloward, R. B. A new method of diagnosis and treatment of cervical disc disease. Clin. Neurosurg., *8:* 93–132, 1962.
6. Connolly, E. S., Seymour, R. J., and Adams, J. E. Clinical evaluation of anterior cervical fusion for degenerative cervical disc disease. J. Neurosurg., *23:* 431–437, 1965.
7. DePalma, A. F., and Cooke, A. I. Results of anterior interbody fusion of the cervical spine. Clin. Orthop., *60:* 169–185, 1968.
8. DePalma, A. F., Rothman, R. H., and Lewinnek, G. E., et al. Anterior interbody fusion for severe cervical disc degeneration. Surg. Gynecol. Obstet., *134:* 755–758, 1972.
9. Dohn, D. F. Anterior interbody fusion for treatment of cervical disc conditions. J.A.M.A. *197:* 897–900, 1966.
10. Hankinson, H. L., and Wilson, C. B. Use of the operating microscope in anterior cervical discectomy with fusion. J. Neurosurg., *43:* 452–456, 1975.

11. Heeneman, H. Vocal cord paralysis following approaches to the anterior cervical spine. Laryngoscope, *83:* 17–21, 1973.
12. Hirsch C. Cervical disc rupture. Diagnosis and treatment. Acta. Orthop. Scand., *30:* 172–186, 1960.
13. Hirsch, C., Wickbom, I., Lidström, A., et al. Cervical disc resection: a follow-up of myelographic and surgical procedure. J. Bone Joint Surg., *46A:* 1811–1821, 1964.
14. Hodgson, A. R., and Stock, F. E. Anterior spine fusion. Br. J. Surg., *44:* 266–275, 1956.
15. Horwitz, W. H., and Rizzoli, H. V. Postoperative complications in neurosurgical practice: *In* Recognition, Prevention, and Management, 427 pp. Williams & Wilkins Co., Baltimore, 1967.
16. Ito, H., Tsuchiya, S., and Asami, G. A new radical operation for Pott's Disease. J. Bone Joint Surg., *16:* 499–515, 1934.
17. Jenkins, J. A. Spondylolisthesis. Br. J. Surg., *24:* 80–85, 1936.
18. Krieger, A. J., and Rosomoff, H. L. Sleep-induced apnea. Part 2: Respiratory failure after anterior spinal surgery. J. Neurosurg., *40:* 181–185, 1974.
19. Mayfield, F. H. Cervical spondylosis: a comparison of the anterior and posterior approaches. Clin. Neurosurg., *13:* 181–188, 1966.
20. Mercer, W. Spondylolisthesis. Edinburgh Med. J., *43:* 545–572, 1936.
21. Murphy, M. G., and Gado, M. Anterior cervical discectomy without interbody bone graft. J. Neurosurg., *37:* 71–74, 1972.
22. Naito, Y. Experimental study on facial nerve paralysis. Jap. J. Otol., *70:* 178–179, 1967.
23. Norrell, H., and Wilson, C. B. Early anterior fusion for injuries of the cervical portion of the spine. J.A.M.A. *214:* 523–530, 1970.
24. Onji, Y., Akiyama, H., Shimomura, Y. and associates. Posterior paravertebral ossification causing cervical myelopathy. A report of eighteen cases. J. Bone Joint Surg., *49A:* 1314–1328, 1967.
25. Phillips, D. C. Surgical treatment of myelopathy with cervical spondylosis. J. Neurol. Neurosurg. Psychiatry, *36:* 879–884, 1973.
26. Riley, L. H., Jr. Robinson, R. A., Johnson, K. A., et al. The results of anterior interbody fusion of the cervical spine; review of 93 consecutive cases. J. Neurosurg., *30:* 127–133, 1969.
27. Robinson, R. A., and Smith, G. W. Anterolateral cervical disc removal and interbody fusion for cervical disc syndrome. (Abstract). Bull. John Hopkins Hosp., *96:* 223–224, 1955.
28. Robinson, R. A., Walker, A. E., Ferlic, D. C., and Wiecking, D. K. The results of anterior interbody fusion of the cervical spine. J. Bone Joint Surg., *44A:* 1569–1586, 1962.
29. Simmons, E. H., Bhalla, S. K. and Butt, W. P. Anterior cervical discectomy and fusion, with note on discography. J. Bone Joint Surg., *51B:* 225–237, 1969.
30. Smith, G. W., and Robinson, R. A. The treatment of certain cervical-spine disorders by anterior removal of the intervertebral disc and interbody fusion. J. Bone Joint Surg., *40A:* 607–624, 1958.
31. Speed, K. Spondylolisthesis. Treatment by anterior bone graft. Arch. Surg., *37:* 175–189, 1938.
32. Susen, A. F. Simple anterior cervical discectomy without fusion. Presented at the American Academy of Neurological Surgery, San Francisco, Calif., 1966.
33. Taheri, Z. E., and Gueramy, M. Experience with calf bone in cervical interbody spinal fusion. J. Neurosurg., *36:* 67–71, 1972.
34. Tew, J. M., and Mayfield, F. H. Anterior cervical disc resection. The treatment of acute herniated cervical disc. Presented at the Joint Meeting of the Society of British

Neurological Surgeons and the American Academy of Neurological Surgery, Bermuda, November 1974.

35. Verbiest, H. Anterolateral operation for fractures or dislocation of the cervical spine due to injuries or previous surgical intervention. Clin. Neurosurg., *20:* 334–366, 1972.
36. White, A. A., Southwise, W. O., and Deporte, R. J., et al. Relief of pain by anterior cervical spine fusion for spondylosis. J. Bone Joint Surg., *55A:* 525–534, 1973.
37. Wilkinson, M. C. Curettage of tuberculous vertebral disease in the treatment of spinal caries. Proc. R. Soc. Med., *43:* 114–115, 1950.
38. Wiltberger, B. R. Resection of vertebral bodies and bone grafting for chronic osteomyelitis of the spine. J. Bone Joint Surg., *34A:* 215–218, 1952.

CHAPTER

32

Complications of Laminectomy

FRANK H. MAYFIELD, M.D., F.A.C.S.

Literally, the word complication means to fold together; medically, it has traditionally identified unfavorable influences upon one system of the body, especially that under treatment, by disorders in another system. Today it identifies any unfavorable clinical result from death to discrepancies in the record which at times lead to malpractice suits which are unjustified.

Continuing review of clinical results is, of course, essential to evaluate risks and to prevent, recognize, and properly treat complications. Fifteen minutes is not sufficient time for me to account for all the trouble I have seen from entering the spinal canal from the rear for more than 40 years.

I have elected, therefore, to use our experience at the Good Samaritan and Christ Hospitals of Cincinnati during the last 4 years to identify the complications which we have recognized before the patient was discharged from the hospital. These I will classify as acute. I will draw upon my experience of the last 25 years to discuss other acute complications and to identify certain late or delayed complications and will report upon them anecdotically. It is not proposed to include the transient complications of other systems unless they modified appreciably the clinical course of the laminectomy.

From July 1, 1971 through June 30, 1975, laminectomy was done by the neurosurgical staff at the Good Samaritan and Christ Hospitals on 1408 patients. The work was done by 12 surgeons, all highly trained, but with varying degrees of experience, and by residents under supervision. At the end of each month, the work done during that period was carefully reviewed with the entire attending and resident staff present and the results analyzed and classified.

The purpose for the operations done is shown in the following table:

Lumbar disc	1104
Cervical disc	76
Spinal cord tumor (not metastatic)	86
Traumatic myelopathy	24
Cordotomy	5
Rhizotomy	54
Other (including 13 metastatic tumors)	59
	1408

The low incidence of cervical laminectomy in this group reflects our preference for the anterior approach for cervical disc disorders. The low incidence of cordotomy results from the increased use of percutaneous techniques.

In this group of 1408 patients, there were 32 major complications of which 26 were nonfatal, and 6 were fatal.

The nonfatal complications included:

Wound infections	14
Cerebrospinal fluid fistula	5
Postoperative hematoma with myelopathy (all in cases of metastatic carcinoma)	3
Postoperative hematoma without myelopathy	1
Monoparesis (position on the table)	1
Monoparesis (root avulsion)	1
Foreign body	1

The fatal complications were due to:

Air embolus	1
Pulmonary embolus	3
Pulmonary complications of postoperative hematomas	2

Other major complications observed between 1950 and 1971 include:

Injury to great vessels of the abdomen	2
Air emboli	3
Dislocation of vertebrae	6
Lumbar—2	
Cervical—4	
Death (unexplained)	3
Myelopathy (postsurgical)	1
Avulsion of root	2

Delayed complications of laminectomy included:

Pseudomeningoceles	11
Spinal stenosis	7
Arachnoiditis	?

Errors of diagnosis and recurrence of herniated disc or tumor have not been considered complications and are not considered within the scope of this paper, important though both are.

Wound infection has been the most common complication. Though the rate is at 1%, a high rate for a short period raised it from a 0.5%. A careful record of wound infection identified the cause and prompted its correction.

Air emboli during cervical laminectomy has been verified on three occasions early in our experience. Fortunately, each of these three was recognized and corrected by prompt change of position before permanent damage to the patient developed. The death referred to in our recent experience, however, requires comment.

When the operator, who was a master surgeon, focused the microscope on the cervical cord for cordotomy, bubbles were noted in the surface veins of the cord. The procedure was quickly terminated with no observable change in the patient's condition. The heart sounds were normal throughout; the blood pressure had not fallen. The patient died 2 days later without awakening. Postmortem was not obtained. The surgeon had been unaware of any vein being open, the bone had been carefully waxed throughout the procedure, the field had been kept wet.

The bubbles were too small to see without the microscope. This experience must suggest that air embolus injury may be subtle and that the point of entrance is obscure at times. We are led, therefore, to wonder if the three unexplained deaths included in our experience in which coma persisted unexplained after cervical laminectomy in the sitting position may have resulted from air emboli.

Two patients have suffered injury to the great vessels of the abdomen. One was to the iliac artery. The surgeon recognized the injury, closed the back, opened the abdomen, and ligated the vessel with no significant residual. The other, which was referred to us, was an injury to the iliac vein from which a major arteriovenous fistula had developed.

It would appear obvious that injury to the major vessels would require prompt exploration of the retroperitoneal space.

Prevention of this type of injury requires adequate exposure to mobilize the root and the dural tube and also an opening into the intervertebral disc space of sufficient size to permit removal of the disc under direct vision. Measured instruments, as has been proposed, may add a factor of safety but will not obviate the requirement of wide visual exposure. Long instruments as developed by McBride are a great aid when operating on patients of large stature or on those who are very obese. The lateral position offers the opportunity in the event of injury to explore the retroperitoneal space without change of position or anesthesia if an accident should occur.

It is to be noted that 13 patients underwent laminectomy for metastatic disease. Two died of hemorrhagic complications in the wound; one with pulmonary embolus in the postoperative period. It should be noted that the field is difficult to dry in patients with metastatic tumor and that perhaps the hemovac should be used more often. Three deaths in 13 cases is a high rate and suggests that restrained judgment should be exercised in planning surgery for metastatic cancer of the spine.

A total of two patients suffered root avulsions during surgery. In each

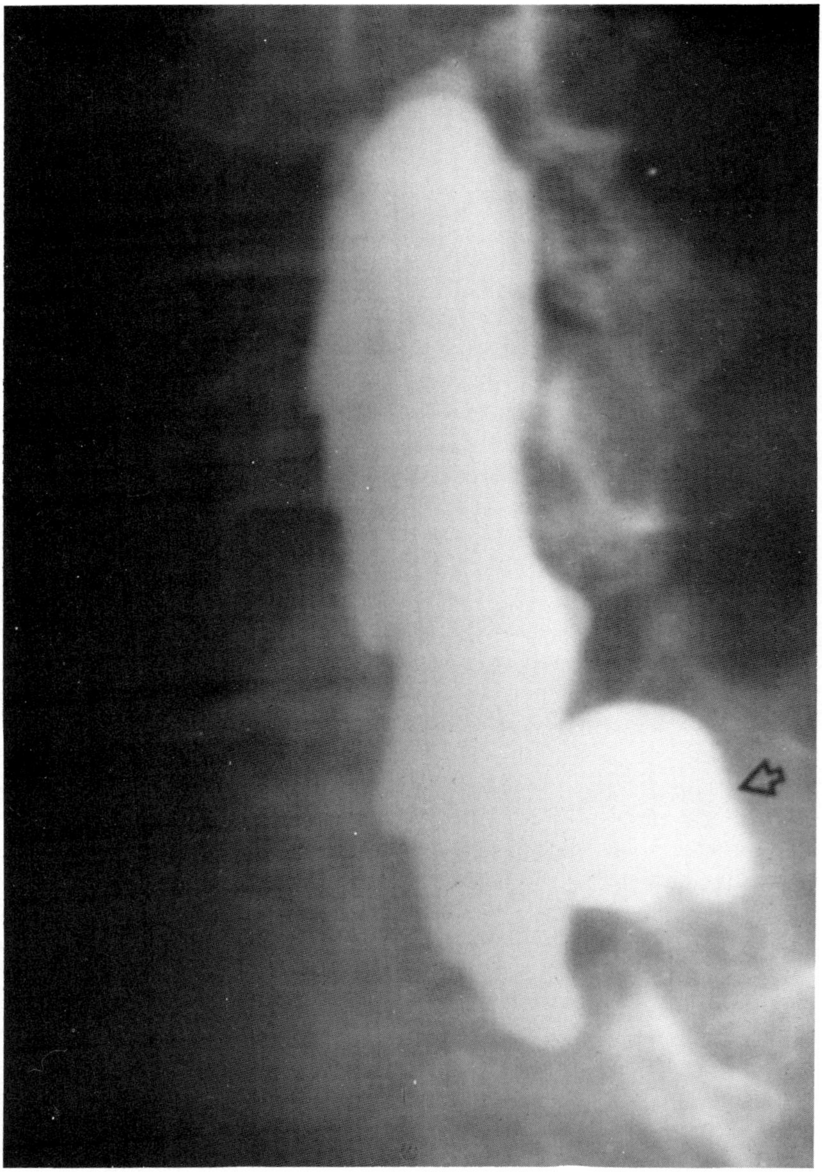

FIG. 32.1. Pseudomeningocele as shown by myelogram. The sac was actually much larger and the fistula much smaller than suggested by the x-ray.

instance the Kerrison-type punch was being used for removal of bone. It is disconcerting to see several centimeters of a root dangling from the instrument when it is withdrawn. It is suggested that after each bone bite with the punch that the instrument be released before lifting the bone out of the field.

One patient had a preexisting myelopathy due to spondylosis which was aggravated when the cord was contused during cervical laminectomy. The importance of great care in removing the lamina in the cervical area for tumor or spondylosis cannot be overemphasized.

The other developed a partial cauda equina syndrome on the sixth postoperative day after disc and fusion in the lumbar region. The partial paralysis appeared to result from serum entrapped under the fascia. Its presence had not been reflected in a recognizable way in the wound as blood usually is.

You will note that six patients had persistent cerebrospinal fluid fistula that required closure. All were in the lumbar area. Eleven patients have returned or have been referred to us with symptomatic postsurgical pseudomeningoceles. (Figure 32.1) is a myelogram of one such case. Most of these have resulted from rents near the dural sleeve. We would propose that every effort be made to close such rents. We have found fat plugs useful for this purpose and have confirmed in the dog that they do actually seal the defect. We also use fat graft to close larger defects in the dura as one patches worn-out garments—that is, placing the graft inside the dural tube and then plicating it.

Stenosis of the spinal canal does occur after laminectomy, especially when the operation has been combined with a spinal fusion. We have verified seven cases of this type. The interval from the original surgical procedure to the onset of symptoms due to stenosis has been quite long, but the picture is quite characteristic.

When myelography is done for persistent or recurring symptoms after laminectomy, filling defects are frequently noted and attributed to adhesions involving the arachnoid. The filling defects are commonly described as arachnoiditis. The defects may occur from compression of the dura by a disc or tumor, by reaction to the manipulation of the dura during operation, or from other causes. When it is segmental and at the level of the surgical procedure, it is important to include the adhesive process in the differential diagnoses. It is believed that postsurgical arachnoiditis is rarely the cause of significant symptoms.

These, then, involve the principal complications that we have observed in carrying out laminectomy over the last 25 years. It is inevitable that some complications occur, I presume, but careful workup, precise planning, and considerable self-restraint will tend to minimize them.

CHAPTER

33

The Role of Vascular Proliferation in the Growth of Brain Tumors*

STEVEN BREM, M.D.

"It was but natural that attention should be focused on the cellular elements of the gliomata rather than on the vessels . . . And yet these vessels tell a story could it be read" (23).

The time elapsed between the origin of a malignant brain tumor and its clinical detection by the neurosurgeon may be several months or years. Whatever its etiology, a brain tumor, like all solid tumors, passes through two distinct phases (1, 17, 18, 40): (1) The *avascular* phase. At this early stage of development, without blood vessels, the tumor is restricted to a minute size, less than a few millimeters in diameter. The tumor must rely on diffusion as the sole means for the procurement of nutrients and the elimination of wastes. Because of the miniscule size of the tumor, this stage is generally asymptomatic and clinically undetectable. (2) The *vascular* phase. The penetration of the tumor by host capillaries leads to rapid, exponential growth. Vascular perfusion provides the tumor with essential metabolites. As the tumor grows faster, it stimulates an increasing number of capillaries, and a synergistic relationship is established between the neoplastic and the vascular elements.

At the center of this vicious circle lies the formation of new blood vessels, *i.e.*, tumor angiogenesis. Vascular proliferation allows the tumor to progress from a harmless, small, avascular nodule to a clinically overt, vascularized mass. Furthermore, for the cerebral astrocytomas, the intensity of capillary proliferation appears to be an indicator of the malignant potential of the neoplastic glial cells.

Because there are no methods available to observe the early, avascular stage within the parenchyma of the brain, the following experiments were performed in the eye. They demonstrate the close interrelationship between the neoplastic cells of the brain tumor and the vascular elements of the host.

---

* Selected for the 1975 Annual Resident Award of the Congress of Neurological Surgeons.

THE VASCULAR PHASE

The Formation of New Blood Vessels in the Cornea

The capacity of a small tumor to induce new blood vessels can be measured by transplanting it to the cornea (21). This procedure anatomically separates the neoplasm from the responding host vessels of the limbus. Prior to vascularization, the cornea is an immune privileged site (21), permitting the study of xenografts such as gliomas taken from humans or mice and transplanted to the rabbit.

A methylcholanthrene-induced ependymoblastoma was maintained by serial subcutaneous and intracerebral passage in C57 mice (41). A subcutaneous nodule was removed aseptically, minced in lactated Ringer's solution, yielding tumor fragments of approximately 4.0 mm. × 1.5 mm. × 0.1 mm. Each fragment was inserted into a pouch created in the corneal stroma of a rabbit eye by a previously described method (21). All of the implants were placed at a distance of 2.0 ± 0.5 mm. from the limbal blood vessels. This distance has been shown to be within a critical diffusion distance, beyond which the chemical mediator of tumor angiogenesis fails to induce new blood vessels in the cornea (21). Observations of vascular length, number of vessels, and tumor size were made every 48 hours. At the end of the experiment, the tumor and the corneal vessels were studied further by light microscopy after fixation in 10% formalin and staining with hematoxylin and eosin.

In six separate experiments, the mouse glioma elicited brisk neovascularization in 34 of 36 eyes. New blood vessels first appeared at the limbus between days 4 and 12 after transplantation (Table 33.1). These vessels grew toward the tumor at an average rate of 0.3 mm per day (Fig. 33.1). Transplants of a human glioblastoma induced a similar response. Neovascularization was absent in all 37 control eyes containing: heat-killed tumor; adult human cortex; adult mouse cortex; and fetal rabbit cortex (Table 33.1).

In these experiments, tumor grafts in the cornea induce neovascularization. If the tumor grafts are immunologically compatible with the

TABLE 33.1
Neovascular Responses of Transplants to the Rabbit Cornea

Test Specimen	Species	No. Eyes Positive	No. Eyes Negative
Ependymoblastoma	Mouse	34	2
Glioblastoma	Human	8	0
Cortex, normal	Human	0	5
Cortex, atrophic	Human	0	9
Cortex, normal	Mouse	0	6
Glioblastoma, boiled	Human	0	9
Cortex, fetus	Rabbit	0	8

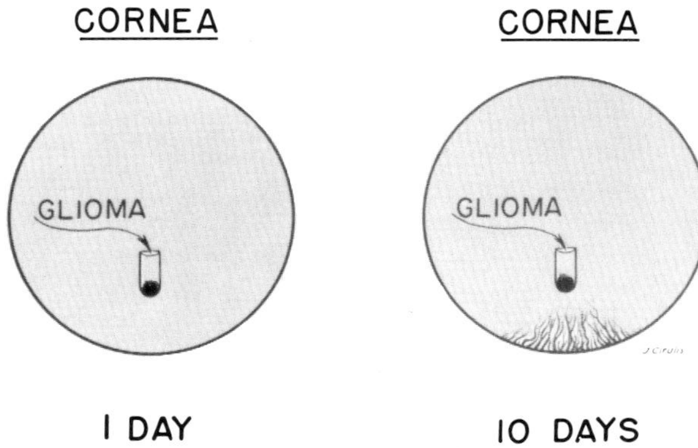

FIG. 33.1. Gliomas transplanted to the rabbit cornea induce a brisk neovascular response. Brain tumors produce a diffusable message to the host capillary bed, eliciting new vessels.

rabbit host, such as a rabbit V2 carcinoma, extremely rapid growth follows vascularization (4, 21). By contrast, vascularization of foreign tumors, such as those derived from mice or humans, leads to a classical immune rejection with corneal clouding and leucocyte infiltration.

These experiments suggest that the glioma secretes a diffusable, vasoformative substance that can induce capillary proliferation even at a distance of approximately 2.0 mm. from the tumor. This ability to elicit new blood vessels distinguishes the gliomas from normal or fetal cerebral tissues.

We next sought a method for interrupting the signal for capillary proliferation, depriving a tumor of its vascular component, thereby studying the behavior of a tumor confined to the avascular phase.

THE AVASCULAR PHASE

Prevention of Vascularization in the Vitreous

A clinical observation led to the selection of the vitreous body of the eye as a transplantation site. In childhood retinoblastomas, the vascularized tumor grows rapidly along the retinal surface as a large, exophytic mass. It sheds minute metastases, however, into the vitreous. These "floaters" or "seeds" are less than 1 mm. and remain dormant for weeks without harming the patient (16).

Experimentally, we therefore have used the vitreous to study tumor dormancy in the avascular phase (10). The vitreous is composed of a transparent, relatively acellular, viscous gel; tumor implants maintain a fixed position and can be repeatedly observed (9). The avascularity of the vitreous confers an immune privileged status, permitting the study of tumor xenografts.

For these experiments. a mouse glioma was maintained as described earlier. A cell suspension containing approximately 2×10^7 cells was prepared by passing the solid tumor through a cytosieve and suspending the cells in 2 ml. of lactated Ringer's solution; viability was greater than 90% by trypan blue exclusion. The cells were transferred to the vitreous using a #27 needle passed through the superiortemporal sclera (10). Approximately 50 μl. (10^6 cells) were inoculated in the midvitreous at a distance between 2.0 and 5.0 mm. anterior to the retinal vessels. In 8 of 12 eyes, the cells aggregated to form a visible, spherical colony. The nodules grew slowly, reaching a maximal diameter of about 0.8 mm. They remained at this small size throughout the entire duration of the experiment, for as long as 180 days (Fig. 33.2). Neovascularization failed to occur while the tumors were suspended in the vitreous. The vitreous remained transparent without any evidence of an immune rejection. Autoradiography after incorporation of ^{3}H-thymidine and histological examination revealed an outer layer of viable tumor cells and an inner necrotic center (Fig. 33.3).

When these experiments were performed with a rabbit carcinoma (10), the tumor likewise remained dormant for weeks with a small, steady state volume as long as it remained suspended in the vitreous. But if the tumor drifted towards the retinal vessels, or if it was placed on the retina, neovascularization occurred, followed by explosive growth with up to a 19,000-fold increase in tumor volume in 2 weeks time.

CLINICAL CORRELATES

Capillary Proliferation and the Malignant Potential of Cerebral Astrocytomas

A glioma arising in the brain, unlike one transplanted to the vitreous, lies in close proximity to host capillaries. Early in its development, it may acquire the capacity to induce angiogenesis and stimulate capillary proliferation.

The striking degree of capillary proliferation observed in histological sections of human brain tumors is well recognized (32). Many authors have suggested a relationship between the extent of capillary changes and the malignant potential of the tumor (2, 3, 12, 26, 30, 33, 36). These workers have provided detailed, descriptive accounts of the microvasculature in brain tumors.

To make comparisons among large numbers of tumors, we developed a quantitative method for histological grading based upon the degree of capillary proliferation (6, 7). The microscopic angiogenesis grading (MAG) system measured endothelial growth by three criteria: (1) vasoproliferation, (2) endothelial hyperplasia, and (3) endothelial cytology.

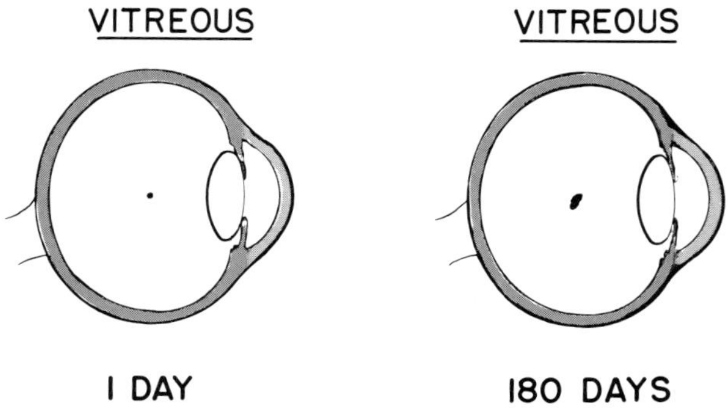

FIG. 33.2. Gliomas transplanted to the rabbit vitreous fail to induce a neovascular response. The vasoformative signal is interrupted; the tumor persists in the avascular state for months. In the avascular phase, growth is slow, the tumor exists as a dormant nodule.

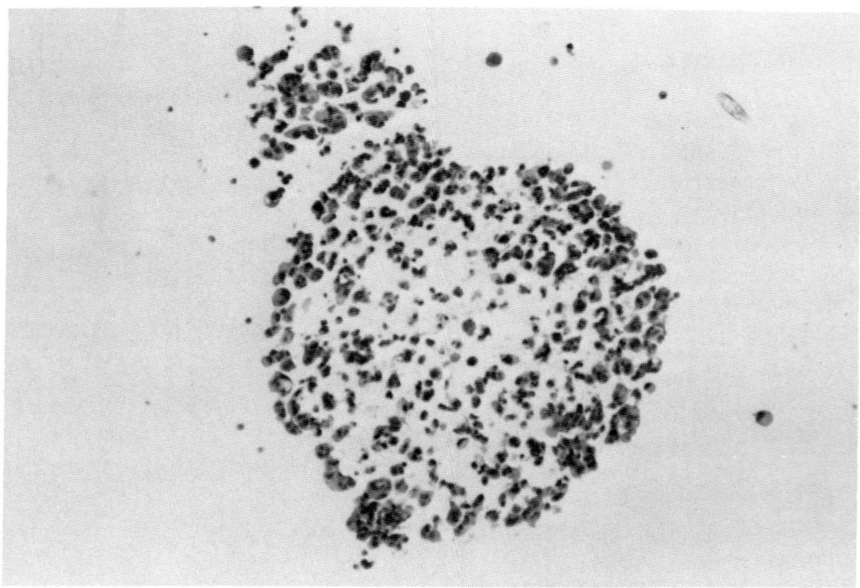

FIG. 33.3. Histological section through an avascular glioma, day #47 of intravitreal growth. Note viable tumor cells at the periphery and necrotic cells in the center of the tumor. Magnification × 64.

Vasoproliferation indicated the capillary density within a defined area. *Endothelial hyperplasia* was the maximal number of endothelial cells lining the cross section of a capillary, from 0 to 10. During neovascularization, a variety of primitive endothelial forms appeared (7). *Endothelial cytology* referred to the appearance of the most primitive endothelial cell within a hyperplastic zone, graded from 0 to 5: 0 = normal endothelial cell—thin, flat, elongated, well differentiated nucleus; 1 = plump, clear nucleus; 2 = plump, clear nucleus plus a prominent nucleolus; 3 = large, hyperchromatic nucleus; 4 = bizarre endothelial cell; and 5 = mitotic figure. A simple equation then gave an over-all index (0 to 100) of endothelial regeneration. Avascular tissues received a score of 0, normal cerebral cortex 20 ± 5, and a glioblastoma with maximal endothelial regeneration, 100.

We applied this method for the histological study of 80 cerebral astrocytomas biopsied at the Massachusetts General Hospital (8). These tumors showed a wide spectrum of endothelial proliferation. When the astrocytomas were grouped according to the conventional classification based upon the degree of anaplasia, Kernohan's grade I to IV, a trend developed: for each consecutive grade of anaplasia there was a corresponding increase in the MAG score (Fig. 33.4). The more malignant the appearance of the tumor cell population, the greater was the degree of endothelial proliferation.

To determine whether the MAG score might correlate with the clinical course of a patient with an astrocytoma, we reviewed the postoperative survival of 31 of these patients (Fig 33.5). Eight patients surviving less than 1 month had a mean MAG score of 71 (S.D. ± 8); 18 patients surviving less than 1 year, 59 (S.D. ± 14); and five patients with up to a 10-year survival, 36 (S.D. ± 7).

The MAG technique has been simplified further by eliminating the measurement of capillary density which correlated poorly with the glial anaplasia and the postoperative survival. Additional data on the

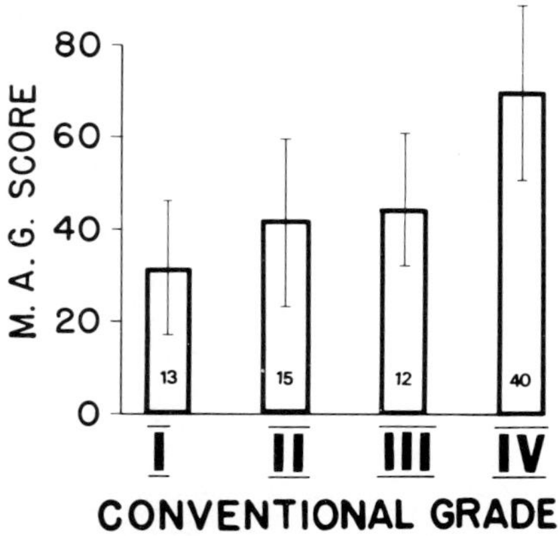

FIG. 33.4. Correlation of capillary proliferation with increasing malignancy of astrocytomas. Intensity of endothelial proliferation (MAG score) is compared to the Kernohan grading of malignancy.

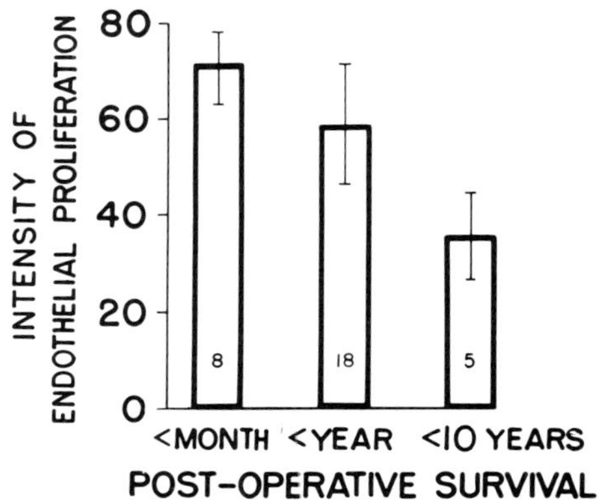

FIG. 33.5. Intense capillary proliferation is associated with a poor prognosis.

vascular grading of cerebral astrocytomas are presented in Tables 33.2 to 33.4. Measurements of either endothelial hyperplasia or endothelial cytology served as useful guides to the clinical and pathological virulence of the tumor. Although there was a wide variation between individual patients (Table 33.2), a good correlation existed between the values for hyperplastic or cytological changes and the postoperative survival for a group of patients (Table 33.3).

Three groups of astrocytomas could be distinguished on the basis of vascular proliferation (Table 33.3). The low grade tumors (astrocytomas I and II) were characterized by well differentiated endothelial cells and minimal hyperplasia. An intermediate group (astrocytomas II–III and III) showed an increase in the number of endothelial cells lining the capillary lumen as well as endothelial cell nuclei that were more primitive in appearance. The anaplastic tumors (astrocytomas III–IV, and IV) showed the most extreme vascular changes.

The most significant sign of vascular proliferation may be the appearance of a mitotic figure in the endothelial cell population of the tumor. Normally, an endothelial mitosis is a rare occurrence on histological sections except in those tissues with actively regenerating endothelium (7). They could be found, however, in a large number of the astrocytomas (Table 33.2). When these tumors were divided into two groups according to whether a mitotic figure could be observed in the capillary endothelium, there was a seven-fold shorter postoperative survival associated with the tumors displaying endothelial mitotic figures (Table 33.4). These observations provide further evidence that the renewal of the endothelial cell population is related to the growth rate of the tumor.

TABLE 33.2
Microvascular Grading and Postoperative Survival in 41 Patients with Cerebral Astrocytomas

Patient (M.G.H.* No.)	Astrocytoma Grade† (I, II, III, IV)	Endothelial Hyperplasia (0–10)	Endothelial Cytology (0–5‡)	Postoperative Survival (Months)
172-68-50	I	1	1	3
131-32-85	I	3	1	240
099-50-50	I	3	1	48
115-44-59	I	3	1	41
128-04-60	I	3	1	13
129-84-03	I	8	1	84
115-28-43	I–II	4	1	99
114-84-42	I–II	10	3	130
128-93-36	II	4	1	57§
140-50-98	II	2	0	2
150-36-06	II	2	2	36
170-71-79	II–III	3	1	24§
108-36-70	II–III	3	1	6
117-68-65	II–III	4	2	3
118-78-19	II–III	8	3	4
100-03-43	II–III	10	5	11
107-65-43	III	2	2	62
170-94-18	III	4	1	9
014-31-61	III	6	3	8
002-01-36	III	10	3	3
112-57-68	III	9	5	4
113-92-63	III	10	5	8
114-36-05	III–IV	4	1	28
116-83-14	III–IV	5	4	8
101-29-78	III–IV	7	1	<1
116-43-77	III–IV	6	3	<1
113-80-72	III–IV	7	4	<1
143-03-27	III–IV	9	3	23
113-51-13	III–IV	9	5	5
113-76-30	III–IV	10	4	<1
117-11-01	III–IV	9	5	3
168-94-61	III–IV	10	5	7
118-13-47	III–IV	10	5	11
118-66-37	III–IV	10	5	6
171-86-45	III–IV	10	5	6
064-06-59	III–IV	10	5	5
115-47-91	III–IV	10	5	3
119-47-75	III–IV	10	5	<1
173-14-82	III–IV	10	5	<1
127-76-58	IV	10	3	13
039-30-93	IV	10	5	<1

* Massachusetts General Hospital.
† Kernohan and associates, 1949 (25).
‡ Mitotic figure = 5.
§ Still alive.

TABLE 33.3
Summary: Tumor Grade, Vascular Histology, and Postoperative Survival (41 Astrocytomas)

Tumor Grade	No. Patients	Endothelial Hyperplasia (0–10)	Endothelial Cytology (0–5)	Mean Survival (Months)
I; II	11	3.5 ± 2.8	1.2 ± 0.7	68.5
II–III; III	11	6.3 ± 3.2	2.8 ± 1.5	12.9
III–IV; IV	19	8.6 ± 1.9	4.2 ± 1.3	6.3

TABLE 33.4
Postoperative Survival Related to the Appearance of Mitotic Figures in the Capillary Endothelial Cells of 41 Astrocytomas

Mitotic Figures	No. Tumors	Mean Survival (Months)
Observed	14	5.0
Not Observed	27	35.0

DISCUSSION

The corneal experiments show that gliomas produce a diffusable, vasoformative substance that acts on the host vascular bed. Feigin and associates postulated that endothelial hyperplasia, so prominent in brain tumors, might be due to a diffusable factor released by the tumor cells (12). Folkman and colleagues have isolated a biochemical mediator of capillary proliferation, called "tumor-angiogenesis-factor", (TAF) (13, 37). Recently, Suddith and associates reported a similar "endothelial growth factor" produced by cell lines derived from neural tumors (34). A wide range of human and experimental neoplasms contain TAF (17), but the most potent source, to date, of TAF has been cell lines derived from a human meningioma and glioblastoma (28).

The finding of a potent vasoformative signal within brain tumors is in agreement with the high levels of capillary proliferation observed histologically. When we examined the histological sections of a wide spectrum of human neoplasms, including sarcomas and carcinomas, the glioblastomas displayed the most intense capillary proliferation (7).

The histological data presented here support the concept that the rate of vascular proliferation parallels that of tumor growth. Tannock, using an isotopic labeling technique, studied the interrelationship between the kinetics of tumor and vascular proliferation (35). He showed that only tumor cells located near capillaries remain in the replicating cell cycle. In addition, the likelihood of a tumor cell entering mitosis decreased the further away it was from an adjacent capillary. At a distance beyond 160 μ from the nearest capillary, cell death occurred. Furthermore, Wright observed that in experimental brain tumors, cell proliferation tends to occur in regions in close proximity to surrounding blood vessels (39).

Thus, there is a mutual dependency between the tumor and its vascular elements. The tumor stimulates capillary proliferation, which in turn, promotes tumor growth. Vascularization allows the tumor to express its maximal growth rate.

Although it is required by malignant tumors, vascularization by itself does not imply malignancy. For example, in cerebellar gliomas of childhood, endothelial proliferation can be seen even in benign tumors (32, 38). It is likely that these cerebellar astrocytomas have the capacity to stimulate capillaries but lack other malignant factors.

The vitreous experiments show that prevention of neovascularization causes a glioma to remain in a dormant state for months at a tiny, innocuous size. Freeman and Zimmerman studied the behavior of brain tumors transplanted to the avascular anterior chamber of the eye. At first, these tumors grew as small, avascular nodules; further growth into large, vascularized masses was associated with recruitment of blood vessels from the iris (19). Greene and Arnold transplanted a human glioblastoma to the anterior chamber and observed it for a period of 6 to 9 months without any change in its size or damage to the host; yet, it remained viable (22). He suggested that the long period of dormancy was a characteristic of gliomas. Gimbrone and associates investigated tumor dormancy in the avascular phase by transplanting a rabbit epithelioma to the anterior chamber of the rabbit eye (20). Growth of the tumors was arrested at a volume of less than 1 mm^3. These small tumors remained viable, and when transferred to the vascular iris, penetration of the tumor by new capillaries resulted in rapid, exponential growth.

The explanation for "dormancy" in the avascular phase is that a population of cells growing in three dimensions reaches a critical diameter in which cells in the center of the mass die for lack of nutrients. Cells at the periphery continue to be metabolically active, and even replicate. Peripheral growth, however, is neutralized by central necrosis. The size of the dormant nodule is determined by the diameter at which this equilibrium occurs (15). These considerations explain the regional differences in growth rates noted in human and experimental gliomas. Metabolic gradients exist with the highest concentration of proteins and nucleic acids at the vascularized periphery (11, 23, 27, 29).

Thus, vascular proliferation, by controlling the supply of metabolites to the tumor, becomes an important control point in the evolution of a cerebral neoplasm.

In neurosurgery, we may someday be able to detect brain tumors and intervene therapeutically while the tumor is still in a dormant or

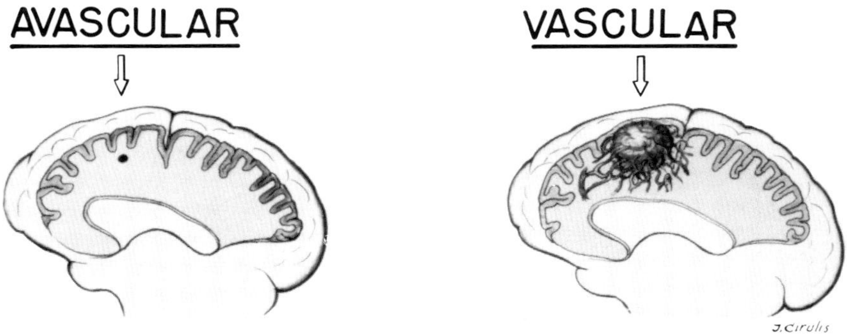

FIG. 33.6. Theoretical model of brain tumor development. Brain tumors arise as an avascular cluster of cells, analagous to *in situ* cancer at other sites. Angiogenesis results in rapid growth and presentation of the tumor as a clinically overt, vascularized mass. Blockade of angiogenesis would be an important therapeutic adjunct because tumors deprived of capillaries exist as tiny, dormant nodules.

avascular phase (Fig. 33.6). We may even begin to recognize *in situ* cancer of the brain. At the present time, only the ophthalmologist, the dermatologist, and the gynecologist possess the necessary technology to observe and treat *in situ* cancer. In the *in situ* stage, tumors are confined to their original location, are not vascularized, and produce no grossly visible alterations (31). The passage of a cluster of malignant cells from the *in situ* stage to a clinically apparent, vascularized mass is characterized by a long quiescent period. For cancer of the cervix, the transitional period has been estimated to be 15 years; furthermore, the vast majority of *in situ* lesions never develop into clinically overt carcinoma (24, 31).

What would the management of brain tumors be like if: (a) we had the ability to diagnose a brain tumor in the avascular phase? or (b) failing that, treating tumors by interrupting the signal for vascular proliferation, thereby forcing the tumor into a prolonged state of dormancy in the avascular phase? It is conceivable that various therapeutic approaches which inhibit angiogenesis will become powerful adjuncts to the surgery of brain tumors (4, 5, 14).

The vitreous experiments demonstrate that by whatever means the signal for capillaries is interrupted, the result is the same: even the most virulent tumor is restricted to a tiny size of less than a few millimeters. Despite its malignant potential, without blood vessels, the tumor acts benign.

SUMMARY

The formation of new blood vessels, *i.e.*, angiogenesis, is a critical step in the evolution of a brain tumor from the earliest avascular phase to the clinically overt, vascular stage. For cerebral astrocytomas, intense capillary proliferation is a poor prognostic sign, associated with rapidly growing tumors. The *in vivo* production of a vasoformative substance can be demonstrated by transplanting human and experimental gliomas to the rabbit cornea. Intense neovascularization is elicited by the tumor and not by control tissues. If the same tumor is transplanted to the vitreous, thereby interrupting the vasoformative signal, the tumor remains in a dormant state for a prolonged period of time, despite its malignant potential. Inhibition of angiogenesis would be an important adjunct to the surgical treatment of gliomas.

ACKNOWLEDGMENT

The author gratefully acknowledges the suggestions and advice of Dr. Judah Folkman, the support of Dr. Michael D. Walker, and the guidance of Dr. William H. Sweet. The diagrams were drawn by Mr. Janis Cirulis.

REFERENCES

1. Ackerman, N. A. The blood supply of experimental liver metastases. IV. Changes in vascularity with increasing tumor growth. Surgery, *15:* 589–596, 1974.
2. Arieti, S. The vascularization of cerebral neoplasms studied with the fuschin method of Eros. J. Neuropathol. Exp. Neurol., *1:* 375–393, 1942.
3. Bertrand, I., and Mannen, H. Etude des reactions vasculaires dans les astrocytomes. Rev. Neurol. (Paris), *102:* 3–19, 1960.
4. Brem, H., and Folkman, J. Inhibition of tumor angiogenesis mediated by cartilage. J. Exp. Med., *141:* 427–439, 1975.
5. Brem, H., Arensman, R., and Folkman, J. Inhibition of tumor angiogenesis by a diffusable factor from cartilage. *In* Extracellular Matrix Influences on Gene Expression, edited by H. C. Slavkin and R. C. Greulich, pp. 767–772. Academic Press, New York, 1975.
6. Brem, S. Studies on the Host Response to a Human Brain Tumor. Thesis, Harvard Medical School, 1972.
7. Brem, S., Cotran, R. S., and Folkman, M. J. Tumor angiogenesis: a quantitative method for histologic grading. J. Natl. Cancer Inst., *48:* 347–356, 1972.
8. Brem, S., Cotran, R. S., and Folkman, M. J. Angiogenesis in brain tumors: a quantitative histologic study. Surg. Forum, *25:* 462–464, 1974.
9. Brem, S., Finkelstein, D., Chen, C., Brem, H., Folkman, J., and Patz, A. Retinal neovascularization: experimental induction by intravitreal tumors. Assoc. Res. Vision Ophthalmol. Abstract #10, p. 21, 1975.
10. Brem, S., Brem, H., Folkman, J., Finkelstein, D., and Patz, A Prolonged tumor dormancy by prevention of vascularization in the vitreous. Cancer Res., in press.
11. Caspersson, T., and Santesson, L. Studies on protein metabolism in cells of epithelial tumors. Acta Radiol. Scand. (Suppl.), *46:* 1–105, 1942.
12. Feigin, I., Allen, L. B., Lipkin, L., and Gross, S. W. The endothelial hyperplasia of the cerebral blood vessels with brain tumors and its sarcomatous transformation. Cancer, *11:* 264–277 1958.
13. Folkman, J., Merler, E., Abernathy, C., and Williams, G. Isolation of a tumor factor responsible for angiogenesis. J. Exp. Med., *133:* 275–288, 1971.
14. Folkman, J. Tumor angiogenesis: therapeutic implications. N. Engl. J. Med., *285:* 1182–1186, 1971.

15. Folkman, J., and Hochberg, M. Self-regulation of growth in three dimensions. J. Exp. Med., *138:* 745–753, 1973.
16. Folkman, J. Proceedings: Tumor angiogenesis factor. Cancer Res., *34:* 2109–2113, 1974.
17. Folkman, J. Tumor angiogenesis. Adv. Cancer Res., *19:* 331–358, 1974.
18. Folkman, J. Tumor angiogenesis: A possible control point in tumor growth. Ann. Intern. Med., *82:* 96–100, 1975.
19. Freeman, D., and Zimmerman, H. M. Experimental brain tumors; behavior in intraocular transplants. Cancer Res., *4:* 273–278, 1944.
20. Gimbrone, M. A., Jr., Leapman, S. B., Contran, R. S., and Folkman, J. Tumor dormancy in vivo by prevention of neovascularization. J. Exp. Med., *136:* 261–276, 1972.
21. Gimbrone, M. A., Jr., Cotran, R. S., Leapman, S. B., and Folkman, J. Tumor growth and neovascularization: An experimental model using rabbit cornea. J. Natl. Cancer Inst., *52:* 413–427, 1974.
22. Greene, H. S. N., and Arnold, H. The homologous and heterologous transplantation of brain and brain tumors. J. Neurosurg., *2:* 315–331, 1945.
23. Hardman, J. The angioarchitecture of the gliomata. Brain, *63:* 91–118, 1940.
24. Johnson, L. D., Easterday, C. L., Gore, H., and Hertig, A. Histogenesis of carcinoma in situ of the uterine cervix. Cancer, *17:* 213–229, 1964.
25. Kernohan, J. W., Mabon, R. F., Svien, H. J., and Adson, A. W. A simplified classification of gliomas. Proc. Staff Meet., Mayo Clin. *24:* 71–75, 1949.
26. Khominsky, B. S., and Schamaev, M. I. Vascularization of neuroectodermal tumors of various malignancy grades. Arch. Geschwulstforsch., *37:* 136–151, 1971.
27. Kirsch, W. M., and Schulz, D. W. Regional bioenergetic events in the experimental glioblastoma. A quantitative histochemical study. J. Neurosurg., *34:* 448–451, 1971.
28. Klagsburn, M., Knighton, D., and Folkman, J. Tumor angiogenesis activity in cells grown in tissue culture. Cancer Res., *36:* 110–114, 1976.
29. Maker, H. S., and Lehrer, G. M. Environmental factors in the structure, metabolism and growth of glial tumors. *In* Experimental Biology of Brain Tumors, edited by W. M. Kirsch, E. Grossi-Paoletti, and P. Paoletti, pp. 519–532. Charles C Thomas, Springfield, Ill., 1971.
30. O'Connor, J. S., and Laws, E. R. Changes in histochemical staining of brain tumor blood vessels associated with increasing malignancy. Acta Neuropathol. (Berl.), *14:* 161–173, 1969.
31. Robbins, S. L. Pathologic Basis of Disease, 4th ed., p. 116. W. B. Saunders Co., Philadelphia, 1974.
32. Russel, D. S., and Rubinstein, L. J. Pathology of Tumours of the Nervous System, 3rd ed., 429 pp. Williams & Wilkins Co., Baltimore, 1971.
33. Sahs, A. L., and Alexander, L. Vascular pattern of certain intracranial neoplasms. Arch. Neurol. Psychiatr., *42:* 44–66, 1939.
34. Suddith, R. L., Kelly, P. J., Hutchison, H. T., and Haber, B. In vitro stimulation of endothelial cell proliferation by tumor cell conditioned media. Fed. Proc., *34:* 731, Abstr. #2898, 1975.
35. Tannock, I. F. The relation between cell proliferation and the vascular system in a transplanted mouse mammary tumor. Br. J. Cancer, *22:* 258–273, 1968.
36. Torack, R. M. Ultrastructure of capillary reaction to brain tumors. Arch. Neurol., *5:* 416–428, 1961.
37. Tuan, D., Smith, S., Folkman, J., and Merler, E. Isolation of the nonhistone proteins of rat Walker carcinoma 256. Their association with tumor angiogenesis. Biochemistry, *12:* 3159–3165, 1973.

38. Winston, K., Gilles, F., Leviton, A., and Fulchiero, A. Cerebellar gliomas in children. Unpublished data, 1975.
39. Wright, R. L. Vascular permeability in experimental brain tumors. Angiology, *18:* 69–75, 1967.
40. Yamaura, H., and Sato, H. Quantitative studies on the developing vascular system of the rat hepatoma. J. Natl. Cancer Inst., *53:* 1229–1240, 1974.
41. Zimmerman, H. M. Experimental Brain Tumors. *In* The Biology and Treatment of Intracranial Tumors, edited by W. S. Fields and P. C. Sharkey, pp. 49–74. Charles C Thomas, Springfield, Ill., 1962.

CHAPTER

34

Complications of Percutaneous Surgery for Pain

JAMES G. WEPSIC, M.D.

In the past 10 years, an increasing number of patients with pain have been treated utilizing percutaneous methods of interrupting the pain pathways in the spinal cord and trigeminal system. The relatively rapid acceptance of these effective techniques is, in large measure, due to their low rates of complications and side effects. This report will focus on the complications seen with these two procedures. Their therapeutic effectiveness has been reported earlier. Considerations of stereotaxic intracranial pain-relieving procedures and the various neurolytic chemical procedures to interrupt function of peripheral nerves or spinal roots will not be discussed here.

PERCUTANEOUS TRIGEMINAL PREGANGLIONIC THERMAL RHIZOTOMY

Although the technical problems and complications encountered by Kirschner (5) in his Gasserian ganglion coagulations led most European and American neurosurgeons to use the subtemporal retrogasserian rhizotomy as their standard method of treating trigeminal neuralgia, modifications in the procedure initiated in Europe by Hubner (4), Piotrowski (14), and Menzel (8) reawakened interest in this method of selectively destroying the sensory innervation to the face. Further modifications of the technique employing careful temperature regulation and control of lesion location have improved upon the results of the earlier workers (22, 23).

The technique of introducing a hollow coagulating cannula capable of bearing a thermister-tipped probe into the region of the preganglionic rootlets has been described in detail earlier (23, 27, 28). As important as the equipment and technique of insertion are the physiological changes obtained upon stimulation of the electrode and the anatomical findings noted on submental-vertex and lateral views of the skull. The use of short acting barbiturates and neuroleptic anesthetic agents improves upon the comfort of the patients and allows their active participation in sensory testing during the sequence of gradually increasing thermal lesions. This gives greater control in the selective destruction of pain fibers in the particular division or divisions required.

A recent survey by Sweet (21) indicates that well over 2000 patients have been treated for idiopathic trigeminal neuralgia in the past 9 years utilizing the radiofrequency thermal technique with an extremely low rate of major and minor complications. Table 34.1 summarizes the experience of eight neurosurgical groups treating facial pain. Although the vast majority of patients treated suffer from idiopathic trigeminal neuralgia, this technique has also been used in treating patients with facial pain due to invasive carcinoma, periodic migrainous neuralgia, atypical trigeminal neuralgia and atypical facial pain. Results in patients with tic douloureux show an extremely low mortality with the primary complication continuing to be unwanted corneal anesthesia and painful dysesthesias in the zone of the lesion. Only one death has occurred as a result of the procedure. This compares very favorably with the mortality rate of 1.3% achieved by White and Sweet (28) in their 805 patients with subtemporal retrogasserian rhizotomies. It also compares favorably with the 4.5% mortality rate for the posterior fossa approach. In a large series of patients described in Table 34.1, the rate of unwanted corneal anesthesia varied from 1.6 to 11%. This also compares favorably to the 6 to 10% noted in the open operation. Painful dysesthesias are much less common with the thermal lesion of the preganglionic rootlets, ranging from 1 to 5%. This is a much lower figure than is generally reported for the open operation.

Analysis of the total experience utilizing percutaneous thermal rhizotomy at the Massachusetts General Hospital over the past 9 years included 700 patients. Table 34.2 summarizes the *intraoperative complications*. They include: arterial bleeding from the radiofrequency-

TABLE 34.1
Major Complications of Trigeminal Rhizotomy

Series	Patients	Deaths	Unwanted Corneal Anesthesia	Painful Dysesthesia
A. Percutaneous Thermal Technique				
	no.	%	%	%
Nugent (11)	292	0.3	5	1.3
Menzel (8)	315	0	—	5
Onofrio (13)	135	0	7.4	1.5
Rich (15)	88	0	7	3
Sweet (21)	484	0	5	1.2
Tew (26)	250	0	11	0.5
Thiry (27)	365	0	4.2	3.5
Wepsic	125	0	1.6	4
B. Open Surgical Techniques				
White and Sweet (28)	305	1.3	6	26
Dandy (1)	88	4.5	9.5	27.7

TABLE 34.2

Intraoperative Complications 816 Trigeminal Radiofrequency Thermal Rhizotomies in 700 Patients

Intraoperative Complication	Patients
Arterial bleeding from cannula	8
Cardiovascular reaction	6
Other cranial nerve paresis	1
Seizure	2

coagulating cannula noted in eight patients; hypotension or cardiac arrhythmias in six patients; transient paresis of cranial nerves II, III, IV, and VI in one patient; and seizure activity at or during the time of lesion making in two patients. When arterial bleeding is encountered, this usually indicates the electrode to lie extracranially in the internal carotid at the foramen lacerum with the cannula posterior to the foramen ovale. For this reason, it is generally wise in initial electrode positioning to aim somewhat anterior and medial to the foramen and to take a sagittal x-ray early to assist in electrode repositioning. If arterial bleeding is seen, the procedure is terminated, the patient observed, and the procedure repeated on the following day. No neurological deficit has accompanied such penetrations. In one case, a tortuous internal carotid artery passed directly over the foramen ovale and it was not possible, on three successive procedures, to enter the foramen without penetrating the carotid artery; therefore, an open subtemporal retrogasserian rhizotomy was done. No lasting sequelae of the hypotension or cardiac arrhythmias were encountered. In this group of elderly and often infirm patients, it is not unusual to have a history of previous myocardial infarctions or serious cardiac disease. Monitoring of cardiac activity throughout the procedure is a useful addition to the standard vital signs observations in these patients. The single case of cranial nerve paresis outside of the trigeminal zone has been described in detail by Sweet (21) as have the two patients who had seizures during the procedure.

The most troublesome *postoperative complications* after trigeminal thermal rhizotomies in these 700 patients have been the disagreeable paresthesias associated with sensory loss. Ten patients have had anesthesia dolorosa and eight patients analgesia dolorosa. Less severe, but disagreeable sensations, have been present in several other patients with less severe sensory loss (Table 34.3). Additional lesions have not been helpful in relieving the patients of their discomfort in those with minor sensory loss if the complaint is an unpleasant paresthesia rather than a recurrence of tic. One patient developed aseptic meningitis with a CSF leucocytosis which cleared in 2 days without treatment. One patient had temporary dysphasia and Sweet (21) has reported on one patient developing a temporal lobe abscess several months following a radiofrequency lesion.

These complications, although disturbing, are far less common than those reported with open surgical retrogasserian rhizotomy (Table 34.4). Anesthesia dolorosa occurs between 1 and 25% in reported series of open surgical treatment, and disturbing dysesthesias are much more common than we note in our series. Intracranial hemorrhage occurs in about 1% of patients as does infection of one type or another. Neuroparalytic keratitis is seen with the open operation between 1 and 15% and ocular paresis is also present. The posterior fossa approach, while appearing to have less preponderance of dysesthesias, has a similarly high incidence of keratitis and ataxia.

Reports from other centers (Table 34.5) on additional complications of percutaneous trigeminal radiofrequency thermal rhizotomies include: individual cases of VI nerve palsy; increase in lacrimation; intratemporal hematoma; subarachnoid hemorrhage; and hemiplegic stroke. The intratemporal hematoma required a craniotomy for evacuation and the subarachnoid hemorrhage cleared spontaneously without neurological deficit.

Although percutaneous lesioning of the trigeminal rootlets is accompa-

TABLE 34.3

Postoperative Complications 816 Trigeminal Radiofrequency Thermal Rhizotomies in 700 Patients

Postoperative Complication	Patients
Abscess, temporal lobe	1
Analgesia dolorosa	8
Anesthesia dolorosa	10
Dysphagia	1
Meningitis, aseptic	1

TABLE 34.4

Other Reported Complications of Open Trigeminal Rhizotomy (28)

Complication	Subtemporal	Posterior Fossa
	%	%
Anesthesia dolorosa	1–25	2
Dysesthesias, disturbing	3–56	3–25
Hematoma, intracranial	0–1	—
Infection	0–0.1	0.4
Keratitis	1–15	1–10
Ocular paresis	0.3–1	—

nied by few major complications, most patients express some unhappiness over a few temporary, but quite common, side effects (Table 34.6). Pains in the ear, "stuffiness" of the ear, or actual hearing impairment have been reported in many cases. These are thought to be due to a partial lesion of the fifth motor nerve with paralysis of the tensor veli palatini causing failure of the opening of the eustachian tube. This generally clears as motor nerve function returns. In patients with unilateral lesions, the masseter weakness is rarely a problem, although for several weeks following the procedure many state that they have difficulty chewing tough foods. The sensory disturbance which necessarily accompanies all preganglionic lesions is almost always interpreted as "numbness" for the first few weeks following the lesion. Although nearly normal tough sensation is often preserved, the patients are aware of a sensory deficit and take some time to adjust to it. A few patients have complained bitterly of the sensory loss despite the sensory examination demonstrating the nearly normal Von Frye hair thresholds over the heated zone. It is important to caution the patient that such sensory loss will be present, and it is our practice to provide the patient with a written description of the procedure which includes an outline of this particular side effect as well as the less common but more severe complications noted above.

Major problems associated with radiofrequency percutaneous thermocoagulation of the trigeminal preganglionic rootlets can be minimized by thoroughly evaluating the patients medically before the procedure. Although we generally administer the anesthetic agents for this procedure ourselves, formal anesthesia consultations are obtained in those

TABLE 34.5
Other Reported Complications of Percutaneous Trigeminal Radiofrequency Thermal Rhizotomy

Complication	Patients
Cranial nerve (VI) palsy	1
Lacrimination	1
Hemorrhage, intratemporal	1
Hemorrhage, subarachnoid	1
Stroke (hemiplegia)	1

TABLE 34.6
Common Minor Side Effects of Trigeminal Radiofrequency Thermal Rhizotomy

Hearing impairment or earache
Masseter/pterygoid weakness
Sensory disturbance

patients with questionable cardiorespiratory status. Coagulation factors are also checked preoperatively.

During the performance of a radiofrequency lesion, one must proceed slowly and cautiously to avoid producing total anesthesia over the zone of interest or unwanted loss of sensation over the first division. A vascular flush in the division being heated often precedes sensory loss there, and if noted in the first division, may herald an unwanted loss of sensation. If one notes a flush in the first division, it is best to discontinue lesion making immediately and withdraw the electrode to a more anterolateral position, away from the first division preganglionic fibers which tend to run more medially. Careful measurements of the position of the coagulating electrode with respect to the posterior edge of the foramen ovale in the submental vertex view of the skull in our first 274 patients demonstrated that first division sensory loss is unlikely if the tip of the electrode is less than 10 mm. medial to the reference point at the posterior medial boundary of the foramen. Paresthesias produced by test electrical stimulation are often not referred to the first division even when modest heating will produce a lesion there. Therefore, one cannot depend on this physiological aid to avoid corneal anesthesia. With care, one can induce the proper degree of general anesthesia so that the patient's cilial reflex remains during the lesion making. Repeated testing of this reflex during lesion making is carried out when an evolving lesion begins to involve the second division. If the observer notes it to decrease in speed or strength, it is best to discontinue the lesion and retest the patient. Recording of the evoked potentials at the supraorbital nerve produced by intermittent stimulation of the coagulating electrode is being investigated as a means of further reducing the incidence of unwanted first divison loss.

Unpleasant dysesthesias seem to be related to the degree of sensory loss and to the patient's cause for pain. Patients with atypical facial pain or atypical trigeminal neuralgia are more prone to find even a modest amount of sensory loss disagreeable. Therefore, in many of these patients, a preliminary lidocaine (Xylocaine) block of the Gasserian ganglion and rootlets is carried out to demonstrate to the patient the sensory loss which may be achieved on a permanent basis with a trigeminal lesion. In addition, in these patients, one also strives to produce minimal loss of touch by making low temperature lesions. It is far better to produce less sensory loss and repeat a trigeminal lesion than it is to create an unwanted anesthesia which can be treated medically with only modest success. We have informed the patients that multiple lesions may be necessary to achieve desired loss of sensation and that these may be required over successive days. Of the 125 patients treated by me in the past 28 months, 11 have required procedures; six of these taking place during the same hospitalization.

To our knowledge, we have not overlooked a treatable intracranial lesion such as fifth nerve neuroma, arteriovenous (AV) malformation, or aneurysm which produces facial pain by compression or traction upon the preganglionic rootlets. Careful Von Fyre hair examination of the face is made in each case, and all patients with atypical trigeminal neuralgia or those in whom historical features, age, or other factors suggesting a surgically treatable lesion are evaluated with appropriate neurodiagnostic procedures.

PERCUTANEOUS SPINOTHALAMIC TRACTOTOMY

Percutaneous cervical cordotomy, introduced by Mullan (9) in 1963 and modified by Rosomoff (17), is a second percutaneous procedure of great utility in treating pain, particularly of malignancy, without the need for an open operation. Anatomical factors make this procedure, done as a stereotaxic maneuver, somewhat more hazardous than the trigeminal lesion. We have modified the procedure as described by Rosomoff (17) by adding a temperature-monitoring probe and utilizing impedance monitoring and electrical stimulation as described by Tasker and Organ (24, 25).

Published reports on the performance of the percutaneous cordotomies are summarized in Table 34.7. Death as a complication of the procedure occurs between 0 and 5%. The major cause of death appears to be sleep-induced apnea produced in the performance of either planned or unintended bilateral anterior quadrant lesions. Recognition of this phenomenon has reduced the incidence of respiratory death in recent years, but a significant number of patients continue to have respiratory distress especially when bilateral lesions are carried out. The influence of percutaneous cervical cordotomy on pulmonary function has been carefully studied by Rosomoff and associates (19). They noted a significant reduction of tidal volume in patients undergoing bilateral cordotomies. There was a reduction of tidal volume as well as minute ventilation and in those with high levels of analgesia, these changes were associated with symptomatic respiratory distress. In the published series, respiratory distress was present between 0 and 9%. In almost all series, bladder abnormalities are present for variable lengths of time. Dysesthesias associated with cordotomy are reported by some groups as high as 6% and corticospinal tract involvement is seen in up to 12%. These figures, however, compare favorably to those for open cervical and unilateral thoracic cordotomies described by Schwartz (20) and Sweet and White (28). Their mortality rates for cervical cordotomies were 9.2

TABLE 34.7
Major Complications of Anterior Spinothalamic Tractotomy

Series	Patients	Deaths	Respiratory Distress	Bladder Paresis	Dysesthesias	Ataxia	Permanent Paresis
A. Percutaneous, Cervical							
	no.	%	%	%	%	%	%
Gildenberg (3)							
C1–2	35	8.6	8.6	—	—	—	0
C5–6	253	0	0	—	—	—	1.2
Mullan (10)	47	2	—	4	—	—	12
Onofrio (12)							
Early series	50	2	—	30	—	—	12
Later series	41	4	7	10	—	—	7
Rosomoff (18) bilateral	100	2	4	2	—	2	3
Lipson (7)	375	5.5	8.7	1.5 (unil.) 58 (bilat.)	5	Rare	2
Tasker (24)	78	1	1	4	3	—	0
Wepsic	34	0	0	6	6	0	0
B. Open High Cervical Cordotomy							
Schwartz (20)	120	9.2	2.5	11 (unil.) 42 (bilat.)	2.5	—	14 (unil.) 15 (bilat.)
White and Sweet (28)	28	21	—	3	3	—	10

and 21%, respectively. Orthostatic hypotension (2) as well as development of a subdural hematoma with third nerve palsy (16) have also been reported following such a procedure.

In order to minimize the respiratory complications associated with bilateral cervical cordotomies, our patients who have bilateral pain requiring bilateral spinothalamic tractotomies have undergone a percutaneous cordotomy on one side and an open lower cordotomy on the other. We have had little experience with the percutaneous cordotomy from the anterior approach described by Lin and associates (6). The intraoperative complications associated with unwanted mechanical trauma to the spinal cord produced by movement of the head in agitated patients can be avoided by either allowing the cordotomy electrode to ride free with the patient's head and neck as suggested by Mullan or by firmly fixing the head and cordotomy electrode assembly to the table in a head holder such as that employed by Rosomoff. However, we have found the Rosomoff head holder does not provide rigid fixation in patients who become severely agitated, and in patients of this type, it may be best to use a skeletal fixation device.

Over the past 8 years, 128 cordotomies performed at the Massachusetts General Hospital, 80 were done by the percutaneous technique. In my group of 34 patients treated with unilateral percutaneous cordotomy for pain due to malignancy, lasting relief of pain was achieved in 25. Initial pain relief with later failure occurred in 6 patients. In the remainder, it was not possible to produce an adequate lesion because of lack of patient cooperation or development of transitory weakness causing termination of the procedure prematurely. As opposed to the trigeminal lesions, we have found patients reluctant to repeat the percutaneous cordotomy. If a second lesion is necessary, they generally request an open operation be performed under general anesthesia.

Monitoring rises in impedance to signal entry into the spinal cord, air and pantopaque myelography, and physiological stimulation have all been used in these patients to assist in localization of the electrode. Our current electrode includes a thermister at its etched sharp tip for monitoring temperature. Because of our concern that electrode localization within the spinal cord is not as precise as we would like, we are now modifying our procedure to permit direct visual observation by fiberoptic means. This may permit more precise placement of the coagulating electrode.

SUMMARY

Percutaneous procedures are proving themselves to be useful additions to the group of neurosurgical procedures for treating pain. They demand a different style of careful operating technique and they place heavy reliance on the gradual production of lesions to achieve the desired degree of denervation. Control of lesion position and extent through further advances in neurophysiological monitoring should give these procedures an even wider margin of safety and reliability.

REFERENCES

1. Dandy, W. E. The treatment of trigeminal neuralgia by cerebellar route. Ann. Surg., *96:* 787–795, 1932.
2. Fox, J. L. Orthostatic hypotension following bilateral percutaneous cordotomy. A case report of treatment with anti-G suit. Acta Neurochir. (Wien), *24:* 219–224, 1971.
3. Gildenberg, P. C. Percutaneous cervical cordotomy. Clin. Neurosurg., *21:* 246–256, 1974.
4. Hübner-Frankfurt, B. Ist Die Elektrokoagulation des Ganglion Gasseri bei der Trigeminusneuralgie Noch Zeitgemäss? Bericht über 524 Operationen and 372 Patienten von 1952–1967. Langenbecks Arch. Chir., *322:* 577–581, 1968.
5. Kirschner, M. Zur Behandlung der Trigeminusneuralgie. Erfahrungen an 250 Fällen. Arch. Klin. Chir., *186:* 325–334, 1936.
6. Lin, P. M., Gildenberg, P. L., and Polakoff, P. P. An anterior approach to percutaneous lower anterior cordotomy. J. Neurosurg., *25:* 553–560, 1966.
7. Lipton, S. Pain control and the management of advanced malignant disease. Proc. R. Soc. Med., *66:* 607–609, 1973.
8. Menzel, J., Piotrowski, W., and Penzholz, H. Long term results of Gasserian ganglion electrocoagulation. J. Neurosurg., *42:* 140–143, 1975.
9. Mullan, S., Harper, P. V., Hekmatpanah, J., Torres, H., and Dobbin, G. Percutaneous interruption of spinal-pain tracts by means of a strontium^{90} needle. J. Neurosurg., *20:* 931–939, 1963.
10. Mullan, S., Hekmatpanah, J., Dobbin, G., and Beckman, F. Percutaneous intramedullary cordotomy utilizing the unipolar anodal electrolytic lesion. J. Neurosurg., *22:* 548–553, 1965.
11. Nugent, G. R., and Berry, B. Trigeminal neuralgia treated by differential percutaneous radiofrequency coagulation of the Gasserian ganglion. J. Neurosurg., *40:* 517–523, 1974.
12. Onofrio, B. M. Recent results with percutaneous cordotomy. Mayo Clin. Proc., *45:* 689–694, 1970.
13. Onofrio, B. M. Radiofrequency percutaneous Gasserian ganglion lesions; results in 140 patients with trigeminal pain. J. Neurosurg., *42:* 132–139, 1975.
14. Piotrowski-Heidelberg, W. Derzeitiger Standbunkt zur Electrokoagulation des Ganglion Gasseri beim Gesichtsschmerz. Langenbecks Arch. Chir., *322:* 573–577, 1968.
15. Rich, R. Trigeminal neuralgia: A comparison of surgical methods of treatment. Presented to the American Association of Neurosurgical Surgeons, April 1973.
16. Roberts, M. Third nerve paresis with contralateral subdural hematoma following cerebrospinal fluid loss. Eye, Ear, Nose, Throat Mon., *50:* 436–439, 1971.
17. Rosomoff, H. L., Carroll, F., Brown, J., and Sheptak, P. Percutaneous radiofrequency cervical cordotomy; technique. J. Neurosurg., *23:* 639–644, 1965.
18. Rosomoff, H. L. Bilateral percutaneous cervical radiofrequency cordotomy. J. Neurosurg., *31:* 41–46, 1969.
19. Rosomoff, H. L., Kriger, A. J., and Kupman, A. S. Effects of percutaneous cervical cordotomy on pulmonary function. J. Neurosurg., *31:* 620–627, 1969.

20. Schwartz, H. High cervical cordotomy–technique and results. Clin. Neurosurg., *8:* 282–293, 1962.
21. Sweet, W. H. Percutaneous differential thermal rhizotomy for the management of facial pain. Presented to the German Neurosurgical Society, Heidelberg, Germany, May 1975.
22. Sweet, W. H., and Wepsic, J. G. Relation of fiber size in trigeminal posterior root to conduction of impulses for pain and touch; production of analgesia in the effective treatment of trigeminal neuralgia. Trans. Am. Neurol. Assoc., *95:* 134–139, 1970.
23. Sweet, W. H., and Wepsic, J. G. Controlled thermocoagulation of trigeminal ganglion and rootlets for differential destruction of pain fibers. I. Trigeminal Neuralgia. J. Neurosurg., *40:* 143–156, 1974.
24. Tasker, R. R., and Organ, L. W. Percutaneous cordotomy; physiological identification of target site. Confin. Neurol., *35:* 110–117, 1973.
25. Tasker, R. R., Organ, L. W., and Smith, K. C. Physiological guidelines for the localization of lesions by percutaneous cordotomy. Acta Neurochir. (Wien)., *210:* 111–117, 1974.
26. Tew, J., and Mayfield, F. H. Trigeminal neuralgia: A new surgical approach. Laryngoscope., *83:* 1096–1101, 1973.
27. Thiry, S., and Hotermans, J. M. Traitment de la névalgie essentielle du trijume au par stéréotaxie et électrocoagulation partielle sélective du ganglion de Gasser. Expérience portant sur 365 cas traités entire 1950 et 1970. Neurochir., *20:* 56–60, 1974.
28. White, J. C., and Sweet, W. H. Pain and the Neurosurgeon; a forty year experience, 1000 pp. Charles C Thomas, Springfield, Ill., 1969.

CHAPTER

35

Complications of Surgery for Subdural Hematoma

GEORGE T. TINDALL, M.D., F.A.C.S., NETTLETON S. PAYNE II, M.D., AND MARK S. O'BRIEN, M.D.

INTRODUCTION

Several different neurosurgical procedures ranging from subdural taps to formal craniotomy are employed in the management of subdural hematoma in infants, children, and adults. Complications of these procedures are not uncommon and are often disabling to patients. In this chapter, the recognition, incidence, and management of complications following various neurosurgical procedures for subdural hematoma will be discussed.

PERCUTANEOUS TAP OF SUBDURAL HEMATOMA IN INFANTS

Acute and Subacute Subdural Hematoma

Subdural tap is probably not indicated in acute head injury because of the limited diagnostic and therapeutic value and the potential hazard of complications.

COMPLICATIONS

The subdural space may be obliterated by the softened and edematous brain, predisposing to laceration of the cortex during the tap. This may give rise to an iatrogenic subdural or intracerebral clot or create an epileptogenic focus (51). False aneurysm formation secondary to subdural taps has been described (50). Also, the needle may fail to enter a subdural accumulation of blood which may be located at a site away from the anterior fontanelle and thus give the physician an erroneous impression as to the diagnosis. In addition, even when the needle enters the hematoma, withdrawal of the clotted blood is not possible.

Chronic Subdural Hematoma

While contraindicated in acute craniocerebral trauma, the subdural tap is an excellent therapeutic procedure in chronic subdural hematoma of infancy. Indeed, when these cases are associated with marked elevations of intracranial pressure, a subdural tap provides an immediate decompression and can be lifesaving. In managing chronic subdural hematoma in infants and children, it is our belief that the reduction of pressure within the hematoma and not the fluid volume determines the quantity of subdural hematoma to remove during a subdural tap. Thus, pressure within these lesions is monitored and used as a guide to therapy. This method has been described in detail in a previous publication (66).

COMPLICATIONS

A notable lack of complications following subdural taps was recorded by McLaurin and associates (31, 40), Mealey (43), and Matson (33).

Although relatively rare, complications do occur and include:

1. Infection. While the possibility of introducing infection into the subdural space has long concerned neurosurgeons (33, 43, 63), a literature search (1, 5, 10, 11, 13–17, 22, 23, 25, 26, 31, 33, 37, 40, 42, 43, 46, 47, 50, 51, 53, 57–60, 63, 66) reveals only a single documented case in which infection of the subdural space followed subdural taps (58). This septic complication consisted of a subdural empyema which developed after needle puncture for drainage of a chronic subdural hematoma. Anderson (1) ascribed the difficulties he experienced with infection and wound healing in 14 of 104 patients who underwent craniotomy and removal of membranes to the trauma of multiple preoperative subdural taps.

2. Seizures. While epilepsy is frequently associated with subdural hematoma in infants and children, occurring in from 35 to 76% of cases (16, 21, 33, 43, 57, 60, 63), the information available in the literature regarding the incidence of seizures initiated by subdural taps is meager. Unintentional puncture and/or laceration of the cortex and leptomeninges has been described (1, 56, 58) and could create epileptogenic foci when repeated taps are performed, particularly in the absence of subdural fluid (23). Rabe and associates (51) reported one patient in whom intractable seizures developed following repeated subdural taps. Yashon and associates (66) described three children who did well following treatment for subdural hematoma but who subsequently died during or following a series of seizures. However, it is not clear from their report whether the seizures were related to the treatment.

3. Acute Deterioration from Brain Stem Hemorrhages. Several authors have cautioned against rapid decompression of subdural hematoma in children (10, 33, 37, 43, 58) because of the potential acute shifts of brain stem structures. Collins (10) described one case of acute deterioration following the removal of a large volume of subdural fluid with consequent shifting of the intracranial contents and brain stem hemorrhages. Similar cases have been reported also by Green (20) and Peet and Kahn (49).

4. Unintentional Ventricular Puncture. In the infant or child with head enlargement the differential diagnosis between obstructive hydrocephalus and subdural hematoma may be difficult to establish prior to subdural taps (1, 58). Salmon (58) reported two instances in which it was believed that the needle was in the subdural space, but a small amount of injected air revealed that a dilated ventricle had been entered. This error in diagnosis can be avoided by using computerized axial tomography (CAT scan) to determine ventricular size and by cautiously inserting the subdural needle only a few millimeters beyond the dural membrane. Verification of the location of the needle may be obtained after removal of several milliliters of fluid by injecting 2 ml. of air and obtaining brow-up skull x-rays.

5. Iatrogenic Subdural Hematoma. Iatrogenic subdural hematoma consequent to subdural taps has been reported by Herzberger and associates (23), Anderson (1), and Rock (56). In a series of 152 cases, Anderson cited 10 cases in whom a subdural hematoma was either caused by or enlarged as a result of subdural taps. He attributed this complication to unexpected laceration of a vessel in the vascularized subdural hematoma membrane.

If a vessel is unintentionally punctured during a subdural tap, the needle should be withdrawn a short distance but left in the subdural space so that it will drain the induced hematoma. The stylet should be replaced periodically to prevent clotting in the needle.

6. Traumatic Intracranial Aneurysm. This is a very rare complication. Overton and Calvin (50) reported a child who developed bilateral subdural hematomas following trauma. Multiple bilateral subdural taps were performed and on one occasion bright red blood dripped from the needle. Eventually, a craniotomy was done to excise the subdural membrane and at surgery a cortical laceration and traumatic aneurysm were discovered.

SHUNTING PROCEDURES FOR SUBDURAL HEMATOMA IN INFANTS AND CHILDREN

In our opinion, a subdural shunting procedure is indicated in those cases in whom subdural taps over 10 to 14 days fail to reduce and maintain the pressure within the subdural hematoma to a level of 100 mm. H_2O or below. Through a burr hole the dura mater and outer membrane are opened. A ventricular catheter is inserted into the subdural hematoma and connected to the proximal end of a very low pressure (5 to 10 mm. H_2O) Hakim valve. A single piece of silastic catheter is connected to the distal end of the valve and tunneled subcutaneously to the peritoneal cavity. If there are bilateral subdural collections, both sides are drained into a common peritoneal catheter with an appropriate "T" or "Y" connector. After 6 to 8 weeks a CAT scan and/or a cerebral angiogram are obtained and if the lesion has cleared, then the complete shunt system is removed.

Some authors (1, 63) have suggested that the status of the subdural membrane and the quantity and appearance of the subdural fluid as visualized through a burr hole should be considered in making the decision for shunting. Anderson (1) recommended that taps or a shunting procedure should be done when the membranes are relatively thin and translucent and subdural fluid is present and that craniotomy with removal of the constricting membranes should be performed if the membranes are thick and inelastic.

COMPLICATIONS

1. Infection. As shown in Table 35.1, the incidence of infection following shunting procedures for chronic subdural hematoma varies considerably among several reported series. The over-all incidence among all series listed is 9 (5.6%) of 160 cases.

Infection should be suspected when signs of neurological deterioration or increasing irritability develop, along with erythema, tenderness, or fluctuance along the shunt tubing. Frequently, spiking fever in an otherwise asymptomatic patient is the only indication of an infected shunt. Bacteriological confirmation of the infection can be obtained by percutaneous needle tap of the reservoir of the shunt device.

TABLE 35.1

Incidence of Infection Following Shunting for Subdural Hematoma

Author	Patients Shunted	Infection
Anderson (1)	24	5
Moyes, Moyes and associates (46, 47)	24	1
Collins (11)	26	1
Ransohoff (53)	8	1
Rock (56)	1	1
Shulman and Ransohoff (60)	11	0
Yashon and associates (66)	6	0
Meacham and associates (42)	2	0
Mealey (43)	20	0
Till (63)	34	0
Emory series	6	0
Total	160	9
Over-all incidence		5.6%

Strict adherence to aseptic technique is particularly important in shunting procedures. It is our policy to administer methicillin 25 mg. per kg. every 6 hours intravenously for 24 hours before and 48 hours after surgery.

2. *Migration of Shunt Tubing.* Displacement, or migration, of the shunt tubing has been reported by Shulman and Ransohoff (60), Moyes and associates (47), and Collins and Pucci (11). The latter authors have emphasized the importance of securing both ends of the shunt tubing in order to prevent this complication.

3. *Obstruction of the Shunt.* In order to manage the subdural collection effectively, the shunt should function from 4 to 8 weeks. Collins and Pucci (11) and Moyes and associates (47) recommended that the shunt system be removed once the hematoma has resolved. However, prior to completing drainage of the lesion the shunt may become kinked or blocked, thus requiring reoperation for replacement. The high protein content of the subdural fluid is believed to be a frequent cause of shunt obstruction. The use of a very low pressure valve (5 to 10 mm. H_2O) and a long smooth tube free from frequent connections and sharp bends should help reduce the chance of obstruction.

CRANIOTOMY AND MEMBRANECTOMY FOR SUBDURAL HEMATOMA IN INFANTS AND CHILDREN

As already mentioned, some neurosurgeons advocate craniotomy and membranectomy in infants in whom repeated subdural taps fail to resolve the hematoma and who have thick, inelastic membranes. There is divergence of opinion among pediatric neurosurgeons regarding the indications for removal of chronic subdural hematoma membranes in early life. As it has not been convincingly demonstrated that thickened subdural membranes either damage or restrict growth of the cerebral cortex, the present authors do not perform subdural membranectomy as a treatment for chronic subdural hematoma. However, it is not the purpose of this publication to evaluate the indications of the various modes of therapy but rather to focus attention on the complications that may accompany each form of treatment.

COMPLICATIONS

1. *Hypovolemic Shock.* During intracranial surgery in infants, meticulous hemostatis is essential as sudden losses of apparent small amounts of blood in these patients with a small total blood volume may be sufficient to precipitate a severe state of hypovolemic shock. Hypovolemic shock is not peculiar to subdural hematoma but may occur during any surgical procedure in infants. Guthkelch (21) experienced one death in 16 patients due to hemorrhage.

2. *Cortical Injury.* Transient minor cortical injury is not uncommon and probably accounted for the hyperactive deep tendon reflexes observed by Matson (33) in many infants postoperatively. The hyperreflexia usually clears in several days to a week. More serious complications have been noted and include acute subdural hematoma (51), acute cerebral edema, and meningocele (56). Till (63) believes that the greatest risk of membranectomy is cortical injury during removal of the inner membrane. When the inner membrane is firmly adhered to the cortical surface, vigorous attempts to remove it should be avoided.

3. *Infection.* Infection in most reported series has been no higher than in any other pediatric group that has undergone craniotomy, ranging from 1% (23) to 13% (1). Although lacking statistical documentation, Matson (33) believed the danger of infection was greater when the subdural hematoma was shunted rather than treated with craniotomy and membranectomy.

4. *Seizures.* This complication occurs relatively infrequently following membranectomy. Postoperative cortical irritation is related to the ease with which the subdural membrane may be separated from the cortical surface. In patients with densely adherent calcified subdural membranes, seizures usually occur when attempts at removal are made (39).

5. *Recurrence of the Subdural Hematoma.* Craniotomy and removal of the membrane often is performed as a definitive procedure and yet, depending on the series reviewed, recurrence of the hematoma occurs in from 10 to 100% of infants (Table 35.2). Craniotomy and membranectomy do not eliminate the hematoma in most cases who have large volumes of subdural fluid associated with significant craniocerebral disproportion (43). Procedures to tailor the dura and calvarium to conform to the brain have been recommended in these instances, but their value is unproven and they may add significant morbidity and mortality to the operative procedure (17, 33).

TWIST-DRILL DRAINAGE OF SUBDURAL HEMATOMAS

Rand and associates (52) described a twist-drill technique which can be used in a variety of situations including subdural hematoma drainage and brain tumor biopsy. After suitable aseptic preparation of the scalp, a 7/64-inch drill bit is used to make an opening in the skull, following which a #16 or #18 Cone ventricular needle is passed into the intracranial cavity.

Rand and associates (52) encountered complications in only 15 (0.18%) cases of the 1834 twist-drill procedures employed. Their complications are summarized in Table 35.3. There were two deaths both of which resulted from bleeding due to laceration of an intracranial artery. In their large series, the twist-drill technique was used for diagnosis and

TABLE 35.2
Recurrence of Subdural Hematoma in Infants Following Craniotomy and Membrane Removal

Series	No. of Sides Treated by Craniotomy	Percentage of Recurrence
Matson (33)	565	10
Collins and Pucci (11)	14	29
Rabe and associates (51)	40	50
Rock (56)	10	100

TABLE 35.3
Complications of Twist Drill Drainage of Subdural Hematomas, Rand and associates (52)

Complication	No. of Cases
Missed subdural or epidural hematoma	5
Intracerebral mistaken for subdural hematoma	3
Subdural empyema	2
Broken drill point	2
False positive	2
Penetration of saggital sinus	1
Total	15

treatment of 106 subdural hematomas of which 49 were chronic. In three of these 106 (2.8%) patients, the clot was missed with their technique.

The present authors have had only a limited experience with this technique in treating subdural hematoma. The complications of Rand and associates' large series have been described above and since the twist-drill procedure is similar in some respects to subdural taps for chronic hematomas in infants, it seems appropriate to assume that many of the complications following subdural taps already discussed would also apply to the technique of twist-drill drainage.

BURR HOLES, CRANIECTOMY AND CRANIOTOMY TREATMENT OF ACUTE, SUBACUTE AND CHRONIC SUBDURAL HEMATOMA

Operative procedures for subdural hematoma vary considerably among neurosurgeons. In general, the size of the cranial opening appears to depend upon whether or not the lesion is acute, subacute, or chronic, and whether clotted or liquid. Large cranial openings, *i.e.*, formal craniotomy or generous craniectomy are usually made and the bone flap often not replaced in acute and subacute subdural hematomas because in these conditions, the hematoma usually consists of solid clot and there may be varying degrees of cerebral contusion and edema. The purpose of the large skull opening is to permit a more thorough removal of the clots and also to provide postoperative decompression of the brain. Smaller skull openings, *i.e.*, either one or two burr holes or a small craniectomy, are adequate to treat the majority of chronic subdural hematomas because these lesions usually have liquefied and are easily drained.

COMPLICATIONS

1. Reaccumulation of Subdural Hematoma. This complication may result from failure to evacuate the hematoma completely; from continued oozing from the incised outer subdural membrane; or from fresh hemorrhage from a cortical vessel and/or a surface contusion. Perhaps the most common cause for recurrence in chronic subdural hematoma is slow and continued bleeding from the incised outer membrane, particularly when this structure is thick and well vascularized. Failure to evacuate the lesion completely through small cranial openings probably accounts for the majority of reaccumulations in subacute subdural hematomas, while diffuse lacerations and cortical contusion lead to further hematoma formation in the acute lesions.

The incidence of significant clinical reaccumulation varies considerably depending upon whether the hematoma is acute, subacute, or chronic; the type of surgical procedure used for removal; whether or not a drain was used postoperatively; and the degree of re-expansion of the brain following evacuation of the hematoma. The incidence of reaccumulation among several reported series is shown in Table 35.4.

Significant degrees of reaccumulation should be suspected whenever a patient either fails to improve clinically or improves and subsequently shows progressive neurological deterioration following surgery. The exceptional group includes many patients with acute subdural hematomas whose failure to improve following operation is due either to underlying brain contusion (29, 55, 62) or associated intracranial lesion such as an intracerebral hematoma (41). Other causes for deepening level of consciousness and the appearance or worsening of neurological signs such as electrolyte imbalance, infection, etc. should be investigated.

The diagnosis of reaccumulation of the subdural hematoma can be made with cerebral angiography. Interpretation of the angiogram may be difficult in that the brain frequently fails to expand completely following surgery. Usually, this avascular extracerebral space seen on the angiogram is smaller than the preoperative subdural hematoma (24). If the postoperative avascular space is as large, or larger than the preoperative lesion, then it may be assumed that a significant reaccumulation is responsible for the patient's adverse change.

The diagnosis of reaccumulation of subdural hematoma following surgery can also be established with the tantalum dust technique (65). In this method, tantalum in the form of fine particles is placed on the

TABLE 35.4
Reaccumulation of Subdural Hematoma Following Treatment by Burr Holes, Craniectomy, and Craniotomy

Age of Hematoma	Series	Treatment	No. of Patients	Reaccumulation
				%
Acute subdural hematoma	McLaurin and Tutor (41)	Craniotomy	34	27
	Richards and Hoff (55)	Craniotomy	100	61
	Hoff and associates (24)	Craniotomy	10	10
	Hoff and associates (24)	Burr holes	11	45
Chronic subdural hematoma	Svien and Gelety (61)	Craniotomy	19	37
	Svien and Gelety (61)	Burr holes	50	20
	Raskind and associates (54)	Burr holes	25	12
	Vieth and associates (65)	Burr holes	38	8
Combined series of acute, subacute and chronic subdural hematoma	Jamieson and Yelland (29)	Burr holes, craniectomy, craniotomy	553	13.5

exposed cerebral cortex and several metal clips are applied to the incised dural edge. Postoperatively, stereoscopic skull x-rays are taken and the size of the subdural space estimated from the separation between the clips and the tantalum particles. Studies have established that tantalum is a relatively inert element in contact with cerebral tissue (65).

Ultimately, CAT scan may provide more information regarding the nature of a fluid accumulation than cerebral angiography or tantalum dust, as the ability of this diagnostic instrument to distinguish between the density of blood and cerebrospinal fluid should allow differentiation between reaccumulation of the subdural hematoma and failure of cerebral re-expansion. A disadvantage of the CAT scan is that a chronic subdural hematoma may have the same density as normal brain and thus may not be demonstrated. In addition, it is necessary for the patient to remain motionless during the procedure in order to obtain an adequate study. Experience with the CAT scan in postoperative reaccumulation of subdural hematoma has not been sufficient to define the exact role of this diagnostic test in the investigation of these patients.

The management of this complication consists of reoperation to evacuate the hematoma. Upon opening the wound, a careful search is made for bleeding points on the cortical surface and along the cut edges of both the dura and the outer membrane. In these cases it is probably best to place drains in the subdural space following reoperation (28, 32).

2. *Infection.* Infection can occur following any type of surgical procedure for subdural hematoma. Fortunately, the reported incidence following burr holes, craniectomy and/or craniotomy is low, usually below 5%. There is relatively little information available regarding the nature of the microorganisms involved; however, staphylococci and streptococci appear to be the most common offenders. Infrequently, involvement by gram negative, microaerophilic and/or anaerobic organisms occurs. Postoperative septic complications include superficial cellulitis, osteomyelitis, epidural abscess, cortical vein thrombosis, meningitis, brain abscess, or a combination of any of these processes.

Out of a total of 69 operated cases for chronic subdural hematoma, Svien and Gelety (61) encountered postoperative wound infection in three cases, all of whom had undergone reoperation for reaccumulation of the hematoma. Vieth and associates (65) reported an infection rate of 4% in 70 cases of subdural hematoma. One of their patients developed a subdural empyema following evacuation of a chronic subdural hematoma. The lesion drained for 6 weeks during which time all cultures were negative. Their two other cases were extradural infections which necessitated removal of the bone flap in each instance. Raskind and associates (54) had a 4% incidence of superficial wound infections in their series of 52 patients with chronic subdural hematoma.

Septic complications following surgery for subdural hematoma can usually be recognized from clinical findings. Patients commonly exhibit temperature elevations (usually 100–102° F) postoperatively, and inspection of the wound reveals varying degrees of cellulitis and drainage from the wound, particularly when the infection is relatively superficial. Patients with epidural or subdural empyema or cortical vein thrombosis may exhibit focal neurological signs, seizures, and impairment in the level of consciousness in addition to a febrile response.

CAT scan and cerebral angiography are beneficial in the diagnosis of septic complications producing mass effect, *e.g.*, epidural or subdural empyema, intracerebral abscess, etc. Interpretation of the angiograms may be difficult because normally there may be a persistent space due to failure of the brain to re-expand after the initial drainage and also, striking clinical findings frequently result from a small empyema collection.

Both aerobic and anaerobic bacterial cultures should be taken in all cases and antibiotic sensitivities determined in order to administer appropriate therapy. After obtaining material (wound swab, purulent drainage, etc.) for bacteriological cultures and sensitivities, the patient is started on intravenous penicillin, 5 million units every 6 hours and chloramphenicol 2 gm. every 6 hours. When the specific microorganism and its sensitivity are determined, the patient can be placed on the appropriate antibiotic(s). Hot compresses and antibiotic treatment are used to treat superficial cellulitis and early suspected osteomyelitis. In cases with frank purulent drainage and cellulitis in whom craniotomy has been performed, additional treatment consists of surgical removal of the bone flap. The wound is irrigated with a topical antibiotic solution such as bacitracin; drained at two or three sites, the galea aponeurotica closed with absorbable sutures, and the skin reapproximated with either monofilament wire or synthetic suture.

3. Cerebral Edema. The compressive effect of subdural hematoma upon the cerebral hemisphere may cause ipsilateral swelling, or edema, of the white matter (3, 8, 12). This pathological change has been attributed to interference with venous drainage caused by the pressure of the extracerebral mass (2).

Whether or not the occurrence of cerebral edema should be considered as part of the natural course of subdural hematoma or a complication of surgery is not always clear. In instances where the surgery fails to evacuate the subdural hematoma adequately, or when there is a significant postoperative reaccumulation, the hematoma itself may be responsible for cerebral edema. Certainly, if pre-existing cerebral edema is made worse and becomes apparent clinically, then it should be considered as a complication of the surgery.

The following case illustrates an example of cerebral edema associated with subdural hematoma:

A 53-year-old female chronic alcoholic was admitted to Grady Memorial Hospital on May 8, 1975, following a fall down a flight of concrete stairs. Initially, she was not unconscious and upon arrival in the emergency ward showed only mild lethargy. Skull x-rays revealed a linear right temporoparietal skull fracture. Shortly after admission the patient developed a left hemiparesis and coma. Five hundred milliliters of 20% mannitol were administered rapidly. Cerebral angiography revealed a left subdural collection with a 1.2-cm. midline shift to the right. The patient underwent a left temporal crainectomy and a large subdural hematoma was evacuated. The underlying cerebral cortex was unremarkable in appearance. Postoperatively, the patient improved as evidenced by regression of the hemiparesis and improvement in her level of consciousness. However, on the 2nd postoperative day the patient's neurological picture rapidly deteriorated into Grade 4 coma with right-sided decerebrate posturing. Repeat angiography revealed a swollen left cerebral hemisphere most marked in the area of the temporal lobe. Reoperation revealed diffuse swelling of the ipsilateral hemisphere with no evidence of recurrent subdural or intracerebral hematoma. A left temporal lobectomy was carried out and postoperatively the patient's level of consciousness improved. A ventricular catheter attached to a Rickham reservoir was placed in the frontal horn of the right lateral ventricle and intracranial pressure (ICP) monitored for 48 hours postoperatively. ICP remained normal over the period of measurement. Over the next 3 weeks the patient gradually improved and she was discharged ambulatory 6 weeks after admission with a mild right spastic hemiparesis.

As no significant reaccumulation of blood was found at reoperation, it is believed that the adverse postoperative clinical picture was a result of the marked cerebral edema which developed subsequent to the initial operative procedure.

Two of the 30 cases showing postoperative deterioration in McKissock and associates' (35) series had cerebral edema at autopsy. These patients were initially improved by surgery but later deteriorated and died. Although several authors (45, 52) have discussed the occurrence of cerebral edema in association with subdural hematomas, the majority do not distinguish between the edema created by the trauma itself and that which may be secondary to the subdural hematoma. McLaurin and Tutor (41) believe that postoperative symptoms indicating possible reaccumulation of subdural hematoma may indeed be related to progression of cerebral swelling beneath a hematoma which was not completely removed.

Recognition of cerebral edema as a major postoperative complication requires that the physician exclude other causes for deterioration of a patient's condition such as reaccumulation of the hematoma, infection, serum and electrolyte abnormalities, etc. The presence and extent of cerebral edema can be determined by CAT scan. If the CAT scan shows an area of decreased density compatible with cerebral edema, then appropriate therapy should be instituted.

Dexamethasone (Decadron, E. Lilly, Indianapolis, Ind.) 10 mg. administered parenterally every 6 hours and furosemide (Lasix, Hoechst

Pharmaceutical Co., Cincinnati, Ohio) 40 mg. administered in a single intravenous bolus may be given concomitantly with 20% mannitol solution administered intravenously in a dose of 1 to 1.5 gm. per kg. of body weight over a 1- to 2-hour period. ICP monitoring may serve as a useful adjunct to determine the effectiveness of the treatment.

4. Seizures. This complication is relatively rare and even when seizures become manifest for the first time during the postoperative period, there is always the probability that the associated brain injury incurred at the time of trauma is responsible for the disorder. In 389 operative cases of subdural hematoma, McKissock and associates (35) observed that 18 patients deteriorated with status epilepticus and eight patients in this group died.

5. Hydrocephalus. Hydrocephalus following surgical treatment of subdural hematoma has been reported by several authors (3, 24, 44, 45, 54). While hydrocephalus frequently accompanies subdural hematoma it has been found in patients both with and without surgery, and there is little evidence in the literature to support the contention that it is a direct complication of the surgery performed to treat the lesion.

Hydrocephalus should be considered in the differential diagnosis of patients who fail to improve or who deteriorate following surgery, particularly when this adverse change develops several days or weeks after operation. The diagnosis of enlarged ventricles can be made by cerebral angiography or CAT scan, and the presence of a CSF absorptive defect may be established by isotope cisternography.

When the diagnosis is clearly established, treatment consists of placement of a ventriculoperitoneal or ventriculoatrial shunt.

6. Failure to Recognize and Treat Associated Lesions of Clinical Significance. In the course of surgically managing patients with subdural hematoma, other clinically significant intracranial lesions due to the trauma may not be recognized and thus, not be appropriately treated. Failure to respond favorably or deterioration postoperatively may occur as a result of the missed lesion. Postoperative deterioration occurred in 30 of the 389 operative cases reported by McKissock and associates (32). Deterioration was more common in cases with acute and subacute hematomas, and in these cases the adverse change was most commonly associated with intracerebral hematomas, the latter occurring in 14 cases of their series. The importance of searching for associated lesions that may require surgery also is emphasized by the study of Jamieson and Yelland (29). These workers reported a series of 553 patients with subdural hematomas, and in 134 of these patients an associated intracranial lesion that warranted surgery was present. These associated lesions included 76 extradural and 73 intracerebral hematomas.

Rupture of cortical vessels may occur with head injuries that produce acute subdural hematomas (27, 34). Moreover, subdural hematomas may harbor a false cortical aneurysm (6, 18, 50) which would be missed if exploratory burr holes were carried out instead of angiography.

Other disease processes including blood dyscrasias (30) and meningeal carcinomatosis (7) may present with subdural hematoma and may not be recognized at the time of surgery. The use of diagnostic techniques including CAT scan, cerebral angiography, and histological examination of subdural hematoma membranes will reduce the incidence of associated lesions which otherwise may be overlooked in the surgical management of subdural hematoma.

7. Associated Serum and Electrolyte Abnormalities. The metabolic response to neurosurgical stress includes retention of both sodium and water and negative nitrogen balance (38). These same phenomena may accompany a variety of types of head injuries including subdural hematoma (9, 36, 64) and predispose to serious postoperative complications. Indiscriminate administration of low sodium parenteral fluid in the postoperative period may lead to water intoxication, a syndrome which may be clinically indistinguishable from recurrent subdural hematoma. Careful monitoring of serum and urinary sodium, and serum and urinary osmolality will allow early identification of dilutional hyponatremia and appropriate sodium administration (48).

The inappropriate secretion of antidiuretic hormone (ADH) (4) may complicate surgery for subdural hematoma. This syndrome may be recognized by the low serum sodium (less than 130 mEq. per liter) and osmolality (less than 380 mOsm. per liter), with an elevated urinary sodium (25 mEq. per liter or greater) and a urine osmolality greater than that of the serum. Clinically, the patient is confused and lethargic and may develop seizures. In such cases it is necessary to exclude a recurrent subdural hematoma with angiography or CAT scan, as both inappropriate ADH secretion and recurrent hematoma may develop concomitantly. Treatment of the former syndrome consists of water restriction to as little as 600 ml. per 24 hours. Occasionally, it may be necessary to administer hypertonic (3 or 5%) sodium chloride. The latter form of therapy is of doubtful value as the total extracellular sodium is normal and most of the additional sodium is excreted in the urine.

Dehydration with hypertonicity of serum and urine, and increased serum sodium may occur with inadequate fluid replacement following surgery for subdural hematoma (9, 48). This is particularly common in infants where subdural taps have been repeated at frequent intervals. It is important to periodically measure fluid intake and output as well as bodyweight in these patients postoperatively. Insensible loss must be estimated and replaced, particularly in the presence of fever, tachypnea, or tracheostomy to prevent dehydration. Diabetes insipidus may follow acute head injury leading to dehydration, but it is a very rare complication following surgery for subdural hematoma.

Removal of a chronic subdural hematoma may be complicated by inadequate wound healing in patients with serum protein depletion. Often these individuals are poorly nourished and have marginal hepatic function. Albumin replacement and rapid return to an adequate nutritional status is mandatory in these patients. In infants, repeated taps for chronic subdural hematoma may dangerously lower serum protein. We believe that the development of iatrogenic hypoproteinemia is an indication for subdural peritoneal shunting.

Disseminated intravascular coagulation has been described in severe acute head injury (19) but has not been a problem in subdural hematoma surgery unless the patient has developed shock during or as a result of the operative procedure. Thus, while this is not a complication unique to subdural hematoma surgery, it may develop in the massively brain-injured patient, the chronically dehydrated patient, and/or an individual with excessive blood loss and inadequate volume replacement.

SUMMARY

In this report we have discussed the complications of surgery for subdural hematoma. The complications are varied and many depend primarily on the type of treatment required by the patient. We have considered the problems associated with: percutaneous tap in infants, subdural shunts in infants and children, craniotomy for membranectomy, twist-drill drainage, and burr holes, craneictomy, and/or craniotomy. Infection, epilepsy, and reaccumulation of the subdural hematoma are common to all forms of therapy, while other complications are related to the specific form of subdural hematoma treatment. In addition, significant serum and electrolyte abnormalities which may occur as a consequence of subdural hematoma surgery have been reviewed. In general, the over-all complication rate of surgery for subdural hematoma is low in relationship to the morbidity and mortality associated with this lesion. Because of the frequency of subdural hematoma, the neurosurgeon should be ever vigilant in the prevention, recognition, and management of these complications.

REFERENCES

1. Anderson, F. M. Treatment of subdural hematoma in infants. Bull. Los Angeles Neurol. Soc., *38:* 103–109, 1973.
2. Aronson, S. M., and Kaplan, H. A. Pathogenesis of cerebral lesions resulting from contact trauma to the head. Bull. N.Y. Acad. Med., *33:* 450–452, 1957.

3. Aronson, S. M., and Okazaki, H. A study of some factors modifying response of cerebral tissue to subdural hematoma. J. Neurosurg., *20:* 89–93, 1963.
4. Bartter, F. C., and Schwartz, W. B. The syndrome of inappropriate secretion of antidiuretic hormone. Am. J. Med., *42:* 790–806, 1967.
5. Benstead, J. G. Infantile subdural hematoma. Br. Med. J., *3:* 114–115, 1971.
6. Bergstron, K., and Hemmingsson, A. False cortical aneurysms in subdural hematoma following head injury without fracture. Acta Radiol. (Diagn.) (Stockh.), *14:* 657–661, 1973.
7. Braun, E. M., Burger, L. J., and Schlong, H. A. Subdural hematoma from metastatic malignant disease. Cancer, *32:* 1370–1373, 1973.
8. Browder, J., and Rabiner, A. M. Regional swelling of the brain in subdural hematoma. Ann. Surg., *134:* 369–375, 1951.
9. Clark, K. Seminar on the management of head injuries. Emergency treatment considerations. Fluid & electrolyte management in head injury. Ariz. Med., *25:* 149–156, 1968.
10. Collins, W. F. Subdural hematoma of infancy. Clin. Neurosurg., *15:* 394–404, 1968.
11. Collins, W. F., and Pucci, G. L. Peritoneal drainage of subdural hematoma in infants. J. Pediatr., *58:* 482–485, 1961.
12. Cook, A. W., Browder, E. J., and Carter, W. B. Cerebral swelling and ventricular alterations following evacuation of intracranial extracerebral hematoma. J. Neurosurg., *19:* 419–423, 1962.
13. Coonrod, J. D., and Dans, P. E. Subdural empyema. Am. J. Med., *53:* 85–91, 1972.
14. Farmer, T. W., and Wise, G. R. Subdural empyema in infants, children, and adults. Neurology (Minneap.), *23:* 254–261, 1973.
15. Faulhauer, K., Herrmann, H. D., and Loew, F. Operative treatment of extremely large bilateral subdural effusions in infancy. Acta Neurochir. (Wien), *28:* 179–187, 1973.
16. Forman, P. M., Chipps, B. E., and Meyer, G. A. Managing chronic subdural hematomas and effusions in infants: a continuing dilemma. Tex. Med. *70:* 62–66, 1974.
17. Gjerris, F., and Schmidt, K. Chronic subdural hematoma. Surgery or mannitol treatment. J. Neurosurg., *40:* 639–642, 1974.
18. Go, K. G., Penning, L., and Oen, T. S. Acute subdural hematoma in connection with angiographically demonstrated traumatic rupture of a cortical cerebral artery (presenting as a false cortical aneurysm); a report of 2 cases. Neuroradiology, *2:* 107–110, 1971.
19. Goodnight, S. H., Kenoyer, G., Rapaport, S. I., Patch, M. J., Lee, J. A., and Kurze, T. Defibrination after brain-tissue destruction. A serious complication of head injury. N. Engl. J. Med., *290:* 1043–1047, 1974.
20. Green, R. M. Intracranial hemorrhage in the newborn. Boston Med. Surg. J., *170:* 682–686, 1914.
21. Guthkelch, A. N. Subdural effusions in infancy; 24 cases. Br. Med. J., *1:* 233–239, 1953.
22. Hendrick, E. B. Subdural hematoma in children. Presented at the Fifth Annual Neurosurgery Postgraduate Course, University of California, San Francisco, May 1975.
23. Herzberger, E., Rotem, Y., and Braham, J. Remarks on 33 cases of subdural effusion in infancy. Arch. Dis. Child., *31:* 44–50, 1956.
24. Hoff, J., Grollmus, J., Barnes, B., and Margolis, M. T. Clinical, arteriographic, and cisternographic observations after removal of acute subdual hematoma. J. Neurosurg., *43:* 27–31, 1975.
25. Ingraham, F. D., and Matson, D. D. Subdural hematoma in infancy. J. Pediatr., *24:* 1–37, 1944.

26. Ingraham, F. D., and Matson, D. D. Subdural hematoma. *In* Neurosurgery of Infancy and Childhood, Ed. 1, pp. 186–200. C. C Thomas, Springfield, Ill. 1954.
27. Ito, J., Ueki, K., and Ishikawa, H. Angiographic extravasation of contrast medium in acute traumatic subdural hematoma from arterial rupture. Case report. J. Neurosurg., *37:* 226–228, 1972.
28. Jackson, F. E., and Pratt, R. A. A silicone rubber suction drain for drainage of subdural hematomas. Surgery, *70:* 578–579, 1971.
29. Jamieson, K. G., and Yelland, J. D. N. Surgically treated traumatic subdural hematomas. J. Neurosurg., *37:* 137–149, 1972.
30. Látr, I., Parızek, J., Cernoch, Z., et al. Hemophilia discovered in the course of treatment of post-traumatic subdural hematoma. Sb. Ved. Pr. Lek. Fak. Karlovy Univ. *16:* 319–322, 1973.
31. LeBeau, J., Croissard, P., Harispe, L., and Redondo, A. Surgical treatment of brain abscess and subdural empyema. J. Neurosurg., *38:* 198–203, 1973.
32. Matricali, B. Subdural suction drainage of hematomas. Surg. Neurol., *3:* 245–246, 1975.
33. Matson, D. D. Subdural hematoma. *In* Neurosurgery of Infancy and Childhood. Ed. 2, pp. 328–347. Charles C Thomas, Springfield, Ill., 1969.
34. Miyazaki, Y., Takayama, H., and Ando, H. Acute exacerbation in the case of chronic subdural hematoma due to arterial bleeding from communicating vascular stalk. Brain Nerve (Tokyo), *25:* 1349–1356, 1973.
35. McKissock, W., Richardson, A., and Bloom, W. H. Subdural hematoma: a review of 389 cases. Lancet, *1:* 1365–1369, 1960.
36. McLaurin, R. L. Metabolic changes accompanying head injury. Clin. Neurosurg., *12:* 143–160, 1966.
37. McLaurin, R. L., Isaacs, E., and Lewis, H. P. Results of nonoperative treatment in 15 cases of infantile subdural hematoma. J. Neurosurg., *34:* 753–759, 1971.
38. McLaurin, R. L., King, L. R., Knowles, H. Jr., and Elam, E. B. Water intoxication following intracranial surgery. Neurology (Minneap.), *11:* 630–638, 1961.
39. McLaurin, R. L., and McLaurin, K. S. Calcified subdural hematoma in childhood. J. Neurosurg., *24:* 648–655, 1966.
40. McLaurin, R. L., and Timperman, A. Management of post-traumatic subdural hematoma in infancy. Clin. Neurosurg., *19:* 271–280, 1972.
41. McLaurin, R. L., and Tutor, F. T. Acute subdural hematoma. Review of ninety cases. J. Neurosurg., *18:* 61–67, 1961.
42. Meacham, W. F., and McPherson, W. F. The diagnosis and treatment of subdural fluid collections in infants. Pediatr. Clin. North Am., *17:* 363–372, 1970.
43. Mealey, J., Jr. Infantile subdural hematomas. Pediatr. Clin. North Amer., *22:* 433–442, 1975.
44. Meredith, J. M., and Rinaldi, I. Obstructive internal hydrocephalus following operative removal of chronic subdural hematoma in infants. Report of two cases. J. Neurosurg., *18:* 19–26, 1961.
45. Morantz, R. A., Abad, R. M., George, A. E., and Rovit, R. L. Hemicraniectomy for acute extracerebral hematoma: an analysis of clinical and radiographic findings. J. Neurosurg., *39:* 622–628, 1973.
46. Moyes, P. D. Subdural effusions in infants. Can. Med. Assoc. J., *100:* 231–234, 1969.
47. Moyes, P. D., Thompson, G. B., and Cluff, J. W. Subdural peritoneal shunts in the treatment of subdural effusions in infants. J. Neurosurg., *23:* 584–587, 1965.
48. Parent, A. D., Meyer, G. A., and Tindall, G. T. The clinical laboratory in the investigation of patients with head injury. South. Med. J., *66:* 579–585, 1973.

49. Peet, M., and Kahn, E. Subdural hematoma in infants. J.A.M.A., *98:* 1851–1856, 1932.
50. Overton, M. C. III, and Calvin, T. H., Jr. Iatrogenic cerebral cortical aneurysm. Case report. J. Neurosurg., *24:* 672–675, 1966.
51. Rabe, E. F., Flynn, R. E., and Dodge, P. R. Subdural collections of fluid in infants and children. A study of 62 patients with special reference to factors influencing prognosis and the efficacy of various forms of therapy. Neurology (Minneap.), *18:* 559–570, 1968.
52. Rand, B. O., Ward, A. A., and White I. E., Jr. The use of the twist drill to evaluate head trauma. J. Neurosurg., *25:* 410–415, 1966.
53. Ransohoff, J. Chronic subdural hematomas treated by subdural-pleural shunt. Pediatrics, *20:* 561–564, 1957.
54. Raskind, R., Glover, M. B., and Weiss, S. R. Chronic subdural hematoma in the elderly; a challenge in the diagnosis and treatment. J. Am. Geriatr. Soc., *20:* 330–334, 1972.
55. Richards, T., and Hoff, J. Factors affecting survival from acute subdural hematoma. Surgery, *75:* 253–258, 1974.
56. Rock, D. A. Subdural effusion and hematoma in infants. J. Maine Med. Assoc., *63:* 35–36, 1972.
57. Russel, P. A. Subdural hematoma in infancy. Br. Med. J., *2:* 446–448, 1965.
58. Salmon, J. H. Subdural hematoma in infancy; suggestions for diagnosis and management. Clin. Pediatr. (Phila.), *10:* 597–599, 1971.
59. Schurr, P. H. Subdural hematomas and effusions in infancy. Dev. Med. Child. Neurol., *11:* 108–111, 1969.
60. Shulman, K., and Ransohoff, J., Subdural hematomas in children; the fate of children with retained membranes. J. Neurosurg., *18:* 175–181, 1961.
61. Svien, H. J., and Gelety, J. E. On the surgical management of encapsulated subdural hematoma; a comparison of the results of membranectomy and simple evacuation. J. Neurosurg., *21:* 172–177, 1964.
62. Tallala, A., and Morin, M. A. Acute traumatic subdural hematoma; a review of 100 consecutive cases. J. Trauma, *11:* 771–777, 1971.
63. Till, K. Subdural hematoma and effusion in infancy. Br. Med. J., *3:* 400–402, 1968.
64. Tindall, G. T., Patton, J. M., Dunion, J. J., and O'Brien, M. S. Monitoring of patients with head injuries. Clin. Neurosurg., *22:* 332–363, 1974.
65. Vieth, R. G., Tindall, G. T., and Odom, G. L. The use of tantalum dust as an adjunct in the postoperative management of subdural hematoma. J. Neurosurg., *24:* 514–519, 1966.
66. Yashon, D., Jane, J. A., White, R. J., and Sugar, O. Traumatic subdural hematoma of infancy; long term follow-up of 92 patients. Arch. Neurol., *18:* 370–377, 1968.

CHAPTER

36

Pulmonary Complications in Neurosurgery

THOMAS B. DUCKER, M.D., F.A.C.S., AND JOSEPH S. REDDING, M.D., F.A.C.P.

DISEASE STATES

Neural Regulatory Dysfunction

With any significant intracranial pathology, there are areas of the brain where metabolic derangement occurs with inadequate oxygen utilization and acidosis. While this can be demonstrated most commonly in both experimental and clinical brain injury, it does occur with any major pathological process that affects the central nervous system. The resultant low tissue oxygen partial pressure and the accumulation of acid by-products are reflected in the cerebrospinal fluid (9, 25, 26). The major fraction of the cerebral spinal fluid acid is lactic; at the same time, there is a concomitant marked reduction in the bicarbonate ion (13). With the flow of cerebrospinal fluid through the 4th ventricle by the respiratory centers in the medulla, there is commonly a change in the neural regulatory drive of respiration. The acid milieu acting on these respiratory centers results in an increased respiratory minute volume. This is reflected initially in a more rapid rate of respiration, but not in an increased tidal volume. In fact, the tidal volume is commonly diminished. Decreased tidal volumes, absence of sighing and coughing, and immobility of the patient so the same areas of lung remain dependent for protracted periods, lead to small airway closure. The result is reduction of residual lung volume and shunting of pulmonary blood flow through extensive areas of unventilated or collapsed lung. Since carbon dioxide is far more diffusible than oxygen, the increased minute volume of ventilation lowers arterial CO_2 tension below normal by hyperventilation of the aereated portions of the lung. Oxygen being less diffusible, the resultant hypoxemia can not be compensated by hyperventilation. Consequently, cerebral acidosis that causes a change in cerebrospinal fluid can result in a respiratory alkalosis and low arterial oxygen levels (2, 7, 8, 24).

While the partial pressure of carbon dioxide is consistently low, the arterial oxygen may be only moderately depressed (12, 23, 25); but if the cerebral damage is associated with intracranial hypertension, then the arterial oxygen tension is likely to be more decreased (1). The systemic hypoxemia is due to pulmonary arteriovenous shunting, either by direct action of the effect of mass sympathetic discharge on the pulmonary vascular bed, or passively, as a consequence of changes in pulmonary blood flow resulting from small airway closure and uneven distribution of pulmonary gas.

While the clinical neurosurgeon most commonly notes these events in the dramatic setting of an acute head injury, the same pulmonary problems readily occur in other central nervous system disorders, such as subarachnoid hemorrhage, brain tumor, and cerebrovascular accident (8, 14, 26).

Mechanical Insufficiency

Mechanical insufficiency is by far the most common problem in central nervous system disease, and obtunded airway reflexes are the most common type of mechanical problem (19). While complete airway obstruction can be corrected immediately, the hazards of partial airway obstruction—that is, heavy snoring—are often overlooked. Partial airway obstruction is usually accompanied by copious saliva production. When these secretions stimulate the vocal cords of an obtunded patient, severe laryngospasm may result. Moderately severe partial obstruction may lead to air swallowing, gastric distension, and explosive vomiting. If the obstruction is so severe that the patient must labor forcefully during inspiration to pull in air, he may generate enough negative airway pressure to pull capillary and interstitial fluid into his alveoli and thus precipitate pulmonary edema.

Another type of mechanical insufficiency is that seen with muscle paralysis from trauma to the spinal cord or the phrenic nerve. Although the patient is usually left with adequate strength to breathe and maintain normal blood gases initially, he may not have enough reserve muscle strength to sigh, take deep breaths, and cough effectively. A monotonous respiratory pattern, unbroken by an occasional sigh or deep breath, will lead to diffuse microatelectasis of the lungs. The chest roentgenogram is normal in such instances, and the only manifestation is hypoxemia. If the patient cannot cough effectively, secretions will accumulate and obstruct small bronchioles. The unventilated areas of lung will subsequently develop macroatelectasis, and later pneumonia. These conditions may be predicted and prevented by measuring the patient's vital capacity upon admission. The vital capacity is an index of the ability to sigh and cough effectively. Awake patients can take their deepest breath and blow into a spirometer; obtunded patients should be intubated and the volume of a forceful cough determined. If the patient's vital capacity is less than 25% of his predicted normal, a mechanical ventilator should be utilized. Percussion of the chest, or pulmonary physiotherapy, is also needed. Even if there is neurological improvement, the vital capacity and respiratory function will improve in a week to 10 days. Initially, the intercostal spaces sink inward as the diaphragm descends during inspiration. As reflex intercostal muscle tone increases, this effect decreases and the patient is able to take deeper breaths and cough more effectively.

A very similar type of problem is seen in patients who have the muscular ability to sigh and cough effectively but who simply fail to do so. Commonly, this is seen in patients during protracted recovery from frontal lobe injuries and cerebrovascular accidents (19). Occasionally, this abnormal pattern is seen in trauma patients with very subtle changes in intracranial pressure (18). While these patients may be responsive to command, they are frequently totally disinterested in their surroundings and well being. The respiratory pattern is marked by a monotonously constant rate and depth of respiration, uninterrupted by sighing, deep breathing, or coughing. The result is diffuse microatelectasis and hypoxemia. Reduction of the intracranial pressure will reverse the abnormal respiratory pattern in some trauma patients. Hourly hyperinflation of the lungs using a self-inflating bag may help others. In the more severe cases, mechanical ventilation for 24 hours, followed by intermittent mandatory ventilation at a rate of two breaths per minute, is effective in preventing microatelectasis.

Acute Pulmonary Edema

In the last 10 years, the occurrence of pulmonary edema in association with central nervous system and multisystem trauma has received much attention. At least one variant of this syndrome appears to be neurogenic in origin: the acute fulminating type of pulmonary edema which may follow within minutes after a sudden rise of intracranial pressure (4). While there are cases where it has occurred in patients who did have a patent airway (endotracheal tube), it now appears that the combination of partial airway obstruction and increased intracranial pressure expedites the pathophysiological process (10). The partial airway obstruction causes labored breathing which, in turn, causes tremendous negative intrathoracic pressure. This pulls fluid out of the vascular bed into lung interstitial tissue and alveoli. At the same time, the increased intracranial pressure causes an increase in cardiac output and a rise in peripheral resistance (vasoconstriction) and engorgement of the pulmonary vascular bed (3, 5, 6). Elevation of pulmonary capillary pressure contributes to the occurrence of pulmonary edema (22). The two events, congested lung and the labored breathing, will cause an overwhelming pulmonary edema which, in many cases is fatal (4). Now that airway problems are quickly corrected, and many neurosurgical patients are treated with positive pressure hyperventilation, the incidence of acute "neurogenic" pulmonary edema has markedly diminished.

(Subacute) Respiratory Distress Syndrome

In addition to the acute form of pulmonary edema just mentioned, there is a less acute variation which is generally referred to as the respiratory distress syndrome of the adult or "shock lung" syndrome. This appears to follow a variety of multisystem traumatic injuries, particularly after hemorrhagic or septic shock has occurred. The etiology remains uncertain, but it has generally been considered a result of various direct influences on the pulmonary capillary endothelium. Certainly, an underventilated and contaminated pulmonary bed contributes to the presence of this pathological state. More recently, an attractive unifying theory has been proposed which blames central nervous system hypoxemia as the initial event (17). Once the central nervous system has been injured, the sympathetic nervous system reacts with constriction of small pulmonary venules as well as increased pulmonary vascular resistance. When the pulmonary venular constriction persists, interstitial pulmonary edema is created. Subsequently, there is increased permeability of the pulmonary capillaries with loss of albumin into the interstitial space, closure of small airways, loss of pulmonary compliance, and hypoxemia. A vicious cycle is set in motion which leads to progressive pulmonary edema and respiratory failure. Oxygen toxicity added to the current problem only further complicates the condition. The edematous lung is more susceptible to infection, and a superimposed pneumonia may obscure the diagnosis, as well as adding further pulmonary damage.

Pulmonary Toxic Reactions

Chemical and bacteria contamination commonly occur in the patient with significant central nervous system disease. It has been common knowledge since the work of Denney-Brown and Russel, in 1941, that in cerebral disorders gag and swallowing reflexes are impaired, and fluid runs freely into the unprotected trachea. Vomiting readily occurs, and the gastric contents may cause a severe inflammatory response in the lung, referred to as Mendelson's syndrome (15). With the acid gastric contents, a severe chemical pneumonitis occurs. In addition, focal atelectasis compounds the problem and accentuates the pulmonary inflammatory response. The damaged pulmonary bed interrupts gas exchange in the lung and can accentuate the existing pathology within the brain or spinal cord.

Bacterial pneumonia can also further complicate the course of a patient with significant neurological disease. In a patient with a depressed state of consciousness carefully treated in a hospital, the respiratory bacterial flora changes to an enteric bacillus, coagulase positive staphylococci, Candida species, *etc*. These pathogens have ready access to the pulmonary bed (21). If the patient's defenses are further lowered, and if the pulmonary bed becomes further congested, a severe infection readily occurs. While it is possible to keep a patient in an unconscious state with either an endotracheal tube or a tracheostomy in supportive ventilation for a prolonged period of time without infection, the slightest break in technique, or change in the patient's internal milieu will allow bacterial contamination which requires therapy.

PATIENT EVALUATION

In a patient with significant central nervous system disease, there are four essential questions to ask concerning that person's pulmonary function:

1. Are the neural mechanisms which insure respiratory drive and protective airway reflexes adequate?
2. Are there limitations in ventilatory function from others causes?
3. Are the patient's oxygen-carrying capacity, arterial oxygen tension, and cardiac output adequate for tissue oxygenation?
4. Are there superimposed chemical and bacterial toxins?

Neural Drive and Reflexes

First, count the respiratory rate and carefully observe the patient's chest and abdominal excursions, noting the pattern of respiration. It is important to realize that the normal person in a basal state has a respiratory rate as low as 12 to 14 breaths per minute. A rate above 20 is distinctly abnormal. Commonly, such patients have a high rate with a low volume exchange, resulting in alveolar hypoventilation. Even when the brain stem reflex drive to respiration maintains a normal rate and volume, it may have a distinctly abnormal pattern. Intermittent sighs, or deep breaths, may be completely absent. Without sighing, there is not intermittent full expansion of all the alveolar spaces, and ventilation/perfusion inequality readily occurs. A very slight change in intracranial pressure may be associated with the presence or absence of normal sighs in the respiratory pattern.

Sufficient neural reflexes to open and close the glottis and control the swallowing mechanism can be readily tested by the clinician. A simple, modified corneal reflex using the eyelash can give important information. This is referred to by anesthesiologists as the lash reflex, and involves the V and VII cranial nerves. If there is involuntary winking when the lash is brushed gently, the gag and swallowing reflexes commonly are also present. Patients with intact medullary reflexes are unlikely to accumulate secretions and gastric material in their pulmonary beds.

Pulmonary Function

The pulmonary function of the patient must be assessed. Pre-existing obstructive or restrictive problems are often present in the elderly patient prior to the onset of significant intracranial disease. In those patients who can cooperate, the measurement of vital capacity is the simplest and quickest way to ascertain ventilatory ability. An accurate and portable ventilometer (Wright respirometer) can be used for an approximation of this determination in intubated or tracheotomized patients. A timed vital capacity (TVC) is a recording of vital capacity as a function of time and can be measured with a portable McKesson Vitalor. The first second forced expiratory volume ($FEV_{1.0}$) is that volume which is recorded during the first second of the total forced expiratory volume measured from the maximal inspiratory position. By reference to standard nomograms calibrated for height and sex of the patient, the total vital capacity can be expressed as a percentage of predicted normal. Reduction of the observed vital capacity below 80% of the predicted normal indicates a restrictive defect of the lungs and/or thorax. Reduction of the $FEV_{1.0}$ below 75% of the *observed* vital capacity indicates existence of obstructive airway disease. Many patients exhibit a mixture of both components (20). Reduction of vital capacity below 25% of predicted normal, or reduction of $FEV_{1.0}$ below 40% of observed vital capacity, will result in ventilatory failure with hypercapnia usually compounded by hypoxemia (20).

The success of the lungs in oxygenation of blood is appreciated by serial measurements of the amount of intrapulmonary shunting. The standard formula which utilizes the relationship between pulmonary alveolar and systemic arterial oxygen tensions can be easily used for such determinations. An expanding gradient between alveolar and arterial oxygen tensions implies deteriorating pulmonary function.

Systemic Condition

The patient's hemoglobin value is just as important as the blood gas determination. While it is not advisable to have an excessively high hemoglobin in a patient with brain disease, it certainly is desirable to have a hemoglobin in the range of 12 gm.% in order to insure adequate oxygenation of the tissues (16).

The delivery of oxygen is, of course, influenced by the arterial blood gas tensions. But high inspired oxygen tensions can be dangerous and are not necessary if the hemoglobin level is normal, if the cerebral blood flow is adequate, and if alveolar ventilation is maintained. The common occurrence of cerebral metabolic acidosis with resultant systemic respiratory alkalosis and hypoxemia can often be corrected by giving the patient respiratory support utilizing tidal volumes of 12 to 15 ml./kg. body weight and frequent sigh volumes of 20 ml./kg., combined with frequent changes in the patient's position. These measures minimize small airway closure with reduced residual lung volume and the resultant hypoxemia. Thus, the respirator rate and volume need to be adjusted first to correct abnormal blood gases. Finally, the inhaled oxygen concentration should be adjusted to correct any hypoxemia which exists in spite of the foregoing measures. The success of long term ventilation (longer than 24 hours) in part depends on the type of ventilator selected and the diligence of the nursing personnel. A pressure guaranteed, volume variable ventilator such as the Bird is often inadequate for patients on long term support and those with abnormal lungs since atelectasis will occur even with large volumes. The gases are not distributed uniformly leading to progressive ventilation perfusion mismatching and hypoxemia. Volume guaranteed, pressure variable ventilators such as Engstrom or Emerson as a class have superior flow characteristics permitting more physiological gas distribution within the lungs. However, regardless of volume or class of ventilator used, long term ventilatory support will lead to progressive hypoxia unless chest physiotherapy is vigorous and unless aseptic technique is strictly adhered to.

Finally, the systemic condition is markedly altered by fat embolization. This can be concomitant with certain traumatic central nervous system disorders. The persistent hypoxemia that may occur even with ventilatory support needs to be corrected by increased inhaled oxygen concentrations. Use of glucocorticosteroids will reduce the inflammatory response associated with this phenomenon.

Chemical and Bacterial Toxins

Chemical and bacterial toxins need immediate and direct treatment. If these conditions are superimposed, the patient has two distinct diagnoses, not just one. The presence of chemical and bacterial toxic pneumonitis can be determined by physical findings, chest x-ray, and pulmonary cultures. These disease states alter the ventilation/perfusion ratio in the lung beds and result in arterial hypoxemia. On occasion, the pneumonitis may cause transient bacteremias and set up infections in devitalized brain to further complicate the course of the patient.

TREATMENT

Treatment of patients with pulmonary disorders secondary to nervous system disease cannot be meaningfully simplified. Initially, however, it is important to answer the five logical questions in the patient's evaluation in order to determine treatment. For example:

1. Must airway obstruction be corrected?
2. Does the patient require ventilatory support and protection against absent protective reflexes?
3. What measures are indicated to improve ventilatory function?
4. What measures will improve the systemic condition?
5. Is treatment of a chemical or bacterial pneumonitis indicated?

An adequate airway and respiratory drive are vital to survival. If airway insufficiency is allowed to continue without active support, respiratory and circulatory exhaustion occur. Severe airway obstruction is most reliably recognized by placing the hand over the nose and mouth and recognizing absent or diminished air flow. Partial airway obstruction is recognized by hearing a "snore" on inspiration or palpating it immediately above the larynx. If a patient is too obtunded to respond to command, he may aspirate if he regurgitates. Not infrequently, a patient will respond to command when stimulated but lapse into a deeper state of unconsciousness when he is left alone.

If the patient has an active lash reflex, a gag reflex, and responds purposeful to pain, he does not require intubation or tracheostomy. If these are not present, then the brain stem reflex centers are depressed, and the patient may readily aspirate and get a chemical pneumonitis. In such cases, either an endotracheal tube or a tracheostomy is required. Oral airways are basically worthless; instead, with transient sedation, a properly placed endotracheal tube will achieve good ventilatory support. Since irritation of the posterior pharynx may precipitate gagging and vomiting, an oral or nasal pharyngeal airway should be used only until a cuffed endotracheal tube is placed. The use of pharyngeal airways should be avoided in slightly unconscious patients because of the risk of vomiting. In these patients proper head and jaw position should be used to maintain airway patency until intubation. The anticipated duration of airway protection will influence the decision regarding use of a tracheostomy or prolonged intubation. Nasogastric intubation should be deferred until after the endotracheal tube is placed. The endotracheal tube cuff should be inflated until there is only a slight leak when the patient is sighed with an Ambu bag. This minimal leak technique should be used continuously until airway reflexes are intact. Humidification and warming of inspired gases, frequent aseptic suctioning of the trachea, and frequent change of the patient's position, and chest percussion, chest vibration, etc. will decrease the incidence of atelectasis followed by superimposed infection. If aspiration has occurred prior to intubation, methylprednisolone is administered in a dose of 250 mg. immediately and repeated every 6 hours for at least 2 days to reduce the inflammatory response. When wheezing is a problem, a bronchodilator such as an intravenous aminophylline drip can be considered. Bronchoscopy is necessary if the chest roentgenogram shows segmental or lobar atelectasis.

Once the patient has a protected airway, the respiratory pattern should be carefully observed. If there is the typical fast rate and low volume exchange. then the patient should be placed on a ventilator utilizing large tidal volumes and frequent sighs. In patients with constant unvarying tidal volumes, a respirator may be required to induce sighing and prevent microatelectasis. Improvement in the patient's clinical condition can be monitored by repeated pulmonary function measurements, such as TVC. If there are problems in obstructive disease or restrictive disease, they require appropriate care. To improve the patient's systemic condition, the most important determination is the hemoglobin concentration. The patient needs sufficient oxygen-carrying capacity to maintain adequate oxygenation of the tissues. Finally, any chemical or bacterial toxin needs direct treatment consisting of the use of steroids and/or specific antibiotics.

As recently pointed out, the syndrome of acute neurogenic pulmonary edema rarely occurs (10). The presence or absence of an adequate airway strongly influences its occurrence (11). When there is partial airway obstruction, tremendous intrathoracic negative pressure occurs. When there is increased intracranial pressure, the pulmonary bed is flooded (3, 6). The combination of events is probably necessary to cause the clinical syndrome. When it does occur, the patient should be intubated, ventilated with 100% O_2, and, if necessary, gradual increments of positive end expiratory pressure (PEEP). Such patients may require sedation so that they do not struggle on the respiratory, even when they are suctioned. If intracranial pressure is elevated, further treatment of the pulmonary edema should be continued during an immediate decompressive procedure. If pulmonary edema persists postoperatively, positive end expiratory pressure must be applied sparingly to minimize its effect on increasing intracranial pressure.

When the subacute respiratory distress syndrome of "shock lung" syndrome occurs, the patient most commonly has been in the hospital for

2 to 3 days. In many cases, the syndrome can be prevented by early, active pulmonary support. The diagnosis is made primarily on the basis of history, a latent period is followed by onset of respiratory alkalosis and a progressively more severe hypoxemia. Usually the presence of interstitial edema on the chest film is noted. Treatment is primarily supportive at this time. Mechanical ventilation with PEEP helps to prevent small airway closure and permits adequate oxygenation with nontoxic oxygen concentrations. An adequate level of PEEP prevents further deterioration and appears to reduce the amount of edema present. Fluid restriction, mild diuresis, and the osmotic activity of albumin help prevent the accumulation of interstitial pulmonary edema. It must be stressed that maintenance of a hemoglobin concentration greater than 12 gm. per cent is essential and helps assure adequate oxygen delivery to the brain and other vital tissues.

CONCLUSION

Hopefully, each neurosurgeon reading this chaper will remember all of it. In reality, that will not occur. Possibly it could be summed up in two ways. First, we are responsible for complete airway assessment. Secondly, aggressive pulmonary support is important for the patient with a serious neurosurgical disease.

Complete airway assessment includes appreciation of the lash reflex, the gag reflex, and purposeful motor response. A patient without these reflexes will develop airway and pulmonary difficulties.

Aggressive pulmonary support is best achieved by a cooperative effort by both anesthesia and neurosurgery. Early intubation is to be encouraged. Regulation of ventilation and maintenance of oxygen-carrying capacity and prevention of pulmonary toxic condition—all are important for the healing of diseased cerebral tissue in any postinjury or postoperative patient.

REFERENCES

1. Berman, I. R., Ducker, T. B., and Simmons, R. L. The effects of increased intracranial pressure upon the oxygenation of blood in dogs. J. Neurosurg., *30:* 532–536, 1969.
2. Brackett, C. E. *In* Head Injuries: Proceedings of an International Symposium on Respiratory Complications of Head Injury, p. 255–265. Williams & Wilkins Co., Baltimore, 1971.
3. Brashear, R. E., and Ross, J. C. Hemodynamic effects of elevated cerebrospinal fluid pressure: Alterations with adrenergic blockade. J. Clin. Invest., *49:* 1324–1333, 1970.
4. Ducker, T. B. Increased intracranial pressure and pulmonary edema, Part I, Clinical study of 11 patients. J. Neurosurg., *78:* 112–117, 1968.
5. Ducker, T. B., Simmons, R. L., and Anderson, R. W. Increased intracranial pressure and pulmonary edema. Part 3: The effects of increased intracranial pressure of cardiovascular hemodynamics of chimpanzees. J. Neurosurg., *29:* 475–483, 1968.
6. Ducker, T. B., Simmons, R. L., Anderson, R. W., and Kempe, L. G. Hemodynamic

cardiovascular response to raised intracranial pressure. Med. Ann. D.C., *37:* 523–525, 1968.

7. Froman, C. Alterations of respiratory function in patients with severe head injuries. Br. J. Anaesth., *40:* 354–360, 1968.
8. Froman, C., and Smith, A. C. Hyperventilation associated with low pH of the cerebrospinal fluid after intracranial hemorrhage. Lancet *1:* 780, 1966.
9. Gordon, E. Some correlations between the clinical outcome of the acid-base status of blood and cerebrospinal fluid in patients with traumatic brain injury. Act. Anaesthesiol. Scand., *15:* 209–228, 1971.
10. Graf, C. J. Pulmonary edema and the central nervous system: A clinico-pathological study. Surg. Neurol., *4:* 319–325, 1975.
11. Graf, C. J. and Rossi, N. P. Cardiovascular and pulmonary effect of increased intracranial pressure. Presented at American Association of Neurological Surgeons Annual Meeting, 1975.
12. Kaste, M., and Troupp, H. Effect of experimental brain injury on blood pressure, cerebral sinus pressure, cerebral venous oxygen tension, respiration, and acid-base balance. J. Neurosurg., *36:* 625–633, 1972.
13. Katsurada, K., Sugimoto, T., and Onju, Y. Significance of cerebrospinal fluid bicarbonate ions in the management of patients with cerebral injury. J. Trauma, *9:* 799–805, 1969.
14. Lassen, N. A. The luxury-perfusion syndrome and its possible relation to acute metabolic acidosis localized within the brain. Lancet, *2:* 1113–1115, 1966.
15. Mendolson, C. L. The aspiration of stomach contents into the lungs during obstetric anaesthesia. Am. J. Obstet. Gynecol., *52:* 191, 1946.
16. Mithoefer, J. O., Keighley, J. F., et al. Response of the arterial Po_2 to oxygen administration in chronic pulmonary dissease: Interpretation of findings in a study of 46 patients with 14 normal subjects. Ann. Intern. Med., **74:** 328–335, 1971.
17. Moss, G., Staunton, C., and Stein, A. A. Cerebral etiology of the "Shock Lung Syndrome". J. Trauma, *12:* 885–890, 1972.
18. North, J. B. and Jannett, S. Abnormal breathing patterns associated with acute brain damage. Arch. Neurol., *31:* 338–344, 1974.
19. Parham, A. M., Ducker, T. B., and Redding, J. S. Lung dysfunction in the presence of central nervous system disease, performed in the procedure of NIH conference on Neurotrauma, March 1975.
20. Redding, J. S., Yakaitis, R. W. Predicting need for ventilatory assistance. Md. State Med. J., *19:* 53–57, 1970.
21. Romig, D. A., Voth, D. W., Liu, Ch., and Brackett, C. E. Bacterial flora and infection in patients with brain injury. J. Neurosurg., **38:** 710–716, 1973.
22. Rudolph, A. M. Cardiac failure in children; a hemodynamic overview. Hosp. Prac., *5:* 44–47, 53–55, 1970.
23. Simmons, R. L., Martin, A. M., Heisterkamp. C. A., and Ducker, T. B. Respiratory insufficiency in combat casualties: II. Pulmonary edema following head injury. Ann. Surg., *170:*(1): 34–44, 1969.
24. Sinha, R. P., Ducker, T. B., Perot, P. L. Arterial oxygenation findings and its significance in central nervous system trauma patients. J. A. M. A., *224:* 1258–1269, 1973.
25. Zupping, R. Cerebral acid-base and gas metabolism in brain injury. J. Neurosurg., **33:** 448–505, 1970.
26. Zupping, R. Cerebral metabolism in patients with intracranial tumors. J. Neurosurg., *36:* 451–462, 1972.

CHAPTER

37

ICP Monitoring: Complications and Associated Factors

MICHAEL J. ROSNER, M.D., AND DONALD P. BECKER, M.D.

The neurosurgical patient may deteriorate with little provocation and less warning. One of the current techniques available to increase the degree of warning prior to this deterioration (and hopefully to avert it) is the use of intracranial pressure (ICP) monitoring in conjunction with monitoring of systemic parameters.

The inability to predict the course of the patient with increased ICP still remains profound and requires greater study of the pathophysiological relationships existing with neurological-neurosurgical disease. This requires intricate and often invasive monitoring techniques to observe an increasingly large number of complex parameters (17, 18, 21, 22, 37, 38).

The essential answer that the physician requires regarding each patient who may be a candidate for some form of monitoring is that of the risk attendant to monitoring as compared with the ultimate return. This return is complex: it may be expanded knowledge of the disease and only be useful to future patients on a long term basis; or it may be immediately beneficial to the patient. The answer to this question must come from each individual physician and his interaction with his unique environment and his patients. There is no *easy* answer to this question.

It is the premise of these investigators that a more thorough knowledge of the complications of monitoring techniques and the factors associated with, and contributing to these risks will help to minimize the dangers, and maximize the return, be it either greater knowledge or better patient management, and, ideally, both.

Most investigators have noted that the complication rate associated with a given procedure increases with the duration of the procedure. Grant noted the development of sterile meningitis when lumbar needles were left in place for as little as 36 hours (13). Ingraham and Campbell used silver ventriculostomy cannulae for constant drainage and intermittent pressure recording. Their only comments regarding infection were that septic complications were absent if drainage was discontinued within 72 hours; they make no reference to the risk of longer monitoring (16).

Poppen reported "well over 500 patients" who had undergone continuous ventricular drainage for up to 12 days " . . . without untoward effects." At the same time he acknowledged the 72-hour limit noted by previous investigators by saying that "rarely is it necessary to decompress the ventricular system for more than three days . . . " (28). Robinson in 1948 put forth the same basic ventricular drainage-monitoring system using a woven silk catheter. He felt that if monitoring should be continued for more than 72 hours, then the collection apparatus (but not the ventricular catheter) should be replaced with a sterile set (30). He failed to mention the risks inherent in the system, or why he felt it necessary that the container, but not the catheter, be changed.

In 1951 Bering reported a continuous drainage-monitoring system of similar design to the above techniques but included reference to three cases of ventriculitis that were secondary to the ventriculostomy. These developed on days 1, 5, and 6 of ventriculostomy drainage. More importantly, he reported several cases, as had others, that had been left on drainage for considerably longer periods of time without complication (3).

Lundberg in 1960 reported 130 patients who had been monitored with a ventricular catheter continuously for up to 8 weeks without serious complication due to the catheter. The majority (54%) of his patients had ICP monitoring for 4 to 14 days. In the original paper Lundberg firmly stated that there were no significant intracranial complications due to the monitoring techniques. Still, all of his patients were on prophylactic antibiotics, the wound was dusted with antibiotic powder, and regular cultures and cell counts of the CSF were taken. If a culture was reported as positive (as it was in 13 patients, or 10% of the sample) then the usual procedure was to remove the ventricular catheter. This was done five times as a result of the culture report. Presumably, the antibiotics which had been started as prophylaxis were not stopped in the face of a positive culture and the patient was treated as if he had an infected CSF. Lundberg further described two cases of craniotomy infection and two cases of postoperative intracranial sepsis. None of these did Lundberg attribute to the ICP monitor, nor did he consider the monitor as a contributing factor in the development of the complication (21).

In toto, Lundberg initially reported 13 cases of positive CSF culture, four cases of craniotomy wound infection or meningitis and six cases of fistulae that developed at the site of the ICP catheter (secondary to the rubber stopper left in the wound). Of 130 monitored cases, there was some type of complication in 23 instances, or 17% to 18% of the total series.

Since then, Sundbärg and associates have continued the Lund series to a total of 938 monitored patients. They report a rate of 1.1% for meningitis, suspected infection in another 3.5% and make no mention of total craniotomy infection rate, nor do they consider the presence or absence of a ventricular catheter as a contributing factor in wound infection (33). The Lund group have generally reported no association between the length of time that ventricular drainage was continued and rate of infection (21, 33). No mention was made of the role of steroids in the development of concurrent monitor complications.

Wright in his review of 2,148 craniotomies done at Massachusetts General Hospital found an over-all infection rate of about 5% (42). This is in the same range as Balch and others have reported (2). These series have generally dealt only with the so-called "clean" surgical case. Re-exploration of the surgical wound, external drainage, and lengthy operation have all been closely associated with operative sepsis. Wyler and Kelly reported that infection rate increased with increased time spent with ventriculostomy in place, and that prophylactic antibiotics significantly decrease the rate of eventual infection (from 27% to 9% after an analysis of 102 cases) and delayed the onset of the complication (43).

Other investigators have also suggested that prophylactic antibiotics are helpful in the face of an implanted foreign body, but details of the results and their role in ICP monitoring are far from clear. Lundberg placed all of his initial series of 130 patients on prophylaxis of some sort, so a clear analysis of their role in his low rate of infection is impossible (5, 9, 21, 27, 32, 42, 43). Sundbärg's report in 1972 acknowledged that many patients were placed on antibiotics for intercurrent infection, disclaims the use of *any* prophylactic antibiotics at all, and fails to analyze the series in terms of the antibiotics that were used and possible relation to infection (33). The question remains unanswered with regard to the role, the type and method of possible antibiotic usage prophylactically with invasive monitoring.

Table 37.1 is a partial list of the many reports and methodologies available in the last several decades for the monitoring of ICP. It also lists the number of each patient in each sample and the number and type of reported complications. There are two main points to be made from this data:

1. While the number of methodologies and reports is vast, the number of those who report any associated complication is a small part of the total.

2. Of those who do report associated complications, the rate of complication is relatively low (1, 3, 4, 6–8, 11, 12, 14–16, 19–25, 28–30, 33–37, 40).

From 1973 through July 1975 more than 250 patients have had ICP monitoring. Records of 112 of these were immediately available for study

TABLE 37.1
*Methodology and Complications of Monitoring and Measuring Intracranial Pressure**

Series	Year	Methodology	Number in series	Complications
Ingraham and Campbell	1941	Ventriculostomy	Not stated	None if drainage stopped by 72 hrs. No comment about rate with longer drainage
Poppen	1943	Ventriculostomy	"Over 500"	None
Robinson	1948	Ventriculostomy	Not stated	Not stated
Bering	1951	Ventriculostomy	26	Ventriculitis--3 cases
Lundberg	1960	Ventriculostomy	130	Wound fistula--6 Positive CSF cultures--15 Craniotomy infection--2 Intracranial infection--2
Hoppenstein	1965	Subdural balloon	Not stated	Not stated
Lundberg, et al	1965	Ventriculostomy	30	None
Rand et al	1966	Subdural twist drill taps	1834	Subdural hematoma--2 Subdural empyema--2 Broken drill bit--2
Atkinson et al	1967	Ventricular "transensor"	1	Not stated
Coe et al	1967	Subdural transducer	2	None
White et al	1969	Ventriculostomy	51	Ventriculitis--1 proven 7 possible
Kaufman and Clark	1970	Forehead frontal twist drill ventriculogram	20	None
Nornes and Serck-Hanssen	1970	Epidural transducer	11	Not stated
Nornes and Magnaes	1971	Epidural transducer	58	None
Brock and Diefenthäler	1972	Epi-or subdural telemeter	Not stated	Not stated
Gobiet et al	1972	Epidural transducer	45	Not stated
Tindall et al	1972	Subdural transducer	36	Not stated
Gobiet et al	1974	Epidural transducer	30	None
Sundbärg et al	1972	Ventriculostomy	938	Meningitis 1.1% Suspected infection--3.5% Mass lesion--1 case
Vander Ark and Stecher	1974	Ventriculostomy	Not stated	Not stated
Cohadon et al	1975	FET microprobes	Not stated	None
Handa et al	1975	Sub-and epidural transducer	Not stated	Not stated
Kindt	1975	Subdural stopcock	"Many"	None
Numoto and Donaghy	1975	Pressure indicating bag	5	None
Rongemont	1975	Epidural pressure chamber	300	Local infection--6 cases
Turner et al	1975	Epidural pressure chamber	16	Not stated

* Partial, but representative list; most investigations have not listed associated complications.

and are considered, for statistical purposes, as a randomly acquired group. They were reviewed in detail with respect to:

1. patient age at the time of admission;
2. principal-admitting diagnosis;
3. length of time monitored, inclusive of the day monitoring began and the day monitoring was discontinued;
4. method of monitoring: ventriculostomy, subarachnoid screw, or both;
5. length of time treated with steroids, inclusive of first and last days of treatment;
6. type of steroid;
7. length of hospitalization on neurosurgical service;
8. development of any cranial, intracranial, or monitor-related complication;
9. cerebral spinal fluid culture reports;
10. eventual outcome in terms of survival *vs.* death;
11. presence or absence of prophylactic antibiotics;
12. development of "early" *vs.* "late" complication.

Complications which were clearly related to the presence of an ICP monitor were categorized as such. A distinction was then made between those complications that were probably *not* due to the monitor, and the remainder of the patients were then placed in the category of "possibly monitor related."

TABLE 37.2
*Distribution by Diagnosis of Patients Monitored in Neurosugical Intensive Care Unit at Medical College of Virginia from mid-1973 to Early 1975**

Diagnosis	N	AGE		DAYS HOSPITALIZED		DAYS MONITORED		DAYS STEROIDS	
		X	S.E.M.	X	S.E.M.	X	S.E.M.	X	S.E.M.
Trauma	55	26.7	16.4	29.9	22.9	7.5	7.2	10.2	7.8
SAH - Aneurysm	16	51.6	21.8	25.6	25.6	10.1	7.0	10.4	8.4
Tumor - Malignant	15	55.3	13.0	22.8	15.0	6.5	2.3	18.1	13.2
Tumor - Benign	12	39.2	18.9	44.6	38.4	6.6	2.5	14.8	9.4
GSW	5	27.6	15.6	19.6	14.2	8.4	7.2	11.4	4.2
Other	9	36.4	21.1	25.7	18.7	9.0	6.5	9.9	7.3
Total	112	36.3	20.5	29.1	24.3	7.8	6.2	11.8	9.1

* SAH, subarachnoid hemorrhage; GSW, gunshot wound.

Where there was some question as to the relationship of the monitoring to a given complication, the distinction was based upon the presence or absence of a number of "risk" factors (*i.e.*, basal or compound skull fracture, craniotomy, excessively long surgery, operative re-exploration). The presence of a complication not clearly related to monitoring was scored as "possibly monitor related" if one of the above factors was present; two or more of these factors with an otherwise unexplained complication were sufficient to categorize the complication as "probably *not* monitor related."

Prophylactic antibiotics were defined as any antibiotic begun *prior* to the development of a septic cranial complication even though it may have had its initial indications on some other basis.

"Early" complications were defined as any complication which became manifest *during* the period of ICP monitoring. A "late" complication was one which became manifest *after* the ICP monitor had been removed.

RESULTS

Characteristics of Sample

Table 37.2 gives some general characteristics of the patients who were monitored in the Neurosurgical Intensive Care Unit. The largest diagnostic category was "trauma" with 49% of the monitored patients. Subarachnoid hemorrhage from aneurysm and malignant tumors (primary and mestastatic) made up 14% and 13% of the total sample, respectively. Benign tumors (which were mostly meningiomas) contributed 11%, gunshot wounds to the head 4.5%, and "others" (intracerebral hemorrhage, metabolic encephalopathy, arteriovenous malformations (AVM)) made up the final 8%.

The average age over-all was 36 years. The trauma group were, on the average, somewhat younger with a mean age of 26.7, which was nearly the same as the gunshot wound (GSW) group. Not surprisingly the subarachnoid hemorrhage (SAH) and malignant tumor categories both had mean ages in the early to mid-fifties. The benign tumors averaged 40 years of age.

Average days hospitalized was 29 days over-all. Trauma, SAH, and the "other" groups were very close to this mean. The mean stays for the GSW and malignant tumor groups were somewhat shorter than the average by 7 to 10 days. The benign tumor group had a mean nearly 2 weeks longer than average; this was due to a single patient with a 158-day hospitalization. The median stay for this group was 32 days.

The length of monitoring was remarkably uniform between groups. The average was about 8 days over-all.

The length of time that patients were treated with steroids had a mean of 12 days. Benign and malignant tumors were both treated with steroids for slightly longer periods of time, 15 and 18 days, respectively. The means are greater partly because preoperative tumor patients were begun on steroids 4 to 5 days prior to surgery and also continued throughout the postoperative period (and during any radiation therapy that the patients may have received).

On the average, patients were on steroids for about 50% longer than their periods of ICP monitoring.

Complication vs. No Complication

There were a total of 24 patients in the series of 112 who developed some form of cranial or monitoring complication (Table 37.3). Of these, four patients developed "fluctuance" at the site of the ICP (subarachnoid screw). In two, this led to reopening of the ICP wound with the finding of only old hematoma and fluid. A third patient underwent needle aspiration of the fluctuant area with the recovery of old hematoma; the fourth patient was merely observed. All cultures of this material were sterile, and there was no other evidence of infection. These four patients therefore are not considered to have suffered a significant complication and have generally been considered within the "no complications" group for statistical purposes (Table 37.4)

There were 92 patients of the 112 who had no complication (82%). Eighteen per cent of the total series suffered a complication of some degree. Analysis of the characteristics of the group suffering a complication when compared to the noncomplication category reveals that the group suffering a complication was an average of 10 years older than those who did not have a complication. This difference was significant at the $p < 0.05$ level.

The complications group averaged an 8-day longer period of hospitalization than those who had no complication; the difference approached, but did not quite attain, statistical significance.

However, those who suffered a complication averaged a period of monitoring twice as long as the noncomplicated group: 14 days *vs.* 6.5 days. This difference was significant at the $p < 0.005$ level. There were *no* complications in those patients who were monitored for *less* than 4 days.

The patients who developed a complication received steroid medication for a significantly longer period of time than those without complications; *i.e.*, 18 days as opposed to 10 days.

The steroid used was almost exclusively dexamethasone phosphate, with only occasional uses of methylprednisolone succinate. Cortisone

TABLE 37.3
Complications

Patient	Age	Sex	Days Hosp.	Days Monitored	Monitoring Method	Days on Steroids	Days Latency to Complication	Type Complication	Culture Results	Comments
1. DC	15	F	30	6	S	10		Fluctuant ICP Site	No Growth	Closed head injury. No craniotomy. Wound became fluctuant at ICP site resolved spontaneously with no evidence of infection. Recovery.
2. RL	9	M	87	14	S	7		Fluctuant ICP Site	No Growth	Closed head injury. No craniotomy. Wound developed fluctuance at ICP site, resolved spontaneously with no evidence of infection. Recovery.
3. HA	34	M	56	14	S	1	10	Craniotomy infection	S. aureus S. epidermidis Klebsiella Pseudomonas aeroginosa	Multiple trauma. Acute subdural hematoma Craniotomy. Developed craniotomy wound infection with multiple organisms; no ICP site infection. Required removal of bone flap. Never developed intracranial infection during prolonged course. Died.
4. HC	21	M	36	7	S	0		Fluctuant ICP Site	No Growth	Closed head injury. No craniotomy. Fluctuance developed at ICP site. Aspiration by needle revealed only old, sterile hematoma. Permanent vegetative.
5. AC	53	M	49	21	SV	25	14	Positive CSF Culture	S. epidermidis P. mirabilis	Cerebellar AVM with SAH. Monitored with ICP screw and ventricular drainage. Developed major pulmonary sepsis requiring tracheostomy. Later developed positive CSF cultures that became sterile with antibiotic treatment. Died shortly after posterior foassa exploration.
6. TS	25	M	11	6	V	10	2	Positive CSF Culture	Alpha streptococcus	Acute subdural hematoma. Craniotomy. Progressive downhill course. Developed positive CSF culture xl. Died.
7. EM	44	F	57	7	S	15	5	Craniotomy infection	S. aureus	Closed head injury with intracerebral hematoma. Burr holes. Craniotomy. Craniotomy wound infeciton. Meningitis. Removal bone flap. No ICP site infection. Recovery.
8. CS	19	F	25	6	S	12		Fluctuant ICP Site	No Growth	Closed head injury. No craniotomy. Developed fluctuance at ICP site. No evidence infection. Recovery.
9. JW	26	M	6	8	S	11	11	Meningitis	E. coli	Closed head injury with long, progressive downhill course. Developed meningitis. Responded to antibiotics. ICP site remained benign. Bronchopleural fistual 2° lung abscess. Died.

TABLE 37.3—*Continued*

Patient	Age	Sex	Days Hosp.	Days Monitored	Monitoring Method	Days on Steroids	Days Latency to Complication	Type Complication	Culture Results	Comments
10. GW	42	M	9	7	SV	8	6	Positive CSF Culture	Gram positive coccus (no further identification)	Left frontal intracerebral hematoma 2° closed head trauma. Craniotomy. Treated with ventricualr drainage and chronic mannitol. Died.
11. EP	20	M	66	55	S	60	21	Craniotomy infection Meningitis	Pseudomonos Sturtzei	Massive multiple trauma. Craniotomy. Developed pleural empyema, broncho-pleural fistual and craniotomy wound infection. CSF with positive cultures. Died.
12. GH	69	M	46	20	S	8	5	Positive CSF Culture	S. aureus	SAH 2° aneurysm. Single positive CSF culture. Died.
13. DS	59	F	29	4	S	20	9	ICP wound infeciton Subdural empyema	S. aureus	Metastatic SCE to R parietal lobe. Craniotomy with radiation and steroid treatment. Developed virulent ICP site infection and subdural empyema on L beneath ICP site. Craniotomy on L. Died.
14. JP	64	M	24	17	SV	4	7	Subdural drains x 2 Positive CSF culture	Alpha strepto-coccus(enteric type)	SAH 2° aneurysm. Craniotomy with two rubber subdural drains left in place. Drains and CSF with positive culture. Responded to antibiotics. Died 2° SAH.
15. PS	73	F	26	18	SV	21	12	Positive CSF culture	Beta strepto-coccus	SAH 2° aneurysm. Craniotomy for aneurysm. Multiple CSF cultures positive. Became sterile with antibiotic treatment. No ICP site infection.Died.
16. JN	10	M	78	22	S	13	21	ICP site infection	S. epidermidis	Closed head trauma with cerebral contusion and acute subdural hematoma. Craniotomy. ICP site infection requiring debridement. No intracranial spread. Later developed infection in lumbo-peritoneal shunt with S. aureus. Cleared after removing shunt.
17. BC	23	F	18	12	SV	18	10	Wound infection	Entero-bacter	GSW left parietal region. Craniotomy. Retained bone fragments. Re-exploration craniotomy. Wound infection. CSF leak closed on ward. Sterile CSF. No ICP site infection. Died.
18. EJ	47	F	30	4	S	10	15	ICP site infection	S. aureus	Closed head injury. No craniotomy. Local ICP site infection requiring debridement x 2. Sterile CSF. Recovery.

TABLE 37.3—*Continued*

Patient	Age	Sex	Days Hosp.	Days Monitored	Monitoring Method	Days on Steroids	Days Latency to Complication	Type Complication	Culture Results	Comments
19. JM	23	M	40	14	S	14	6	Meningitis	E. coli	Closed head injury and anterior fossa basal fracture with rhinorrhea; massive abrasions, hemopneumothorax, flail chest. Acute neurologic deterioration on hospital day 5. Craniotomy for frontal lobe swelling and high ICP: Dx. acute meningitis at surgery. Responded to systemic and intrathecal antibiotics. Late wound infection and L frontal abscess. Removal of bone flap and abscess. No ICP site infection. Recovery.
20. MM	62	F	158	10	S	19	29	Wound infection Meningitis	S. spidermidis	Craniotomy for meningioma. Wound infection with meningitis. Removal of bone flap. Post-operative subdural hematoma. Re-operation. Infection cleared with antibiotic. No ICP local infection. Recovery.
21. FM	72	F	19	11	V	19	9	Positive smear	Gram positive coccus seen on smear only--sterile culture	SAH 2° aneurysm. No craniotomy. Monitored with ventriculostomy drainage. Gram positive organism seen on smear. Culture negative. Died.
22. RF	26	M	29	19	V	14	5	Facial wound infection	Alpha streptococcus	Transfacial biopsy "mass" ethmoid-sphenoid sinus "mass". In advertent entry into anterior fossa, with "brain" returned on frozen section. Much hemorrhage with eventual blockage L internal carotid artery, neurological deterioration. Eventual decompressive craniotomy. Facial wound infection and positive CSF cultures. No ICP site or craniotomy infections. Died.
23. LL	62	F	60	8	S	56	12	Wound infection Meningitis	S. epidermidis Klebsiella	L Frontal glioblastoma IV. Craniotomy with Rickham reservior and tube left in tumor bed. Radiation therapy. Meningitis with positive CSF culture. Wound infection. Removal Rickham. Removal of bone flap. No ICP site infection. Died.
24. EB	55	F	27	4	S	10	6	Wound infection	S. aureus	L CPA meningioma removed via transmastoid approach in 10 hr. surgery. Later wound breakdown and infection. CSF leak. Wound debrided and reclosed. No ICP site infection. Recovery.

acetate was used only for replacement therapy. Methylprednisolone was used less than 5% of the time and judgments concerning its relationship to development of infective complications were not possible.

Monitor Related Complications

It was felt that five of the complications were clearly and solely due to the presence of the monitor, or 25% of the total complications were related to the ICP monitor (four secondary to the subarachnoid screw, one to the ventriculostomy). Thus, the complication rate unequivocally related to monitoring was 4.5% of the total series (Table 37.5). Eight cases were categorized as "possibly monitor related" or 40% of the

TABLE 37.4
*Comparison of Patients with Complications to Those Without**

	N	Age		Hosp. Days		Days Monitored		Days Steroids	
		$\bar{X}$	S.E.M.	$\bar{X}$	S.E.M.	$\bar{X}$	S.E.M.	$\bar{X}$	S.E.M.
No Complication	92	34.5	20.3	27.7	23.3	6.5	2.3	10.3	6.7
Complication	20	44.4	19.8	35.7	27.7	14.0	11.3	18.3	14.5
t		2.01		1.2		2.94		2.41	
p		$p < .05$		Not Significant		$p < .005$		$p < .025$	

* Those patients who developed only localized wound fluctuance (4) are considered in the "No Complication" group.

TABLE 37.5
*Complications Likely Related to Monitoring**

Relation to Monitor	N	% of Complication	% of Total (N = 112)
Definitely Monitor Related	5	25%	4.5%
Possibly Monitor Related	8	40%	7.1%
Probably Not Monitor Related	7	35%	6.2%

* In this series, 4.5% of the 112 patients suffered a complication clearly related to the monitor; 25% of the total number of complications are related to monitoring.

TABLE 37.6
*Diagnostic Categories of Complicated vs. Noncomplicated Patients**

Diagnosis			Complication		No Complication	
	N	% Total	N	% Total	N	% Total
Trauma	55	49%	8	40%	47	51%
Tumor - Benign	12	11%	2	10%	10	11%
Tumor - Malignant	15	13%	2	10%	13	14%
GSW	5	4.5%	1	5%	4	4.7%
SAH	16	14%	4	20%	12	13%
MISC.	9	8%	3	15%	6	6.5%
TOTAL	112	100%	20	100%	92	100%

* These data demonstrate that there was roughly the same proportion of each diagnostic category suffering a complication as had no complication, i.e., there is no diagnostic category that is more likely to have a complication.

complications; these represented about 7% of the total series. An additional seven cases were categorized as *probably not* due to the monitoring procedure and account for 6% of the total series and 35% of the complications.

Diagnosis vs. Complication

Table 37.6 examines the distribution of those suffering complications as opposed to those not having complications according to diagnostic categories. There is no difference between the "complication" and "no complication" groups of distribution in their diagnostic categories. That is, no particular diagnosis was more likely to lead to a complication. The differences between the mean ages, days monitored, and days treated with steroids between the complication and no complication groups (Table 37.4) cannot be explained on the basis of a preponderance of a single diagnostic category or disease state.

Complications: Survivors and Nonsurvivors

Table 37.7 compares the characteristics of the group having complications when they are divided according to whether they survived or

TABLE 37.7
Characteristics of Those Surviving and Those Deceased with Complications

	N	AGE		Days Hospitalized		Days Monitored		Days Steroids	
	20	X̄	S.E.M.	X̄	S.E.M.	X̄	S.E.M.	X̄	S.E.M.
Survivors	6 30%	40.2	19.8	65.0	49.3	10.2	6.94	13.5	3.39
Deceased	14 70%	46.3	20.6	34.9	20.0	15.4	12.7	20.4	17.0
t		0.623		1.444		1.118		1.451	
p		< 0.4 NS*		<0.1 NS*		<0.25 NS*		< 0.1 NS*	

*NS = Not significant

expired. There is no statistically significant difference between the two groups along any of the variables reviewed; however, the mean age was somewhat higher among those expiring than surviving by 6 years, but this could be due to chance variation.

The length of hospitalization of the deceased with complications was nearly 30 days less than those who survived, this difference (which could have been due to chance) approached but did not reach statistical significance at the 0.1 level. The length of monitoring was also greater in the deceased group, but not statistically significant. The same relationship held for the duration of steroid treatment comparing the deceased and surviving groups with complications.

Survivors vs. Nonsurvivors

This data illustrate that the mean age of those dying is greater than for the survivors for the over-all series by about 15 years (Table 37.8). Those patients who died while being monitored spent 2 weeks less in the hospital than did the survivors. Both of these differences were significant at the 0.001 level and follow the same trends as seen among the "complications" group where the differences were not quite significant (Table 37.7). There was no difference between the survivors and nonsurvivors in terms of the length of time they were monitored or in the duration of steroid treatment.

Death vs. Complication

The death rate among those *not* having complications was about 33%; it was 70% among those suffering a complication (Table 37.9). The difference by chi-square test is significant at the $p < 0.005$ level. Thus,

Table 37.8
*Monitoring Characteristics of Survivors vs. Nonsurvivors**

Group N=112		Age $\bar{X}$	S.E.M.	Days Hospitalized $\bar{X}$	S.E.M.	Days Monitored $\bar{X}$	S.E.M.	Days Steroids $\bar{X}$	S.E.M.
Survivors	67	30	18.7	35	25.6	7.2	3.6	11.8	7.0
Non-Survivors	45	46	19.6	21	19.3	8.7	8.6	11.7	11.6
t		4.29		3.3		1.1		0.05	
p		0.001		0.001		NS		NS	

* Those who succumbed while being monitored were on the average older (45.8 years *vs.* 29.9 years) and were hospitalized for a shorter period of time than those who survived. There was no difference between the length of time each group was monitored or treated with steroids.

Table 37.9
Relationship between Outcome (Death vs. Surviving) and Complications

	No Complications	Complications	Total
Deceased	31	14	45
Survivors	61	6	67
Total	92	20	112
$x^2 = 9.008$		$p < 0.005$	

those monitored patients who develop a complication are twice as likely to die as those who do not suffer a complication.

Only one patient died (Case 13, Table 37.3) as a direct result of a complication resulting from ICP monitoring. All of the remaining complications were successfully controlled by local debridement, bone flap removal, and/or antibiotics.

Type of Complication

Table 37.10 lists the complications according to specific type. The most frequent complication was meningitis and/or positive CSF culture. There were two patients who developed meningitis while being monitored who had *not* had a previous craniotomy, basal skull fracture, or some other reason for developing meningitis. Both of these episodes were successfully treated with antibiotics, though both patients eventually

TABLE 37.10
*Frequency of Complications by Type (112 Patients)**

ICP wound fluctuance (sterile)	4	3.6%
ICP site infection only	2	1.8%
ICP site infection with subdural empyema	1	0.9%
Craniotomy wound infection	3	2.7%
Meningitis or positive CSF culture	9	8.0%
Craniotomy wound infection and positive CSF culture	5	4.5%
Total	24	21.4%
Total (when "ICP wound fluctuance" is eliminated as a category of complication	20	17.8%
Confidence limits at 0.95 level	11% - 25%	

* If the four patients who developed the sterile, fluctuant wounds are considered as not having had a significant complication, then the over-all complication rate is 20 complications in 112 monitored patients of all categories (17.8%).

succumbed to their basic disease entity, one due to a severe head injury (Case 9), the other due to SAH from aneurysm (Case 21).

Clearly, both local wound infections at the ICP site were due to the monitor (subarachnoid screw); one patient had had a craniotomy (Case 16), while the other had suffered moderately severe closed head injury (Case 18). Both required bony debridement before healing; both patients recovered. The third local infection (Case 13) developed a subdural empyema beneath the ICP site. This was treated by craniotomy; however, the patient expired. The actual cause of death was an anesthetic complication at the time of craniotomy for the subdural empyema.

All local ICP site infections were secondary to the subarachnoid screw. Ventriculostomy sites had no associated wound infections. The rate of meningitis and other complications was basically the same for the subarachnoid screw (92 cases), the subarachnoid screw plus ventriculostomy (10 cases), and ventriculostomy alone (10 cases). Still, the rate of complication was low enough and the use of ventriculostomies rare enough that valid statistical comparisons of the two methods were impossible.

Organism vs. Complication

Table 37.11 lists the various flora cultured from the contaminated loci. With the exception of the six reports of S. epidermidis, nearly all of the organisms are pathogenic (89%).

"*Late*" *vs.* "*Early*" *Infection*

This table focuses on the time element in the development of the given complication (Table 37.12). Those who developed their complication while monitoring was still under way comprise 65% (early) of the total, while the remaining 35% developed their complication at some time after monitoring had been discontinued (late infection). Those developing "late" infection had their complication become evident about 2 weeks after initiating monitoring, or about 7 days after the monitor was removed.

TABLE 37.11
*Organism Isolated from Wounds and Cerebrospinal Fluid**

Organism	CSF	Craniotomy wound	ICP site	Total	
S. aureus	2	2	2	6	21%
S. epidermidis	3	2	1	6	21%
Klebsiella	1	3		4	14%
E. coli	2	1		3	10%
Pseudomonas	2	1		3	10%
Alpha streptococcus (enteric type)	2			2	7%
Gram positive coccus (not identified)	2			2	7%
Alpha streptococcus	1			1	3%
Enterobacter	1			1	3%
Beta streptococcus	1			1	3%
Total	17	9	3	29	100%

* Figures represent only the *different* organism cultured from each site—not the number of times the organism was recultured from the same site of a given individual.

TABLE 37.12
*Late vs. Early Infection**

Infection manifest:	Days monitored		Day complication manifest		N	%
	$\bar{X}$	S.E.M.	$\bar{X}$	S.E.M.		
Early	15.8	12.8	8.6	5.0	13	65%
Late	7.7	4.39	14.7	7.89	7	35%
t	2.07		1.99		20	100%
p	< 0.05		< 0.05			

* Comparison of the length of monitoring *vs.* the concurrent development of a septic complication (*i.e.*, "early" infection) and the development of a complication after monitoring has been discontinued (*i.e.*, "late" infection). Those developing their complication "late" had been monitored for a significantly *shorter* period of time than those who developed "early" infections.

The group developing "early" infection continued to be monitored for an additional 7 days after the development of their complication. They were eventually monitored for twice as long as the group developing "late" infection. This difference was significant at the $p < 0.05$ level for both parameters: days until complication and duration of monitoring.

The distribution of organisms cultured from the two groups was essentially the same; this did not account for the difference in "early" *vs.* "late" infection. However, most of the patients categorized as developing "early" infection were grouped as "probably *not* monitor related"; this was in contradistinction to the "late" infection group of seven patients, four of whom were definitely monitor related (80% of this category). Two of the remaining three were "possibly monitor related" and the third was "not related."

Prophylactic Antibiotics

Table 37.13 demonstrates that the use of antibiotics in the prophylactic sense was unrelated to the development of "early" *vs.* "late" infection. The chi-square test demonstrated no association between these parameters.

Using the chi-square test for association between prophylactic antibiotics and the development of a complication for the entire series (Table 37.14), we find that there is no association between the two. Half of the patients who developed a complication had been treated with prophylactic antibiotics, while the remaining 50% had not been so treated.

DISCUSSION

General Characteristics

In the analysis of the over-all complication rate, we are struck first by the basic statistics describing the population of this series of 112

TABLE 37.13
*Early or Late Infection vs. Prophylactic Antibiotics**

	"Early" infectior	"Late" infection	Total
Prophylactic antibiotics	8	2	10
No prophylactic antibiotics	5	5	10
Total	13	7	20
$\chi^2 = 1.978$	$0.1 < p < 0.25$		

* Data demonstrate no association between antibiotics with early and late infection.

TABLE 37.14
Complications vs. Prophylactic Antibiotics

	Complications	No Complications	Total
Prophylactic Antibiotics	10	40	50
No Prophylactic Antibiotics	10	52	62
Total	20	92	112

$X^2 = 0.28$ Not significant

patients. The average age of our sample was 36 years, and the mean length of time hospitalized on the neurosurgical service was 29 days. Each patient was monitored for an average of 7.8 days, and 90% of the time this was carried out by the subarachnoid screw. The remaining 10% were made up of ventriculostomies or screw combined with a ventriculostomy. The average length of time that each patient was maintained on steroid medication was about 12 days, or an average of 4 days longer than the monitoring device remained in place.

Complication Rate

There were a total of 24 complications of all sorts in the series with four considered to be of a trivial nature. The remaining 20 complications were septic in nature; the rate was 17.8% of the total. This compares very closely with a rate of 17 to 18% over-all complication rate that Lundberg reported in his 1960 series when all types and classes of his complications are included (as defined by the present authors in this series).

Age

In the present series, the mean age of the group comprising the complications is both clinically and statistically significantly higher than the noncomplicated group (44.4 years compared to 34.5 years). The relationship of age to complication/infection rate has been somewhat variable in the experience of previous investigators. Wright in his review of 2,148 surgically "clean" craniotomies found no relationship with patient age; the British studies of Forbes, and Williams and associates both found a relationship of increasing infection rate with increasing age (9, 41, 42). Certainly this is true in our series. One might suppose that this could be due to a preponderance of a diagnostic group that tended to be older (such as malignant tumors or SAH) in the makeup of the complication group. This was not the case (Table 37.6). The distribution of diagnostic category within the complication group was the same as that within the noncomplication category and the series as a whole. We have no immediate explanation for the difference in age, but we suppose that it must relate to a change within the individual associated with the aging process itself that makes the older patient more susceptible to infection.

Length of Hospitalization

The patients developing a complication in the series also were noted to be hospitalized somewhat longer, though the difference was not quite statistically significant and might have been produced by chance. However, this finding is consistent with that of others who have found that a complication of any sort leads to longer hospitalization: it seems logical that it would (42).

Length of Monitoring

Interestingly, the group suffering a complication was monitored for a considerably longer period of time, (about a full week longer), than the group that had no complication. This is in conflict with Lundberg's series where he felt that the rate of complication was not particularly related to the period of monitoring (21). Our data do agree with several other investigators who have related length of time of surgical procedures to infection, and more appropriately to length of time that ventriculostomies were left in place (2, 39, 42, 43).

Certainly, it seems logical that the time of exposure to a complicating factor must increase the likelihood of developing a complication: our data are consistent with this thesis.

Steroids

Equally as important, the group of our patients who developed a significant complication had been treated with steroids for an average of 8 days longer than the noncomplicated group. Not all investigators have found a relationship of infection to steroid treatment, but the physiological basis is present in the mechanism of action of the drug, and an increased incidence of infection has been related to steroids by some (10, 31, 42).

However, the exact interaction of the steroid treatment with age and length of monitoring is not clear, and any statement of the pathophysiology seems premature. Interestingly, Table 37.6 reveals that there is no difference between the diagnostic categories in terms of infection rate including tumors; since tumors were treated with steroids somewhat longer than the other diagnostic groups, one might expect this to increase their rate of complication: it did not.

Likewise, the tumor group was nearly 20 years older than the average, and this also would tend to increase the rate of complications which it did not. The only explanation at this point is that the malignant tumor patients actually had a 62% in hospital *mortality* rate, in conjunction with a period of hospitalization that was 22 days on the average—1 week less than the average for the series. This suggests that the complication rate might have been higher had this group of patients survived longer, particularly with regard to "late" infection. There were no deaths among the benign tumor patients.

Relation of Infection to Monitoring

There was great difficulty in deciding which of the complications in this series were likely related to ICP monitoring, which were representative of the normal operative infection rate, and which were complications of the disease state, *e.g.*, meningitis in the presence of basal skull fracture or GSW.

However, out of the total complication rate of 17.8% for this series, only 4.5% of the total, and 25% of the complications were thought to be directly related to ICP monitoring. Six per cent of total, and 35% of our complications were thought not to be related to monitoring and were readily explained either on the basis of the basic disease process or a combination of other predisposing factors (such as those discussed by Wright and by Balch) (2, 42).

This figure compares very closely with the over-all infection rate for "surgically clean" craniotomies of 5 to 6% described by Wright, and the 3 to 4% of Balch. We feel that this compares very favorably with our figure of 6% which is composed of nearly 50% "dirty" cases. The above authors do not give complication rate for the so-called "dirty case." Most likely, this immediate explanation accounts for the intermediate group of 7% (or 40% of our complications) who had complications which were not readily attributed to either the monitoring or to other risk factors. Some of these complications were due to monitoring and some were due to other factors; and perhaps there was interaction of multiple factors with monitoring to produce a complication that might not have otherwise occurred, but not due solely to the monitor.

Therefore, we feel that the actual rate of complication related to ICP monitoring or exacerbated by it is at least 4.5%, at most 11.5%, and most reasonably somewhere between these values.

Death and Complications

There was only one death directly attributable to monitoring; the remainder of the complications were readily controlled by routine methods, such as the removal of foreign bodies (monitors), debridement, drainage, and antibiotics. Still, the death rate of those patients who were monitored and also developed a complication was about 70%—more than twice that of the patients who did not undergo a complication. The high over-all death rate is due in part to the high proportion of severe trauma (49%), SAH from aneurysm (14%), and malignant tumors (13%) for a total of 76% of the entire series. These groups had death rates from 50 to 65%.

The association between death and monitoring is quite statistically significant (Table 37.9). Yet the distribution of diagnostic categories among the patients with a complication is the same as among those patients who did not have a complication and the entire series. Thus, one cannot explain the longer periods of steroid treatment or of the duration of monitoring among those with complications by stating that these were the patients more seriously ill, who, therefore, were monitored longer and treated with steroids longer. Rather, we infer that steroids and monitoring both contributed to the development of a complication, just as age seems to have increased the risk of complication.

Yet, when one examines the characteristics of the survivors *vs.* the nonsurvivors, one is impressed that the surviving group and the expiring group were both monitored and treated with steroids for the same period of time: there is no difference. Yet the dying patients were 16 years older on the average than were the survivors, and had spent nearly 2 weeks less in the hospital (while not significant, the same trends were seen, in Table 37.7, between those dying with complications and without complications).

These data suggest that while age probably contributes to the likelihood of dying from a serious disease (and if the patient dies, his period of hospitalization is actually shorter) that monitoring and steroids are not related to the likelihood of dying. To an extent this is supported by our experience that only one patient succumbed as a direct result of monitoring (and had actually succumbed by virtue of an anesthetic complication—Case 13), and that the remaining 95% had their complications successfully treated and controlled prior to their death.

Type of Complication

The distribution in terms of types of complication is given in Table 37.10. The essential point of discussion is that we found it impossible to retrospectively differentiate "meningitis" and a positive CSF culture from a patient who at the time was often very ill and had an intracranial foreign body. This distinction is often difficult at the bedside with complete information and the patient himself. Therefore, we included in this category any patient whose records indicated a clinical meningitis as well as any patient whose CSF culture results were positive (regardless of the CSF analysis which often was distributed between lumbar puncture and ventricular fluid). Previous investigators have not taken this more conservative approach to the evaluation of the complications (21).

When one examines the delay in the manifestation of a complication when defined in terms of the number of days after the initiation of monitoring, an interesting finding emerges: There are indeed two groups of patients both clinically and statistically. The first, or two-thirds of the total complications developed their complication *while* being monitored and are distinct from the remainder who developed their complication "late", nearly a week after the "early" group have manifested their infection. The surprising finding is that while the "early" infection group had manifested their complication on day 8.6 (mean time), they were monitored for an additional 7 days. The only ready explanation for this is that the clinicians caring for the patients at the time that the complication became manifest were of the opinion that the complication was *not* due directly to the monitor and that there was still useful information to be gained by leaving it in place.

Corroborative data are available in the form of the distribution of those who developed "early" as opposed to "late" infection. Four of the seven patients who developed a "late" infection were directly related to the monitor (Cases 13, 16, 18, and 21). Two of the remaining three were "possibly monitor related" and the last was thought "probably not monitor related." All but one of the 13 cases in the remainder were either not monitor related or only possibly monitor related.

Prophylactic Antibiotics

When we looked at the relationship of prophylactic antibiotics to the development of early *vs.* late infection, we found no association between them. We also found no statistical association by chi-square for the entire series between the use of "prophylactic" antibiotics and the development of infection. However, since the patients were not *randomly* treated with antibiotics, and frequently what we considered "prophylactic" in terms of a monitor was not prophylactic in terms of initial indication, it may be that the complication rate would have been higher had not antibiotics been used as frequently as they were. We believe that only a carefully controlled study will ever answer this question. Wyler did report a drop from 27% to 9% incidence of infection when prophylactic antibiotics were used in the routine management of ventriculostomy, and others have advocated prophylaxis (5, 27, 44). Lundberg initially used antibiotics on all of his patients, and later, apparently, discontinued their routine use according to Sundbärg, so these data are not helpful in this question (21, 33).

If prophylactic antibiotics are to be used, then the general trend of the literature beginning with Burke's study is that they should be begun *prior* to the introduction of a foreign body so that tissue level of the antibiotic is present at the time of contamination (2).

The distribution of organisms found in our review was essentially that reported by other investigators for surgical wound infection and by the Lund group for ICP related infection (21, 31, 33, 41–43). Seventy per cent of the organisms are Gram positive, primarily S. aureus, S. epidermidis, and streptococcal species. Therefore, the greatest success with prophylactic antibiotics ought to be with narrow spectrum antibiotics that are effective against Gram positive organisms. The Gram negative infections encountered were similar in distribution to general surgical sepsis. While prophylactic antibiotics may decrease the rate of complication with Gram positive organisms, care must be exercised that superinfection with fast growing Gram negative organisms are not encouraged. Thus, the length of time prophylaxis is used should be kept to a minimum.

SUMMARY

1. Patients with complications when compared with those not developing a complication:
   a. Were older, 44.4 *vs.* 34.5 years;
   b. Were monitored longer, 14.0 *vs.* 6.5 days;
   c. Were treated with steroids longer, 18.3 *vs.* 10.3 days;
   d. Were hospitalized longer, 35.7 *vs.* 27.7 days;
   e. Are twice as likely to die;
   f. Average age of those dying is older, 46 *vs.* 30 years;
   g. Have no clear relationship to antibiotics;
   h. Do not have a preponderance of single diagnostic category to account for these differences;
   i. Complications were always controlled with standard therapy;
   j. An ICP complication was almost never responsible, *per se*, for death.
2. Over-all complication rate was 18%; due to monitoring was 4.5 to 11.5%.
3. Monitoring was responsible for, or contributed to, 25 to 60% of the complications.
4. No complications occurred when monitoring was discontinued within 3 days.
5. Long periods of treatment with steroids increased the risk of a complication developing.

6. Long periods of monitoring were associated with an increased risk of complication.
7. "Individual" factors are partly responsible for the development of a complication, and death.
8. There are two groups of complications: "early" and "late."
   a. Those most *likely* to be monitor related occur "late" and account for 35% of the complications.
   b. Those developing "early" infection account for 65% of the complications and are most likely caused by factors *other* than monitoring.

While there are complications directly attributable to monitoring, the rate is low and they are readily controlled by standard neurosurgical management. While monitoring may increase the morbidity, it does not increase the mortality. We feel that the over-all risk is small and that the returns are great—both in terms of knowledge and patient benefit.

REFERENCES

1. Atkinson, J. R., Shurtleff, D. B., and Foltz, E. L. Radio telemetry for the measurement of intracranial pressure. J. Neurosurg., *27:* 428–432, 1967.
2. Balch, R. E. Wound infections complicating neurosurgical procedures. J. Neurosurg., *26:* 41–45, 1967.
3. Bering, E. A. A simplified apparatus for constant ventricular drainage. J. Neurosurg., *8:* 450–452, 1951.
4. Brock, M., and Diefenthäler, K. A modified equipment for the continuous telemetric monitoring of epidural or subdural pressure. *In* Intracranial Pressure: Experimental and Clinical Aspects, edited by M. Brock and H. Dietz, pp. 21–26. Springer-Verlag, Berlin/Heidelberg/New York, 1972.
5. Burke, J. F. The effective period of preventive antibiotic action in experimental incisions and dermal lesions. Surgery, *50:* 161–168, 1961.
6. Coe, J. E., Nelson, W. J., Rudenberg, F. H., and Garza, R. Technique for continuous intracranial pressure recording. Technical Note. J. Neurosurg., *27:* 370–375, 1967.
7. Cohandon, F., LaBalme, M., Castel, J. P., and Vandendriessche, M. ICP microprobe series microfet. *In* Intracranial Pressure II, edited by N. Lundberg, U. Ponten, and M. Brock, pp. 375–376. Springer-Verlag, Berlin/Heidelberg/New York, 1975.
8. DeRougemont, J., Benabid, A. L., and Barge, M. Intracranial pressure measurement by epidural technique. A simple solution. *In* Intracranial Pressure II, edited by N. Lundberg, U. Ponten, and M. Brock, pp. 384–385. Springer-Verlag, Berlin/Heidelberg/New York, 1975.
9. Forbes, G. B. Staphylococcal infection of operation wounds with special reference to topical antibiotics prophylaxis. Lancet, *2:* 505–509, 1961.
10. Fuenfer, M. M., Grant, E. O., and Polk, H. C. Effect of various corticosteroids upon the phagocytic bactericidal activity of neutrophils. Surgery, *78:* 27–33, 1975.
11. Gobiet, W., Bock, W. J., Liesegang, J., and Grote, W. Experience with an intracranial pressure transducer readjustable in vivo. J. Neurosurg., *40:* 272–276, 1974.
12. Gobiet, W., Bock, W. J., Liesegang, J., and Grote, W. Long-time monitoring of epidural pressure in man. *In* Intracranial Pressure: Experimental and Clinical Aspects, edited by M. Brock and H. Dietz, pp. 17–17. Springer-Verlag, Berlin/Heidelberg/New York, 1972.

13. Grant, F. C. The value of hypertonic solutions by mouth, by rectum, or by intravenous injection for the reduction of increased intracranial pressure. *In* "The intracranial pressure in health and disease." Res. Publ. Assoc. Res. Nerv. Ment. Dis., *8:* 437–454, 1929.
14. Handa, H., Yoneda, M., Matsuda, M., and Handa, J. A miniature SFT transducer for continuous monitoring of intracranial pressure. *In* Intracranial Pressure II, edited by N. Lundberg, U. Ponten, and M. Brock, pp. 378–379. Springer-Verlag, Berlin/Heidelberg/New York, 1975.
15. Hoppenstein, R. A device for measuring intracranial pressure. Lancet, *1:* 90–91, 1965.
16. Ingraham, F. D., and Campbell, J. B. An apparatus for closed drainage of the ventricular system. Ann. Surg., *114:* 1096–1098, 1941.
17. Johnston, I. H., and Jennett, B. The place of continuous intracranial pressure monitoring in neurosurgical practice. Acta Neurochirurgica, *29:* 53–63, 1973.
18. Johnston, I. H., Johnston, J. A., and Jennett, B. Intracranial pressure changes following head injury. Lancet, *2:* 433–436, 1970.
19. Kaufman, G. E., and Clark, K. Emergency frontal twist drill ventriculostomy. J. Neurosurg., *33:* 226–227, 1970.
20. Kindt, W. Simplification of intracranial pressure monitoring. *In* Intracranial Pressure II, edited by N. Lundberg, U. Ponten, and M. Brock, pp. 381–383. Springer-Verlag, Berlin/Heidelberg/New York, 1975.
21. Lundberg, N. Continuous recording and control of ventricular fluid pressure in neurosurgical practice. Acta Psychiatr. Scand., *36* (Suppl. *149*): 1–193, 1960.
22. Lundberg, N., Troupp, H., and Lorin, H: Continuous recording of the ventricular-fluid pressure in patients with severe acute traumatic brain injury. J. Neurosurg., *22:* 581–590, 1965.
23. Nornes, H., and Magnaes, B. Supratentorial epidural pressure recorded during posterior fossa surgery. J. Neurosurg., *35:* 541–549, 1971.
24. Nornes, H., and Serck-Hanssen, F. Miniature transducer for intracranial pressure monitoring in man. Acta Neurol. Scand., *46:* 203–214, 1970.
25. Numoto, M., and Donaghy, R. M. P. Pressure indicating bag. *In* Intracranial Pressure II, edited by N. Lundberg, U. Ponten, and M. Brock, pp. 382–383. Springer-Verlag, Berlin/Heidelberg/New York, 1975.
26. Numoto, M., Slater, J. P., and R. M. P. Donaghy. An implantable switch for monitoring intracranial pressure. Lancet, *1:* 528, 1966.
27. Pennybacker, J. B., Taylor, M., and Cairns, H. Penicillin in the prevention of infection during operations on the brain and spinal cord. Lancet, *2:* 159–162, 1947.
28. Poppen, J. L. Ventricular drainage as a valuable procedure in neurosurgery: report of a satisfactory method. Arch. Neurol. Psychiatr., *50:* 587–589, 1943.
29. Rand, B. O., Ward, A. A., and White, L. E. The use of the twist drill to evaluate head trauma. J. Neurosurg., *25:* 410–415, 1966.
30. Robinson, F. An apparatus for continuous ventricular drainage and intraventricular therapy. J. Neurosurg., *5:* 320–323, 1948.
31. Romig, D. A., Voth, D. W., Liu, C., and Brackett, C. E. Bacterial flora and infection in patients with brain injury. J. Neurosurg., *38:* 710–716, 1973.
32. Schimkf, R. T., Black, P. H., Vernon, H. M., and Swartz, M. N. Indolent staphylococcus albus or aureus bacteremia after ventriculoatriostomy: role of foreign body in its initiation and perpetuation. N. Engl. J. Med., *264:* 264–270. 1961.
33. Sundbärg, G., Kjällquist, A., Lundberg, N., and Pontén, U. Complications due to prolonged ventricular fluid pressure recording in clinical practice. *In* Intracranial Pressure: Experimental and Clinical Aspects, edited by M. Brock, and H. Dietz, pp. 348–352, Springer-Verlag, Berlin/Heidelberg/New York, 1972.

34. Tindall, G. T., McGraw, C. P., and Iwata, K. Subdural pressure monitoring in head-injured patients. *In* Intracranial Pressure: Experimental and Clinical Aspects, edited by M. Brock, and H. Dietz, pp. 9–13. Springer-Verlag, Berlin/Heidelberg/New York, 1972.
35. Turner, J. M., Bibson, R. M., McDowell, D. G., and Nahhas, F. Further experiences with extradural pressure monitoring. *In* Intracranial Pressure II, edited by N. Lundberg, U. Ponten, and M. Brock, pp. 397–402. Springer-Verlag, Berlin/Heidelberg/New York, 1975.
36. Vander Ark, G. D., and Stecher, K. A disposable ventriculostomy apparatus. Technical Note. J. Neurosurg., *41:* 399–400, 1974.
37. Vries, J. K., Becker, D. P., and Young, H. F. A subarachnoid screw for monitoring intracranial pressure. J. Neurosurg., *39:* 416–419, 1973.
38. Vries, J. K., Becker, D. P., Young, H. F., Sakalas, R., Greenberg, R. F., and Rosner, M. J. The hollow screw technique for monitoring intracranial pressure. *In* Intracranial Pressure II, edited by N. Lundberg, U. Ponten, M. Brock, p. 386. Springer-Verlag, Berlin/Heidelberg/New York, 1975.
39. Weiss, Martin. Personal communication, 1975.
40. White, R. J., Dakters, J. G., Yashon, D., and Albin, M. S. Temporary control of cerebrospinal fluid volume and pressure by means of an externalized valve-drainage system. J. Neurosurg., *30:* 264–269, 1969.
41. Williams, R. E. O., McDonald, J. C., and Blowers, R. Incidence of the surgical wound infection in England and Wales. A report of the Public Health Laboratory Service. Lancet, *2:* 659–663, 1960.
42. Wright, R. L. A survey of possible etiologic agents in postoperative craniotomy infections. J. Neurosurg., *25:* 125–132, 1966.
43. Wyler, A. R., and W. A. Kelly. Use of antibiotics with external ventriculostomies. J. Neurosurg., *37:* 185–187, 1972.

CHAPTER

38

The Law of Medical Professional Liability

WALTER H. BECKHAM, JR., A.B., J.D.

Since many treatises have been written on this subject and we are under time limitations, of necessity, we must paint here with a broad brush. Accordingly, we will limit ourselves to a generalized discussion of some of the basic and some of the controversial legal principles involved in the hope that it may stimulate you to more detailed study in the copious literature at your leisure.

The physician-patient relationship is normally regarded as a contractual one to which each party gives his consent, express or implied. In return for the patient's promise to pay compensation, the physician agrees to treat him. It is, of course, possible though not usual, that a physician for a consideration expressly contracts with his patient to guarantee a certain result by his care and treatment. If such a contract is proved and it is breached by the physician, he may be held liable as in other cases of breach of contract.

A basic principle of our law is that: "Every human being of adult years and sound mind has the right to determine what shall be done with his own body . . . " Schoendorff *vs.* Society of New York Hospital, 211 N.Y. 125, 129; 105 N.E. 92, 93 (1914). Likewise, one who intentionally, and without a privilege or consent, brings about a harmful or offensive touching of another's body is guilty of a battery. If, prior to the touching, the party touched is put in reasonable apprehension of the unlawful touching, then an assualt has also been committed. Therefore, it is only the patient's consent, express or implied, which permits the physician intentionally to touch, or to cause something else to touch, the patient's body.

In addition, once the physician-patient relationship is established, there exists, in law, a fiduciary relationship—that is, a relationship of trust and confidence—between them. Such a legal relationship carries with it an affirmative duty to disclose all relevant facts which are pertinent to it, for, legally, the parties are no longer dealing with each other at arms' length.

Once the physician-patient relationship is established, the physician also has the legal duty in his care and treatment of the patient to exercise that degree of care and skill which is usually exercised, or which the courts declare should be exercised, by similar practitioners under the same or similar circumstances. This standard is normally a matter to be established by expert testimony of practitioners in the field unless the matter involved is so elementary that a lay person can understand it without the necessity of expert testimony. Likewise, it is normally for a jury of lay people to determine whether or not the practitioner was negligent in allowing his performance to fall below the acceptable standard and whether the patient as a proximate result thereof sustained damages. In negligence actions it is only for conduct resulting in damage that there is liability.

If there is a breach of contract, or an assault and/or battery, or negligence resulting in damage, a lay jury assesses an amount of money which represents reasonable compensation for the damages which have proximately resulted. If a tort is intentional or if there is gross negligence, which is usually defined as willful and wanton misconduct evidencing a reckless disregard for human life, a lay jury may also be asked to assess punitive damages against the wrongdoer.

There are some additional legal principles that have evolved from these basic principles we have been discussing. One of these is the doctrine of informed consent. This doctrine addresses itself to the problem of whether or not at the time the patient purportedly gave consent to an operation or treatment by the physician such consent was given under such a mistake as to either its essential nature or as to the risks involved in it, that the consent will be declared invalid with consequent liability for harmful or offensive touching caused by the physician. Though this doctrine originated through the law of assault and battery, it was later recognized that the physician's standard of professional conduct requires him to make to his patient a reasonable disclosure of the available choices open to him and of the dangers involved in each. He must disclose enough so that the normally nonmedically oriented patient can make an intelligent choice on which to base his consent. With this recognition the courts found it was negligent for the physician not to conform to this standard of professional conduct. Most informed consent cases now proceed on the legal basis of negligence although assault and battery may still be applied if the procedure or treatment is clearly one to which the patient has not consented. The nature and extent of the required disclosure is now in the process of being codified and, hopefully, clarified by legislation in several states. Since these matters have traditionally been governed by the law of each state, you must look to the statutes and to the opinions of the highest court in the state where you practice medicine to determine the nature and extent of your individual duty as a physician.

Though there are relatively few cases where patients claim a breach of a contract to guarantee a certain result by their physician, several states have recently added this kind of a contract to those included in the protection of their Statute of Frauds. The result of this legislation is to require that such a contract to be enforceable must be in writing and signed by the physician to be charged.

The law recognizes that there should be some time limit within which a person may exercise his legal remedy. Statutes of Limitations in the various states specify the time within which different kinds of actions must be brought or else be barred from enforcement in the courts. One of the problems here has been to determine when the statute should begin to run in a negligence case. The basic issue is whether the statute should begin to run from the date of the act or omission which gives rise to the cause of action, or whether it should begin to run from the date when the injured party discovers or reasonably should discover that there has been such an act or omission, and he has been damaged thereby. Legislation in this field today is taking the form of: (a) reducing the number of years for bringing the action under either rule, (b) adopting the date of the act or omission as the date when the statute begins to run, and (c) providing that no matter which test is used, in no event will action be allowed beyond a certain number of years after the date of the act or omission giving rise to the cause of action.

In an action for negligence, the plaintiff has the burden of proving by a preponderance of the credible evidence both that the defendant was negligent and that the defendant's negligence was a proximate cause of injury to the plaintiff. If the agency or instrumentality causing the injury is totally within the control of the defendant, it is frequently very difficult for the plaintiff to meet this burden. As a result of this difficulty, with the inequitable results which it many times produced, the courts evolved a doctrine to assist the plaintiff to get to a jury in a case of this sort. This doctrine says that if the agency or instrumentality causing the injury to the plaintiff is totally within the control of the defendant and the occurrence is of a kind that ordinarily does not happen in the absence of negligence, then the jury may, though they are not required to, draw an inference of negligence by the defendant proximately causing the injury to the plaintiff from the occurrence itself. This doctrine has been given the name *res ipsa loquitur*, the thing speaks for itself. Though this doctrine did not originate in medical negligence cases, it also has been applied in these cases, at least where the negligence is so clear that expert testimony is not required to establish it. There is some agitation today to abolish or limit this doctrine in its application to medical negligence cases by appropriate legislation.

When one by his negligent conduct proximately causes injury to another, he is required to compensate the injured party for the injuries and damages which he has proximately caused. In arriving at the amount of this compensation our courts have traditionally felt it unfair for the defendant to receive any credit because of any benefits which the plaintiff has received from a collateral source not connected with the defendant. Examples of such collateral source benefits are workmen's compensation, medical and hospitalization insurance, sick leave, etc. The rationale behind this rule of law is that these benefits are benefits which the plaintiff has secured from his own resources and relationships and that the wrongdoer defendant should not be allowed to reduce his liability to the plaintiff because of them. Defendants on the other hand have argued that the plaintiff is in some cases being allowed to recover double compensation for some of his losses albeit as a result of his own thrift or foresight. Of course if the defendant can get such a credit, it will reduce what he has to pay the plaintiff, and this in turn will reduce his own losses or those of his insurance company. As a result the suggestion has been made that legislation should be enacted which would allow the defendant this credit.

It has been the rule that the amount of compensation, if any, to which the plaintiff might be entitled from the defendant should be decided by a jury of his peers which theoretically represents the conscience of the community. The only limitation on this has been the power of a court to enter a remittitur or additur, or to grant a new trial by another jury where the amount which has been awarded by the jury under the evidence submitted is such that on that evidence it shocks the judicial conscience; this usually means that it is an amount which the court feels is more or less than any reasonable person could award on that evidence. There is some pressure being exerted today to fix, by legislation, a maximal amount which the law will not allow to be exceeded no matter what the evidence is in a medical negligence case.

In our legal system, negligence cases, including medical negligence cases, have been tried to lay juries and have been decided by them with the aid of expert testimony and opinions where appropriate. Those whose liability has been determined in this way have sometimes complained that a lay jury is not sufficiently able to comprehend all the complex technical evidence and testimony in today's complex society. In the field of medical negligence, a few state legislatures have now set up screening or mediation panels to which a claimant must submit his case before going to court. This screening or mediation panel usually includes one or more physicians. It is further provided by some that the liability findings of the panel, while not binding on the parties or on the courts may be admitted into evidence at any subsequent trial on the claim involved if either party proceeds to litigate rather than to accept the findings of the panel.

As an alternative to the jury system, voluntary binding arbitration pursuant to contractual agreement between the patient and the physician is being proposed. The idea behind this appears to be that it will not take as long as the traditional jury trial process, the fact finders and judges will be more sophisticated and learned in the field of medicine than the lay jury, and hopefully the awards given, will be less on the average than recent jury awards. The rules for arbitration proceedings are also less rigorous concerning the evidence that is admissible on the issue being decided than they are in the law courts.

Negligence cases have traditionally been handled by claimant's attorneys on a contingent fee basis. Under this system if the case is lost, there is no fee to the attorney; and if the case is won, the attorney receives a percentage of the recovery. This type fee system has been called the poor man's key to the court house and, historically, clients of attorneys handling cases on this basis have registered very few complaints. In the final analysis, the reasonableness of every attorney's fee is subject to regulation by the court of which the attorney is an officer. When awards were very low in negligence cases, there was very little criticism of this system. As awards have increased, there has been increased criticism of the amounts earned under contingent fee contracts by attorneys. This criticism, for the most part, has been by nonclients and mostly by defendants and their insurance carriers. Our limitations here do not permit a full discussion of this matter. Recently, however, some courts and some legislatures have been imposing limitations on the percentages of the recovery for which a claimant's attorney may contract. Although this is many times put on the ground that it will give the injured person a greater share of the proceeds of the recovery, one may be permitted to wonder if, in the absence of client discontent, the real reason is to discourage the successful prosecution of these cases by competent attorneys.

In order to avoid publicity about suits being filed for large amounts of money, some legislatures have eliminated the statement of the amount being claimed from the allegations of the claimant's complaint when it is filed in the court to initiate a court action. How effective this will be in reducing the size of jury awards remains to be seen.

There is much that we have not discussed. Hopefully, what we have said may be of some help in understanding some of the law that applies in medical negligence cases and some of the changes in that body of law which are being made or proposed. There is much to be said as to whether these changes and proposals are desirable or not. Indeed, there is doubt as to the constitutionality of some of them if applied only to medical negligence and not to negligence in other fields. My task has been to try to inform you. The law is the lubricant of society. It must change to conform to the changing needs and desires of the society in which it operates. It is like a pendulum which swings back and forth. Since it reflects human desires and institutions, it is not perfect. The measure of its success at any given time is its ability to gain acceptance by those it governs and to assist them in an acceptable ordering of their affairs and relationships with each other and with their government. The present law in this field and the proposed changes must be evaluated in this light and not in the light of only what is in the best interests of any one segment or group.

CHAPTER

39

Prophylaxis and Therapy of Malpractice Litigation

JAMES LEWIS GRIFFITH, ESQ.

There are few physicians, particularly those practioners within the so-called high risk specialities, who have not been exposed to malpractice litigation. Hopefully, their experience has been limited to that of a treating physician or perhaps as an expert witness on behalf of a colleague. Others still have been named as defendants in cases either pending or concluded. No physician I have interviewed ever enjoyed the experience even when the cases were successfully defended. Such factors as adverse publicity, the emotional stress of pretrial discovery and the trial itself, the time spent away from practice, and the ever present concern that this case might cause the carrier to refuse to renew coverage all combine to make the malpractice experience particularly distasteful to the physician. Having spent the last 10 years defending malpractice cases, I have concluded that although the medicine tastes terrible, it need not follow that it also does no good for the patient. The longer the physicians choose to cast themselves as the innocent victims of a hostile society manipulated by those archdemons, the plaintiffs' lawyers, the longer it will be before the experience value of past cases is realized. What then, it might be appropriate to ask, are these so-called benefits of the past cases?

The first benefit would be the realization that there are no more sacred cows in our society. The people today are no longer the ignorant, believing masses that adhere without question to whatever is told to them. This is true not only of Presidents, but also of physicians. Not only are patients capable of understanding the truth, they demand it. The physician is accountable to himself, his peers, and most important, to the patient. Therefore, no matter what occurs in the course of a patient's treatment, put it down on the chart and tell the patient exactly how it is. I have had physicians call me from an operating room to report an unfortunate occurrence and to inquire how this can be explained away. My advice has always been to confront the patient and/or the family with a factual explanation placing responsibility where it lies. In a surprising number of cases, no suit ever followed. In those instances where suit did follow, there was no jury backlash because the patient could not introduce any suggestion of physician deceit to incite the jury against the physician. The awards in these cases were surprisingly moderate and in several instances below what had been offered in settlement prior to trial.

Likewise, it will aid in the defense of a suit brought beyond the usual statute of limitations. The only justification for asserting a cause of action beyond the statute period is either physician concealment of the injury or the proven inability of the patient to discover the injury within the statutory period. A concise, frank explanation to the patient, the substance of which is preserved in an appropriate progress note is clearly the best policy.

The second benefit could be called the "Death of a Boy Scout." If you have not learned by now, let me be the first to assure you that patients, like all other classes of people, do lie. They do distort their memories when the opportunity for economic enrichment is present. They resolve all doubts caused by the passage of time in their favor and against the physician. If they believe the physician has lied to them, this is taken as a carte blanche to so testify in whatever manner is best for their case and most detrimental to the defendent physician. I cannot tell you that I have some magical cure for the disease of tumacity but I would like to suggest a prophylaxis. The physician must view his office notes and hospital charts as the first line of defense. There is no way a physician can expect to win a question of credibility with the patient when he must rely solely on his memory many years after the event when he has seen hundreds, perhaps thousands, of patients in the interim. I invite you to get in the habit of recording in the initial office notes or admission history some catch word or description that will aid you in identifying the patient and the events that surrounded his treatment. Such entries as "likes sailing"; "friend of Mr. X"; "has British accent" might be just enough to restore your recollection as to the patient who is now suing you. More significantly, I invite you to educate your entire staff and particularly the nurses to record all visits by physician to the patients by date and time. I invite you, your staff,and your hospital personnel to record what you are doing and forget telling us how well the patient is doing. A nursing note rewritten at the end of his or her shift which states that a patient had a bowel movement, ate, drank, and slept does not tell your defense counsel 5 years later that she checked hourly on circulatory changes, I.V. solution, and possible extravasations, etc. Examine your own records the next time you are signing out charts. Do they accurately reflect what you did, what you noted about the patient; what changes occurred in the patient's condition, or the therapy administered? It is far more effective in a courtroom to say "yes, I noted that fact and so recorded it at 9:00 a.m., October 24, 1975 on page 12 of the chart" than to say "I'm sure I must have realized that fact but when and where I first realized it, I do not know."

Examine your charts and note if you ever bothered to record your discharge instructions on levels of activity, return for follow-up care, discharge medications, etc. I cannot tell you the number of times I have heard in a courtroom the question as to what instructions were given to the patient at discharge. Invariably, the answer is that the doctor told them nothing. A clear chart entry would make the job of defending the case a lot easier.

Lawyers use briefs to set forth arguments as to the law and the facts. Our briefs, however, are always retrospective. Why not write your brief concurrently by making meaningful entries in your charts. Generally speaking, lawyers, judges, and juries really do not care what the patient ate or whether the bowel movement was dark and firm as opposed to yellow and soft. We might be very interested, however, as to precisely when an EEG, for example, was ordered, performed, and interpreted. In addition, please do not overlook the importance of recording significant patient conversations particularly those relating to informed consent, past medical history, and statements as to the probable outcome of surgery. Wherever possible or appropriate, get the patient to sign the entry or at least have some other member of the family sign it.

The third benefit is that "hide and seek" is not the way to defend a malpractice case. By that I mean that too many doctors after receiving service of a suit paper immediately go and hide. The theory seems to be that if the physician does not know what is going on in the case, he must not be involved in the matter and it is just a little detail for the carrier and defense counsel to solve. The second aspect of this syndrome is that it is defense counsel's job to seek out an expert and the other materials essential to a liability defense. I remind you that the person who should be most concerned with the defense of *your* case is you. I always get a little rigid when I hear physicians, as I have heard at this annual meeting of the Congress, woefully rue that their defense attorney really did not understand the medical aspects of the case or that the physician he selected as a witness was inadequate, and it goes on and on. My response to this is always to inquire where the defendant physician was hiding when the trial preparations were in progress. I urge you to become directly involved in *your* case right from day one. As soon as the attorney who is to defend you has been retained, make an appointment to see him. It is critical that counsel be told immediately of all the strengths and weaknesses of the medical care given. Do not be offended if counsel appears by his questions to be challenging you; he is simply being a "devil's advocate." Any information as to the personality of the patient and/or the family members should be given. Information relating to any rumors either from the hospital staff, other patients, or the community as to the cause of the patient's dissatisfaction can be very helpful.

The physician should be prepared at this initial conference to discuss the selection of qualified experts and to suggest references from the medical literature so that the attorney can educate himself as to the medical aspects of the case. Finally, the meeting should end with a firm understanding that the physician is to receive copies of all relevant depositions, answers to interrogatories, opinion letters from opposing experts, and periodic status reports.

Following the meeting, the physician should be alert for all journal articles relevant to the case and send either the reference or preferably a xerox copy of the article. This not only aids counsel but reminds the physician to inquire about the case if he has not received any recent reports from counsel. The defense of a malpractice case is a *team* effort and not the sole responsibility of counsel.

Once the identity of the opposing expert is known, try to find out from other physicians at annual meetings, etc. as much information as possible as to prior cases where the same expert has testified, the nature of his practice, the extent of his experience with the procedure or technique involved, his association with the family, or the plaintiff's attorney. This information is extremely important and can only come from the defendant physician. There is no defendable excuse for an attorney to be unprepared in any case, but in a malpractice case, only the physician can insure that it does not happen.

A fourth benefit is the awareness of the need to eliminate "casual" conferences or conversations. As an experiment, I invite you to listen to discussions in the hallways, elevators, etc. of your hospital or office building. As you are listening, put yourself in the position of a family friend or relative.

> "Did you hear about that appendectomy case this morning? We had a tough time with the bleeding and that nurse anesthetist really blew the anesthesia."

If the fellow passenger on the elevator overheard this conversation and was going to visit an appendectomy patient, I do not think any of us could be surprised if the visitor felt obliged to tell the patient that he had better investigate what happened to him in the O.R. The visitor has no way of knowing that there might have been any number of patients operated upon on that day for the same procedure. Many cases get started because of critical comments made by nurses, aids, medical students, interns, residents, or even fellow staff members. All too often such comments are devoid of merit or even a factual basis. Start an educational program in your hospital of the need to maintain professional discipline. Criticism of a physician, nurses, or any other medical support person should be made either to the person involved directly or through the appropriate channels. Resist the temptation to prove how caring, knowledgeable, dedicated, educated, etc. you are by blasting someone else to the assembled hospital staff or the occupants of the visitors lounge. This suggestion has nothing to do with a cover-up or the concealment of medical error. This is designed to avoid suits based on patient/family misunderstandings, error in the identification of the patient and/or physician, rumor, vindictiveness of a rejected or reprimanded nurse, etc. It is unprofessional and a violation of a patient's rights of privacy to discuss that patient in the hearing range of a third person. It is also a statistically high source of litigation.

A fifth factor is what I call the "when in doubt" rule. Basically stated, the proposition is that whenever you are in doubt about doing something, there is most likely something about the clinical picture that concerns you. Accordingly, unless there is some grave risk to the patient associated with the proposed test or procedure, you should always resolve that doubt in favor of the patient and not his pocketbook.

If the history given to you *via* the telephone raises some doubt about the accuracy of the patient's condition or diagnosis, go and see the patient. If the clinical picture raises a doubt about a developing condition, resolve the doubt by ordering that additional test or diagnostic procedure. Some critics call this defensive medicine. If resolving all doubts in favor of the patient so that the patient has nothing to complain about because he received the best possible medical care is defensive medicine, then I, and I hope all of you, will go on record as supporting defensive medicine. Ask yourself the question: "Am I electing to do or not do this because I believe there is a clinical basis for it, or am I electing to *run the risk* of doing or not doing it?" If the true reason is the latter alternative, you are a gambler; and losers should not cry if they get burned by being sued.

In conclusion, there are obviously other lessons which have been learned from all of the malpractice cases to date. My discussion here is not intended, nor would time permit me, to catalogue all of these hard taught lessons. Rather, I would hope that the factors I have touched upon would trigger an approach, a thought process if you will, to the question of malpractice and the prophylaxis of cases in the future. The time was never more ripe for an analytical examination by the physician of his role, *vis-a-vis* the patient, his peers, and the legal process.

The tremendous effort in progress by the physicans to create legislation to insure a fund to meet future claims is, in my opinion, neither prophylactic nor therapeutic. As such, it is a departure from historical medical practice. For myself, I think it better to stop bad or poor practice than to simply find a way to pay for it. I think the second best step is to stop moaning about future malpractice cases and to get serious about winning the ones which are already pending.

CHAPTER

40

The Prognosis of Medical Malpractice Insurance

WILLIAM L. MARTIN

The "crisis" in medical malpractice, as we all know, came on in full force early in 1975. Our interest now is in the future since we cannot do more than learn from our recent experiences. But any look at the future can be meaningful in terms of what is happening now and what has gone before.

The unavailability of insurance coverage for the professional liability of physicians is quite unlike the usual market shortage. The manufacture of buggy whips came to a halt a few decades ago simply because few people continued to want buggy whips; the automobile had made horse-drawn carriages obsolete.

There is no lack of customers for medical professional liability coverage. On the contrary, the demand is great; never before have physicians needed this financial protection more. At the same time liability insurers, in contrast to the buggy whip manufacturers, are increasingly reluctant to sell their services insofar as medical professionals are concerned.

We have seen the number of insurers engaged actively in selling this form of coverage decline from well over a hundred some 20 years ago to perhaps a dozen today. And, most remaining insurers of medical malpractice coverages are seeking to reduce their share of the market. Why?

Early in the crisis there was a lot of finger pointing. Doctors blamed the lawyers and the courts; lawyers claimed that there was simply more malpractice and the doctors should get their houses in order; some of each blamed insurers, saying insurers were trying to reap exhorbitant profits or to recoup their stock market losses.

Every serious study today suggests there is sufficient blame for all of us but the facts are that (1) there is more malpractice in a legal sense, (2) medical malpractice insurance has been highly unprofitable and threatens to get worse, much worse, and (3) the problem is serious, complex and will demand substantive changes in our system of compensating victims of negligence in medical treatment. But no one, no single group in fact, is, as yet, close to a solution or solutions.

Parenthetically, I should point out that those who accuse the industry of seeking unconscionable profits through recent rate filings must have poor regard for the intelligence of the vast majority of insurers for having abandoned or seeking to abandon the field. Quite obviously, an insurer cannot make a profit from medical malpractice coverages when it ceases writing those coverages; they can only minimize their losses from that source when they cease business. And, there is no way the property and casualty business can recoup reduced surpluses of some 8 billion dollars suffered since 1972. If recoupment of the depreciated value of an insurer's stock and bond holdings were possible by engaging in writing medical malpractice insurance, we would have several hundred insurers competing actively for that business rather than a handful.

The situation became intolerable to insurers in 1975 when because of declining surpluses, over-all unprofitability, and an increasingly unfavorable outlook for medical malpractice insurance, some insurers of state medical society plans decided to terminate those plans. In most of those instances, no other insurer was willing to pick up the terminated plan—at any price. Insurers quite naturally wanted to choose those lines of business which offered a greater chance of making a profit—the indispensable element of any business.

Although the amount of an insurer's surplus will vary from time to time and is *not* an element of rate making, it does bear upon the total amount of insurance any company may insure. Only a few years ago many insurers had a dollar or more of surplus for each dollar of premium written by it. This means they are in a very stable condition so far as their solvency is concerned. Under today's unfavorable conditions, many insurers are writing large amounts of insurance as compared to their surplus. Some large insurers today are writing five dollars of business to each dollar of surplus; that is, their surplus condition has changed from 1:1 to a ratio of 5:1.

This is not to say that the crisis in medical malpractice was caused by factors extraneous to the medical profession, but the industry's current surplus position, not to mention underwriting experience, helps explain the reluctance of insurers to run the very large risks which are part of writing medical professional liability lines of insurance.

Thus, in the past it was often possible to get another insurer to take over an unprofitable plan—at increased premiums—because its business in the aggregate was profitable. In an unprofitable period, insurers seek to write potentially profitable lines and to eliminate those which appear to guarantee losses.

And recent changes in medical malpractice experience are very real. From 1969 to 1974 the experience of doctors insured by the St. Paul Fire and Marine Insurance Company worsened from 1 claim pending per 23 doctors insured to 1 in 10. In California today, the number of claims pending is about 1 in 5 doctors.

During the same 5-year period the St. Paul has seen the average cost of a claim go from $6,705 to $12,534. In New York their average claim cost grew from $6,000 to $23,400 in 10 years. A study of Jury Verdict Research, Inc., shows that the *average* malpractice award granted by juries (excluding those awards in excess of $1 million) increased from $62,151 in 1965 to approximately $350,000 in 1974. Last year in California alone there were 15 awards for more than $1 million.

Given these and other statistical evidence does not help us in determining *why* the problem is so acute. Unfortunately, there is a paucity of underlying evidence as to the reasons for the medical malpractice crisis although the American Insurance Association is sponsoring a closed claim study which we hope will supply many of the answers. There has been much speculation as to the basic causes for our problem and some of these undoubtedly do contribute either to the nature or extent of the problem.

Today's social climate of concern for individual rights undoubtedly is a factor. We are in the midst of a social revolution which impacts upon all our institutions. We see this in other lines of insurance, especially liability insurance. If you have the opinion that medical malpractice is unique (except perhaps in the *extent* of impact), you could not be more mistaken. Increasingly troublesome lines of insurance include products liability, owners-landlords and tenants coverage, other professional liability lines (accountants, architects, lawyers, dentists, officers, and directors coverages, and so on).

Insurance has been called a measure of the extent of order in a society. This fact may help explain the over-all underwriting loss for the property/casualty business of $2.4 *billion* during the first 6 months of 1975 on top of the most unprofitable year in history in 1974.

The current concentration on social change has been reflected in bulging law schools' enrollments. The law schools of the nation have recently enrolled sufficient students to replace the supply of practicing lawyers every 6 years.

Also, it is undoubtedly true that attorneys specializing in personal injury litigation have become increasingly competent in obtaining awards and in magnifying the size of those awards. Faced with a current average jury award of $350,00 in malpractice cases, an insurer will go to extreme lengths to avoid allowing such a case to go to trial.

In addition to the litigious nature of today's society we have seen many defenses eroded and destroyed by court decision. An example would be statutes of limitation which have been extended by court decision to exclude periods of minority or other disability and until actual discovery by the patient. In cases where proof was lacking or inconclusive, the courts have determined that the facts of the injury speak for themselves in establishing negligence or that the burden is upon the physician to prove he was not at fault.

Medically, many people believe that the public has acquired a Doctor Welby complex, having been educated to expect miracles from modern medicine. There are indications that the recent publicity about medical malpractice has caused an increase in the number of such claims. In addition, the doctor-patient relationship has suffered from increasing specialization. [The author has been operated upon by a surgeon whom he met neither before, during, or after the surgery.] Undoubtedly, too, the practice of medicine is complex and becoming more so; the choices available for treatment, increasingly sophisticated, bring new risks to the practitioner.

We have then a complex problem the exact scope of which is not completely known, the causes of which are the subject of speculation, and for which a variety of solutions, mostly palliative in nature, have been proposed. A modern day Moses surely is needed.

The American Insurance Association established a special committee early this year primarily to deal with long range solutions. That committee is composed of senior executives of members insurers, both those writing malpractice and those who do not, and with a senior staff officer to coordinate their efforts. In addition, representatives of other insurance trade associations and unaffiliated insurers were invited to participate.

Unfortunately, the immediate crises, state by state, as they arose tended to divert the group from their task of formulating long range solutions. Before any efforts at solving the problem could be undertaken, it was essential that a market be maintained. While there was substantial sentiment among insurers for no private solution in favor of a state solution, such as a state fund as the market for medical malpractice coverages, the majority of our insurers opted for a market to be provided by the industry as a whole.

From this decision our committee developed the framework for a joint underwriting association (JUA). It should be understood that this was intended as strictly a temporary solution to keep open a market for coverages until long range answers could be developed. A JUA cannot provide the coverge cheaper or in an improved manner than a private insurer.

The JUA, as proposed, had certain special features which you should understand.

1. To be successful, it had to have the mandatory participation of all liability insurers. If malpractice insurers alone were to be included, this would be an additional incentive for insurers to abandon malpractice as a line of coverage.

2. The JUA would come into being only after a finding that coverage was unavailable in the voluntary market. Separate decisions would be required for medical practitioners and for hospitals. This requirement avoids introducing the JUA where there is no market problem or a problem, say, only for hospital coverages.

3. The JUA would be the exclusive provider of coverage for physicians if it were established. Otherwise, the JUA would serve only the risks which insurers had rejected. The greatest nonsolution to be feared by medical specialists is the nonexclusive JUA (which has been proposed as a permanent market mechanism in Florida). This gives the voluntary market or medical society insurer, as the case may be, the right to cream the market by accepting only those low rated risks. Obviously, the high rated specialists will see their rates in the JUA climb to possibly unaffordable levels since only the risks with the greatest loss potential would be rejected by insurers. In addition, the permanent JUA tends to delay or avoid any solution to the underlying problem.

4. The JUA would be self-supporting. Obviously, malpractice insureds cannot expect to be supported by other lines of insurance such as homeowners insureds or insurers' surpluses (especially in their presently depleted state). One of the major provisions designed to prevent such subsidization is the stabilization fund which is created through a surcharge on premiums. If anticipated deficits do not occur, the stabilization reserve would be returned to malpractice policyholders.

5. Another major feature of our JUA would be that it would pay no operating profit to insurers. Any profits, including investment income from medical malpractice premiums and the stabilization fund, would insure to the benefit of policyholders.

Again, I want to emphasize that the JUA is merely a temporary measure and in no way attempts to treat the underlying causes. It is a solution which is unsatisfactory to the industry and should be unsatisfactory to the medical profession except as a temporary expedient. A number of state medical societies have sponsored the organization of medical mutuals in order to keep a market—but, again, this does little or nothing to deal with the underlying problem.

We come now to long range solutions. Such a solution ideally would provide prompt and adequate reimbursement to compensate injured patients; medical malpractice insurance would be readily available at a reasonable cost; and the medical profession would provide supervision of health care so as to reduce injury from medical malpractice or mishap to the lowest possible level. At this moment that seems to be a large order, and as I have suggested, we do not have any such system to offer you, but we are working to that end.

One of the steps being taken by our organization is that of seeking improved statistical data. An all industry study, sponsored by the American Insurance Association, of medical malpractice claim files closed in 1974 is being made. This study should give us useful information relative to the injured patient's extent of injury and the basis of settlement. Hopefully, it will help us in designing and costing a system which will approach the goals of an ideal system.

Such data have not been available in the past for a number of reasons. An insurer settles claims at the lowest possible amount; to collect information as to the components of a settlement or the cause of the injury do not help it in determining its loss experience. Moreover, collecting such information would add to its costs. The paucity of industry wide data is due, in part at least, to the fact that state medical societies have tended to sponsor plans which involve a single insurer. The result of course is that only a single insurer would have the bulk of data for those states where it insured the medical society members.

We believe that some favorable impact can be expected from modification of tort laws and we are cooperating with other insurers, public officials, and with medical groups to develop effective tort law amendments. We have drafts of bills in the following areas: informed consent, burden of proof, statute of limitations, medical malpractice hearing panels, contingent fees, limitation of damages, elimination of punitive damages, advance payments, notice of intent to sue, elimination of ad damnum clause, and peer review immunity.

Our actuaries, however, tell us that it is not possible to predict what impact such measures will have on the cost and availability of medical malpractice insurance. In any event, it would take several years to measure any impact in view of the "long tail" on malpractice claims. The likelihood, however, is that they will have some favorable impact upon both cost and availability. On the whole, however, such changes do not represent a long range answer to the problem.

Our special committee continues to meet frequently and continues to investigate all likely avenues toward ultimate solutions. Advocates of solutions such as Professor Jeffrey O'Connell and Clark Havighurst are being given the opportunity to explain their proposals in detail. Following are some of the "solutions" being studied.

1. National health insurance which would presumably pay most hospital and medical bills. Of course, in the absence of legislative prohibition, patients could still institute a tort suit to recover these expenses as well as other damages. There are many problems to resolve in coordinating a health insurance system with the liability system, and medical malpractice may not be able to await that development.

2. Channeling of liability through hospitals is one proposed answer. This contemplates a single benefit provider and a single premium payer (the hospital) since 80% of all medical treatment mishaps which result in claims occur in hospitals. While this would facilitate the handling of claims, it would not touch incidents which occur outside hospitals. Moreover, it would tend to encourage additional treatment within hospitals and increase the cost of health care.

3. Early in the game some advocates suggested no fault systems as the answer. Unfortunately, the parallel to automobile reparations is inept since a no fault system suggests payment for every injury whether negligence was involved or not. The number of injuries to be compensated is most important to the costing of such a system. In an automobile accident, generally negligence of one or both parties is involved; in the case of patient care, a poor result may be one that was unavoidable. We have no data as yet which indicate that such a "no fault" system for medical malpractice would reduce insurance costs.

4. Workers' compensation furnishes one obvious model. This would involve administrative awards, payment of medical expenses in defined instances, other payments according to a schedule, and limitation of general damages. Such a system has been argued as of doubtful constitutionality since it would abolish tort suits without expanding the area of recovery as is done in no fault automobile systems.

5. Arbitration, especially by specially qualified panels, has been put forth as another answer. Nonbinding arbitration, however, may add to rather than limit costs inasmuch as the claimant would still be entitled to a trial by a common law jury. Binding arbitration is considered of doubtful validity by some legal experts.

In short, a great deal of work is being done by a great many sources, but we are not on the precipice of the ideal system. The likelihood is that 1976 will see us still attempting to make the old system work. Rates will continue to increase substantially and coverage may be unavailable in some states. Many efforts will be made to amend the tort laws which affect malpractice cases, and those efforts hopefully will succeed even though we do not believe they are more than a small part of any solution.

While I do not suggest that the answer to malpractice is eliminating malpractice, it is likely that there will be increasing efforts to strengthen supervision of health care providers. Current peer review is understandably weak. In many instances, no immunity from liability is given to medical society disciplinary procedures. We will support efforts to make supervision more effective, and we believe it must become effective. Our health care system cannot tolerate professional incompetence of whatever nature.

It is hoped that 1976 will see the development and presentation of a reshaped system. Enactment of such a system into law may not be easy, however, in the face of an entrenched and powerful group which has profited from the present system; but the present system has proved its lack of merit and cannot stand as an obstacle and as a threat to quality medical care.

CHAPTER

41

Clinical Evaluation of Strokes and Threatened Strokes

H. J. M. BARNETT, M.D., F.R.C.P. (C.)

INTRODUCTION

The early descriptive neurologists studied strokes from an anatomical perspective. Focus was on the territory of damage in relation to blood supply and reflected their searchings for functional localization in the brain. Stroke prevention was ignored and the natural history of the evolution of stroke and of its prodromata were overlooked.

Today's evaluation of stroke, by contrast, must be very dynamic. The prodromata, their prognostic significance, their pathogenesis, and thus their rational therapy are the keys to stroke prevention. The varieties of vascular stroke have come into much clearer focus. Three out of four are of thromboembolic origin while hemorrhage, due to a ruptured abnormal artery or of the hypertensive intracerebral variety, accounts for most of the other 25%.

This communication will concern itself with some of the factors which need to be considered in embarking on therapy for the treatment of threatened thromboembolic stroke and which must be carefully reviewed either in evaluating reputed therapeutic measures or in descriptions of the natural history of stroke. The following will be discussed in this brief survey.

1. Pathogenesis and symptomatology of threatened stroke: transient ischemic attack (TIA) and partial nonprogressive stroke (PNPS);
2. Certain difficulties in identifying TIA's;
3. Ischemic events beyond arteries already known to be occluded;
4. Cerebral and retinal ischemic events with prolapsing mitral valve.

Large areas of stroke evaluation will not be touched, including that very vexed and ill defined condition referred to as "progressing stroke," nor will much be said of the major calamitous stroke with its large fixed deficit.

Pathogenesis and Symptomatology of Threatened Stroke and Partial Nonprogressive Stroke

A TIA is defined conventionally as an event of swift onset developing over a few seconds and producing a focal neurological deficit lasting commonly a few minutes and not more than 24 hours. It has to be recognized that PNPS's and major catastrophic strokes will have the same pathogenetic bases. The difference comes from the size and location of the pathological process and many patients progress from the minor events to the more formidable in a continuum of ischemic episodes. For this reason it is not reasonable to discuss TIA , PNPS, or major stroke as events isolated from each other whether one is considering pathogenesis, natural history, or preventive measures.

It is important in utilizing terms that some conventional arrangement be adapted so that comparisons between reports can be made. It is to be noted in reviewing the literature of this subject that the terms now in commonest usage are TIA, TIA with residua, PNPS, reversible ischemic neurological disability (RIND), and major, or catastrophic, or completed stroke. There would appear to be no essential difference among the conditions described under the terms "TIA with residua," "PNPS," and "RIND." For the rest of this communication, "ischemic events" will be used as a generic term to describe any of these occurrences.

Ischemic events, including the simple variety, TIA, may result from one of three major pathogenetic mechanisms. Failure to recognize this will lead to institution of erroneous preventive therapy. They are listed in Table 41.1.

The *hemodynamic attacks* result from low cerebral perfusion, are frequently accompanied by diffuse cerebral symptoms most closely imitating vertebral-basilar symptomatology, often with loss of consciousness, quite frequently with convulsions, and rarely with focal ischemic symptoms. During the past 4 years we have been studying the possible value of platelet-inhibiting drug therapy and 524 cases of presumed artery-to-artery emboli have been entered into the trial. Fifty-six cases have appeared in our exclusion list judged to be inappropriate to our trial since hemodynamic mechanisms appeared the probable source of their ischemic events (Table 41.2).

The proportion of cases is not a true reflection of the total incidence of hemodynamic ischemic events relative to artery-to-artery emboli since many of the former would not be referred for neurological opinion and since our experience indicates that the reporting of "exclusions" from our trial is less scrupulously attended to than the documentation of the accepted "entries." Nevertheless, it gives a reasonable guide to the

TABLE 41.1
Pathogenesis of Ischemic Events

Hemodynamic
Cardiac embolic
Artery-to-artery embolic

TABLE 41.2
Hemodynamic Attacks (56)

Orthostatic hypotension		14
Arrhythmias—	bradyarrhythmia—8	13
	Auricular flutter—1	
	Unclassified—4	
Carotid sinus hypersensitivity		4
Severe hypertension		4
Polycythemia rubra vera		3
Unspecified		18

variety and relative incidence of conditions mimicking artery-to-artery emboli that are to be diligently sought in the evaluation of cerebral and retinal ischemic events.

The territory of ischemia in these cases was 3:1 vertebral-basilar *cf.* carotid artery. The number with TIA with residual was small (1:4 *cf.* those without residual). The occurrrence of classical focal TIA was uncommon. It occurred once in the orthostatic hypotensive group, in the 4 cases with serious sustained diastolic hypertension (diastolic pressures above 125 mm Hg) and in the three instances of TIA with polycythemia. These findings are in keeping with the report from the Mayo Clinic (13) respecting the rarity of transient focal cerebral ischemia in cardiac dysrhythmia wherein only 1.4% of 290 patients who had a pacemaker inserted for bradyarrhythmia described focal ischemic events.

In a negative fashion it is to be noted that no instances of "steal" mechanisms were recorded from these centers in the 4 years of this study, no "low perfusion syndromes" were described unless other factors were also contributing, and there were no instances of recurrent ischemic events produced by extracranial kinking of the carotid or vertebral arteries in relation to bony structures.

It is beyond the scope of this communication to elaborate on *cardiac embolic phenomenon* in detail. A particular variety will be synopsized under "Cerebral Ischemic Events with Prolapsing Mitral Valve."

The concept of *artery-to-artery emboli*, either of platelet-fibrin origin or from fragments of atheromatous debris has emerged as the most significant cause of TIA with and without residua. Such emboli to intracranial branches when sufficiently large or appropriately located will result in major strokes in just the same way as will complete obliteration of the major external channels. The symptoms of these ischemic events are too well known to require detailed elaboration. However, an analysis of such symptoms in 524 patients entered into our collaborative trial in the six categories of acceptable subgroups (carotid, with and without residua; vertebral-basilar, with and without residua; both carotid and vertebral-basilar, with and without residua) reflects the fact that vague and poorly defined symptoms are uncommon even in the setting of a collection of more readily recognizable symptoms (Tables 41.3, 41.4, and 41.5). For example, carotid disease is rarely associated with vertigo and nonspecific dizziness, mental changes rarely reflect early manifestations of vertebral-basilar and carotid disease. Headache, generally of a localized nature, is a recognized feature of TIA, partial stroke, and major stroke. It was originally described by Willis in 1684 (18), reviewed as "Willis' headache" by Edmeads and Barnett (7), and recently reviewed by Grindal and Toole (9) in a series of TIA patients. Alone it is not possible to identify it as a reflection of ischemia.

There is no doubt from our experience that patients will experience symptoms that are related to both carotid arteries within the same period of weeks and months. Furthermore, they will experience symptoms that reflect carotid plus vertebral-basilar disturbance again within the same period of weeks and months. Rather than indicating "intracranial steal" phenomenon, these symptoms frequently reflect disease in

TABLE 41.3
Carotid Symptomatology

Symptoms	TIA Only (208 cases)	PNPS (103 cases)
	%	%
Monocular visual	34	21
Paresis (mono, hemi)	59	88
Paraesthesia (mono, hemi)	57	62
Paresis (facial)	22	43
Paraesthesia (facial)	30	26
Dysphasia	21	30
Dysarthria	14	18
Headache	11	11
Binocular visual (hemianopsia)	7	10
"Dizzy"—nonspecific	6	2
Mental change	1	—
Convulsion (focal) (grand mal)	1.5	2
Loss of consciousness	—	1
Visual hallucination	1	—

TABLE 41.4
Vertebral-basilar Symptomatology

Symptoms	TIA Only (78 cases)	PNPS (46 cases)
	%	%
Binocular visual	50	30
Vertigo	51	35
Diplopia	44	48
"Dizzy"	22	13
Ataxia	41	46
Paraesthesia	44	54
Paresis	33	59
Dysarthria	21	37
Headache	18	33
Nausea/vomiting	14	17
Hearing loss	3	7
Mental change	8	9
Dysphagia	4	4
Dysphasia	3	4
Visual hallucination	5	2
"Drop attacks"	4	4
Convulsion	—	2
Drowsiness	1	2

TABLE 41.5
Both Carotid and Vertebral-basilar Symptomatology

Symptoms	TIA Only (26 cases)	PNPS (22 cases)
	%	%
Paraesthesia	88	77
Paresis	35	86
Binocular visual	42	27
Vertigo	27	41
Ataxia	34	32
"Dizzy"–nonspecific	35	32
Monocular visual	27	27
Dysphasia	19	23
Diplopia	19	18
Headache	19	23
Dysarthria	15	23
"Drop attacks"	4	14
Nausea/vomiting	4	14
Loss of consciousness	—	10
Convulsion	—	5
Visual hallucination	—	9
Mental change	4	5

more than one site productive of artery-to-artery emboli developing within a reasonable limit of time.

The relationship of ischemic events to lesions that are radiologically identifiable is a reasonable, but not a complete, measure of the causal relationship between the ischemia and the arterial lesion. In an analysis of a random selection of 151 of the patients entered into the Canadian TIA trial, lesions of readily recognizable atheromatous disease either smooth, ulcerative, or significantly stenotic (more than 30% encroachment on the lumen in two planes) have been recognized in locations appropriate to the symptoms in 134 of 151 cases. In 86 there was such a lesion in more than one site on the vessel appropriate to the symptoms (Table 41.6).

Stenosis occurred 81 times, in 73 cases, 64 extracranially and 17 intracranially. In 8 instances there was stenosis appropriate to the symptoms both extra- and intracranially (Table 41.7).

Appropriate ulcerative atheroma ("ulcer") was recognized or was suspicious on 40 occasions, 36 extracranially and 4 intracranially, one of the latter in the basilar artery. We recognize that this rather positive correlation between TIA symptoms and angiographic lesions is at variance with the negative correlation reported by Alter and associates (1). The difference here may be related to the intensity with which cardiac sources or hemodynamic mechanisms are sought and excluded to follow our protocol requirements. We are engaged in an analysis of an age-matched group of cases undergoing angiography for aneurysm,

TABLE 41.6

Relationship of Angiography to Clinical (150 Cases)

Potentially appropriate lesion	132
More than one potentially appropriate	86
Not appropriate	8
Normal angiography	11

TABLE 41.7

Relationship of Angiography to Clinical (151 Cases)

Potentially Appropriate Lesions	Total	E/C	I/C
Stenosis (more than 30%)*	81	64	17
Atheroma (without stenosis)	134	71	63
Occlusion	38	26	12
Ulcer	29	26	3
Suspect ulcer	11	10	1

* Eight had appropriate stenosis both E/C (extracranially) and I/C (intracranially).

tumor, and epilepsy to determine the incidence of similar lesions interpreted by the same individuals and investigated by the same people. This information is not yet available.

Certain Difficulties in Identifying TIA's

SYMPTOMS WHOSE ISOLATED OCCURRENCE CANNOT BE ATTRIBUTED TO ISCHEMIA

There are a number of symptoms which occur within the framework of the presentation of a threatened stroke which cannot be accepted as diagnostic when they occur by themselves. These include, for the most part, symptoms which arise from structures within the vertebral-basilar territory (Table 41.8).

So many other disorders can be productive of these recurrent symptoms that it is wrong to attribute their origins to vascular disease even in the presence of neck bruits and demonstrable radiographic abnormalities. Other common, frequently insignificant, and even occult causes may be operating to produce them. If they are of isolated occurrence or recurrence, carotid stenosis is a most improbable explanation for them, and even vertebral-basilar insufficiency cannot be diagnosed definitely despite potentially appropriate arteriographic lesions.

DEMENTIA AND AMNESIA AS ISCHEMIC PHENOMENA

Forgetfulness and some vague nonentities called the "chronic brain syndrome" are loosely and carelessly equated with cerebral vascular disease. They are purported especially by commercial proponents of a variety of drugs which are said to influence brain blood supply and metabolism to be early evidences of cerebral vascular disease. These claims must be examined very critically. Dementing and amnestic states will be produced in circumstances as recorded in Table 41.9 as a consequence of arteriosclerosis.

Amnestic episodes occurring in isolation have a variety of causes, including temporal lobe seizures. They cannot be equated either with cerebral ischemia (with its threat of further and major stroke) nor yet identified with reasonable certainty as to their cause unless other related

TABLE 41.8
Symptoms not Diagnostic of TIA when of Isolated Occurrence or Recurrence

Diplopia
Vertigo
Unconscious episodes
Amnestic attacks
Drop attacks

TABLE 41.9
Dementia Due to Arteriosclerosis

Major cerebral infarctions
Multiple major extracranial arterial occlusion
Bilateral posterior cerebral infarction
Severe persistent hypertension (État Lacunaire)

symptoms, signs, historical data, and investigative results are considered. Transient global amnesia at first was presumed to be always nonvascular. Time has determined that this is not the case and recent convincing evidence is available that in a given instance it may be a reflection of transient ischemia and with further episodes a transient amnesia has converted to a persistent amnesia. Twice in our TIA trial cases, an episode of transient and severe amnesia of several hours' duration has punctuated the course of vertebral-basilar symptomatology, once as an initial event followed by other vertebral-basilar ischemic features, and once intermediate in the evolution of a recurrent tendency to a variety of such symptoms. Before other symptoms or signs develop, however, it is only a presumption to attach an ischemic pathogenesis to the isolated occurrence of amnestic attacks. The occurrence of a persistent amnestic state has now been reported on a few occasions on a vascular basis. Such patients preserving or relatively sparing consciousness, perception, intellectual, and other neurological function, but with severe persistent amnestic state, have been studied in seven cases in our institution and reported more completely elsewhere (17). All were able to recall remote events in full detail but lacked the ability to imprint and recall new information. By a combination of radiological and brain-scanning data and clinical information, unequivocal evidence of interference with bilateral posterior cerebral artery circulation was available in four cases and was evident in one who had been subjected to a contralateral temporal lobectomy 2 years previously (Table 41.10).

It was unilateral in the posterior cerebral artery supply to the dominant hemisphere by angiography and on scan in the other two cases (Table 41.11).

The suspicion is strong, however, that pre-existing occult damage had been afflicted to the nondominant hemisphere in these two cases. No example is available where pathological examination substantiates the continuation of persistent amnesia as a sequel to a unilateral hippocampal-temporal lobe lesion. Penfield and Mathieson (11), in a very late pathological postmortem follow-up to one of their dominant hemisphere temporal lobectomies with persistent amnesic deficit, were able to record contralateral damage which had been clinically undetectable.

TABLE 41.10
Amnesic Stroke (Bilateral Evidence of Posterior Cerebral Artery (PCA) Ischemia)

Case	Angiography	Scan	Clinical
1	Bilateral PCA occlusion*	Normal	Bilateral visual
2	Not done	Normal	Bilateral visual
3	Left PCA occlusion*	L. occipital	Bilateral visual
4	Left PCA occlusion	L. parietal	Previous contralateral temporal lobectomy–2 yrs
5	No filling PCA's from basilar; from carotid, left PCA stenosed; right carotid occluded	Normal	Nil visual

a * No PCA filling from basilar or carotid.

TABLE 41.11
Unilateral Evidence of Posterior Cerebral Artery (PCA) Ischemia

Case	Angiography	Scan	Clinical
6	Left PCA occlusion* (right internal carotid occlusion)	Left parieto-occipital	Right hemianopia
7	Not done	Left occipital	Right hemianopia

* No PCA filling from basilar or carotid.

The evidence that has accumulated now respecting amnestic attacks allows us to draw the following conclusions.

1. They may occur in isolation as TIA's—in this case their ischemic origin is speculative.

2. They may occur within the framework of cerebral ischemic attacks in which case they are part of the vertebral-basilar variety.

3. TIA of amnestic type may be the forerunner of persistent amnesic stroke, in which case the evidence strongly indicates that the posterior cerebral artery blood supply has been interfered with bilaterally.

AMAUROSIS FUGAX IS NOT NECESSARILY ISCHEMIC

An important phenomenon in the diagnosis of carotid artery ischemia is amaurosis fugax. Although readily described by patients it cannot be accepted uncritically as a certain consequence of artery-to-artery embolism. Care must be exercised to exclude other conditions whose therapy may be quite different or who have no need of any therapy. Again, the possibility of the coincidental and insignificant occurrence of an asymptomatic carotid bruit may confuse the issue. We are aware of unnecessary angiography attending the study of some of the conditions stated in Table 41.12.

Table 41.12
Differential Diagnosis of Amaurosis Fugax

Primary ocular conditions—glaucoma, retinal detachment
Muscae volitantes (floaters)
Transient oculomotor imbalance
Migraine aura
Giant cell arteritis
Papilledema

The most likely condition to mislead the unwary in our experience has been muscae volitantes (floaters) occurring in highly miopic individuals and brought to the patient's attention as a sequel to bending and exertion. The floaters, if large enough, will obscure the macula, temporarily causing a frightening amaurosis. In one instance (Fig. 41.1), a partial retinal vein thrombosis developed in a prodromatal phase of an occult malignancy. The patient, a surgeon, became aware of transient monocular amaurosis as often as the small vitreous hemorrhage complicating the retinal vein thrombosis passed in front of the macula. Despite other arteriopathy, his carotid vessels were normal on angiography.

VAGUE AND MISLEADING EVIDENCES OF CEREBRAL ISCHEMIA

Critical analysis of what truly constitutes threatened, early, or even well developed manifest cerebral ischemia will avoid much unnecessary and disappointing therapy. A product reputed to improve cerebral circulation by virtue of an effect on cerebral vascular tone is widely advertised in Canada, and probably more widely elsewhere. The criteria of entry of the 37 cases in the basic trial (4) referred to in the advertisement had symptoms (shown in Table 41.13) that were not elaborated upon.

The end points for the trial were judged to be as shown in Table 41.14.

What conditions were being treated and what interpretation we can place on such a collection of alterations of function are difficult to ascertain. This type of uncritical assessment characterizes many of the reports on all the drugs which are claimed to improve on cerebral function in alleged cerebral vascular disease by purporting to increase its blood supply or improve its metabolism. Evidence is accumulating giving us reason to hope that significant treatment of threatened stroke may be within our grasp in the near future. Uncritical appraisal of therapies designed to treat it must not be allowed to confuse the picture.

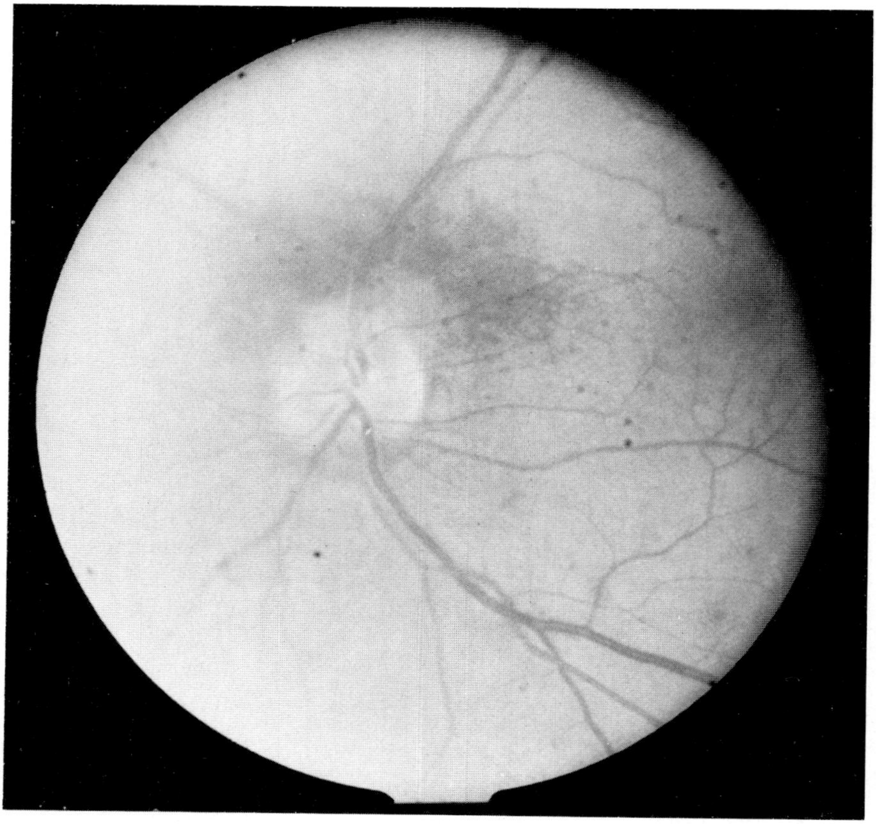

Fig 41.1. Dark cloud representing resolving vitreous hemorrhage mimicked amaurosis fugax in passage over macula.

Table 41.13
Cerebral Vascular Disorders—37 Cases

Entry criteria:
Diffuse brain damage (nature not specified)
Mild paresis (no further description given)
Reduced brain performance
Avoiding social contact
Psychic disorders of impulse

TIA and Ischemic Events beyond an Occluded Artery

The cessation of transient cerebral ischemia after occlusion of a stenosed artery is a commonly accepted phenomenon. However, deliberate follow-up of patients considered for and also entered into our platelet-inhibiting drug trial has led us to a modification of this

TABLE 41.14
Cerebral Vascular Disorders—37 Cases

End points
Activation of psychic impulses
Open and active behaviour
Seeking social contacts
Increased tenacity of will (Kraeplin-Pauli performance test)

proposition. During a 4-year period, four cooperating neurological units in London, Ontario have entered 154 patients presumed by detailed study to have had cerebral or retinal ischemic events on an artery-to-artery embolic basis. At the same time, 218 cases have been excluded for a variety of mandatory factors described in the protocol. From these 372 patients with TIA and PNPS, or suspected of having TIA and PNPS, have come 19 examples of ischemia beyond a known arterial occlusion, and two further patients have been added to this report from other collaborating centers. Nineteen of the ischemic attacks have occurred in carotid and two in vertebral-basilar territory. TIA has occurred in 16, PNPS in 4, and a major catastrophic stroke in one case. Eleven of the patients had amaurosis fugax.

The detail of these cases is recorded elsewhere (3), but the situation will be summarized here. They were carefully scrutinized to determine, if possible, the pathogenesis of the ischemia. It was concluded that in 11 instances an ulcerative atheroma in the appropriate ipsilateral anastomotic external and/or common carotid artery territory, (six cases), or an ulcerative atheromatous lesion on the opposite common or internal carotid artery, (seven cases), could have been responsible for the embolic ischemic phenomena.

In four there was less remarkable nonulcerative atheroma in a position to provide embolic lesions to brain or retina. In eight of these cases there was some further substantiation of the embolic hypothesis in that the attacks ceased in six when anticoagulants were administered, ceased in one when an endarterectomy of the external carotid—common carotid lesion was effected, and in one when the occlusion extended down to include the common carotid artery, a fact fortuitously determined by a repeat angiography. A hemodynamic pathogenesis was probable in a few cases, also fully described elsewhere.

To surgeons, these delayed ischemic events may be of particular interest for another reason. An extensive review of the literature on carotid ligation for aneurysm treatment has produced 11 examples with delay in the ischemia in the territory of the ligation from 8 days to 13 years (Table 41.15).

TABLE 41.15
Delayed Ischemic Events Following Carotid Ligation

Author	Date	Time After Ligation
Astley Cooper (6)	1812	8 days
Seigrist (15)	1900	12 days
Cauchoix (5)	1922	3 months
German and Black (8)	1965	25 months
Oldershaw and Voris (10)	1966	13 years
		1 year
Cooperative Study (14)	1969	6, 11, 12, 18, 48 months

In the cooperative study on intracranial aneurysms and subarachnoid hemorrhage (14), 233 of 814 patients with carotid ligation occlusion for aneurysm had an ischemic neurological deficit. Seventy-nine per cent developed within the first 48 hours, and 10% in the second 48 hours. Five of the 233, however, developed a severe neurological deficit months and years later at 6 months, 11 months, 12 months, 18 months, and 4 years, respectively. Three were younger (ages 13, 30, and 41) and two older (ages 60 and 72). Six similar delayed single ischemic events from the literature are summarized in Table 41.15. None of these recorded cases had amaurosis fugax. Important distinctions between the majority of patients who experience ischemic episodes after carotid ligation and those after spontaneous thrombosis is that the former have isolated events, as a rule, without amaurosis, the latter are frequently recurrent, often with amaurosis. It is apparent that patients with cerebral arteries occluded by atheroma are more prone to subsequent recurrent TIA's than patients who have had deliberate carotid ligature. Therapeutic programs designed for patients with threatened stroke should consider the possibility of these postocclusion ischemic events. This should include not only drug trials, but also microvascular surgical experiments.

Cerebral Ischemic Events with Prolapsing Mitral Valve

Cardiogenic emboli from traditional sources such as mitral stenosis with auricular fibrillation, and from mural thrombi as a sequel to infarction, have been recognized as capable of producing TIA, PNPS, as well as calamitous embolic stroke. Technological advances, including the ability to perform prolonged electrocardiographic monitoring, echocardiography, and left ventricular angiocardiography have added new dimensions to the cardiologist's ability to study the heart. It has become essential to an accurate assessment of the pathogenesis of TIA, PNPS, as well as major stroke to utilize these capabilities. All patients in our treatment trial who have had negative angiography to explain their cerebral or retinal symptoms have been subjected to detailed cardiac scrutiny. During a 3½-year period, nine cases have been identified who have been afflicted with such ischemic events who have had prolapsing mitral valve determined by clinical examinations by echocardiography and confirmed by left ventricular angiocardiography. None had hypertension, none had histories suggestive of hemiplegic migraine, and none of the four females were taking the contraceptive pill. Three gave a history of palpitations, and on 24- to 72-hour monitoring, two had paroxysms of atrial fibrillation, one of ventricular tachycardia, two of sinus tachycardia, two junctional extra systoles, one frequent premature ventricular contractions (PVC's), and only two had perfectly normal rhythms.

The neurological ischemic events occurred singly in two cases and were multiple in seven. Five had residual signs ranging from minimal to severe, and three had evidence of ischemia alternating between the hemispheres.

Again the detail of these cases is fully set out elsewhere and the question of coincidental occurrence is fully discussed. For the time being it appears reasonable to be strongly suspicious of a cause and effect relationship between the TIA and some pathological process initiated by the existence of a myxomatous degeneration of the mitral valve. The patients in this series average 19 years younger than those in our other TIA series where atheroma in the major vessels has been judged to be the source of the TIA. Furthermore, none of the prolapsing mitral valve (PMV) cases have had atheromatous disease in the major extracranial vessels, while 89.3% of those in the trial series have such lesions appropriate to their symptoms.

It is difficult to put the blame on the arrhythmias for these focal ischemic events. The pathological review of 35 cases of PMV conducted by Pomerance (12) may provide a basis in thromboembolism for the ischemia. In 10 of the 35 a superficial tearing of the myxomatously degenerative valve was detected with a 'fibrinous endocarditis' of red cells and fibrin in the superficial zone of the mitral valve attachment. Two had bacterial endocarditis. Silver has illustrated a valvular lesion with macroscopic evidence of adherent premortem thrombus (16).

Until such time as postmortem material is available from a patient who has had ischemic cerebral symptoms associated with PMV, the mechanisms of symptoms produced, and indeed the exact identification of a cause and effect relationship remains speculative. The observations, however, underscore the need to make careful and detailed cardiac examination in all cases of TIA, PNPS, and major stroke.

REFERENCES

1. Alter, M., Kieffer, S., Resch, J., and Ansari, K. Cerebral infarction: clinical and angiographic correlations. Neurology (Minneap.), *22:* 590–602, 1972.
2. Barnett, H. J. M., Jones, M. W., Boughner, D. R., and Kostuk, W. J. Cerebral ischemic events occurring in patients with prolapsing mitral valve. In press, 1976.
3. Barnett, H. J. M., Peerless, S. J., and Aldis, A. E. Delayed cerebral ischemic episodes distal to occlusion of major cerebral arteries. In press, 1976.
4. Birckmayer, W., and Mentasti, M. Clinical experiences with a new vasodilator in neurological diseases. Wien. Med. Wochenschr., *108:* 395–396, 1958.
5. Cauchoix, A. La ligature de la veine ophtalmique dans le traitement de l'exophtalmas pulsatile. Bull. Mem. Soc. Chir. Paris, *48:* 20–23, 1922.
6. Cooper, A. P. Med.-Chir. Tr. Lond., 1912.
7. Edmeads, J., and Barnett, H. J. M. La cefalea en las afecciones cerebrov asculares oclusive as. *In* Cefaleas y jaquecas, edited by A. P. Friedman, and G. E. Poch, pp. 89–100. Eudeba, Rivadavia, 1971/73.
8. German, W. J., and Black, S. P. W. Cervical ligation for internal carotid aneurysms. An extended follow-up. J. Neurosurg., *23:* 572–577, 1965.
9. Grindal, A. B., and Toole, J. F. Headache and transient ischemic attacks. Stroke, *5:* 603–606, 1974.
10. Oldershaw, J. B., and Voris, H. C. Internal carotid artery ligation. A follow-up study. Neurology, *16:* 937–938, 1966.
11. Penfield, W., and Mathieson, G. Memory: Autopsy findings and comments on the role of hippocampus in experimential recall. Arch. Neurol., *31:* 145–154, 1974.
12. Pomerance, A. Ballooning deformity (mucoid degeneration) of atrioventricular valves. Br. Heart J., *31:* 343–351, 1969.
13. Reed, R. L., Siekert, R. G., and Merideth, J. Rarity of transient focal cerebral ischemia in cardiac dysrhythmia. J.A.M.A., *223:* 893–895, 1973.
14. Sahs, A. L., Perret, G. E., Locksley, H. B., and Nishioka, H. Intracranial aneurysms and subarachnoid hemorrhage; a cooperative study. 296 pp. J. B. Lippincott Co., Philadelphia and Toronto, 1969.
15. Siegrist, A. Arch. f. Ophthalmol., *50:* 511, 1900.
16. Silver, M. D. Rheumatic carditis: Acute and chronic atrioventricular valve disease. *In* The Heart, International Academy of Pathology, Monograph No. 15, pp. 87–109. Williams & Wilkins Co., Baltimore, 1974.
17. Spence, D., and Barnett, H. J. M. Amnestic strokes. In press, 1976.
18. Willis, Thomas. The Anatomy of the Brain and Nerves, edited by Wm. Feindel, Vol. II, Tercentenary Edition, 1664–1964, pp. 192. McGill University Press, Montreal, 1965.

Index